EUROPEAN PHARMACOPOEIA - SUPPLEMENT 6.2 TO THE 6th EDITION

published 11 December 2007

The 6th Edition of the European Pharmacopoeia consists of volumes 1 and 2 of the publication 6.0, and Supplements 6.1 and 6.2. These will be complemented by **non-cumulative supplements** that are to be kept for the duration of the 6th Edition. 3 supplements will be published in each of the years 2008 and 2009. A cumulative list of reagents will be published in supplements 6.4 and 6.7.

If you are using the 6th Edition at any time later than 1 April 2008, make sure that you have all the published supplements and consult the index of the most recent supplement to ensure that you use the latest versions of the monographs and general chapters.

EUROPEAN PHARMACOPOEIA - ELECTRONIC VERSION

The 6th Edition is also available in an electronic format (CD-ROM and online version) containing all of the monographs and general chapters found in the printed version. With the publication of each supplement the electronic version is replaced by a new, fully updated, cumulative version.

In addition to the official English and French online versions, a Spanish online version (5th Edition) is also available for the convenience of users.

PHARMEUROPA

Quarterly Forum Publication

Pharmeuropa contains preliminary drafts of all new and revised monographs proposed for inclusion in the European Pharmacopoeia and gives an opportunity for all interested parties to comment on the specifications before they are finalised. Pharmeuropa also contains information on the work programme and on certificates of suitability to monographs of the European Pharmacopoeia issued by the EDQM, and articles of general interest. Pharmeuropa is available on subscription from the EDQM. The subscription also includes Pharmeuropa Bio and Pharmeuropa Scientific Notes (containing scientific articles on pharmacopoeial matters). Pharmeuropa Online is also available as a complementary service for subscribers to the printed version of Pharmeuropa.

INTERNATIONAL HARMONISATION

See the information given in chapter *5.8. Pharmacopoeial Harmonisation*.

WEBSITE

http://www.edqm.eu

http://www.edqm.eu/store (for prices and orders)

HELPDESK

To send a question or to contact the EDQM, use the HELPDESK, accessible through the EDQM website (visit http://www.edqm.eu/site/page_521.php).

KNOWLEDGE

Consult KNOWLEDGE, the new free database at http://www.edqm.eu to obtain information on the work programme of the European Pharmacopoeia, the volume of Pharmeuropa and of the European Pharmacopoeia in which a text has been published, trade names of the reagents (for example, chromatography columns) that were used at the time of the elaboration of the monographs, the history of the revisions of a text since its publication in the 5th Edition, representative chromatograms, the list of reference standards used, and the list of certificates granted.

COMBISTATS

CombiStats is a computer program for the statistical analysis of data from biological assays in agreement with chapter *5.3* of the 6th Edition of the European Pharmacopoeia. For more information, visit the website (http://www.edqm.eu/combistats).

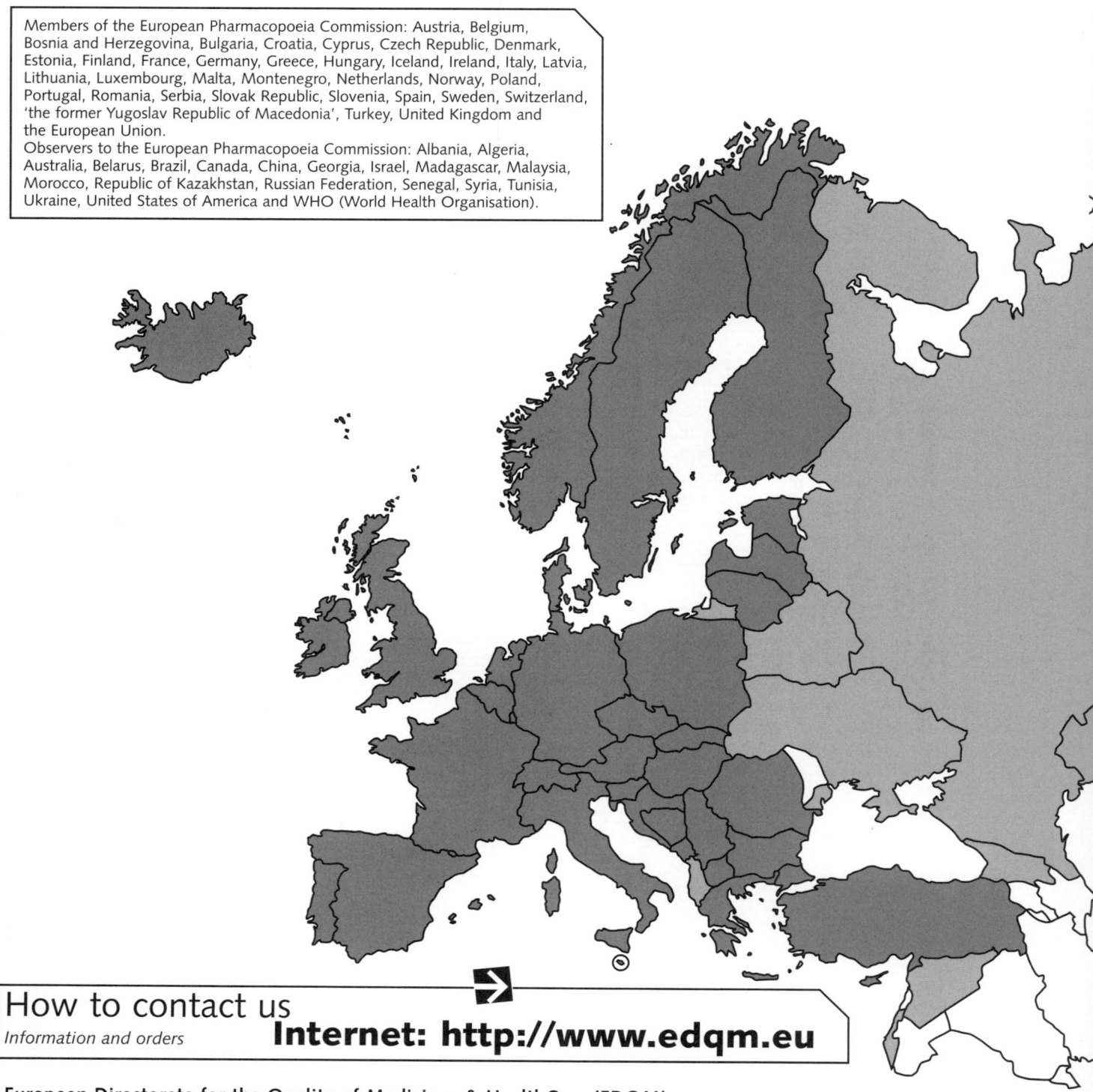

Members of the European Pharmacopoeia Commission: Austria, Belgium, Bosnia and Herzegovina, Bulgaria, Croatia, Cyprus, Czech Republic, Denmark, Estonia, Finland, France, Germany, Greece, Hungary, Iceland, Ireland, Italy, Latvia, Lithuania, Luxembourg, Malta, Montenegro, Netherlands, Norway, Poland, Portugal, Romania, Serbia, Slovak Republic, Slovenia, Spain, Sweden, Switzerland, 'the former Yugoslav Republic of Macedonia', Turkey, United Kingdom and the European Union.
Observers to the European Pharmacopoeia Commission: Albania, Algeria, Australia, Belarus, Brazil, Canada, China, Georgia, Israel, Madagascar, Malaysia, Morocco, Republic of Kazakhstan, Russian Federation, Senegal, Syria, Tunisia, Ukraine, United States of America and WHO (World Health Organisation).

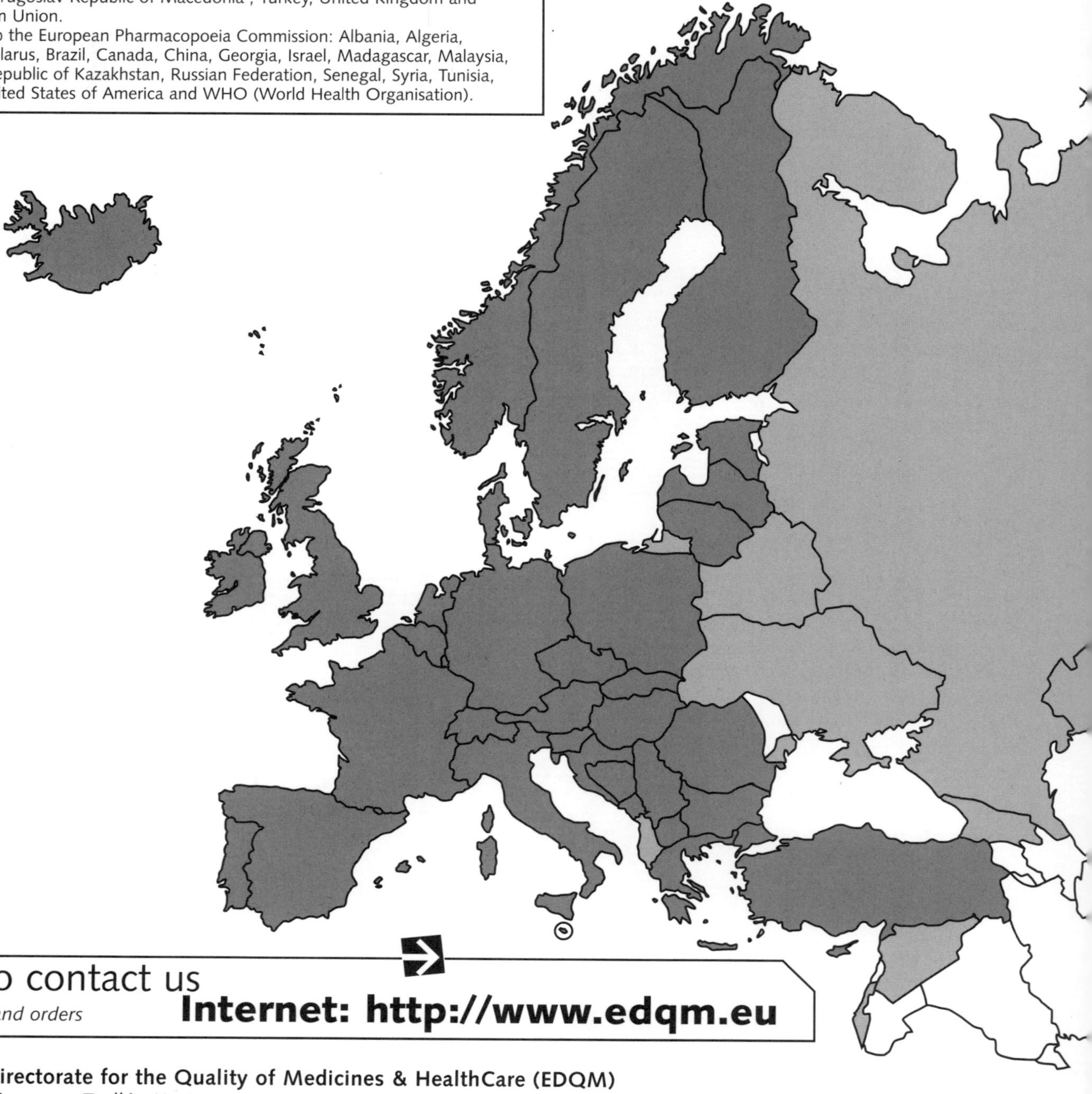

How to contact us

Information and orders

Internet: http://www.edqm.eu

European Directorate for the Quality of Medicines & HealthCare (EDQM)
Council of Europe - 7 allée Kastner
CS 30026, F-67081 STRASBOURG, FRANCE
Tel: +33 (0)3 88 41 30 30*
Fax: +33 (0)3 88 41 27 71*
**Do not dial 0 if calling from outside of France*

Correspondence .... Via the online HELPDESK (http://www.edqm.eu/site/page_521.php)

How to place an order

Publications .... http://www.edqm.eu/store
Reference standards .... http://www.edqm.eu
Reference standards online order form .... http://www.edqm.eu/site/page_649.php

Further information, including answers to the most frequently asked questions regarding ordering, is available via the HELPDESK.

All other matters ....info@edqm.eu

All reference standards required for application of the monographs are available from the EDQM.
A catalogue of reference standards is available on request; the catalogue is included in the Pharmeuropa subscription; it can also be consulted on the EDQM website.

EUROPEAN PHARMACOPOEIA

SIXTH EDITION

Supplement 6.2

EUROPEAN PHARMACOPOEIA

SIXTH EDITION

Supplement 6.2

Published in accordance with the
Convention on the Elaboration of a European Pharmacopoeia
(European Treaty Series No. 50)

European Directorate for the
Quality of Medicines & HealthCare

Council of Europe
Strasbourg

The European Pharmacopoeia is published by the Directorate for the Quality of Medicines & HealthCare of the Council of Europe (EDQM).

ISBN: 978-92-871-6059-1

CONTENTS

CONTENTS OF SUPPLEMENT 6.2 xxxiii

GENERAL CHAPTERS 3621

2. Methods of Analysis 3621

2.4. Limit tests 3621

2.4.29. Composition of fatty acids in oils rich in omega-3 acids 3623

2.6. Biological tests 3625

2.6.26. Test for anti-D antibodies in human immunoglobulin for intravenous administration 3627

2.7. Biological assays 3629

2.7.25. Assay of human plasmin inhibitor 3631

2.7.30. Assay of human protein C 3631

2.7.31. Assay of human protein S 3632

2.7.32. Assay of human α-1-proteinase inhibitor 3633

2.8. Methods in pharmacognosy 3635

2.8.13. Pesticide residues 3637

2.9. Pharmaceutical technical procedures 3639

2.9.9. Measurement of consistency by penetrometry 3641

2.9.23. Gas pycnometric density of solids 3642

2.9.32. Porosity and pore size distribution of solids by mercury porosimetry 3643

2.9.34. Bulk density and tapped density of powders 3646

2.9.35. Powder fineness 3648

2.9.38. Particle-size distribution estimation by analytical sieving 3649

3. Materials for Containers and Containers 3653

3.1. Materials used for the manufacture of containers 3653

3.1.13. Plastic additives 3655

4. Reagents 3659

4.1.1. Materials used for the manufacture of containers 3661

MONOGRAPHS ON VACCINES FOR VETERINARY USE 3663

MONOGRAPHS ON RADIOPHARMACEUTICAL PREPARATIONS 3675

MONOGRAPHS 3681

INDEX 3857

Note: on the first page of each chapter/section there is a list of contents.

CONTENTS OF SUPPLEMENT 6.2

A vertical line in the margin indicates where part of a text has been revised or corrected. A horizontal line in the margin indicates where part of a text has been deleted. It is to be emphasised that these indications, which are not necessarily exhaustive, are given for information and do not form an official part of the texts. Editorial changes are not indicated.

Individual copies of texts will not be supplied.

NEW TEXTS

GENERAL CHAPTERS

2.7.25. Assay of human plasmin inhibitor

2.7.30. Assay of human protein C

2.7.31. Assay of human protein S

2.7.32. Assay of human α-1-proteinase inhibitor

2.9.32. Porosity and pore-size distribution of solids by mercury porosimetry

2.9.34. Bulk density and tapped density of powders

2.9.35. Powder fineness

MONOGRAPHS

*The monographs below appear for the first time in the European Pharmacopoeia. They will be implemented on **1 July 2008** at the latest.*

Vaccines for veterinary use

Coccidiosis vaccine (live) for chickens (2326)

Monographs

Adrenaline (2303)

Altizide (2185)

Carprofen for veterinary use (2201)

Clodronate disodium tetrahydrate (1777)

Flucloxacillin magnesium octahydrate (2346)

Fluvoxamine maleate (1977)

Fresh bilberry fruit dry extract, refined and standardised (2394)

Human α-1-proteinase inhibitor (2387)

Nilutamide (2256)

Racecadotril (2171)

Spanish sage oil (1849)

St. John's wort dry extract, quantified (1874)

Telmisartan (2154)

REVISED TEXTS

GENERAL CHAPTERS

2.6.26. Test for anti-D antibodies in human immunoglobulin for intravenous administration

2.8.13. Pesticide residues

2.9.9. Measurement of consistency by penetrometry

2.9.23. Gas pycnometric density of solids

2.9.38. Particle-size distribution estimation by analytical sieving

4. Reagents (*new, revised, corrected*)

MONOGRAPHS

*The monographs below have been technically revised since their last publication. They will be implemented on **1 July 2008**.*

Vaccines for veterinary use

Vibriosis (cold-water) vaccine (inactivated) for salmonids (1580)

Vibriosis vaccine (inactivated) for salmonids (1581)

Furunculosis vaccine (inactivated, oil-adjuvanted, injectable) for salmonids (1521)

Swine-fever vaccine (live, prepared in cell cultures), classical (0065)

Radiopharmaceutical preparations

Chromium (^{51}Cr) edetate injection (0266)

Fludeoxyglucose (^{18}F) injection (1325)

Monographs

Acacia (0307)

Acacia, spray-dried (0308)

Aceclofenac (1281)

Alginic acid (0591)

Birch leaf (1174)

Calcium carbonate (0014)

Calcium dobesilate monohydrate (1183)

Capsicum (1859)

Cellulose, microcrystalline (0316)

Cellulose, powdered (0315)

Cinchona bark (0174)

Cyclizine hydrochloride (1092)

Devil's claw root (1095)

Dihydrostreptomycin sulphate for veterinary use (0485)

Etamsylate (1204)

Ginger (1522)

Glucose, liquid (1330)

Human anti-D immunoglobulin (0557)

Human normal immunoglobulin (0338)

Human plasma (pooled and treated for virus inactivation) (1646)

Human plasma for fractionation (0853)

Hydroxypropylbetadex (1804)

Imipramine hydrochloride (0029)

Magnesium carbonate, heavy (0043)

Methyltestosterone (0410)

Metoclopramide (1348)

Naproxen (0731)

Norfloxacin (1248)

Ofloxacin (1455)

Orciprenaline sulphate (1033)
Oxacillin sodium monohydrate (2260)
Oxfendazole for veterinary use (1458)
Paraffin, white soft (1799)
Paraffin, yellow soft (1554)
Pseudoephedrine hydrochloride (1367)
Ramipril (1368)
Sodium hyaluronate (1472)
Soya-bean oil, refined (1473)
St. John's wort (1438)
Streptokinase concentrated solution (0356)
Sulfacetamide sodium (0107)
Tinidazole (1051)

CORRECTED TEXTS

The texts below have been corrected and are republished in their entirety. These corrections are to be taken into account from the publication date of Supplement 6.2.

GENERAL CHAPTERS

2.4.29. Composition of fatty acids in oils rich in omega-3 acids
3.1.13. Plastic additives

MONOGRAPHS

Monographs

Agnus castus fruit (2147)
Aprotinin concentrated solution (0579)
Arachis oil, hydrogenated (1171)
Cetirizine dihydrochloride (1084)
Cetostearyl alcohol (type A), emulsifying (0801)
Cetostearyl alcohol (type B), emulsifying (0802)
Cottonseed oil, hydrogenated (1305)
Dimeticone (0138)
Ipratropium bromide (0919)
Maize oil, refined (1342)
Methacrylic acid - ethyl acrylate copolymer (1:1) (1128)
Morphine sulphate (1244)
Moxifloxacin hydrochloride (2254)
Olive oil, refined (1456)
Olive oil, virgin (0518)
Pancreas powder (0350)
Poly(vinyl acetate) dispersion 30 per cent (2152)
Potassium chloride (0185)
Rapeseed oil, refined (1369)
Soya-bean oil, hydrogenated (1265)
Sulbactam sodium (2209)
Sunflower oil, refined (1371)
Tobramycin (0645)

TEXTS CONVERTED TO THE NEW EDITORIAL STYLE

The monographs below have been converted to the new editorial style, which does not entail any changes to their technical content, unless otherwise stated in the above section Corrected texts.

MONOGRAPHS

Monographs

Agar (0310)
Aloes dry extract, standardised (0259)
Arachis oil, hydrogenated (1171)
Belladonna leaf dry extract, standardised (1294)
Belladonna, prepared (0222)
Cassia oil (1496)
Cinnamon bark oil, Ceylon (1501)
Coconut oil, refined (1410)
Cottonseed oil, hydrogenated (1305)
Eucalyptus oil (0390)
Frangula bark dry extract, standardised (1214)
Guar (1218)
Guar galactomannan (0908)
Ipecacuanha, prepared (0093)
Liquorice ethanolic liquid extract, standardised (1536)
Maize oil, refined (1342)
Matricaria liquid extract (1544)
Nitric oxide (1550)
Nitrogen (1247)
Nutmeg oil (1552)
Olive oil, refined (1456)
Olive oil, virgin (0518)
Oxygen (0417)
Peru balsam (0754)
Rapeseed oil, refined (1369)
Senna leaf dry extract, standardised (1261)
Shellac (1149)
Soya-bean oil, hydrogenated (1265)
Stramonium, prepared (0247)
Sunflower oil, refined (1371)
Tragacanth (0532)

TEXTS WHOSE TITLE HAS CHANGED

The title of the following texts has been changed in Supplement 6.2.

GENERAL CHAPTERS

2.9.23. Gas pycnometric density of solids (*previously Pycnometric density of solids*)

MONOGRAPHS

Vaccines for veterinary use

Swine-fever vaccine (live, prepared in cell cultures), classical (0065) (*previously Swine-fever vaccine (live), classical, freeze-dried*)

Monographs

Streptokinase concentrated solution (0356) (*previously Streptokinase bulk solution*)

DELETED TEXTS

The following texts are deleted as of ***1 April 2008***.

MONOGRAPHS

Vaccines for human use

Pertussis vaccine (0160)

Monographs

Stanozolol (1568)

2.4. LIMIT TESTS

01/2008:20429
corrected 6.2

2.4.29. COMPOSITION OF FATTY ACIDS IN OILS RICH IN OMEGA-3 ACIDS

The assay may be used for quantitative determination of the EPA and DHA content in omega-3-containing products of fish oil in different concentrations. The method is applicable to triglycerides or ethyl esters and the results are expressed as triglycerides or ethyl esters, respectively.

EPA AND DHA

Gas chromatography (*2.2.28*). *Carry out the operations as rapidly as possible, avoiding exposure to actinic light, oxidising agents, oxidation catalysts (for example, copper and iron) and air.*

The assay is carried out on the methyl or ethyl esters of (all-*Z*)-eicosa-5,8,11,14,17-pentaenoic acid (EPA; 20:5 n-3) and (all-*Z*)-docosa-4,7,10,13,16,19-hexaenoic acid (DHA; 22:6 n-3) in the substance to be examined.

Internal standard. Methyl tricosanoate R.

Test solution (a)

A. Dissolve the mass of sample to be examined according to Table 2.4.29.-1 and about 70.0 mg of the internal standard in a 50 mg/l solution of *butylhydroxytoluene R* in *trimethylpentane R* and dilute to 10.0 ml with the same solution.

Table 2.4.29.-1.

Approximate sum EPA + DHA (per cent)	Mass of sample to be examined (g)
30 - 50	0.4 - 0.5
50 - 70	0.3
70 - 90	0.25

Ethyl esters are now ready for analysis. For triglycerides continue as described in step B.

B. Introduce 2.0 ml of the solution obtained in step A into a quartz tube and evaporate the solvent with a gentle current of *nitrogen R*. Add 1.5 ml of a 20 g/l solution of *sodium hydroxide R* in *methanol R*, cover with *nitrogen R*, cap tightly with a polytetrafluoroethylene-lined cap, mix and heat on a water-bath for 7 min. Allow to cool. Add 2 ml of *boron trichloride-methanol solution R*, cover with *nitrogen R*, cap tightly, mix and heat on a water-bath for 30 min. Cool to 40-50 °C, add 1 ml of *trimethylpentane R*, cap and shake vigorously for at least 30 s. Immediately add 5 ml of a *saturated sodium chloride solution R*, cover with *nitrogen R*, cap and shake thoroughly for at least 15 s. Transfer the upper layer to a separate tube. Shake the methanol layer once more with 1 ml of *trimethylpentane R*. Wash the combined trimethylpentane extracts with 2 quantities, each of 1 ml, of *water R* and dry over *anhydrous sodium sulphate R*. Prepare 3 solutions for each sample.

Test solution (b). Dissolve 0.300 g of the sample to be examined in a 50 mg/l solution of *butylhydroxytoluene R* in *trimethylpentane R* and dilute to 10.0 ml with the same solution. Proceed as described for test solution (a).

Reference solution (a). Dissolve 60.0 mg of *docosahexaenoic acid ethyl ester CRS*, about 70.0 mg of the internal standard and 90.0 mg of *eicosapentaenoic acid ethyl ester CRS* in a 50 mg/l solution of *butylhydroxytoluene R* in *trimethylpentane R* and dilute to 10.0 ml with the same solution. Proceed as described for test solution (a) step A when analysing ethyl esters. For analysis of triglycerides, continue with step B in the same manner as for test solution (a) and prepare 3 solutions for each sample.

Reference solution (b). Into a 10 ml volumetric flask dissolve 0.3 g of *methyl palmitate R*, 0.3 g of *methyl stearate R*, 0.3 g of *methyl arachidate R* and 0.3 g of *methyl behenate R*, in a 50 mg/l solution of *butylhydroxytoluene R* in *trimethylpentane R* and dilute to 10.0 ml with the same solution.

Reference solution (c). Into a 10 ml volumetric flask dissolve a sample containing about 55.0 mg of *docosahexaenoic acid methyl ester R* and about 5.0 mg of *tetracos-15-enoic acid methyl ester R* in a 50 mg/l solution of *butylhydroxytoluene R* in *trimethylpentane R* and dilute to 10.0 ml with the same solution.

Column:
- *material*: fused silica,
- *dimensions*: *l* = at least 25 m, Ø = 0.25 mm,
- *stationary phase*: bonded *macrogol 20 000 R* (film thickness 0.2 μm).

Carrier gas: *hydrogen for chromatography R* or *helium for chromatography R*.

Flow rate: 1 ml/min.

Split ratio: 1:200, alternatively splitless with temperature control (sample solutions need to be diluted 1/200 with a 50 mg/l solution of *butylhydroxytoluene R* in *trimethylpentane R* before injection).

Temperature:

	Time (min)	Temperature (°C)
Column	0 - 2	170
	2 - 25.7	170 → 240
	25.7 - 28	240
Injection port		250
Detector		270

Detection: flame ionisation.

Injection: 1 μl, twice.

System suitability:
- in the chromatogram obtained with reference solution (b), the area per cent composition increases in the following order: methyl palmitate, methyl stearate, methyl arachidate, methyl behenate; the difference between the percentage area of methyl palmitate and that of methyl behenate is less than 2.0 area per cent units,
- *resolution*: minimum of 1.2 between the peaks due to docosahexaenoic acid methyl ester and to tetracos-15-enoic acid methyl ester in the chromatogram obtained with reference solution (c),
- in the chromatogram obtained with test solution (a), the peaks due to methyl tricosanoate and any heneicosapentaenoic acid methyl ester or ethyl ester (C21:5) present when compared with the chromatogram obtained with test solution (b) are clearly separated (if not, a correction factor has to be used).

Calculate the percentage content of EPA and DHA using the following expression and taking into account the assigned value of the reference substances:

$$A_x \times \frac{A_3}{m_3} \times \frac{m_1}{A_1} \times \frac{m_{x,r}}{A_{x,r}} \times \frac{1}{m_2} \times C \times 100$$

m_1 = mass of the internal standard in test solution (a), in milligrams,

m_2 = mass of the sample to be examined in test solution (a), in milligrams,

m_3 = mass of the internal standard in reference solution (a), in milligrams,

$m_{x,r}$ = mass of *eicosapentaenoic acid ethyl ester CRS* or *docosahexaenoic acid ethyl ester CRS* in reference solution (a), in milligrams,

A_x = area of the peak due to eicosapentaenoic acid ester or docosahexaenoic acid ester in the chromatogram obtained with test solution (a),

$A_{x,r}$ = area of the peak due to eicosapentaenoic acid ester or docosahexaenoic acid ester in the chromatogram obtained with reference solution (a),

A_1 = area of the peak due to the internal standard in the chromatogram obtained with test solution (a),

A_3 = area of the peak due to the internal standard in the chromatogram obtained with reference solution (a),

C = conversion factor between ethyl ester and triglycerides,

C = 1.00 for ethyl esters,

C = 0.954 for EPA,

C = 0.957 for DHA.

TOTAL OMEGA-3 ACIDS

From the assay for EPA and DHA, calculate the percentage content of the total omega-3 acids using the following expression and identifying the peaks from the chromatograms:

$$EPA + DHA + \frac{A_{n-3}\,(EPA + DHA)}{A_{EPA} + A_{DHA}}$$

EPA = percentage content of EPA,

DHA = percentage content of DHA,

$A_{n\text{-}3}$ = sum of the areas of the peaks due to C18:3 n-3, C18:4 n-3, C20:4 n-3, C21:5 n-3 and C22:5 n-3 methyl esters in the chromatogram obtained with test solution (b),

A_{EPA} = area of the peak due to EPA ester in the chromatogram obtained with test solution (b),

A_{DHA} = area of the peak due to DHA ester in the chromatogram obtained with test solution (b).

2.6. BIOLOGICAL TESTS

07/2008:20626

2.6.26. TEST FOR ANTI-D ANTIBODIES IN HUMAN IMMUNOGLOBULIN FOR INTRAVENOUS ADMINISTRATION

MATERIALS

Phosphate-buffered saline (PBS). Dissolve 8.0 g of *sodium chloride R*, 0.76 g of *anhydrous disodium hydrogen phosphate R*, 0.2 g of *potassium chloride R* and 0.2 g of *potassium dihydrogen phosphate R* in *water R* and dilute to 1000 ml with the same solvent. If the solution has to be kept for several days, 0.2 g of *sodium azide R* may be added in order to avoid microbial contamination.

Papain solution. Use serological-grade papain from a commercial source, the activity of which has been validated.

Red blood cells. Use pooled D-positive red blood cells from not fewer than 3 donors, preferably of group OR_2R_2. D-positive red blood cells may also be obtained from OR_1R_1 or OR_1R_2 donors. Mixing phenotypes has not been tested and is therefore not recommended.

Use pooled D-negative red blood cells, preferably from 3 donors of group Orr. When only 1 donor of group Orr is available, D-negative red blood cells from only 1 donor may be used.

Wash the cells 4 times with PBS or until the supernatant is clear. Centrifuge the cells at 1800 *g* for 5 min to pack. Treat the packed cells with papain solution according to the manufacturer's instructions. Store in Alsever's solution for not more than 1 week.

Microtitre plates. Use V-bottomed rigid micro-titre plates.

Reference standards. Immunoglobulin (anti-D antibodies test) BRP and *Immunoglobulin (anti-D antibodies test negative control) BRP* are suitable for use as the reference preparation and negative control, respectively.

METHOD

The test described in this chapter is performed at room temperature on the reference solutions, the negative control solutions and the test solutions at the same time and under identical conditions.

Reference solutions and negative control solutions. Reconstitute the reference preparation and the negative control according to instructions. The immunoglobulin G (IgG) concentration is 50 g/l in each of the reconstituted preparations. Make a 2-fold dilution of each reconstituted preparation with PBS containing *bovine albumin R* at 2 g/l, to give solutions containing IgG at 25 g/l. Prepare 7 further serial 2-fold dilutions of each preparation using PBS containing *bovine albumin R* at 2 g/l to extend the dilution range to 1/256 (0.195 g/l IgG). Add 20 µl of each dilution to the microtitre plate.

Test solutions. Dilute the preparation to be examined with PBS containing *bovine albumin R* at 2 g/l to give a starting IgG concentration of 25 g/l. For 50 g/l products, this is a 2-fold dilution; adjust the dilution factor accordingly for samples that are not 50 g/l to give a starting concentration of 25 g/l for testing. This 25 g/l solution is assigned a nominal 2-fold dilution factor for comparison with the reference preparations, even if this does not reflect the true dilution factor used to achieve 25 g/l. Prepare 7 further serial 2-fold dilutions of each preparation using PBS containing *bovine albumin R* at 2 g/l to extend the nominal dilution range to 1/256 (0.195 g/l IgG) for comparison with the reference preparations over the same IgG concentration range. Make 2 independent sets of dilutions. Add 20 µl of each dilution to the microtitre plate.

Prepare 3 per cent *V/V* suspensions of papain-treated D-positive (preferably OR_2R_2, but OR_1R_1 or OR_1R_2 may also be used) and D-negative (Orr) red blood cells in PBS containing *bovine albumin R* at 2 g/l. Add 20 µl of D-positive cells to 1 dilution series of each of the preparation to be examined, the reference preparation and the negative control, and 20 µl of D-negative cells to the other dilution series of each of the preparation to be examined, the reference preparation and the negative control. Mix by shaking the plate on a shaker for 10 s.

Centrifuge the plate at 80 *g* for 1 min to pack the cells. Place the plate at an angle of approximately 70°. Read after at least 3 min and once the cells have streamed in the wells containing the negative control and the wells where the D-negative cells have been added. A cell button at the bottom of the well indicates a positive result. A stream of cells represents a negative result.

Record the endpoint titre as the reciprocal of the highest dilution that gives rise to a positive result.

The negative control must have a titre not greater than 2, otherwise an investigation of the test reagents and conditions has to be performed.

The titre of the preparation to be examined is not greater than the titre of the reference preparation when all preparations are titrated from 25 g/l.

2.7. BIOLOGICAL ASSAYS

07/2008:20725

2.7.25. ASSAY OF HUMAN PLASMIN INHIBITOR

Human plasmin inhibitor, also called human α_2-antiplasmin, is a plasma protein that inhibits the plasmin (a serine protease) pathway of fibrinolysis by rapidly forming a complex with free plasmin. Furthermore, upon blood coagulation, human plasmin inhibitor is cross-linked to fibrin strands by factor XIII, and interferes with binding of the proenzyme plasminogen to fibrin.

The potency of human plasmin inhibitor is estimated by comparing the ability of the preparation to be examined to inhibit the cleavage of a specific chromogenic substrate by plasmin with the same ability of a reference standard of human plasmin inhibitor. Plasmin cleavage of the chromogenic substrate yields a chromophore that can be quantified spectrophotometrically.

The individual reagents for the assay may be obtained separately or in commercial kits. Both end-point and kinetic methods are available. Procedures and reagents may vary between different kits and the manufacturer's instructions are followed. The essential features of the procedure are described in the following example of a microtitre-plate kinetic method.

REAGENTS

Dilution buffer pH 7.5. According to the manufacturer's instructions, a suitable buffer is used. Adjust the pH (*2.2.3*) if necessary.

Plasmin. A preparation of human plasmin that does not contain significant amounts of other proteases is preferably used. Reconstitute and store according to the manufacturer's instructions.

Plasmin chromogenic substrate. A suitable specific chromogenic substrate for plasmin is used: H-D-cyclohexylalanyl-norvalyl-lysyl-*p*-nitroaniline hydrochloride (H-D-CHA-Nva-Lys-*p*NA.HCl) or L-pyroglutamyl-L-phenylalanyl-L-lysine-*p*-nitroaniline hydrochloride (Glp-Phe-Lys-*p*NA.HCl). Reconstitute in *water R* to give a suitable concentration according to the manufacturer's instructions.

METHOD

Varying quantities of the preparation to be examined are mixed with a given quantity of plasmin and the remaining plasmin activity is determined using a suitable chromogenic substrate.

Reconstitute or thaw the preparation to be examined according to the manufacturer's instructions. Dilute with dilution buffer pH 7.5 and prepare at least 2 independent series of 3 or 4 dilutions for both the preparation to be examined and the reference standard.

Mix 0.020 ml of each dilution with 0.020 ml of dilution buffer pH 7.5 and warm to 37 °C. Add 0.040 ml of a plasmin solution (test concentration in the range of 0.2 nkat/ml to 1.6 nkat/ml) previously heated to 37 °C and leave at 37 °C for 1 min. Add 0.020 ml of the chromogenic substrate solution, previously heated to 37 °C, to each mixture and measure the optical density at a wavelength of 405 nm. Substract the optical density of the blank (prepared with dilution buffer pH 7.5) from the optical density of the preparation to be examined. Check the validity of the assay and calculate the potency of the preparation to be examined by the usual statistical methods (*5.3*).

07/2008:20730

2.7.30. ASSAY OF HUMAN PROTEIN C

1. CHROMOGENIC ASSAY

Human protein C is a vitamin K-dependent plasma protein that, upon activation to activated protein C (APC), can inhibit blood coagulation through the proteolytic cleavage of factors Va and VIIIa. Human protein C activity is estimated using a two-step method: in the 1st step, human protein C in the preparation is activated by a specific activator from snake venom; in the 2nd step, APC cleaves a specific chromogenic substrate to form a chromophore that can be quantified spectrophotometrically.

Step 1

$$\text{human protein C} \xrightarrow{\text{human protein C activator}} \text{APC}$$

Step 2

$$\text{chromogenic substrate} \xrightarrow{\text{APC}} \text{peptide + chromophore}$$

The potency of human protein C is estimated by comparing the ability of the preparation to be examined to cleave a chromogenic substrate with the same ability of a reference standard of human protein C calibrated in International Units. The International Unit is the activity of a stated amount of the International Standard for human protein C. The equivalence in International Units of the International Standard is stated by the World Health Organisation.

Individual reagents may be obtained separately or in commercial kits. Both end-point and kinetic methods are available. Procedures and reagents may vary between different kits and the manufacturer's instructions are followed. The essential features of the procedure are described in the following example of a microtitre plate end-point method.

REAGENTS

Dilution buffer pH 8.4. Dissolve 6.055 g of *tris(hydroxymethyl)aminomethane R* and 16.84 g of *caesium chloride R* in *water R* and adjust the pH (*2.2.3*) if necessary. Dilute to 1000.0 ml with *water R*.

Human protein C activator. Protein isolated from the venom of the viper *Agkistrodon contortrix contortrix* that specifically activates human protein C. Reconstitute and store according to the manufacturer's instructions. Dilute to 0.25 U/ml with *water R* before use in the assay.

Activated protein C chromogenic substrate. Specific chromogenic substrate for APC, for example L-pyroglutamyl-L-prolyl-L-arginine-paranitroaniline hydrochloride (pyroGlu-Pro-Arg-pNA.HCl). Reconstitute with *water R* to give a concentration of 4.5 mmol/l. Further dilute to 1.1 mmol/l with dilution buffer pH 8.4 before use in the assay.

METHOD

Reconstitute or thaw the preparation to be examined according to the manufacturer's instructions. Dilute with *water R* to produce at least 3 separate dilutions for each preparation in the range 0.050-0.200 IU/ml, preferably in duplicate.

Step 1. Mix 0.025 ml of each dilution with 0.050 ml of the human protein C activator, both previously heated to 37 °C, and leave at 37 °C for exactly 10 min. For each dilution, prepare a blank in the same manner, using *water R* instead of the human protein C activator.

Step 2. Add 0.150 ml of diluted chromogenic substrate, previously heated to 37 °C, to each mixture and leave at 37 °C for exactly 10 min. The incubation time must be adjusted, if necessary, to ensure a linear development of chromophore with time. Terminate the reaction by adding 0.050 ml of a 50 per cent *V/V* solution of *glacial acetic acid R*.

Cleavage of the chromogenic substrate by APC causes release of the chromophore pNA, in proportion to the concentration of human protein C in the preparation. Measure the optical density at a wavelength of 405 nm. Subtract the optical density of the blank from the optical density of the test sample. Check the validity of the assay and calculate the potency of the preparation to be examined using the usual statistical methods (*5.3.*).

2. CLOTTING ASSAY

Human protein C activity is estimated following cleavage to APC by a specific activator extracted from the venom of the viper *Agkistron contortrix contortrix*. The resulting APC inactivates factors Va and VIIIa, and thus prolongs the APTT (Activated Partial Thromboplastin Time) of a system in which all the coagulation factors are present, constant and in excess, except for human protein C, which is derived from the preparation being tested. Prolongation of the clotting time is proportional to the concentration of human protein C in the preparation.

The potency of human protein C is estimated by comparing the ability of the preparation to be examined to prolong the clotting time with the same ability of a reference standard of human protein C calibrated in International Units. The International Unit is the activity of a stated amount of the International Standard for human protein C. The equivalence in International Units of the International Standard is stated by the World Health Organisation.

Individual reagents may be obtained separately or in commercial kits. Procedures and reagents may vary between different kits and the manufacturer's instructions are followed. The essential features of the procedure are described in the following example.

REAGENTS

Dilution buffer pH 7.4. Isotonic non-chelating buffer.

Human protein C-deficient plasma. Citrated human plasma with no measurable human protein C content. Reconstitute and store according to the manufacturer's instructions.

Human protein C activator. Protein isolated from the venom of the viper *Agkistrodon contortrix contortrix* that specifically activates human protein C. Reconstitute and store according to the manufacturer's instructions.

Coagulation activator. A suitable APTT reagent containing phospholipids and a contact activator may be used. It may be combined with the human protein C activator.

METHOD

Reconstitute or thaw the preparation to be examined according to the manufacturer's instructions. Dilute with dilution buffer pH 7.4 to produce at least 3 separate dilutions for each preparation in the range 0.010-0.150 IU/ml, preferably in duplicate.

Mix 1 volume of each dilution with 1 volume of human protein C-deficient plasma and 1 volume of the human protein C activator (combined with the APTT reagent where appropriate), all previously heated to 37 °C. Add 1 volume of *calcium chloride R* previously heated to 37 °C, and record the clotting time.

The clotting time is proportional to the concentration of human protein C in each dilution. Check the validity of the assay and calculate the potency of the preparation to be examined using the usual statistical methods (*5.3*).

07/2008:20731

2.7.31. ASSAY OF HUMAN PROTEIN S

Human protein S is a vitamin K-dependent plasma protein that acts as a cofactor for the anticoagulant functions of activated protein C (APC). Human protein S activity may be determined by the clotting assay described below, which is sensitive to the ability of human protein S to accelerate the inactivation of factor Va by APC. In practice, the assay involves the addition of human protein S to a reagent mixture containing APC, factor Va and human protein S-deficient plasma. Prolongation of the clotting time is proportional to the concentration of human protein S in the preparation. Methods in which APC is added directly as a reagent are preferred to those in which APC is generated during the assay by the addition of a specific human protein C activator purified from snake venom. Activation of coagulation is initiated by the addition of an activating reagent such as thromboplastin or activated factor X, together with phospholipids and calcium chloride. During the assay, factor Va is generated from factor V in the human protein S-deficient plasma following the activation of coagulation. The assay procedure must ensure that human protein S is the only limiting factor.

The potency of human protein S is estimated by comparing the ability of the preparation to be examined to prolong the clotting time with the same ability of a reference standard of human protein S calibrated in International Units. The International Unit is the activity of a stated amount of the International Standard for human protein S. The equivalence in International Units of the International Standard is stated by the World Health Organisation.

Individual reagents may be obtained separately or in commercial kits. Procedures and reagents may vary between different kits and the manufacturer's instructions are followed. The essential features of the procedure are described in the following example.

REAGENTS

Dilution buffer pH 7.4. Isotonic non-chelating buffer prepared as follows: dissolve 6.08 g of *tris(hydroxymethyl)-aminomethane R* and 8.77 g of *sodium chloride R* in *water R* and adjust the pH (*2.2.3*) if necessary; add 10 g of *bovine albumin R* or *human albumin R* and dilute to 1000.0 ml with *water R*.

Human protein S-deficient plasma. Citrated human plasma with no measurable human protein S content and, preferably, also free of C4b-binding protein.

Coagulation activator. This reagent is used to initiate coagulation in the human protein S-deficient plasma, and thereby also provides a source of activated factor V. The activator may consist of tissue factor, activated factor X, or an agent capable of directly activating factor X that may be purified from the venom of Russell's viper (*Vipera russelli*). The reagent also contains APC, phospholipids and *calcium chloride R*, or, alternatively, calcium chloride may be added separately after a timed activation period.

METHOD

Reconstitute or thaw the preparation to be examined according to the manufacturer's instructions. Dilute with dilution buffer pH 7.4 to produce at least 3 separate dilutions for each preparation in the range 0.020-0.100 IU/ml, preferably in duplicate.

Mix 1 volume of each dilution with 1 volume of human protein S-deficient plasma, both previously heated to 37 °C. Add 2 volumes of the coagulation activator, previously heated to 37 °C, and record the clotting time.

Alternative procedures may use a coagulation activator without calcium chloride, and require a precisely timed activation period before the addition of calcium chloride and the measurement of clotting time.

The clotting time is proportional to the concentration of human protein S in each dilution. Check the validity of the assay and calculate the potency of the preparation to be examined using the usual statistical methods (*5.3*).

07/2008:20732

2.7.32. ASSAY OF HUMAN α-1-PROTEINASE INHIBITOR

Human α-1-proteinase inhibitor (also known as α-1-antitrypsin or α-1-antiproteinase) content is determined by comparing the ability of the preparation to be examined to inactivate the serine protease elastase (porcine pancreatic elastase or human neutrophil elastase) with the same ability of a reference standard of human α-1-proteinase inhibitor calibrated in milligrams of active (functional) α-1-proteinase inhibitor. Varying quantities of the preparation to be examined are mixed with a given quantity of elastase and the remaining elastase activity is determined using a suitable chromogenic substrate. The method described below is given as an example.

REAGENTS

Tris-albumin buffer solution. Dissolve 24.23 g of *trometamol R* in *water R*, adjust to pH 8.0 ± 0.3 using *hydrochloric acid R1* and dilute to 1000 ml with *water R*. To 100 ml of this solution add 0.5 ml of a 20 per cent solution of *human albumin R* or *bovine albumin R*.

Buffer solution containing human or bovine albumin must be prepared fresh on the day of its use; otherwise, it can be conserved by sterile filtration (0.2 μm) and stored at 2-8 °C for up to 2 weeks.

METHOD

Prepare 2 series of 4 or 5 dilutions in an appropriate human α-1-proteinase inhibitor concentration range, for both the preparation to be examined and the reference standard, using the tris-albumin buffer solution.

Transfer 50 μl of the reference solution dilutions into the wells of a microtitre plate and to each well, add 150 μl of a porcine pancreatic elastase solution diluted to an appropriate concentration with the tris-albumin buffer solution. Incubate for a defined period of time, 3-10 min, at room temperature. Since the activity of the solutions of the different porcine pancreatic elastases may vary, the concentration of elastase can be adjusted by evaluation of blank values containing elastase but no human α-1-proteinase inhibitor, to exhibit a suitable change of absorbance at 405 nm under the actual assay conditions.

Add to each well 100 μl of a solution of chromogenic substrate *N*-succinyl-tri-L-alanyl 4-p-nitroanilide (Suc-Ala-Ala-Ala-pNA), reconstituted in *dimethyl sulphoxide R* to give a solution containing 4.5 mg/ml, then further diluted with the tris-albumin buffer solution to a concentration of 0.45 mg/ml. Immediately start measurement of the change in absorbance (*2.2.25*) at 405 nm using a microtitre plate reader, continuing the measurement for at least 5 min. Calculate the rate of change of absorbance (ΔA/min). Alternatively, an end-point assay may be used by stopping the reaction with acetic acid and measuring the absorbance at 405 nm. If the assay is performed in test tubes using spectrophotometers for monitoring the change in absorbance at 405 nm, the volumes of reagent solutions are changed proportionally.

The rate of change of absorbance (ΔA/min) is inversely proportional to human α-1-proteinase inhibitor activity.

Check the validity of the assay and calculate the potency of the test preparation by the usual statistical methods (*5.3*).

2.8. METHODS IN PHARMACOGNOSY

07/2008:20813

2.8.13. PESTICIDE RESIDUES

Definition. For the purposes of the Pharmacopoeia, a pesticide is any substance or mixture of substances intended for preventing, destroying or controlling any pest, unwanted species of plants or animals causing harm during or otherwise interfering with the production, processing, storage, transport or marketing of herbal drugs. The item includes substances intended for use as growth-regulators, defoliants or desiccants and any substance applied to crops, either before or after harvest, to protect the commodity from deterioration during storage and transport. Pesticide residues can be present and are controlled in herbal drugs and herbal drug preparations.

Limits. Unless otherwise indicated in the monograph, the herbal drug to be examined at least complies with the limits indicated in Table 2.8.13.-1. The limits applying to pesticides that are not listed in Table 2.8.13.-1 and whose presence is suspected for any reason comply with the limits (levels) cross referred to by Regulation (EC) No. 396/2005, including annexes and successive updates. Limits for pesticides that are not listed in Table 2.8.13.-1 nor in European Union texts are calculated using the following expression:

$$\frac{ADI \times M}{MDD_{HD} \times 100}$$

ADI = acceptable daily intake, as published by FAO-WHO, in milligrams per kilogram of body mass,

M = body mass in kilograms (60 kg),

MDD_{HD} = daily dose of the herbal drug, in kilograms.

The limits for pesticides in herbal drug preparations are calculated using the following expressions:

If DER ≤ 10:

$$MRL_{HD} \times DER$$

If DER > 10:

$$\frac{ADI \times M}{MDD_{HP} \times 100}$$

MRL_{HD} = maximum residue limit of the pesticide in the herbal drug as given in Table 2.8.13.-1 or in EU texts or calculated using the expression mentioned above;

DER = drug/extract ratio, i.e. the ratio between the quantity of herbal drug used in the manufacture of a herbal drug preparation and the quantity of herbal drug preparation obtained;

MDD_{HP} = daily dose of the herbal drug preparation, in kilograms.

The competent authority may grant total or partial exemption from the test when the complete history (nature and quantity of the pesticides used, date of each treatment during cultivation and after the harvest) of the treatment of the batch is known and can be checked precisely according to good agricultural and collection practice (GACP).

Table 2.8.13.-1

Substance	**Limit (mg/kg)**
Acephate	0.1
Alachlor	0.05
Aldrin and dieldrin (sum of)	0.05
Azinphos-ethyl	0.1
Azinphos-methyl	1
Bromide, inorganic (calculated as bromide ion)	50
Bromophos-ethyl	0.05
Bromophos-methyl	0.05
Brompropylate	3
Chlordane (sum of *cis*-, *trans* - and oxychlordane)	0.05
Chlorfenvinphos	0.5
Chlorpyriphos-ethyl	0.2
Chlorpyriphos-methyl	0.1
Chlorthal-dimethyl	0.01
Cyfluthrin (sum of)	0.1
λ-Cyhalothrin	1
Cypermethrin and isomers (sum of)	1
DDT (sum of *o,p'*-DDE, *p,p'*-DDE, *o,p'*-DDT, *p,p'*-DDT, *o,p'*-TDE and *p,p'*-TDE)	1
Deltamethrin	0.5
Diazinon	0.5
Dichlofluanid	0.1
Dichlorvos	1
Dicofol	0.5
Dimethoate and omethoate (sum of)	0.1
Dithiocarbamates (expressed as CS2)	2
Endosulfan (sum of isomers and endosulfan sulphate)	3
Endrin	0.05
Ethion	2
Etrimphos	0.05
Fenchlorophos (sum of fenchlorophos and fenchlorophos-oxon)	0.1
Fenitrothion	0.5
Fenpropathrin	0.03
Fensulfothion (sum of fensulfothion, fensulfothion-oxon, fensulfothion-oxonsulfon and fensulfothion-sulfon)	0.05
Fenthion (sum of fenthion, fenthion-oxon, fenthion-oxon-sulfon, fenthion-oxon-sulfoxid, fenthion-sulfon and fenthion-sulfoxid)	0.05
Fenvalerate	1.5
Flucytrinate	0.05
τ-Fluvalinate	0.05
Fonophos	0.05
Heptachlor (sum of heptachlor, *cis*-heptachlorepoxide and *trans*-heptachlorepoxide)	0.05
Hexachlorbenzene	0.1
Hexachlorocyclohexane (sum of isomers α-, β-, δ- and ε)	0.3

Substance	Limit (mg/kg)
Lindan (γ-hexachlorocyclohexane)	0.6
Malathion and malaoxon (sum of)	1
Mecarbam	0.05
Methacriphos	0.05
Methamidophos	0.05
Methidathion	0.2
Methoxychlor	0.05
Mirex	0.01
Monocrotophos	0.1
Parathion-ethyl and Paraoxon-ethyl (sum of)	0.5
Parathion-methyl and Paraoxon-methyl (sum of)	0.2
Pendimethalin	0.1
Pentachloranisol	0.01
Permethrin and isomers (sum of)	1
Phosalone	0.1
Phosmet	0.05
Piperonyl butoxide	3
Pirimiphos-ethyl	0.05
Pirimiphos-methyl (sum of pirimiphos-methyl and *N*-desethyl-pirimiphos-methyl)	4
Procymidone	0.1
Profenophos	0.1
Prothiophos	0.05
Pyrethrum (sum of cinerin I, cinerin II, jasmolin I, jasmolin II, pyrethrin I and pyrethrin II)	3
Quinalphos	0.05
Quintozene (sum of quintozene, pentachloraniline and methyl penthachlorphenyl sulfide)	1
S-421	0.02
Tecnazene	0.05
Tetradifon	0.3
Vinclozolin	0.4

Sampling of herbal drugs. Sampling is done according to the general chapter *2.8.20*.

Herbal drugs: sampling and sample preparation.

Qualitative and quantitative analysis of pesticide residues. The analytical procedures used are validated (e.g. according to Document N° SANCO/10232/2006). In particular, they satisfy the following criteria:

- the chosen method, especially the purification steps, is suitable for the combination pesticide residue/substance to be examined, and not susceptible to interference from co-extractives;
- natural occurrence of some constituents is considered in the interpretation of results (e.g. disulfide from Cruciferaceae);
- the concentration of test and reference solutions and the setting of the apparatus are such that the responses used for quantification of the pesticide residues are within the dynamic range of the detector. Test solutions containing pesticide residues at a level outside the dynamic range, may be diluted within the calibration range, provided that the concentration of the matrix in the solution is adjusted in the case where the calibration solutions must be matrix-matched;
- between 70 per cent to 110 per cent of each pesticide is recovered;
- repeatability of the method: RSD is not greater than the values indicated in Table 2.8.13.-2;
- reproducibility of the method: RSD is not greater than the values indicated in Table 2.8.13.-2.

Table 2.8.13.-2

Concentration range of the pesticide (mg/kg)	Repeatability (RSD) (per cent)	Reproducibility (RSD) (per cent)
0.001 - 0.01	30	60
> 0.01 - 0.1	20	40
> 0.1 - 1	15	30
> 1	10	20

2. Methods of analysis

2.9. PHARMACEUTICAL TECHNICAL PROCEDURES

07/2008:20909

2.9.9. MEASUREMENT OF CONSISTENCY BY PENETROMETRY

This test is intended to measure, under determined and validated conditions, the penetration of an object into the product to be examined in a container with a specified shape and size.

APPARATUS

The apparatus consists of a penetrometer made up of a stand and a penetrating object. A suitable apparatus is shown in Figure 2.9.9.-1.

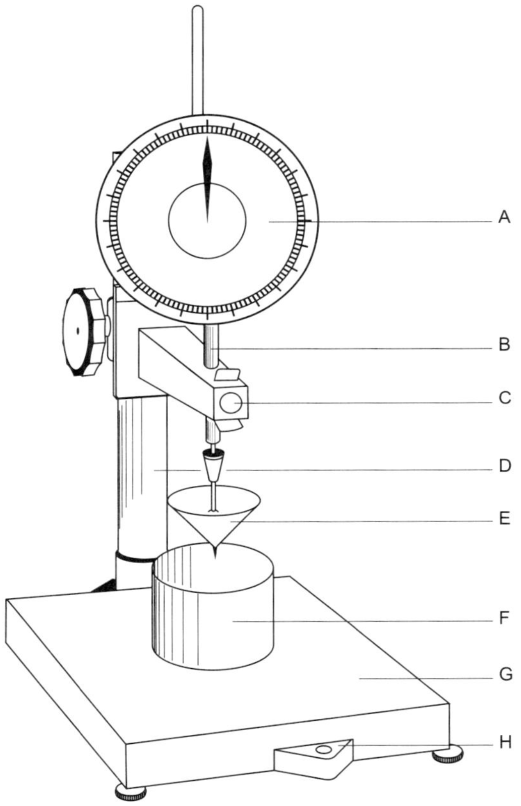

Figure 2.9.9.-1. – *Penetrometer*

A. Scale showing the depth of penetration, graduated in tenths of millimetres.

B. Vertical shaft to maintain and guide the penetrating object.

C. Device to retain and to release the penetrating object automatically and for a constant time.

D. Device to ensure that the penetrating object is vertical and that the base is horizontal.

E. Penetrating object (see Figures 2.9.9.-2 and 3).

F. Container.

G. Horizontal base.

H. Control for the horizontal base.

The stand is made up of:

– a vertical shaft to maintain and guide the penetrating object;

– a horizontal base;

– a device to ensure that the penetrating object is vertical;

– a device to check that the base is horizontal;

– a device to retain and release the penetrating object;

– a scale showing the depth of penetration, graduated in tenths of a millimetre.

The penetrating object, made of a suitable material, has a smooth surface, and is characterised by its shape, size and mass (m).

Suitable penetrating objects are shown in Figures 2.9.9.-2 and 2.9.9.-3.

PROCEDURE

Prepare the test samples according to one of the following procedures.

A. Carefully and completely fill 3 containers, without forming air bubbles. Level if necessary to obtain a flat surface. Store the samples at 25 ± 0.5 °C for 24 h, unless otherwise prescribed.

B. Store 3 samples at 25 ± 0.5 °C for 24 h, unless otherwise prescribed. Apply a suitable shear to the samples for 5 min. Carefully and completely fill 3 containers, without forming air bubbles, and level if necessary to obtain a flat surface.

C. Melt 3 samples and carefully and completely fill 3 containers, without forming air bubbles. Store the samples at 25 ± 0.5 °C for 24 h, unless otherwise prescribed.

Determination of penetration. Place the test sample on the base of the penetrometer. Verify that its surface is perpendicular to the vertical axis of the penetrating object. Bring the temperature of the penetrating object to 25 ± 0.5 °C and then adjust its position such that its tip just touches the surface of the sample. Release the penetrating object and hold it free for 5 s. Clamp the penetrating object and measure the depth of penetration. Repeat the test with the 2 remaining containers.

EXPRESSION OF THE RESULTS

The penetration is expressed in tenths of a millimetre as the arithmetic mean of the 3 measurements. If any of the individual results differ from the mean by more than 3 per cent, repeat the test and express the results of the 6 measurements as the mean and the relative standard deviation.

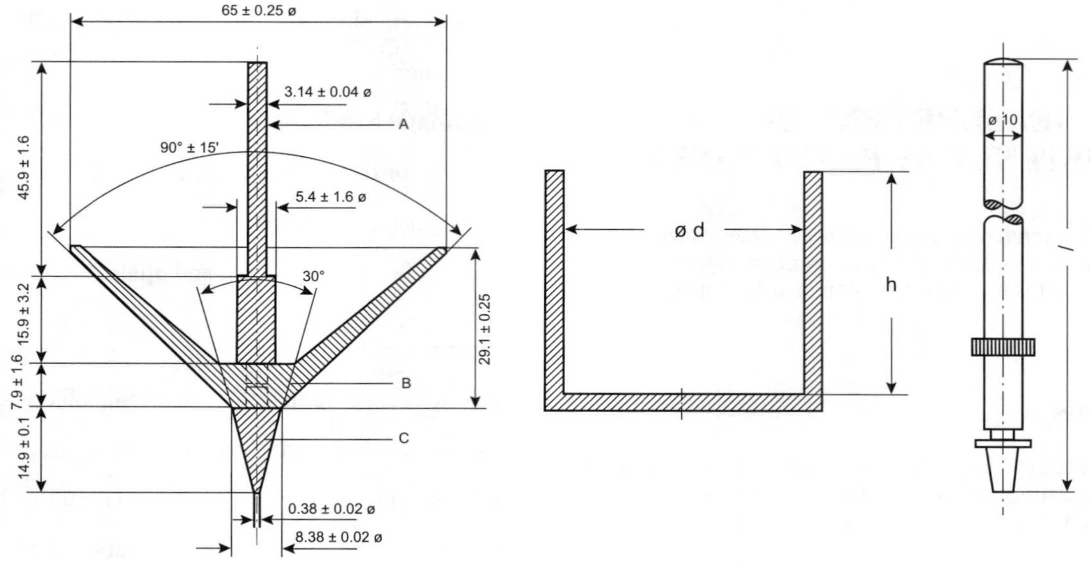

Figure 2.9.9.-2. – *Cone (m = 102.5 ± 0.05 g), suitable container (d = 102 mm or 75 mm; h ≥ 62 mm) and shaft (l = 162 mm; m = 47.5 ± 0.05 g).*

Dimensions in millimetres

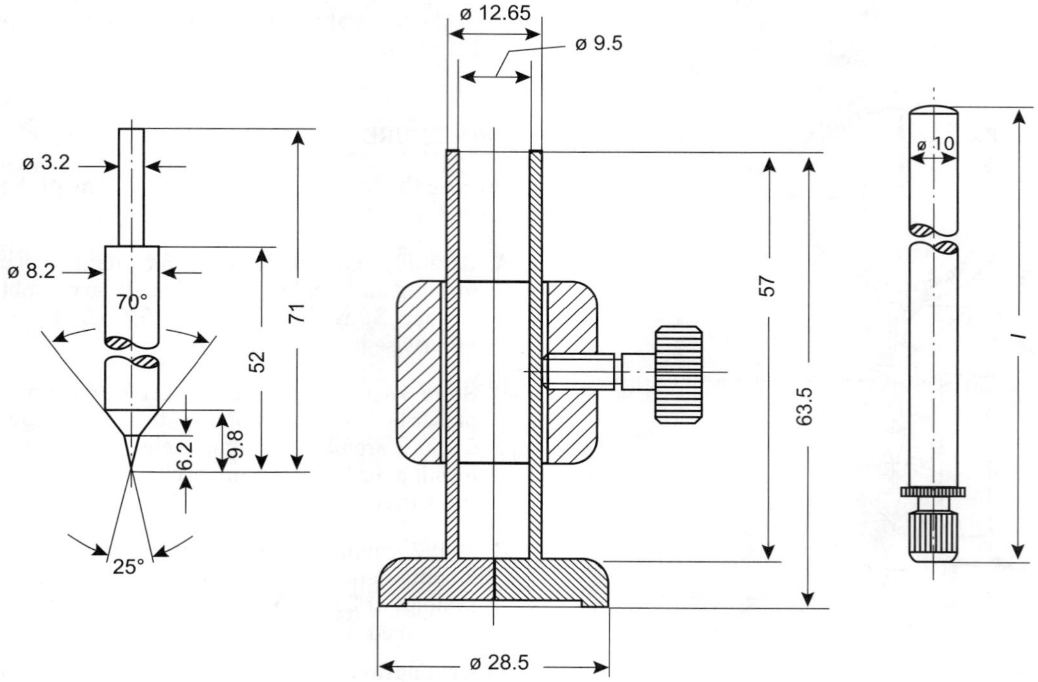

Figure 2.9.9.-3 – *Micro-cone (m = 7.0 g), suitable container and shaft (l = 116 mm; m = 16.8 g)*

Dimensions in millimetres

07/2008:20923

2.9.23. GAS PYCNOMETRIC DENSITY OF SOLIDS

Gas pycnometric density is determined by measuring the volume occupied by a known mass of powder, which is equivalent to the volume of gas displaced by the powder using a gas displacement pycnometer. In gas pycnometric density measurements, the volume determined excludes the volume occupied by open pores; however, it includes the volume occupied by sealed pores or pores inaccessible to the gas.

Usually, helium is used as a test gas due to its high diffusivity into small open pores. If gases other than helium are used, different values would be obtained, since the penetration of the gas is dependent on the size of the pore as well as the cross-sectional area of the gas molecules.

The measured density is a volume-weighted average of the densities of individual powder particles. It is called the particle density, distinct from the true density of a solid or the bulk density of a powder. The density of solids is expressed in grams per cubic centimetre (g/cm^3), although the International Unit is the kilogram per cubic meter ($1\ g/cm^3 = 1000\ kg/m^3$).

APPARATUS

The apparatus (see Figure 2.9.23.-1) consists of the following:

- a sealed test cell, with empty cell volume V_c, connected through a valve to an expansion cell, with volume V_r;
- a system capable of pressurising the test cell with the measurement gas until a defined pressure (P) indicated by a manometer;
- the system is connected to a source of measurement gas, preferably helium, unless another gas is specified.

The gas pycnometric density measurement is performed at a temperature between 15 °C and 30 °C that does not vary by more than 2 °C during the course of measurement.

The apparatus is calibrated, which means that the volumes V_c and V_r are determined using a suitable calibration standard whose volume is known to the nearest 0.001 cm^3. The procedure described below is followed in 2 runs, firstly with an empty test cell, and secondly with the calibration standard placed in the test cell. The volumes V_c and V_r are calculated using the equation for the sample volume (V_s), taking into account that V_s is zero in the first run.

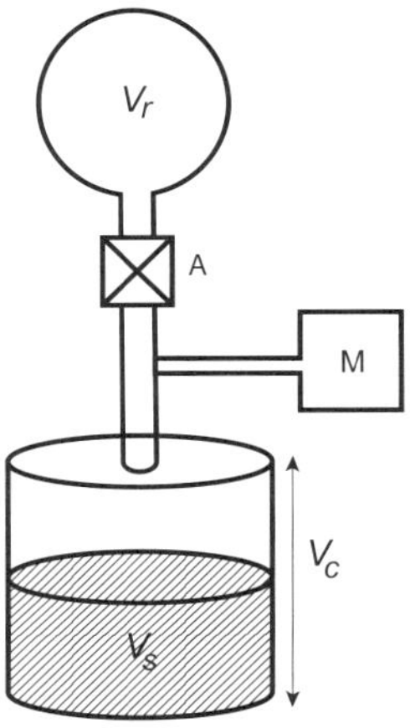

A = valve;

V_r = expansion volume, in cubic centimetres;

V_c = cell volume, in cubic centimetres;

V_s = sample volume, in cubic centimetres;

M = manometer.

Figure 2.9.23.-1. – *Schematic diagram of a gas pycnometer*

METHOD

Volatile contaminants in the powder are removed by degassing the powder under a constant purge of helium prior to the measurement. Occasionally, powders may have to be degassed under vacuum. Because volatiles may be evolved during the measurement, weighing of the sample is carried out after the pycnometric measurement of volume.

Weigh the test cell of the pycnometer and record the mass. Fill the test cell with a given mass of powder of the substance to be examined. Seal the test cell in the pycnometer. Record the system reference pressure (P_r) as indicated by the manometer while the valve that connects the expansion cell with the test cell is open. Close the valve to separate the expansion cell from the test cell. Pressurise the test cell with the gas to an initial pressure (P_i) and record the value obtained. Open the valve to connect the expansion cell with the test cell. Record the final pressure (P_f). Repeat the measurement sequence for the same powder sample until consecutive measurements of the sample volume (V_s) agree to within 0.2 per cent. Unload the test cell and measure the final powder mass (m), expressed in grams. If the pycnometer differs in operation or construction from the one shown in Figure 2.9.23.-1, follow the instructions of the manufacturer of the pycnometer.

EXPRESSION OF THE RESULTS

The sample volume (V_s) is given by the equation:

$$V_s = V_c - \frac{V_r}{\dfrac{P_i - P_r}{P_f - P_r} - 1}$$

The density (ρ) is given by the equation:

$$\rho = \frac{m}{V_s}$$

The sample conditioning is indicated with the results. For example, indicate whether the sample was tested as is or dried under specific conditions such as those described for loss on drying.

07/2008:20932

2.9.32. POROSITY AND PORE-SIZE DISTRIBUTION OF SOLIDS BY MERCURY POROSIMETRY

INTRODUCTION

In general, different types of pores may be pictured as apertures, channels or cavities within a solid body, or as space (i.e. interstices or voids) between solid particles in a bed, compact or aggregate. Porosity is a term that is often used to indicate the porous nature of solid material, and is more precisely defined as the ratio of the volume of accessible pores and voids to the total volume occupied by a given amount of the solid. In addition to the accessible pores, a solid may contain closed pores, which are isolated from the external surface and into which fluids are not able to penetrate. The characterisation of closed pores, i.e. cavities with no access to an external surface, is not covered in this chapter.

Porous materials may take the form of fine or coarse powders, compacts, extrudates, sheets or monoliths. Their characterisation usually involves the determination of the total pore volume or porosity as well as the pore-size distribution.

It is well established that the performance of a porous solid (e.g. its strength, reactivity, permeability or adsorbent power) is dependent upon its pore structure. Many different methods have been developed for the characterisation of pore structure. In view of the complexity of most porous solids, it is not surprising to find that the results obtained are not always in agreement and that no single technique can be relied upon to provide a complete picture of the pore structure. The choice of the most appropriate method depends on the application of the porous solid, its chemical and physical nature and the range of pore-size.

This chapter provides guidance for measurement of porosity and pore-size distribution by mercury porosimetry. It is a comparative test, usually destructive, in which the volume of mercury penetrating a pore or void is determined as a function of an applied hydrostatic pressure, which can be related to a pore diameter. Other information such as pore shape and inter-connectivity, the internal and external surface area, powder granulometry, bulk and tapped density could also be inferred from volume-pressure curves; however, these aspects of the technique do not fall under the scope of this chapter.

Practical considerations presently limit the maximum applied absolute pressure reached by some equipment to about 400 MPa, corresponding to a minimum equivalent pore diameter of approximately 0.003 μm. The maximum diameter will be limited for samples having a significant depth due to the difference in hydrostatic head of mercury from the top to the bottom of the sample. For most purposes this limit may be regarded as 400 μm.

Inter-particle and intra-particle porosity can be determined, but the method does not distinguish between these porosities where they co-exist.

The method is suitable for the study of most porous materials. Samples that amalgamate with mercury, such as certain metals, may be unsuitable for this technique or may require a preliminary passivation. Other materials may deform or compact under the applied pressure. In some cases it may be possible to apply sample-compressibility corrections and useful comparative data may still be obtained.

Mercury porosimetry is considered to be comparative, as for most porous media a theory is not available to allow an absolute calculation of results of pore-size distribution. Therefore this technique is mainly recommended for development studies.

Mercury is toxic. Appropriate precautions must be observed to safeguard the health of the operator and others working in the area. Waste material must also be disposed of in a suitable manner, according to local regulations.

PRINCIPLE

The technique is based on the measurement of the mercury volume intruded into a porous solid as a function of the applied pressure. The measurement includes only those pores into which mercury can penetrate at the pressure applied.

A non-wetting liquid penetrates into a porous system only under pressure. The pressure to be applied is in inverse proportion to the inner diameter of the pore aperture. In the case of cylindrical pores, the correlation between pore diameter and pressure is given by the Washburn equation:

$$d_p = -\frac{4 \cdot \sigma}{p} \cos \theta$$

d_p = pore diameter, in metres;

σ = surface tension, in newtons per metre;

θ = contact angle of mercury on the sample, in degrees;

p = applied pressure, in pascals.

APPARATUS

The sample holder, referred to as penetrometer or dilatometer, has a calibrated capillary tube, through which the sample can be evacuated and through which mercury can enter. The capillary tube is attached to a wider tube in which the test sample is placed. The change in the volume of mercury intruded is usually measured by the change in capacitance between the mercury column in the capillary tube and a metal sleeve around the outside of the capillary tube. If precise measurements are required the expected total void and pore volume of the sample should be between 20 per cent and 90 per cent of the internal volume of the capillary tube. Since different materials exhibit a wide range of open porosities, a number of penetrometers with different capillary tube diameters and sample volumes may be required. A typical set-up for a mercury porosimeter instrument is given in Figure 2.9.32.-1. The porosimeter may have separate ports for high- and low-pressure operation, or the low-pressure measurement may be carried out on a separate unit.

The pressure range is typically 4-300 kPa for low-pressure operation and above 300 kPa for high-pressure operation, depending on the design of the particular apparatus and on the intended use.

METHOD

Sample preparation

The sample is pre-treated to remove adsorbed material that can obscure its accessible porosity, for example by heating and/or evacuation, or by flowing inert gas. It may be possible to passivate the surface of wettable or amalgam-forming

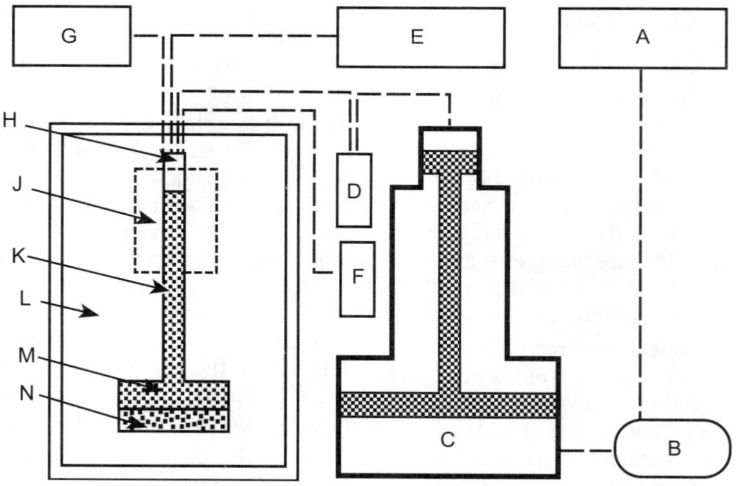

A. Low-pressure hydraulic fluid reservoir
B. Hydraulic pump
C. Pressure multiplier
D. Pressure transducer
E. High-pressure hydraulic fluid reservoir
F. Vacuum pump with gauge
G. Mercury reservoir
H. Oil
J. Penetration volume indicator
K. Capillary tube
L. High-pressure chamber
M. Mercury
N. Sample

Figure 2.9.32.-1. – *Example of the set-up of a mercury porosimeter instrument* solids, for example by producing a thin layer of oxide, or by coating with stearate.

The sample of the pre-treated solid is weighed and transferred to the penetrometer. The pore system of the sample is then degassed in a vacuum to a maximum residual pressure of 7 Pa.

Filling the penetrometer with mercury

The mercury used is of analytical quality. Overlay the sample with mercury under vacuum. The vacuum is required to ensure the transfer of mercury from the reservoir to the penetrometer. In a filled penetrometer the filling pressure comprises the applied pressure plus the pressure contribution created by the head of mercury contacting the sample. A typical filling pressure would be about 4 kPa. The hydrostatic pressure of the mercury over the sample may be minimised by filling the penetrometer in the horizontal position.

Low-pressure measurement

Admit air or nitrogen in a controlled manner to increase the pressure either in stages corresponding to the particular pore sizes of interest, or continuously at a slow rate. The concomitant change in the length of the mercury column in the capillary tube is recorded. When the maximum required pressure has been reached, return to atmospheric pressure.

High-pressure measurement

After measurement at low pressure, the penetrometer filled with mercury is transferred to the high-pressure port or unit of the instrument and overlaid with hydraulic fluid. Mercury is intruded into the pore system via the hydraulic fluid. Increase the pressure in the system to the maximum pressure reached in the low-pressure measurement and record the intrusion volume at this pressure, since subsequent intrusion volumes are calculated from this initial volume. Increase the pressure either in stages corresponding to the particular pore sizes of interest, or continuously at a slow rate. The fall in the mercury column is measured up to the maximum required pressure. If required the pressure may be decreased either in stages or continuously at a slow rate to determine the mercury extrusion curve.

Corrections are made to take account of changes in the volume of the mercury, the penetrometer and other components of the volume detector system under elevated pressure. The extent of the corrections may be determined by means of blank measurements under the same conditions.

An experimentally determined volume-pressure curve is shown in Figure 2.9.32.-2.

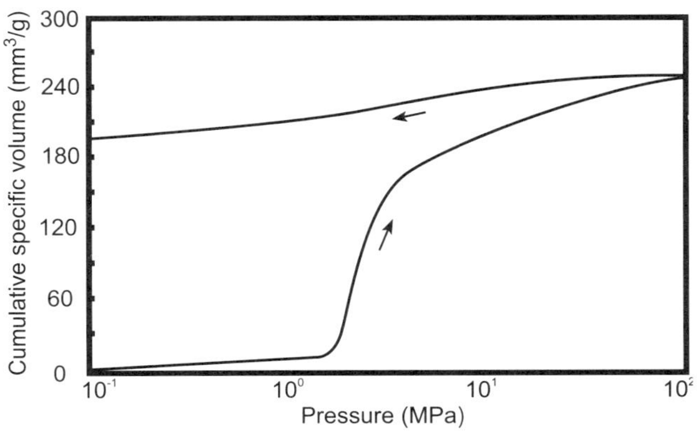

Figure 2.9.32.-2. – *Volume-pressure curve as semilogarithmic plot*

REPORTING OF RESULTS

The pressure readings can be converted to pore diameters by means of the Washburn equation or by another model.

The surface tension of mercury (σ) depends not only on the temperature, but also, in the case of markedly curved surfaces areas, on the radius of curvature. In general, values between 0.41 $N{\cdot}m^{-1}$ and 0.52 $N{\cdot}m^{-1}$ are measured at room temperature. If the value is not known, σ = 0.48 $N{\cdot}m^{-1}$ can be used.

The contact angle of mercury (θ) in most cases is more than 90°. It may be determined using a contact angle instrument. If the value is not known, θ = 130° can be used. The values of contact angle and surface tension and the model used in the calculation are reported.

Visualisation of the data can be done with several types of graphs. Frequently, in a graphical representation the pore diameter is plotted on the abscissa and the intruded volume per sample mass on the ordinate to give the pore-size distribution. It is appropriate here to choose a logarithmic scale for the abscissa (see Figure 2.9.32.-3). The spaces between the particles of the solid sample are included as pores in the calculation. If the pores differ in size from the voids, the latter can be separated by choosing the appropriate pore-size range.

Extrusion curves may not be used for calculating the pore-size distribution (for hysteresis, see Figure 2.9.32.-2), because an intruded part of the mercury always remains in the pore system. The retention ratio may however be useful for the qualitative characterisation of pores that are only accessible via narrow openings ('ink-bottle pores').

Most common characteristic values, such as the total intruded specific volume and the mean and median pore diameters, are calculated from the pore-size distribution. Moreover, sufficient information must be documented about the sample, the sample preparation, the evacuation conditions and the instrument used.

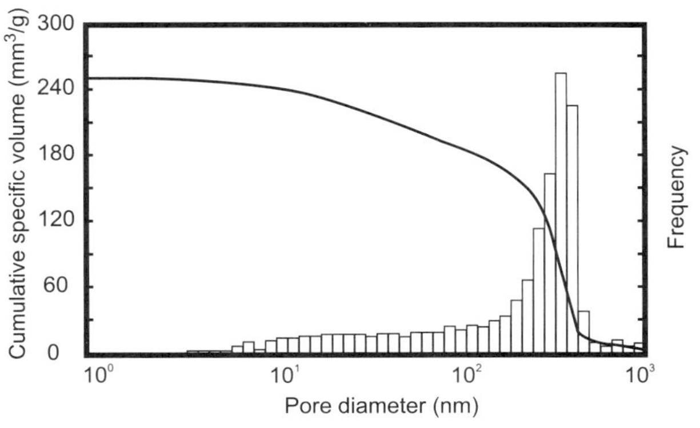

Figure 2.9.32.-3. – *Pore-size distribution as semilogarithmic plots of the cumulative and the normalised density distribution*

CONTROL OF INSTRUMENT PERFORMANCE

As mercury porosimetry is considered to be used as a comparative test, no details are given in this chapter. However, it is recommended that a stable comparison material is tested on a regular basis to monitor instrument calibration and performance.

07/2008:20934

2.9.34. BULK DENSITY AND TAPPED DENSITY OF POWDERS

Bulk density

The bulk density of a powder is the ratio of the mass of an untapped powder sample to its volume, including the contribution of the interparticulate void volume. Hence, the bulk density depends on both the density of powder particles and the spatial arrangement of particles in the powder bed. The bulk density is expressed in grams per millilitre despite the International Unit being kilogram per cubic metre (1 g/ml = 1000 kg/m^3), because the measurements are made using cylinders. It may also be expressed in grams per cubic centimetre.

The bulking properties of a powder are dependent upon the preparation, treatment and storage of the sample, i.e. how it has been handled. The particles can be packed to have a range of bulk densities and, moreover, the slightest disturbance of the powder bed may result in a changed bulk density. Thus, the bulk density of a powder is often very difficult to measure with good reproducibility and, in reporting the results, it is essential to specify how the determination was made.

The bulk density of a powder is determined either by measuring the volume of a known mass of powder sample, which may have been passed through a sieve, in a graduated cylinder (Method 1), or by measuring the mass of a known volume of powder that has been passed through a volumeter into a cup (Method 2) or has been introduced into a measuring vessel (Method 3).

Methods 1 and 3 are favoured.

METHOD 1: MEASUREMENT IN A GRADUATED CYLINDER

Procedure. Pass a quantity of powder sufficient to complete the test through a sieve with apertures greater than or equal to 1.0 mm, if necessary, to break up agglomerates that may have formed during storage; this must be done gently to avoid changing the nature of the material. Into a dry, graduated, 250 ml cylinder (readable to 2 ml), gently introduce, without compacting, approximately 100 g (m) of the test sample weighed with 0.1 per cent accuracy. If necessary, carefully level the powder without compacting, and read the unsettled apparent volume (V_0) to the nearest graduated unit. Calculate the bulk density in grams per millilitre using the formula m/V_0. Generally, replicate determinations are desirable for the determination of this property.

If the powder density is too low or too high, such that the test sample has an untapped apparent volume of more than 250 ml or less than 150 ml, it is not possible to use 100 g of powder sample. In this case, a different amount of powder is selected as the test sample, such that its untapped apparent volume is between 150 ml and 250 ml (apparent volume greater than or equal to 60 per cent of the total volume of the cylinder); the mass of the test sample is specified in the expression of results.

For test samples having an apparent volume between 50 ml and 100 ml, a 100 ml cylinder readable to 1 ml can be used; the volume of the cylinder is specified in the expression of results.

METHOD 2: MEASUREMENT IN A VOLUMETER

Apparatus. The apparatus (Figure 2.9.34.-1) consists of a top funnel fitted with a 1.0 mm sieve, mounted over a baffle box containing 4 glass baffles over which the powder slides and bounces as it passes. At the bottom of the baffle box is a funnel that collects the powder and allows it to pour into a cup mounted directly below it. The cup may be cylindrical (25.00 ± 0.05 ml volume with an internal diameter of 30.00 ± 2.00 mm) or square (16.39 ± 2.00 ml volume with internal dimensions of 25.4 ± 0.076 mm).

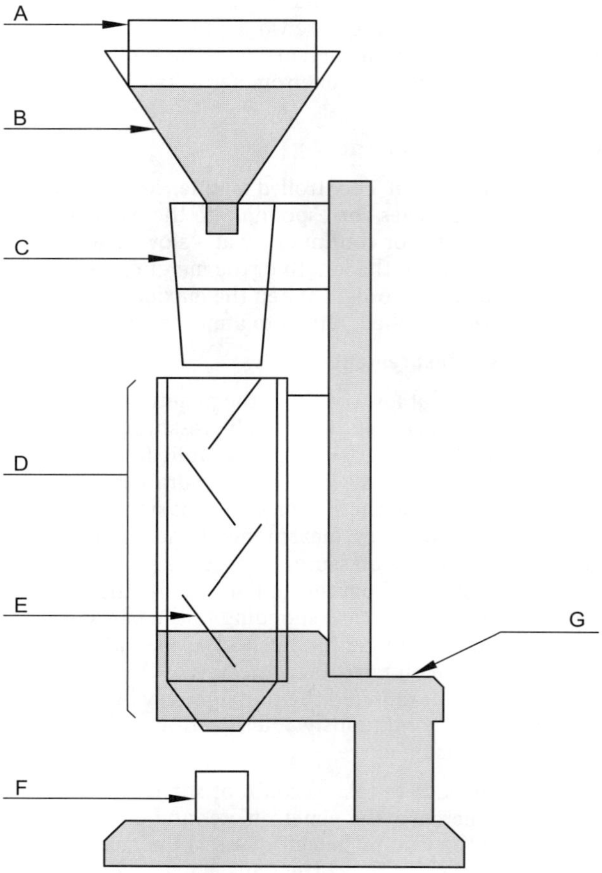

A. 1.0 mm sieve
B. powder funnel
C. loading funnel
D. baffle box
E. glass baffle
F. cup
G. stand

Figure 2.9.34.-1. – *Volumeter*

Procedure. Allow an excess of powder to flow through the apparatus into the sample receiving cup until it overflows, using a minimum of 25 cm^3 of powder with the square cup and 35 cm^3 of powder with the cylindrical cup. Carefully, scrape excess powder from the top of the cup by smoothly moving the edge of the blade of a spatula perpendicular to and in contact with the top surface of the cup, taking care to keep the spatula perpendicular to prevent packing or removal of powder from the cup. Remove any material from the side of the cup and determine the mass (M) of the powder to the nearest 0.1 per cent. Calculate the bulk density in grams per millilitre using the formula M/V_0 where V_0 is the volume of the cup) and record the average of 3 determinations using 3 different powder samples.

METHOD 3. MEASUREMENT IN A VESSEL

Apparatus. The apparatus consists of a 100 ml cylindrical vessel of stainless steel with dimensions as specified in Figure 2.9.34.-2.

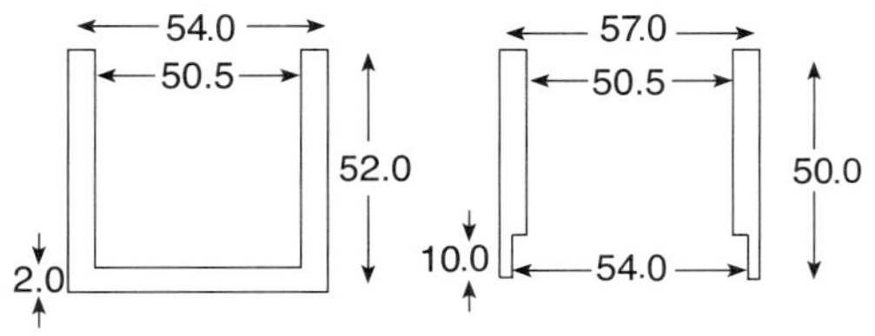

Figure 2.9.34.-2. – *Measuring vessel (left) and cap (right) Dimensions in millimetres*

Procedure. Pass a quantity of powder sufficient to complete the test through a 1.0 mm sieve, if necessary, to break up agglomerates that may have formed during storage, and allow the obtained sample to flow freely into the measuring vessel until it overflows. Carefully scrape the excess powder from the top of the vessel as described under Method 2. Determine the mass (M_0) of the powder to the nearest 0.1 per cent by subtracting the previously determined mass of the empty measuring vessel. Calculate the bulk density in grams per millilitre using the formula $M_0/100$ and record the average of 3 determinations using 3 different powder samples.

Tapped density

The tapped density is an increased bulk density attained after mechanically tapping a receptacle containing the powder sample.

The tapped density is obtained by mechanically tapping a graduated measuring cylinder or vessel containing the powder sample. After observing the initial powder volume or mass, the measuring cylinder or vessel is mechanically tapped, and volume or mass readings are taken until little further volume or mass change is observed. The mechanical tapping is achieved by raising the cylinder or vessel and allowing it to drop, under its own mass, a specified distance by one of 3 methods as described below. Devices that rotate the cylinder or vessel during tapping may be preferred to minimise any possible separation of the mass during tapping down.

METHOD 1

Apparatus. The apparatus (Figure 2.9.34.-3) consists of the following:

- a 250 ml graduated cylinder (readable to 2 ml) with a mass of 220 ± 44 g;
- a settling apparatus capable of producing, per minute, either nominally 250 ± 15 taps from a height of 3 ± 0.2 mm, or nominally 300 ± 15 taps from a height of 14 ± 2 mm. The support for the graduated cylinder, with its holder, has a mass of 450 ± 10 g.

Procedure. Proceed as described above for the determination of the bulk volume (V_0). Secure the cylinder in the support. Carry out 10, 500 and 1250 taps on the same powder sample and read the corresponding volumes V_{10}, V_{500} and V_{1250} to the nearest graduated unit. If the difference between V_{500} and V_{1250} is less than 2 ml, V_{1250} is the tapped volume. If the difference between V_{500} and V_{1250} exceeds 2 ml, repeat in increments of, for example, 1250 taps, until the difference between successive measurements is less than 2 ml. Fewer taps may be appropriate for some powders, when validated. Calculate the tapped density in grams per millilitre using the

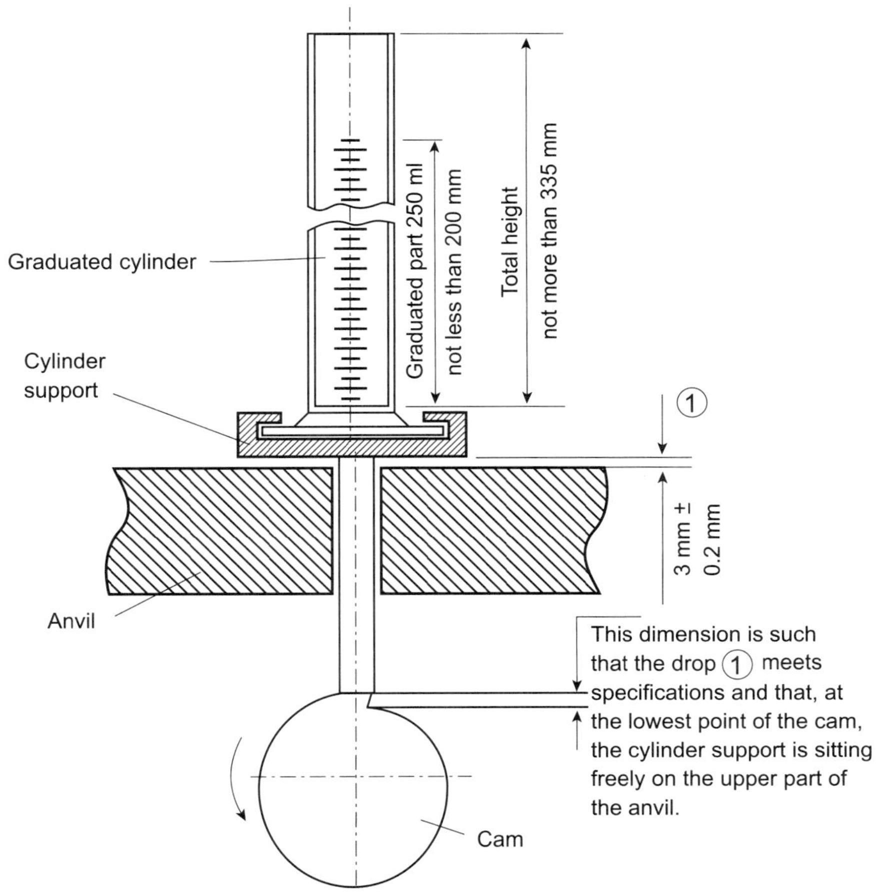

Figure 2.9.34.-3 – *Settling device for powder samples Dimensions in millimetres*

formula m/V_f, where V_f is the final tapped volume. Generally, replicate determinations are desirable for the determination of this property. Specify the drop height with the results.

If it is not possible to use a 100 g test sample, use a reduced amount and a suitable 100 ml graduated cylinder (readable to 1 ml) weighing 130 ± 16 g and mounted on a support weighing 240 ± 12 g. Specify the modified test conditions with the results.

METHOD 2

Procedure. Proceed as directed under Method 1 except that the mechanical tester provides a fixed drop of 3 ± 0.2 mm at a nominal rate of 250 taps per minute.

METHOD 3

Procedure. Proceed as described under Method 3 for measuring the bulk density, using the measuring vessel equipped with the cap shown in Figure 2.9.34.-2. The measuring vessel with the cap is lifted 50-60 times per minute by the use of a suitable tapped density tester. Carry out 200 taps, remove the cap and carefully scrape excess powder from the top of the measuring vessel as described under Method 3 for measuring the bulk density. Repeat the procedure using a further 200 taps. If the difference between the 2 masses obtained after 200 and 400 taps exceeds 2 per cent, repeat the test using 200 additional taps until the difference between successive measurements is less than 2 per cent. Calculate the tapped density in grams per millilitre using the formula $M_f/100$, where M_f is the mass of powder in the measuring vessel. Generally, replicate determinations are desirable for the determination of this property.

Measures of powder compressibility

Because the interparticulate interactions influencing the bulking properties of a powder are also the interactions that interfere with powder flow, a comparison of the bulk and tapped densities can give a measure of the relative importance of these interactions in a given powder. Such a comparison is often used as an index of the ability of the powder to flow, for example the compressibility index or the Hausner ratio.

The compressibility index and Hausner ratio are measures of the propensity of a powder to be compressed as described above. As such, they are measures of the powder's ability to settle, and they permit an assessment of the relative importance of interparticulate interactions. In a free-flowing powder, such interactions are less significant, and the bulk and tapped densities will be closer in value. For more-poorly flowing materials, there are frequently greater interparticulate interactions, and a greater difference between the bulk and tapped densities will be observed. These differences are reflected in the compressibility index and the Hausner ratio.

Compressibility index:

$$\frac{100\,(V_0 - V_f)}{V_0}$$

V_0 = unsettled apparent volume;

V_f = final tapped volume.

Hausner Ratio:

$$\frac{V_0}{V_f}$$

Depending on the material, the compressibility index can be determined using V_{10} instead of V_0.

07/2008:20935

2.9.35. POWDER FINENESS

Particle-size distribution is estimated by analytical sieving (*2.9.38*) or by application of other suitable methods where appropriate. A simple descriptive classification of powder fineness is provided in this chapter. For practical reasons, sieves are commonly used to measure powder fineness. Sieving is most suitable where a majority of the particles are larger than about 75 µm, although it can be used for some powders having smaller particle sizes where the method can be validated. Light diffraction is also a widely used technique for measuring the size of a wide range of particles.

Where the cumulative distribution has been determined by analytical sieving or by application of other methods, particle size may be characterised in the following manner:

x_{90} = particle size corresponding to 90 per cent of the cumulative undersize distribution;

x_{50} = median particle size (i.e. 50 per cent of the particles are smaller and 50 per cent of the particles are larger);

x_{10} = particle size corresponding to 10 per cent of the cumulative undersize distribution.

It is recognised that the symbol *d* is also widely used to designate these values. Therefore, the symbols d_{90}, d_{50}, d_{10} may be used.

The following parameters may be defined based on the cumulative distribution.

$Q_r(x)$ = cumulative distribution of particles with a dimension less than or equal to x where the subscript r reflects the distribution type.

r	**Distribution type**
0	Number
1	Length
2	Area
3	Volume

Therefore, by definition:

$Q_r(x) = 0.90$ when $x = x_{90}$

$Q_r(x) = 0.50$ when $x = x_{50}$

$Q_r(x) = 0.10$ when $x = x_{10}$

An alternative but less informative method of classifying powder fineness is by use of the descriptive terms in Table 2.9.35.-1.

Table 2.9.35.-1.

Classification of powders by fineness		
Descriptive term	**x_{50} (µm)**	**Cumulative distribution by volume basis, $Q_3(x)$**
Coarse	> 355	$Q_3(355) < 0.50$
Moderately fine	180 - 355	$Q_3(180) < 0.50$ and $Q_3(355) \geq 0.50$
Fine	125 - 180	$Q_3(125) < 0.50$ and $Q_3(180) \geq 0.50$
Very fine	≤ 125	$Q_3(125) \geq 0.50$

07/2008:20938

2.9.38. PARTICLE-SIZE DISTRIBUTION ESTIMATION BY ANALYTICAL SIEVING

Sieving is one of the oldest methods of classifying powders and granules by particle-size distribution. When using a woven sieve cloth, the sieving will essentially sort the particles by their intermediate size dimension (i.e. breadth or width). Mechanical sieving is most suitable where the majority of the particles are larger than about 75 μm. For smaller particles, their light weight provides insufficient force during sieving to overcome the surface forces of cohesion and adhesion that cause the particles to stick to each other and to the sieve, and thus cause particles that would be expected to pass through the sieve to be retained. For such materials other means of agitation such as air-jet sieving or sonic-sifter sieving may be more appropriate. Nevertheless, sieving can sometimes be used for some powders or granules having median particle sizes smaller than 75 μm where the method can be validated. In pharmaceutical terms, sieving is usually the method of choice for classification of the coarser grades of single powders or granules. It is a particularly attractive method in that powders and granules are classified only on the basis of particle size, and in most cases the analysis can be carried out in the dry state.

Among the limitations of the sieving method are the need for an appreciable amount of sample (normally at least 25 g, depending on the density of the powder or granule, and the diameter of the test sieves) and the difficulty in sieving oily or other cohesive powders or granules that tend to clog the sieve openings. The method is essentially a two-dimensional estimate of size because passage through the sieve aperture is frequently more dependent on maximum width and thickness than on length.

This method is intended for estimation of the total particle-size distribution of a single material. It is not intended for determination of the proportion of particles passing or retained on 1 or 2 sieves.

Estimate the particle-size distribution as described under Dry sieving method, unless otherwise specified in the individual monograph. Where difficulty is experienced in reaching the endpoint (i.e. material does not readily pass through the sieves) or when it is necessary to use the finer end of the sieving range (below 75 μm), serious consideration must be given to the use of an alternative particle-sizing method.

Sieving is carried out under conditions that do not cause the test sample to gain or lose moisture. The relative humidity of the environment in which the sieving is carried out must be controlled to prevent moisture uptake or loss by the sample. In the absence of evidence to the contrary, analytical test sieving is normally carried out at ambient humidity. Any special conditions that apply to a particular material must be detailed in the individual monograph.

Principles of analytical sieving. Analytical test sieves are constructed from a woven-wire mesh, which is of simple weave that is assumed to give nearly square apertures and is joined to the base of an open cylindrical container. The basic analytical method involves stacking the sieves on top of one another in ascending degrees of coarseness, and then placing the test powder on the top sieve. The nest of sieves is subjected to a standardised period of agitation, and then the mass of material retained on each sieve is accurately determined. The test gives the mass percentage of powder in each sieve size range.

This sieving process for estimating the particle-size distribution of a single pharmaceutical powder is generally intended for use where at least 80 per cent of the particles are larger than 75 μm. The size parameter involved in determining particle-size distribution by analytical sieving is the length of the side of the minimum square aperture through which the particle will pass.

TEST SIEVES

Test sieves suitable for pharmacopoeial tests conform to the current edition of *ISO 3310-1: Test sieves – Technical requirements and testing - Part 1: Test sieves of metal wire cloth* (see Table 2.9.38.-1). Unless otherwise specified in the monograph, use those ISO sieves listed as principal sizes in Table 2.9.38.-1 that are recommended in the particular region.

Table 2.9.38.-1.

ISO Nominal Aperture			US Sieve No.	Recommended USP Sieves (μm)	European Sieve No.	Japanese Sieve No.
Principal sizes	Supplementary sizes					
R 20/3	R 20	R 40/3				
11.20 mm	11.20 mm	11.20 mm			11 200	
	10.00 mm					
		9.50 mm				
	9.00 mm					
8.00 mm	8.00 mm	8.00 mm				
	7.10 mm					
		6.70 mm				
	6.30 mm					
5.60 mm	5.60 mm	5.60 mm			5600	3.5
	5.00 mm					
		4.75 mm				4
	4.50 mm					
4.00 mm	4.00 mm	4.00 mm	5	4000	4000	4.7
	3.55 mm					
		3.35 mm	6			5.5
	3.15 mm					
2.80 mm	2.80 mm	2.80 mm	7	2800	2800	6.5
	2.50 mm					
		2.36 mm	8			7.5
	2.24 mm					
2.00 mm	2.00 mm	2.00 mm	10	2000	2000	8.6
	1.80 mm					
		1.70 mm	12			10
	1.60 mm					
1.40 mm	1.40 mm	1.40 mm	14	1400	1400	12
	1.25 mm					
		1.18 mm	16			14
	1.12 mm					
1.00 mm	1.00 mm	1.00 mm	18	1000	1000	16
	900 μm					

ISO Nominal Aperture			US Sieve No.	Recommended USP Sieves (μm)	European Sieve No.	Japanese Sieve No.
Principal sizes R 20/3	Supplementary sizes R 20	R 40/3				
		850 μm	20			18
	800 μm					
710 μm	710 μm	710 μm	25	710	710	22
	630 μm					
		600 μm	30			26
	560 μm					
500 μm	500 μm	500 μm	35	500	500	30
	450 μm					
		425 μm	40			36
	400 μm					
355 μm	355 μm	355 μm	45	355	355	42
	315 μm					
		300 μm	50			50
	280 μm					
250 μm	250 μm	250 μm	60	250	250	60
	224 μm					
		212 μm	70			70
	200 μm					
180 μm	180 μm	180 μm	80	180	180	83
	160 μm					
		150 μm	100			100
	140 μm					
125 μm	125 μm	125 μm	120	125	125	119
	112 μm					
		106 μm	140			140
	100 μm					
90 μm	90 μm	90 μm	170	90	90	166
	80 μm					
		75 μm	200			200
	71 μm					
63 μm	63 μm	63 μm	230	63	63	235
	56 μm					
		53 μm	270			282
	50 μm					
45 μm	45 μm	45 μm	325	45	45	330
	40 μm					
		38 μm			38	391

Sieves are selected to cover the entire range of particle sizes present in the test sample. A nest of sieves having a $\sqrt{2}$ progression of the area of the sieve openings is recommended. The nest of sieves is assembled with the coarsest screen at the top and the finest at the bottom. Use micrometres or millimetres in denoting test sieve openings.

Test sieves are made from stainless steel or, less preferably, from brass or another suitable non-reactive wire.

Calibration and recalibration of test sieves is in accordance with the current edition of ISO 3310-1. Sieves are carefully examined for gross distortions and fractures, especially at their screen frame joints, before use. Sieves may be calibrated optically to estimate the average opening size, and opening variability, of the sieve mesh. Alternatively, for the evaluation of the effective opening of test sieves in the size range of 212-850 μm, standard glass spheres are available. Unless otherwise specified in the individual monograph, perform the sieve analysis at controlled room temperature and at ambient relative humidity.

Cleaning test sieves. Ideally, test sieves are cleaned using only a low-pressure air jet or a liquid stream. If some apertures remain blocked by test particles, careful gentle brushing may be used as a last resort.

Test sample. If the test sample mass is not given in the monograph for a particular material, use a test sample having a mass of 25-100 g, depending on the bulk density of the material, for test sieves having a 200 mm diameter. For 76 mm sieves, the amount of material that can be accommodated is approximately 1/7 that which can be accommodated by a 200 mm sieve. Determine the most appropriate mass for a given material by test sieving accurately weighed samples of different masses, such as 25 g, 50 g and 100 g, for the same time period on a mechanical shaker (note: if the test results are similar for the 25 g and 50 g samples, but the 100 g sample shows a lower percentage through the finest sieve, the 100 g sample size is too large). Where only a sample of 10-25 g is available, smaller diameter test sieves conforming to the same mesh specifications may be substituted, but the endpoint must be redetermined. The use of test samples having a smaller mass (e.g. down to 5 g) may be needed. For materials with low apparent particle density, or for materials mainly comprising particles with a highly iso-diametrical shape, sample masses below 5 g for a 200 mm screen may be necessary to avoid excessive blocking of the sieve. During validation of a particular sieve-analysis method, it is expected that the problem of sieve blocking will have been addressed.

If the test material is prone to absorbing or losing significant amounts of water with varying humidity, the test must be carried out in an appropriately controlled environment. Similarly, if the test material is known to develop an electrostatic charge, careful observation must be made to ensure that such charging does not influence the analysis. An antistatic agent, such as colloidal silicon dioxide and/or aluminum oxide, may be added at a 0.5 per cent (*m/m*) level to minimise this effect. If both of the above effects cannot be eliminated, an alternative particle-sizing technique must be selected.

Agitation methods. Several different sieve and powder-agitation devices are commercially available, all of which may be used to perform sieve analyses. However, the different methods of agitation may give different results for sieve analyses and endpoint determinations because of the different types and magnitudes of the forces acting on the individual particles under test. Methods using mechanical agitation or electromagnetic agitation, and that can induce either a vertical oscillation or a horizontal circular motion, or tapping or a combination of both tapping and horizontal circular motion are available. Entrainment of the particles in an air stream may also be used. The results must indicate which agitation method was used and the agitation parameters used (if they can be varied), since changes in the agitation conditions will give different results for the sieve analysis and endpoint determination, and may be sufficiently different to give a failing result under some circumstances.

Endpoint determination. The test sieving analysis is complete when the mass on any of the test sieves does not change by more than 5 per cent or 0.1 g (10 per cent in the case of 76 mm sieves) of the previous mass on that sieve. If less than 5 per cent of the total sample mass is present on a given sieve, the endpoint for that sieve is increased to a mass change of not more than 20 per cent of the previous mass on that sieve.

If more than 50 per cent of the total sample mass is found on any one sieve, unless this is indicated in the monograph, the test is repeated, but with the addition to the sieve nest of a more coarse sieve intermediate between that carrying the excessive mass and the next coarsest sieve in the original nest, i.e. addition of the ISO series sieve omitted from the nest of sieves.

SIEVING METHODS

Mechanical agitation (Dry sieving method). Tare each test sieve to the nearest 0.1 g. Place an accurately weighed quantity of test sample on the top (coarsest) sieve, and replace the lid. Agitate the nest of sieves for 5 min, then carefully remove each sieve from the nest without loss of material. Reweigh each sieve, and determine the mass of material on each one. Determine the mass of material in the collecting pan in a similar manner. Re-assemble the nest of sieves, and agitate for 5 min. Remove and weigh each sieve as previously described. Repeat these steps until the endpoint criteria are met (see Endpoint determination under Test sieves). Upon completion of the analysis, reconcile the masses of material. Total loss must not exceed 5 per cent of the mass of the original test sample.

Repeat the analysis with a fresh sample, but using a single sieving time equal to that of the combined times used above. Confirm that this sieving time conforms to the requirements for endpoint determination. When this endpoint has been validated for a specific material, then a single fixed time of sieving may be used for future analyses, providing the particle-size distribution falls within normal variation.

If there is evidence that the particles retained on any sieve are aggregates rather than single particles, the use of mechanical dry sieving is unlikely to give good reproducibility, and a different particle-size analysis method must be used.

Air-entrainment methods (Air-jet and sonic-sifter sieving). Different types of commercial equipment that use a moving air current are available for sieving. A system that uses a single sieve at a time is referred to as air-jet sieving. It uses the same general sieving methodology as that described under Dry sieving method, but with a standardised air jet replacing the normal agitation mechanism. It requires sequential analyses on individual sieves starting with the finest sieve to obtain a particle-size distribution. Air-jet sieving often includes the use of finer test sieves than used in ordinary dry sieving. This technique is more suitable where only oversize or undersize fractions are needed.

In the sonic-sifter method, a nest of sieves is used, and the test sample is carried in a vertically oscillating column of air that lifts the sample and then carries it back against the mesh openings at a given number of pulses per minute. It may be necessary to lower the sample amount to 5 g when sonic sifting is employed.

The air-jet sieving and sonic-sifter sieving methods may be useful for powders or granules when the mechanical sieving techniques are incapable of giving a meaningful analysis.

These methods are highly dependent upon proper dispersion of the powder in the air current. This requirement may be hard to achieve if the method is used at the lower end of the sieving range (i.e. below 75 μm), when the particles tend to be more cohesive, and especially if there is any tendency for the material to develop an electrostatic charge. For the above reasons endpoint determination is particularly critical, and it is very important to confirm that the oversize material comprises single particles and is not composed of aggregates.

INTERPRETATION

The raw data must include the mass of the test sample, the total sieving time, the precise sieving methodology, and the set values for any variable parameters, in addition to the masses retained on the individual sieves and in the pan.

It may be convenient to convert the raw data into a cumulative mass distribution, and if it is desired to express the distribution in terms of a cumulative mass undersize, the range of sieves used must include a sieve through which all the material passes. If there is evidence on any of the test sieves that the material remaining on it is composed of aggregates formed during the sieving process, the analysis is invalid.

3.1. MATERIALS USED FOR THE MANUFACTURE OF CONTAINERS

01/2008:30113
corrected 6.2

3.1.13. PLASTIC ADDITIVES

NOTE: the nomenclature given first is according to the IUPAC rules. The synonym given in bold corresponds to the name given in the texts of Chapter 3. The synonym corresponding to the rules of the texts of "Chemical Abstracts" is also given.

add01. $C_{24}H_{38}O_4$. [117-81-7]. PM RN 74640.

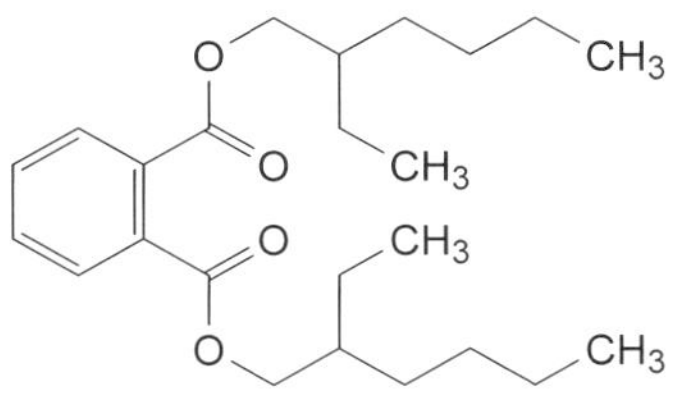

(2*RS*)-2-ethylhexyl benzene-1,2-dicarboxylate

synonyms: – **di(2-ethylhexyl) phthalate,**
– 1,2-benzenedicarboxylic acid, bis(2-ethylhexyl) ester.

add02. $C_{16}H_{30}O_4Zn$. [136-53-8]. PM RN 54120.

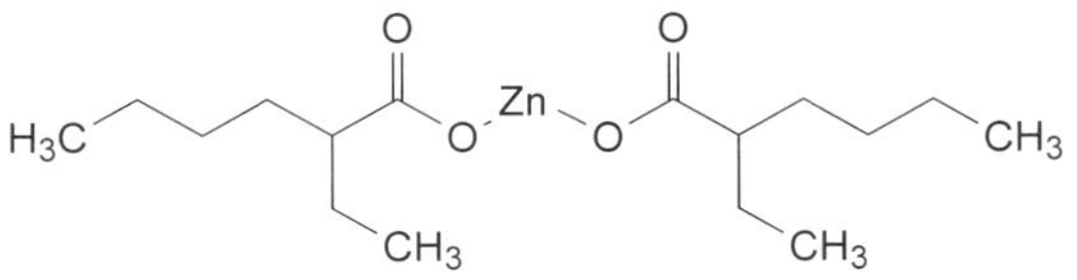

zinc (2*RS*)-2-ethylhexanoate

synonyms: – **zinc octanoate,**
– 2-ethylhexanoic acid, zinc salt (2:1),
– zinc 2-ethylcaproate.

add03. [05518-18-3]/[00110-30-5]. PM RN 53440/53520.

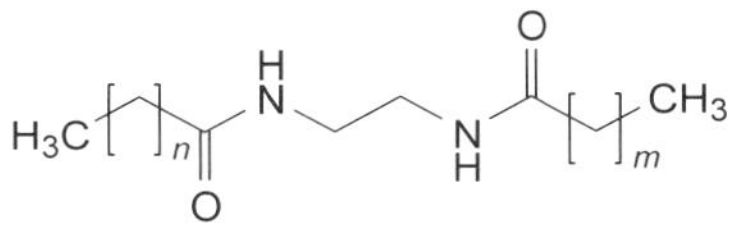

N,N'-ethylenedialcanamide (with *n* and *m* = 14 or 16)

synonyms: – ***N,N'*-diacylethylenediamines,**
– *N,N'*-diacylethylenediamine (in this context acyl means in particular palmitoyl and stearoyl).

add04. [8013-07-8]. PM RN 88640.

epoxidised soya oil

add05. [8016-11-3]. PM RN 64240.

epoxidised linseed oil

add06. [57455-37-5](TSCA)/[101357-30-6] (EINECS)/Pigment blue 29 (CI 77007)

ultramarine blue

add07. $C_{15}H_{24}O$. [128-37-0] PM RN 46640.

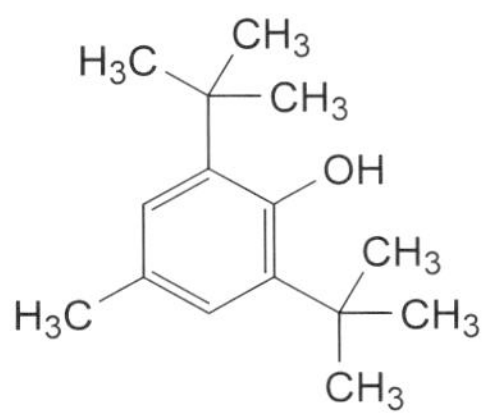

2,6-bis(1,1-dimethylethyl)-4-methylphenol

synonyms: – **butylhydroxytoluene,**
– 2,6-bis(1,1-dimethylethyl)-4-methylphenol,
– 2,6-di-*tert*-butyl-4-methylphenol.

add08. $C_{50}H_{66}O_8$. [32509-66-3]. PM RN 53670.

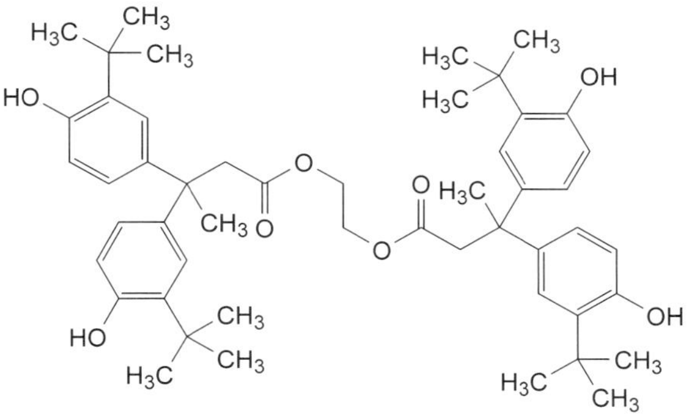

ethylene bis[3,3-bis[3-(1,1-dimethylethyl)-4-hydroxyphenyl]butanoate]

synonyms: – **ethylene bis[3,3-bis[3-(1,1-dimethylethyl)-4-hydroxyphenyl]butanoate],**
– butanoic acid, 3,3-bis[3-(1,1-dimethylethyl)-4-hydroxyphenyl]-, 1,2-ethanediyl ester,
– ethylene bis[3,3-bis(3-*tert*-butyl-4-hydroxyphenyl)butyrate].

add09. $C_{73}H_{108}O_{12}$. [6683-19-8]. PM RN 71680.

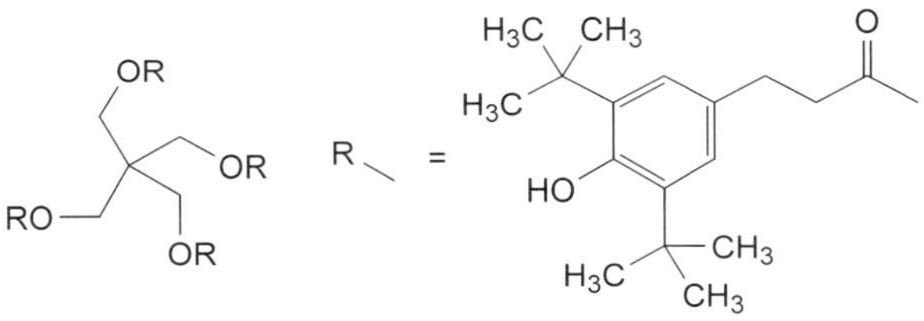

methanetetryltetramethyl tetrakis[3-[3,5-bis(1,1-dimethylethyl)-4-hydroxyphenyl]propanoate]

synonyms: – **pentaerythrityl tetrakis[3-(3,5-di-*tert*-butyl-4-hydroxyphenyl)propionate],**
– 2,2-bis[[[3-[3,5-bis(1,1-dimethylethyl)-4-hydroxyphenyl]propanoyl]oxy]methyl]propane-1,3-diyl 3-[3,5-bis(1,1-dimethylethyl)-4-hydroxyphenyl]propanoate,
– benzenepropanoic acid, 3,5-bis(1,1-dimethylethyl)-4-hydroxy-2,2-bis(hydroxymethyl)propane-1,3-diol ester (4:1),
– 2,2-bis(hydroxymethyl)propane-1,3-diol tetrakis[3-(3,5-di-*tert*-butyl-4-hydroxyphenyl)propionate].

add10. $C_{54}H_{78}O_3$. [1709-70-2]. PM RN 95200.

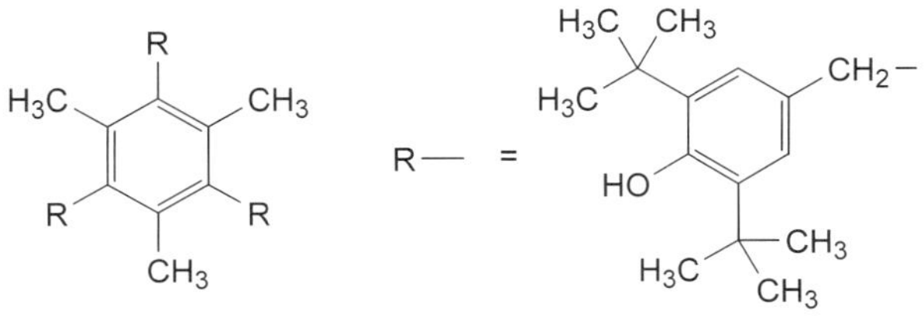

4,4′,4″-[(2,4,6-trimethylbenzene-1,3,5-triyl)tris(methylene)]tris[2,6-bis(1,1-dimethylethyl)phenol]

synonyms: – **2,2′,2″,6,6′,6″-hexa-*tert*-butyl-4,4′,4″-[(2,4,6-trimethyl- 1,3,5-benzenetriyl)trismethylene]triphenol,**

– 1,3,5-tris[3,5-di-*tert*-butyl-4-hydroxybenzyl]-2,4,6-trimethylbenzene,

– phenol,4,4′,4″-[(2,4,6-trimethyl-1,3,5-benzenetriyl)tris(methylene)]tris[2,6-bis(1,1-dimethylethyl)-.

add11. $C_{35}H_{62}O_3$. [2082-79-3]. PM RN 68320.

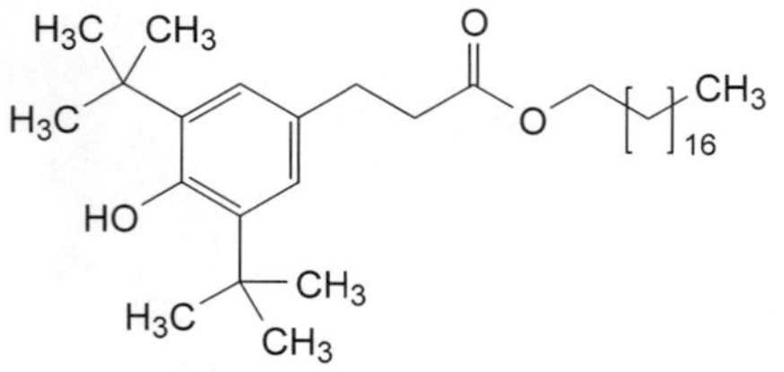

octadecyl 3-[3,5-bis(1,1-dimethylethyl)-4-hydroxyphenyl]propanoate

synonyms: – **octadecyl 3-(3,5-di-*tert*-butyl-4-hydroxyphenyl)propionate,**

– propanoic acid, 3-[3,5-bis(1,1-dimethylethyl)-4-hydroxyphenyl]-, octadecyl ester.

add12. $C_{42}H_{63}O_3P$. [31570-04-4]. PM RN 74240.

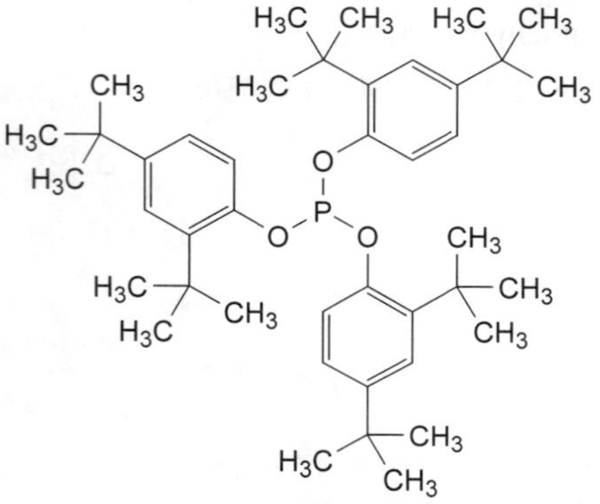

tris[2,4-bis(1,1-dimethylethyl)phenyl] phosphite

synonyms: – **tris(2,4-di-*tert*-butylphenyl) phosphite,**

– phenol, 2,4-bis(1,1-dimethylethyl)-, phosphite (3:1),

– 2,4-bis(1,1-dimethylethyl)phenyl, phosphite.

add13. $C_{48}H_{69}N_3O_6$. [27676-62-6]. PM RN 95360.

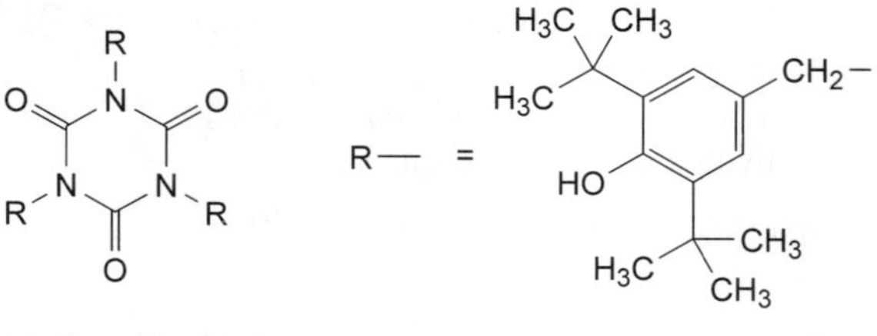

1,3,5-tris[3,5-bis(1,1-dimethylethyl)-4-hydroxybenzyl]-1,3,5-triazine-2,4,6(1*H*,3*H*,5*H*)-trione

synonyms: – **1,3,5-tris(3,5-di-*tert*-butyl-4-hydroxybenzyl)-*s*-triazine-2,4,6(1*H*,3*H*,5*H*)-trione,**

– 1,3,5-triazine-2,4,6(1*H*,3*H*,5*H*)-trione, 1,3,5-tris[[3,5-bis(1,1-dimethylethyl)-4-hydroxyphenyl]methyl]-.

add14. $C_{41}H_{82}O_6P_2$. [3806-34-6]. PM RN 50080.

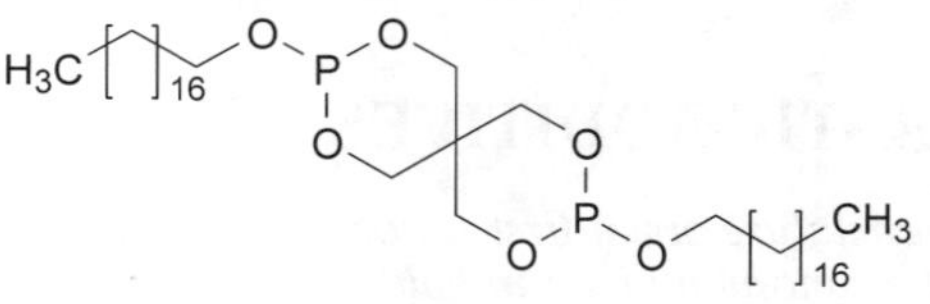

3,9-bis(octadecyloxy)-2,4,8,10-tetraoxa-3,9-diphosphaspiro[5.5]undecane

synonyms: – **2,2′-bis(octadecyloxy)-5,5′-spirobi[1,3,2-dioxaphosphinane],**

– 2,4,8,10-tetraoxa-3,9-diphosphaspiro[5.5]undecane, 3,9-bis(octadecyloxy)-.

add15. $C_{36}H_{74}S_2$. [2500-88-1]. PM RN 49840.

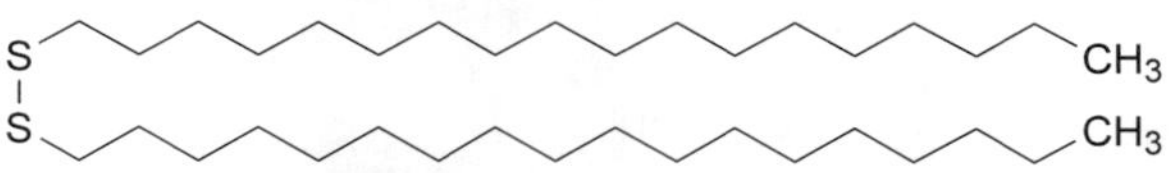

1,1′-disulphanediyldioctadecane

synonyms: – **dioctadecyl disulphide,**

– octadecane, 1,1′-dithio-.

add16. $C_{30}H_{58}O_4S$. [123-28-4]. PM RN 93120.

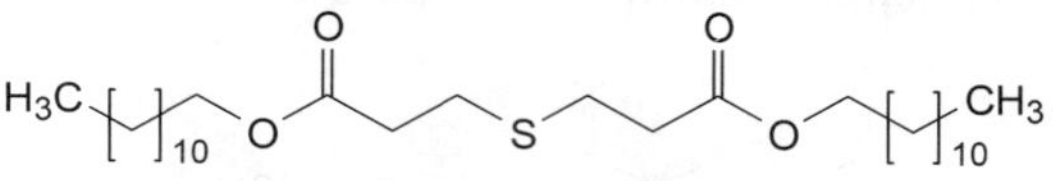

didodecyl 3,3′-sulphanediyldipropanoate

synonyms: – **didodecyl 3,3′-thiodipropionate,**

– didodecyl 3,3′-sulfanediyldipropanoate,

– propanoic acid, 3,3′-thiobis-, dodecyl diester,

– lauryl thiodipropionate.

add17. $C_{42}H_{82}O_4S$. [693-36-7]. PM RN 93280.

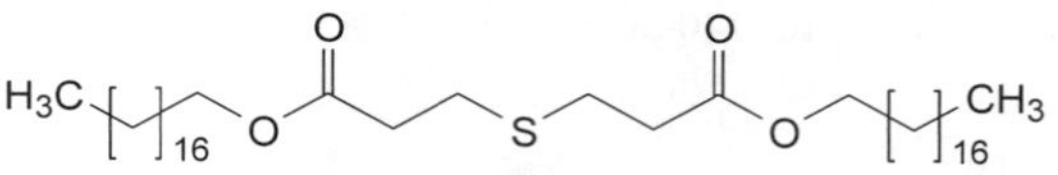

dioctadecyl 3,3′-sulphanediyldipropanoate

synonyms: – **dioctadecyl 3,3′-thiodipropionate,**

– dioctadecyl 3,3′-sulfanediyldipropanoate,

– propanoic acid, 3,3′-thiobis-, octadecyl diester,

– stearyl thiodipropionate.

add18. [119345-01-6]. PM RN 92560.

mixture of seven products corresponding to reaction product of di-*tert*-butyl phosphonite with biphosphorous trichloride, reaction products with biphenyl and 2,4-bis(1,1-dimethylethyl)phenol:

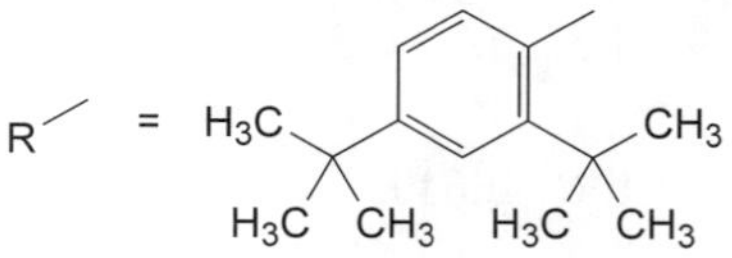

component I

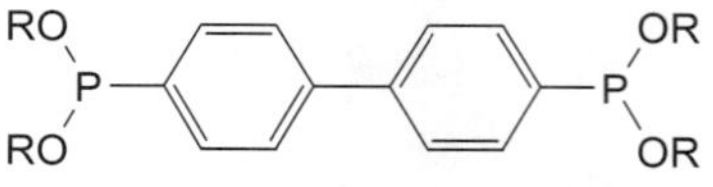

2,4-bis(1,1-dimethylethyl)phenyl biphenyl-4,4′-diyldiphosphonite

component II

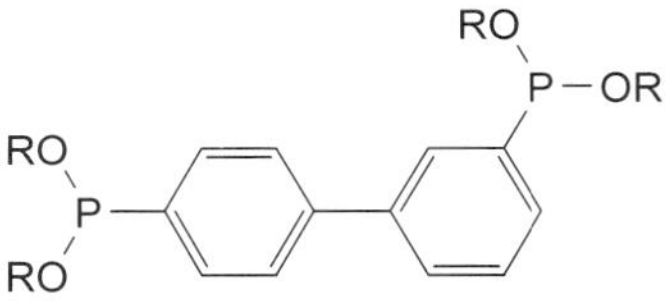

2,4-bis(1,1-dimethylethyl)phenyl biphenyl-3,4′-diyldiphosphonite

component III

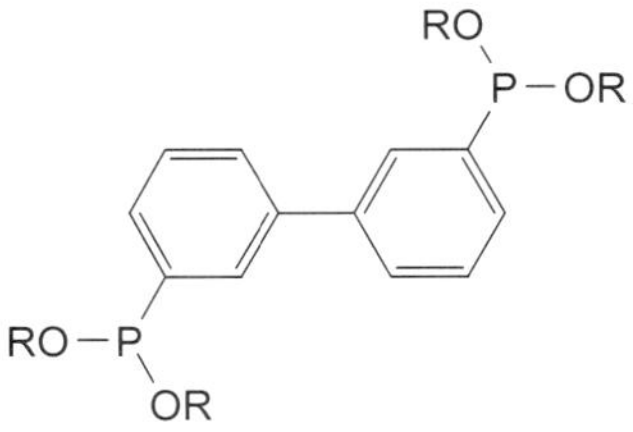

2,4-bis(1,1-dimethylethyl)phenyl biphenyl-3,3′-diyldiphosphonite

component IV

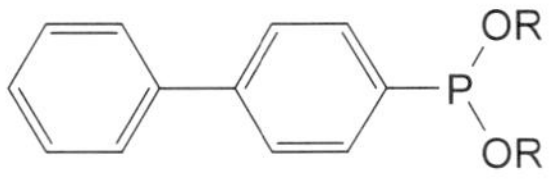

2,4-bis(1,1-dimethylethyl)phenyl biphenyl-4-ylphosphonite

component V

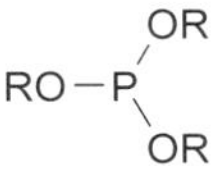

2,4-bis(1,1-dimethylethyl)phenyl phosphite

component VI

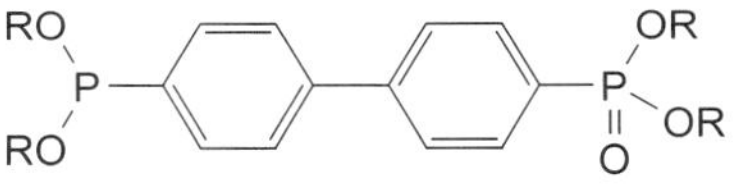

2,4-bis(1,1-dimethylethyl)phenyl 4′-[bis[2,4-bis(1, 1-dimethylethyl)phenoxy]phosphanyl]biphenyl-4-ylphosphonate

component VII

R-OH: 2,4-bis(1,1-dimethylethyl)phenol

add19. $C_{18}H_{36}O_2$. [57-11-4]. PM RN 24550.

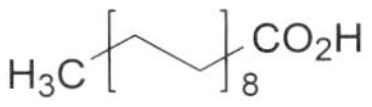

octadecanoic acid

synonyms: – **stearic acid,**
– octadecanoic acid.

add20. $C_{18}H_{35}NO$. [301-02-0]. PM RN 68960.

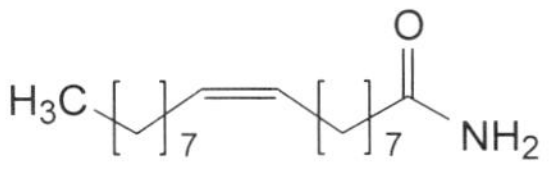

(*Z*)-octadec-9-enamide

synonyms: – **oleamide,**
– 9-octadecenamide, (*Z*)-,
– 9-*cis*-oleamide.

add21. $C_{22}H_{43}NO$. [112-84-5]. PM RN 52720.

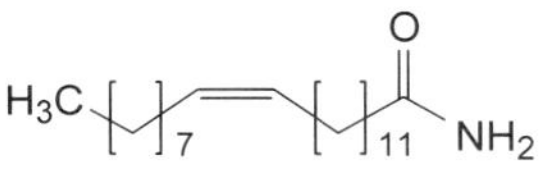

(*Z*)-docos-13-enamide

synonyms: – **erucamide,**
– 13-docosenamide, (*Z*)-,
– 13-*cis*-docosenamide.

add22. [65447-77-0]. PM RN 60800.

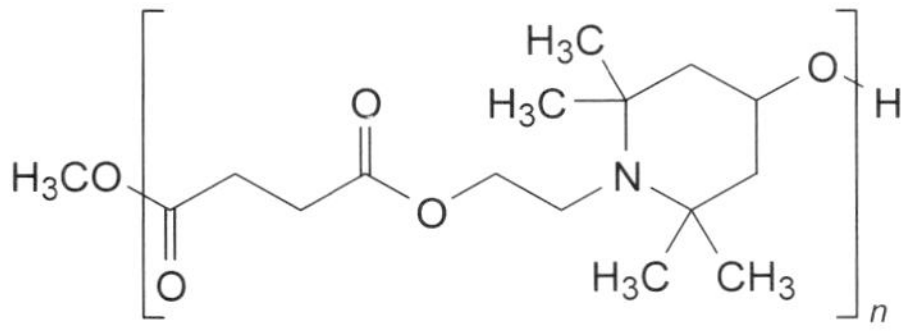

copolymer of dimethyl butanedioate and 1-(2-hydroxyethyl)-2,2,6,6-tetramethylpiperidin-4-ol

synonyms: – **copolymer of dimethyl succinate and (4-hydroxy-2,2,6,6-tetramethylpiperidin-1-yl)ethanol.**

add23.

mixture of component I and about 27 per cent of component II

component I [26401-97-8]

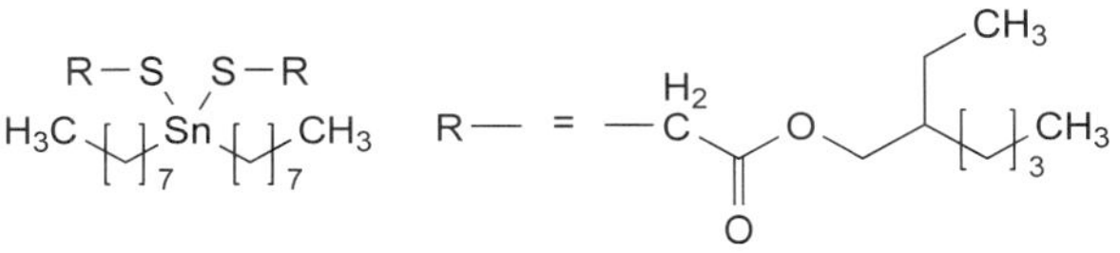

bis[(2*RS*)-2-ethylhexyl] 2,2′-[(dioctylstannanetriyl)bis-(sulfanediyl)]diacetate

synonyms: – **di(isooctyl) 2,2′-[(dioctylstannylene)-bis(thio)]diacetate,**
– bis(isooctyloxycarbonylmethylthio)-dioctylstannane.

component II [26401-86-5]

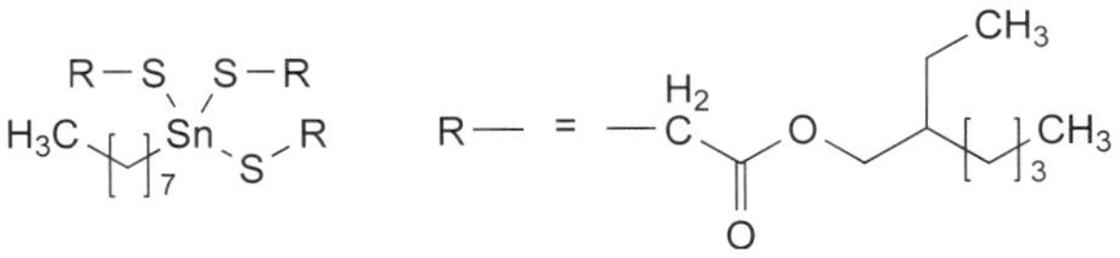

tris[(2*RS*)-2-ethylhexyl] 2,2′,2″-[(octylstannanetriyl)tris-(sulfanediyl)]triacetate

synonyms: – **tri(isooctyl) 2,2′,2″-[(monooctyl-stannylidyne)tris(thio)]triacetate,**
– 2,2′,2″-[(octylstannylidyne)tris(thio)]tri-acetic acid, triisooctyl ester.

4. REAGENTS

07/2008:40101

4.1.1. REAGENTS

Chrysanthemin. $C_{21}H_{21}ClO_{11}$. (M_r 485.8). *1134800.* [7084-24-4]. Cyanidin 3-*O*-glucoside chloride. Kuromanin chloride. 2-(3,4-Dihydroxyphenyl)-3-(β-D-glucopyranosyl)oxy-5,7-dihydroxy-1-benzopyrylium chloride.

Reddish-brown crystalline powder, soluble in water and in ethanol (96 per cent).

Absorbance (*2.2.25*). A 0.01 g/l solution in a mixture of 1 volume of *hydrochloric acid R* and 999 volumes of *methanol R* shows a maximum at 528 nm.

2-Fluoro-2-deoxy-D-mannose. $C_6H_{11}FO_5$. (M_r 182.1). *1172100.* [38440-79-8].

Colourless semi-solid.

Iodoplatinate reagent R1. *1172200.*

Mix 2.5 ml of a 50 g/l solution of *chloroplatinic acid R*, 22.5 ml of a 100 g/l solution of *potassium iodide R* and 50 ml of *water R.*

Storage: protected from light, at a temperature of 2 °C to 8 °C.

Lavandulyl acetate. $C_{12}H_{20}O_2$. (M_r 196.3). *1114200.* [25905-14-0]. 2-Isopropenyl-5-methylhex-4-en-1-yl acetate.

Colourless liquid with a characteristic odour.

Lavandulyl acetate used in gas chromatography complies with the following additional test.

Assay. Gas chromatography (*2.2.28*) as prescribed in the monograph on *Lavender oil (1338).*

Test solution. The substance to be examined.

The area of the principal peak is not less than 93.0 per cent of the area of all the peaks in the chromatogram obtained.

4-(4-Methylpiperidin-1-yl)pyridine. $C_{11}H_{16}N_2$. (M_r 176.3). *1114400.* [80965-30-6].

Clear liquid.

n_D^{20} : about 1.565.

Myrtillin. $C_{21}H_{21}ClO_{12}$. (M_r 500.8). *1172300.* [6906-38-3]. Delphinidin 3-*O*-glucoside chloride.

Silica gel for chromatography, hexadecylamidylsilyl, end-capped. *1172400.*

A very finely divided (5 μm) silica gel, chemically modified at the surface by the introduction of hexadecylcarboxamidopropyldimethylsilyl groups. To minimise any interaction with basic compounds it is carefully end-capped to cover most of the remaining silanol groups.

Sodium pentanesulphonate monohydrate R1. $C_5H_{11}NO_3,H_2O$. (M_r 192.2). *1172500.*

Content: minimum 99 per cent of $C_5H_{11}NO_3,H_2O$.

1,2,3,4-Tetra-*O*-acetyl-β-D-glucopyranose. $C_{14}H_{20}O_{10}$. (M_r 348.3). *1172600.* [13100-46-4].

White or almost white powder, soluble in water with gentle heating.

$[\alpha]_D^{20}$: + 11, determined on a 6 g/l solution in *chloroform R.*

mp: 126 °C to 128 °C.

Thromboplastin. *1090300.*

A preparation containing the membrane glycoprotein tissue factor and phospholipid, either purified from animal brain (usually rabbit) or human placenta or manufactured using recombinant DNA technology with added phospholipid. The preparation is formulated for routine use in the prothrombin time test and may contain calcium.

TLC silica gel plate for aminopolyether test. *1172700.*

Immerse a *TLC silica gel plate R* in *iodoplatinate reagent R1* for 5-10 s. Dry at room temperature for 12 h, protected from light.

Storage: protected from light, in an open container; use within 30 days after preparation.

VACCINES FOR VETERINARY USE

Vaccines

07/2008:2326

COCCIDIOSIS VACCINE (LIVE) FOR CHICKENS

Vaccinum coccidiosidis vivum ad pullum

1. DEFINITION

Coccidiosis vaccine (live) for chickens is a preparation of sporulated oocysts of a suitable line or lines of species of coccidial parasites (*Eimeria* spp.). This monograph applies to vaccines intended for administration to chickens for active immunisation.

2. PRODUCTION

2-1. *PREPARATION OF THE VACCINE*

Oocysts are produced in chickens from a flock free from specified pathogens (SPF) (*5.2.2*) or in embryonated hens' eggs from an SPF flock (*5.2.2*). The eggs must be subject to disinfection and/or incubation conditions validated to ensure the inactivation of any *Eimeria* that may be on the shells. The hatched chickens must then be reared in disinfected premises, in isolation conditions that ensure no infection with *Eimeria*. The chickens must not have been treated with coccidiostats. Oocysts are collected from faeces or contents of the intestinal tract of infected chickens during the patent period. Oocysts of different *Eimeria* lines are produced separately. Oocysts are isolated, purified, disinfected, sporulated and counted. The vaccine is produced by blending defined numbers of sporulated oocysts of each line in a suitable medium.

2-2. *SEED LOTS*

2-2-1. **Identification**. The identity of each *Eimeria* master seed is established from the characteristics of the coccidia produced from it, based on an appropriate selection of the following characteristics: size and shape of the oocyst; localisation of the developmental stages in the chicken intestine; pathognomonic lesions (*E. tenella, E. acervulina, E. necatrix, E. maxima* and *E. brunetti*) and lack of macroscopic lesions (*E. praecox* and *E. mitis*); size of schizonts in the intestinal mucosa; size of gametocytes in the mucosa; differences in the electrophoretic mobilities of certain isoenzymes, e.g. lactate dehydrogenase and glucose phosphate isomerase; and by the use of molecular biology techniques. Artificially attenuated lines may be distinguished from the parent strains by studying parameters appropriate to the method of attenuation.

2-2-2. **Extraneous agents**. Carry out tests 1-6 of chapter *2.6.24. Avian viral vaccines: tests for extraneous agents in seed lots*. General provisions *a-d, f* and *h* and section 7 of chapter *2.6.24* are also applicable. In these tests on the master seed lot, use organisms that are not more than 5 passages from the master seed lot at the start of the tests. Each master seed lot complies with the requirements of each test.

2-3. *CHOICE OF VACCINE COMPOSITION*

Only coccidial lines shown to be satisfactory with respect to residual pathogenicity and increase in virulence may be used in the preparation of the vaccine, and the tests described below (sections 2-3-2 and 2-3-3) may be used to demonstrate this. The vaccine shall be shown to be satisfactory with respect to safety (*5.2.6*) and efficacy (*5.2.7*) for the chickens for which it is intended. The following tests under Specific test for the safety of the vaccine composition (section 2-3-1) and Immunogenicity (section 2-3-4) may be used during the demonstration of safety and efficacy.

2-3-1. **Specific test for the safety of the vaccine composition.** Carry out the test with a preparation containing oocysts of each species at the least attenuated passage level that will be present in a batch of vaccine. Use not fewer than 20 chickens from an SPF flock (*5.2.2*). The chickens must be hatched and reared as described in section 2-1 and must not have been treated with coccidiostats. Use chickens of the category that is expected to be the most sensitive, i.e. 14-day-old chickens. During the test, chickens are housed in suitable conditions with the use of floor pens or cages with solid floors to favour reinfection with oocysts. Administer by gavage or another suitable route to each chicken a quantity of vaccinal oocysts consisting of the equivalent of not less than 10 times the maximum quantity of oocysts of each coccidial species likely to be contained in 1 dose of the vaccine. Observe the chickens at least daily for 21 days. The test is not valid if more than 10 per cent of the vaccinated chickens die from causes not attributable to the vaccinal oocysts. The vaccine complies with the test if no vaccinated chicken shows notable clinical signs of coccidiosis or dies from causes attributable to the vaccine.

2-3-2. **Test for residual pathogenicity**. Carry out a separate test with each coccidial species and line to be included in the vaccine. Use in each case a preparation containing oocysts at the least attenuated passage level that will be present between the master seed lot and a batch of the vaccine. For each test use not fewer than 20 chickens from an SPF flock (*5.2.2*). The chickens must be hatched and reared as described in section 2-1 and must not have been treated with coccidiostats. Use chickens of the category that is expected to be the most sensitive, i.e. 14-day-old chickens. During the test, the chickens are placed in cages (or any other suitable accomodation that prevents reinfection and allows collection of faeces). Administer by gavage or another suitable route to each chicken the equivalent of not less than 10 times the maximum quantity of the vaccinal oocysts likely to be contained in 1 dose of the vaccine. Observe the chickens at least daily for 14 days. The test is not valid if more than 10 per cent of the chickens die from causes not attributable to the vaccinal oocysts. Collect faeces and determine oocyst production daily from day 3 until day 14. On one day between days 4 and 8, depending on the length of the pre-patent period, when lesions are expected to be maximal, and on day 14, euthanise not fewer than 9 chickens and examine the intestinal tract for specific lesions indicative of infection with the coccidial species or, for species known not to induce macroscopic lesions (*E. mitis* and *E. praecox*), microscopic evidence of infection such as demonstration of oocysts or developing oocysts in the intestinal contents or scrapings of the intenstinal wall. For species that have the potential to produce relevant macroscopic pathological changes if not attenuated, a scoring system with a scale from 0 to 4 is used to record the species-specific lesions visible in the intestine as follows.

Eimeria acervulina

0 No gross lesions.

1 Scattered, white, plaque-like lesions containing developing oocysts are confined to the duodenum. These lesions are elongated with the longer axis transversely oriented on the intestinal walls like the rungs of a ladder. They may be seen on either the serosal or mucosal intestinal surfaces. There may be up to a maximum of 5 lesions per square centimetre.

Vaccines

2 Lesions are much closer together, but not coalescent; lesions may extend as far posterior as 20 cm below the duodenum in 3-week-old birds. The intestinal walls show no thickening. Digestive tract contents are normal.

3 Lesions are numerous enough to cause coalescence with reduction in lesion size and give the intestine a coated appearance. The intestinal wall is thickened and the contents are watery. Lesions may extend as far posterior as the yolk sac diverticulum.

4 The mucosal wall is greyish with completely coalescent colonies. Congestion may be confined to small petechiae or, in extremely heavy infections, the entire mucosa may be bright red in colour. Individual lesions may be indistinguishable in the upper intestine. Typical ladder-like lesions appear in the middle part of the intestine. The intestinal wall is very much thickened and the intestine is filled with a creamy exudate, which may bear large numbers of oocysts. Birds dying of coccidiosis are scored as 4.

Eimeria brunetti

0 No gross lesions.

1 No gross lesions. In the absence of distinct lesions, the presence of parasites may go undetected unless scrapings from suspicious areas are examined microscopically.

2 The intestinal wall may appear grey in colour. The lower portion may be thickened and flecks of pink material sloughed from the intestine are present.

3 The intestinal wall is thickened and a blood-tinged catarrhal exudate is present. Transverse red streaks may be present in the lower rectum and lesions occur in the caecal tonsils. Soft mucous plugs may be present in this latter area.

4 Extensive coagulation necrosis of the mucosal surface of the lower intestine may be present. In some birds a dry necrotic membrane may line the intestine and caseous cores may plug the entrance to the caeca. Lesions may extend into the middle or upper intestine. Birds dying of coccidiosis are scored as 4.

Eimeria maxima

0 No gross lesions.

1 Small red petechiae may appear on the serosal side of the mid-intestine. There is no ballooning or thickening of the intestine, though small amounts of orange mucous may be present.

2 The serosal surface may be speckled with numerous red petechiae. The intestine may be filled with orange mucous, but there is little or no ballooning of the intestine. There is thickening of the wall.

3 The intestinal wall is ballooned and thickened. The mucosal surface is roughened. Intestinal contents are composed of pinpoint blood clots and mucous.

4 The intestinal wall may be ballooned for most of its length. It contains numerous blood clots and digested red blood cells giving a characteristic colour and putrid odour. The wall is greatly thickened. Birds dying of coccidiosis are scored as 4.

Eimeria necatrix

0 No gross lesions.

1 Small scattered petechiae and white spots are easily seen on the serosal surface. There is little, if any, damage apparent on the mucosal surface.

2 Numerous petechiae are seen on the serosal surface. Slight ballooning confined to the midgut area may be present.

3 There is extensive haemorrhage into the lumen of the intestine. The serosal surface is covered with red petechiae and/or white plaques, and is rough and thickened with many pinpoint haemorrhages. Normal intestinal contents are lacking. Ballooning extends over the lower half of the small intestine.

4 Extensive haemorrhage gives the intestine a dark colour, and the intestinal contents consist of red or brown mucous. Ballooning may extend throughout much of the length of the intestine. Birds dying of coccidiosis are scored as 4.

Eimeria tenella

0 No gross lesions.

1 Very few scattered petechiae are seen on the caecal wall, and there is no thickening of the caecal walls. Normal caecal contents are present.

2 Lesions are more numerous with noticeable blood in the caecal contents, and the caecal wall is somewhat thickened. Normal caecal contents are present.

3 Large amounts of blood or caecal cores are present, and the caecal walls are greatly thickened. There is little if any normal faecal content in the caeca.

4 The caecal wall is greatly distended with blood or large caseous cores. Faecal debris is lacking or included in the cores. Birds dying of coccidiosis are scored as 4.

The species and line comply with the test for attenuation if no more than mild coccidial lesions or limited signs of infection are observed; where the scoring system described above is appropriate, the average lesion score on the day of sampling between days 4 and 8 and on day 14 is not greater than 1.5 points and no individual score is greater than 3 points. The quantity and time of oocyst production is determined.

2-3-3. **Increase in virulence**. Carry out a separate test with each coccidial species and line to be included in the vaccine. Use a preparation containing oocysts at the least attenuated passage level that will be present between the master seed lot and a batch of the vaccine. For each test use 14-day-old chickens from an SPF flock (*5.2.2*). The chickens must be hatched and reared as described in section 2-1 and must not have been treated with coccidiostats. During the test, the chickens are placed in cages (or any other suitable accomodation that prevents reinfection and allows collection of faeces). Administer by gavage or another suitable route to each of 5 chickens a quantity of oocysts that will allow recovery of the oocysts for the passages described below. Collect faeces daily from day 2 to day 14 after infection and prepare a pooled suspension of sporulated oocysts from the 5 chickens. Administer a suitable quantity by gavage or another suitable route to each of 5 further chickens. Carry out this passage operation not fewer than 5 times, verifying the presence of oocysts at each passage. Repeat the test for residual pathogenicity (section 2-3-2), using the maximally passaged oocysts that have been recovered and administering a similar quantity of sporulated oocysts per chicken to that used in the test with unpassaged oocysts. Compare the results obtained for signs of lesions or infection in the intestinal tract and oocyst output from administration of passaged and unpassaged oocysts. The line complies with the test if no indication of an increase in virulence of the maximally passaged oocysts compared with the unpassaged oocysts is observed. The test is invalid if oocysts are not recovered at any passage level.

2-3-4. **Immunogenicity**. The efficacy of each coccidial species and line included in the vaccine is determined in a separate study with an appropriate challenge strain. For each component, a test is carried out with vaccine administered by each route and method of administration to be recommended, using in each case chickens not older than the youngest age to be recommended for vaccination. The quantity of each of the components in the batch of vaccine administered to each chicken is not greater than the minimum number of oocysts to be stated on the label and the oocysts are at the most attenuated passage level that will be present in a batch of vaccine. Use for the test not fewer than 40 chickens from an SPF flock (*5.2.2*). The chickens must be hatched and reared as described in section 2-1 and must not have been treated with coccidiostats. Vaccinate not fewer than 20 chickens and maintain not fewer than 20 chickens as controls. For the evaluation of weight gain with *Eimeria* strains showing a low pathogenicity, the number of chickens used may be higher. The test may require different challenge doses for different test parameters and so may be assessed as separate challenge groups. For example, a lower challenge dose may be needed to determine the effect on oocyst output than the dose needed to determine the effect on weight gain and lesion scoring. After vaccination, the chickens are housed in suitable conditions with the use of floor pens or cages with solid floors to favour reinfection with oocysts. On a suitable day between days 14 and 21 after vaccination, weigh each chicken, move them to cages (or any other suitable accomodation that prevents reinfection and allows collection of faeces) and challenge each chicken by gavage or another suitable route with a sufficient quantity of virulent coccidia to induce in the unvaccinated controls signs of disease characteristic of the *Eimeria* challenge species. Observe the chickens at least daily until the end of the test. Record deaths and the number of surviving chickens that show clinical signs of disease. Collect faeces and determine oocyst production from day 3 after challenge until the end of the test. On an appropriate day between days 4 and 8 after challenge, depending on the length of the pre-patent period of the challenge species, weigh each chicken. Euthanise 10 chickens from each group and examine them for lesions in the intestinal tract. Where appropriate, record the specific lesions indicative of the coccidial challenge species (using the scoring system described in section 2-3-2). For species known not to induce macroscopic lesions (*E. mitis* and *E. praecox*), examine the chickens for microscopic evidence of infection such as demonstration of oocysts or developing oocysts in the intestinal contents or scrapings of the intestinal wall. On day 14 after challenge, weigh each of the remaining chickens.

The test is invalid if:

- during the period between vaccination and challenge, more than 10 per cent of the vaccinated or control chickens show abnormal clinical signs or die from causes not attributable to the vaccine;
- for challenges with *E. tenella*, *E. acervulina*, *E. necatrix*, *E. maxima* or *E. brunetti*, fewer than 80 per cent of the control chickens euthanised between days 4 and 8 have marked characteristic lesions of the challenge infection in the intestine at post-mortem examination (e.g. lesion scores not less than 2);
- for challenges with *E. mitis* or *E. praecox*, fewer than 80 per cent of the control chickens euthanised between days 4 and 8 are infected.

The vaccine complies with the test if:

- for all the *Eimeria* challenge species, the production of the oocysts is significantly decreased in vaccinates compared with controls;
- for all the *Eimeria* challenge species, no vaccinated chicken dies due to the challenge infection;
- for challenge with *E. tenella*, *E. acervulina*, *E. necatrix*, *E. maxima* or *E. brunetti*, at least 80 per cent of the vaccinates show no more than mild signs of disease and these are less marked than those in the controls;
- for challenges with *E. tenella*, *E. acervulina*, *E. necatrix*, *E. maxima* or *E. brunetti*, at least 80 per cent of the vaccinates have no or minimal lesions in the intestine (e.g. mean lesion scores not greater than 1) and no bird has a lesion score of 4;
- for challenges with *E. tenella*, *E. acervulina*, *E. necatrix*, *E. maxima*, *E. brunetti*, *E. mitis*, or *E. praecox*, the growth rate in the vaccinates is significantly greater than in the controls.

2-4. *MANUFACTURER'S TESTS*

2-4-1. **In-process test for sporulation rate and oocyst count.** A sample of each oocyst bulk is examined microscopically after the sporulation step and before blending to determine the percentage of sporulated oocysts and the oocyst count. The values obtained are within the limits shown to allow preparation of a satisfactory vaccine.

2-4-2. **Batch potency test for each *Eimeria* species in the vaccine**. It is not necessary to carry out the potency test (section 3-7) for each batch of the vaccine if it has been carried out using a batch or batches of vaccine with minimum potency and sporulated oocyst content. Where the test is not carried out, an alternative validated method is used, the criteria for acceptance for each component being set with reference to a batch of vaccine that has given satisfactory results in the test described under Potency.

2-4-3. **Freedom from extraneous agents**. The disinfection method applied during the preparation of the final product from the harvested oocysts may be validated to show effective inactivation of certain potential extraneous agents. Where relevant validation data is available and where justified and authorised, some or all of the tests indicated under Extraneous agents (section 3-4) may be omitted as routine tests on each batch.

3. BATCH TESTS

3-1. **Identification**

3-1-1. Microscopical examination is used to confirm the presence of coccidial oocysts in the batch of vaccine.

3-1-2. The potency test (or batch potency test) is used to confirm the presence of oocysts of each of the *Eimeria* species stated on the label.

3-2. **Bacteria and fungi**. The vaccine and where applicable the liquid supplied with it comply with the test for sterility prescribed in the monograph *Vaccines for veterinary use (0062)* and comply with the test with a medium selective for *Campylobacter* spp.

3-3. **Mycoplasmas**. The vaccine complies with the test for mycoplasmas (*2.6.7*).

3-4. **Extraneous agents**. Carry out tests 1-6 of chapter *2.6.25. Avian live virus vaccines: tests for extraneous agents in batches of finished product*. General provisions *a-d*, *g* and *h* are also applicable. The vaccine complies with the requirements of each test.

3-5. **Safety**. Use not fewer than 10 chickens from an SPF flock (*5.2.2*) and of the minimum age recommended for vaccination. The chickens must be hatched and reared as described in section 2-1 and must not have been treated with coccidiostats. Administer by a recommended route and method to each chicken preferably 10 doses of vaccine. If the volume of 10 doses is too large, administer the largest volume possible. After vaccination, the chickens are housed in suitable conditions with the use of floor pens or cages with solid floors to favour reinfection with oocysts. Observe the chickens at least daily for 21 days. The test is not valid if more than 20 per cent of the chickens show abnormal clinical signs or die from causes not attributable to the vaccine. The vaccine complies with the test if no chicken shows notable clinical signs of disease or dies from causes attributable to the vaccine.

3-6. **Sporulated oocyst count**. The sporulated oocysts content per dose is determined by counting the sporulated oocysts in a suitable counting chamber, under the microscope. The contents are not less than the minimum and not more than the maximum content of sporulated oocysts stated on the label.

3-7. **Potency**. The vaccine complies with the requirements of the test prescribed under Immunogenicity (section 2-3-4) using 1 dose of the vaccine administered by a recommended route.

Vaccines

4. LABELLING

The label states the minimum and maximum number of sporulated oocysts per dose.

07/2008:1521

FURUNCULOSIS VACCINE (INACTIVATED, OIL-ADJUVANTED, INJECTABLE) FOR SALMONIDS

Vaccinum furunculosidis inactivatum ad salmonidas cum adiuvatione oleosa ad iniectionem

1. DEFINITION

Furunculosis vaccine (inactivated, oil-adjuvanted, injectable) for salmonids is prepared from cultures of one or more suitable strains of *Aeromonas salmonicida* subsp. *salmonicida*, inactivated while maintaining adequate immunogenic properties. This monograph applies to vaccines intended for the active immunisation of salmonids against furunculosis.

2. PRODUCTION

2-1. *PREPARATION OF THE VACCINE*

The strains of *A. salmonicida* are cultured and harvested separately. The harvests are inactivated by a suitable method. They may be purified and concentrated. Whole or disrupted cells may be used and the vaccine may contain extracellular products of the bacterium released into the growth medium. The vaccine contains an oily adjuvant.

2-2. *CHOICE OF VACCINE STRAIN*

The strains included in the vaccine are shown to be suitable with respect to production of antigens of assumed immunological importance. The vaccine is shown to be satisfactory with respect to safety (*5.2.6*) and efficacy (*5.2.7*) in the species of fish for which it is intended.
The following tests for safety (section 2-2-1) and immunogenicity (section 2-2-2) may be used during the demonstration of safety and efficacy.

2-2-1. **Safety**

2-2-1-1. *Laboratory test.* Carry out the test in each species of fish for which the vaccine is intended, using fish of the minimum body mass to be recommended for vaccination. Use a batch of vaccine containing not less than the maximum potency that may be expected in a batch of vaccine.

Use not fewer than 50 fish from a population that does not have specific antibodies against *A. salmonicida* subsp. *salmonocida* and has not been vaccinated against or exposed to furunculosis. The test is carried out in the conditions to be recommended for the use of the vaccine with a water temperature not less than 10 °C. Administer to each fish by the intraperitoneal route a double dose of the vaccine per mass unit. Observe the fish at least daily for 21 days.

The test is invalid if more than 6 per cent of the fish die from causes not attributable to the vaccine. The vaccine complies with the test if no fish shows abnormal local or systemic reactions or dies from causes attributable to the vaccine.

2-2-1-2. *Field studies.* Safety is also demonstrated in field trials by administering the intended dose to a sufficient number of fish in not fewer than 2 sets of premises. Samples of 30 fish are taken on 3 occasions (after vaccination, at the middle of the rearing period and at slaughter) and examined for local reactions in the body cavity. Moderate lesions involving localised adhesions between viscera or between viscera and the abdominal wall and slight opaqueness and/or sparse pigmentation of the peritoneum are acceptable. Extensive lesions including adhesions between greater parts of the abdominal organs, massive pigmentation and/or obvious thickening and opaqueness of greater areas of the peritoneum are unacceptable if they occur in more than 10 per cent of the fish in any sample. Such lesions include adhesions that give the viscera a 'one-unit' appearance and/or lead to manifest laceration of the peritoneum following evisceration.

2-2-2. **Immunogenicity**. Carry out the test according to a protocol defining limits of body mass for the fish, water source, water flow and temperature limits, and preparation of a standardised challenge. A test is carried out for the route and method of administration to be recommended. The vaccine administered to each fish is of minimum potency.

Use for the test not fewer than 200 fish. Vaccinate not fewer than 100 fish according to the instructions for use. Perform mock vaccination on a control group of not fewer than 100 fish; mark vaccinated and control fish for identification. Keep all the fish in the same tank or mix equal numbers of controls and vaccinates in each tank if more than one tank is used. Challenge each fish, by injection, at a fixed interval after vaccination, defined according to the statement regarding development of immunity, with a sufficient quantity of a culture of *A. salmonicida* subsp. *salmonicida* whose virulence has been verified. Observe the fish at least daily until at least 60 per cent specific mortality is reached in the control group. Plot for both vaccinates and controls a curve of specific mortality against time from challenge and determine by interpolation the time corresponding to 60 per cent specific mortality in controls.

The test is invalid if the specific mortality is less than 60 per cent in the control group 21 days after the first death in the fish. Read from the curve for vaccinates the mortality (*M*) at the time corresponding to 60 per cent mortality in controls. Calculate the relative percentage survival (RPS) using the following expression:

$$\left(1 - \frac{M}{60}\right) \times 100$$

The vaccine complies with the test if the RPS is not less than 80 per cent.

2-3. *MANUFACTURER'S TESTS*

2-3-1. **Batch potency test**. The potency test (section 3-4) may be carried out for each batch of vaccine, using groups of not fewer than 30 fish of one of the species for which the vaccine is intended. Where the test is not carried out, an alternative validated method based on antibody response may be used, the criteria for acceptance being set with reference to a batch of vaccine that has given satisfactory results in the test described under Potency. The following test may be used.

Use not fewer than 35 fish from a population that does not have specific antibodies against *A. salmonicida* subsp. *salmonicida* and that are within specified limits for body mass. Carry out the test at a defined temperature. Inject intraperitoneally into each of not fewer than 25 fish one dose of vaccine, according to the instructions for use. Perform mock vaccination on a control group of not fewer than 10 fish. Collect blood samples at a defined time after vaccination. Determine for each sample the level of specific antibodies against *A. salmonicida* subsp. *salmonicida* by a suitable immunochemical method (*2.7.1*). The test is invalid if the control group shows antibodies against *A. salmonicida* subsp. *salmonicida*. The vaccine complies with the test if the mean level of antibodies in the vaccinates is not significantly lower than that found for a batch that gave satisfactory results in the test described under Potency.

3. BATCH TESTS

3-1. **Identifcation**. When injected into fish that do not have specific antibodies against *A. salmonicida*, the vaccine stimulates the production of such antibodies.

3-2. **Bacteria and fungi**. The vaccine and, where applicable, the liquid supplied with it comply with the test for sterility prescribed in the monograph *Vaccines for veterinary use (0062)*.

3-3. **Safety**. Use not fewer than 10 fish of one of the species for which the vaccine is intended, having, where possible, the minimum body mass recommended for vaccination; if fish of the minimum body mass are not available, use fish not greater than twice this mass. Use fish from a population that preferably does not have specific antibodies against *A. salmonicida* subsp. *salmonicida* or, where justified, use fish from a population with a low level of such antibodies as long as they have not been vaccinated against or exposed to furunculosis and administration of the vaccine does not cause an anamnestic response. Carry out the test in the conditions recommended for the use of the vaccine with a water temperature not less than 10 °C. Administer to each fish by the intraperitoneal route a double dose of the vaccine per mass unit. Observe the fish at least daily for 21 days.

The test is invalid if more than 10 per cent of the fish die from causes not attributable to the vaccine. The vaccine complies with the test if no fish shows notable signs of disease or dies from causes attributable to the vaccine.

3-4. **Potency**. The vaccine complies with the requirements of the test mentioned under Immunogenicity (section 2-2-2) when administered by the recommended route and method.

4. LABELLING

The label states information on the time needed for development of immunity after vaccination under the range of conditions corresponding to the recommended use.

07/2008:0065

SWINE-FEVER VACCINE (LIVE, PREPARED IN CELL CULTURES), CLASSICAL

Vaccinum pestis classicae suillae vivum ex cellulis

1. DEFINITION

Classical swine-fever vaccine (live, prepared in cell cultures) is a preparation obtained from a strain of classical swine-fever virus that has lost its pathogenicity for the pig by *in vivo* and/or *in vitro* passage and has been adapted to growth in cell cultures.

2. PRODUCTION

2-1. *PREPARATION OF THE VACCINE*

The vaccine virus is grown in cell cultures.

2-2. *SUBSTRATE FOR VIRUS PROPAGATION*

Cell cultures. Cell cultures comply with the requirements for cell cultures for production of veterinary vaccines (*5.2.4*).

2-3. *CHOICE OF VACCINE VIRUS*

The vaccine virus is shown to be satisfactory with respect to safety (*5.2.6*) and efficacy (*5.2.7*) for the swine for which it is intended.

The following tests described under Safety test in piglets (section 2-3-1), Safety test in pregnant sows and test for transplacental transmission (section 2-3-2), Non-transmissibility (section 2-3-3), Increase in virulence (2-3-4) and Immunogenicity (2-3-5) may be used during the demonstration of safety and immunogenicity.

2-3-1. **Safety test in piglets**. Carry out the test for each recommended route using in each case piglets not older than the minimum age recommended for vaccination. Use vaccine virus at the least attenuated passage level that will be present in a batch of the vaccine.

Use not fewer than 10 healthy piglets that do not have antibodies against pestiviruses. Administer to not fewer than 10 piglets a quantity of the vaccine virus equivalent to not less than 10 times the maximum virus titre likely to be contained in 1 dose of the vaccine. Observe the piglets at least daily for 21 days. The body temperature of each vaccinated piglet is measured on at least the 3 days preceding administration of the vaccine, at the time of administration, 4 h after and then daily for at least 14 days. The vaccine complies with the test if the average body temperature increase for all piglets does not exceed 1.5 °C, no piglet shows a temperature rise greater than 1.5 °C for a period exceeding 3 days, and no piglet shows notable signs of disease or dies from causes attributable to the vaccine.

2-3-2. **Safety test in pregnant sows and test for transplacental transmission**. Carry out the test by a recommended route using not fewer than 10 healthy sows or gilts of the same age and origin, between the 55th and

Vaccines

80th days of gestation, and that do not have antibodies against pestiviruses. Use vaccine virus at the least attenuated passage level that will be present in a batch of the vaccine.

Administer to not fewer than 10 sows or gilts a quantity of the vaccine virus equivalent to not less than the maximum virus titre likely to be contained in 1 dose of the vaccine. Record the body temperature on at least the 3 days preceding administration of the vaccine, at the time of administration, 4 h after and then daily for at least 15 days. Observe until farrowing.

Carry out tests for serum antibodies against classical swine-fever virus. No antibodies against classical swine-fever virus are found in sera taken from the newborn piglets before ingestion of colostrum. The test is invalid if the vaccinated sows do not seroconvert. The vaccine virus complies with the test if no abnormalities in the gestation or in the piglets are noted, no sow or gilt shows a temperature rise greater than 1.5 °C for a period exceeding 5 days, and no sow or gilt shows notable signs of disease or dies from causes attributable to the vaccine.

2-3-3. **Non-transmissibility**. Keep together for the test not fewer than 12 healthy piglets, 6-10 weeks old and of the same origin, and that do not have antibodies against pestiviruses. Use vaccine virus at the least attenuated passage level that will be present between the master seed lot and a batch of the vaccine. Administer by a recommended route to not fewer than 6 piglets a quantity of the vaccine virus equivalent to not less than the maximum virus titre likely to be contained in 1 dose of the vaccine. Maintain not fewer than 6 piglets as contact controls. The mixing of vaccinated piglets and contact piglets is done 24 h after vaccination.

After 45 days, euthanise all piglets. Carry out appropriate tests on the piglets to detect antibodies to classical swine-fever. Carry out appropriate tests on the control piglets to detect classical swine-fever virus in the tonsils. The vaccine complies with the test if antibodies are found in all vaccinated piglets and if no antibodies and no virus are found in the control piglets.

2-3-4. **Increase in virulence**. The test for increase in virulence consists of the administration of the vaccine virus at the least attenuated passage level that will be present between the master seed lot and a batch of the vaccine to piglets that do not have antibodies against pestiviruses.

Administer to each of 2 healthy piglets, 6-10 weeks old, by a recommended route, a quantity of the vaccine virus equivalent to not less than the maximum virus titre likely to be contained in 1 dose of the vaccine. Collect an appropriate quantity of blood from each piglet daily between day 2 and day 7 after administration of the vaccine virus, and pool the samples taken on the same day. Administer 2 ml of the pooled blood with the highest virus titre by a recommended route to each of 2 other piglets of the same age and origin. If no virus is found, repeat the test once again with another 2 piglets. If virus is found, carry out a 2nd series of passages by administering 2 ml of positive blood by a recommended route to each of 2 other piglets of the same age and origin. Carry out this passage operation not fewer than 5 times, verifying the presence of the virus at each passage. Care must be taken to avoid contamination by virus from previous passages.

The vaccine virus complies with the test if no indication of increasing virulence of the maximally passaged virus compared with the unpassaged virus is observed. If virus is not recovered at any passage level in the 1st and 2nd series of passages, the vaccine virus also complies with the test.

2-3-5. **Immunogenicity**

2-3-5-1. *Protective dose.* The efficacy of the vaccine is expressed by the number of 50 per cent protective doses (PD_{50}) for pigs contained in the vaccinal dose as indicated on the label. The vaccine contains at least 100 PD_{50} per dose.

Use 1 or more groups of piglets aged 6-10 weeks and that do not have antibodies against pestiviruses, and use an additional group of piglets of the same age and origin as controls. Each group of piglets is vaccinated with 1 dilution of the vaccine dose. 14 days after the single injection of vaccine, challenge the piglets by a suitable route with a suitable strain of virulent virus and a dose that kills not fewer than 50 per cent of the non-vaccinated piglets in less than 21 days. Observe the piglets for 21 days and record the body temperature 3 days before challenge and daily after challenge for 21 days. The PD_{50} is calculated by the usual statistical methods (for example, *5.3*), taking into account the surviving piglets that have no clinical signs of swine fever, including cutaneous lesions or an increase in body temperature.

The test is invalid if fewer than 50 per cent of the control piglets display typical signs of serious infection with swine-fever virus, including cutaneous lesions, or die, and if fewer than 100 per cent of the control piglets show clinical signs of disease within the 21 days following challenge. The vaccine complies with the test if the minimum dose stated on the label corresponds to not less than 100 PD_{50}.

2-3-5-2. *Protection against transplacental infection.* Use 8 sows that do not have antibodies against pestiviruses, randomly allocated to either the vaccine group (n = 6) or the control group (n = 2).

Between the 40th and 50th day of gestation, all sows allocated to the vaccine group are vaccinated once with 1 dose of vaccine containing not more than the minimum titre stated on the label. On day 60 of gestation, all sows are challenged by a recommended route with a suitable strain of virulent virus. Just before farrowing and about 5-6 weeks after challenge, the sows are euthanised and their foetuses are examined for classical swine-fever virus. Serum samples from sows and foetuses are tested for the presence of antibodies against classical swine-fever virus. Isolation of classical swine-fever virus is carried out from blood of the sows (collected 7 and 9 days after challenge and at euthanasia), and from homogenised organ material (spleen, kidneys, lymph nodes) of the foetuses.

The test is invalid if one or more of the vaccinated sows do not seronconvert after the vaccination and the control sows do not seroconvert after the challenge, or if no virus is found in more than 50 per cent of the foetuses from the control sows (excluding mummified foetuses).

The vaccine complies with the test if no virus is found in the blood of vaccinated sows and in foetuses from the vaccinated sows, and no antibodies against classical swine-fever virus are found in the serum of the foetuses from the vaccinated sows.

3. BATCH TESTS

3-1. **Identification**

Specific classical swine-fever monoclonal antibodies are used to identify the vaccinal strain.

3-2. **Bacteria and fungi**. The vaccine complies with the test for sterility prescribed in the monograph *Vaccines for veterinary use (0062)*.

3-3. **Mycoplasmas** (*2.6.7*). The vaccine complies with the test for mycoplasmas.

3-4. **Extraneous agents**. Neutralise the vaccine virus using monoclonal antibodies to the vaccine virus. Inoculate into cell cultures known to be sensitive to viruses pathogenic for pigs and to pestiviruses. Maintain these cultures for not less than 14 days and carry out at least 3 passages during this period. The vaccine complies with the test if no cytopathic effect is produced; the cells show no evidence of the presence of haemadsorbing agents.

Use monoclonal antibodies that can identify possible contamination with pestiviruses. No virus is detected by an appropriate method.

3-5. **Safety**. Use 2 healthy piglets, 6-10 weeks old, that do not have antibodies against pestiviruses. Administer to each piglet by a recommended route 10 doses of the vaccine. Observe the piglets at least daily for 14 days. The vaccine complies with the test if no piglet shows notable signs of disease or dies from causes attributable to the vaccine.

3-6. **Virus titre**. Titrate the vaccine virus in suitable cell cultures (*5.2.4*). The vaccine complies with the test if 1 dose contains not less than the minimum virus titre stated on the label.

3-7. **Potency**. The vaccine complies with the requirements of the test prescribed under Immunogenicity (section 2-3-5) when administered by a recommended route and method. It is not necessary to carry out the potency test for each batch of the vaccine if it has been carried out on a representative batch using a vaccinating dose containing not more than the minimum virus titre stated on the label.

07/2008:1580

VIBRIOSIS (COLD-WATER) VACCINE (INACTIVATED) FOR SALMONIDS

Vaccinum vibriosidis aquae frigidae inactivatum ad salmonidas

1. DEFINITION

Cold-water vibriosis vaccine (inactivated) for salmonids is prepared from cultures of one or more suitable strains of *Vibrio salmonicida,* inactivated while maintaining adequate immunogenic properties. This monograph applies to vaccines intended for the active immunisation of salmonids against cold-water vibriosis.

2. PRODUCTION

2-1. *PREPARATION OF THE VACCINE*

The strains of *V. salmonicida* are cultured and harvested separately. The harvests are inactivated by a suitable method. They may be purified and concentrated. Whole or disrupted cells may be used and the vaccine may contain extracellular products of the bacterium released into the growth medium.

2-2. *CHOICE OF VACCINE COMPOSITION*

The strain or strains of *V. salmonicida* used are shown to be suitable with respect to production of antigens of assumed immunological importance. The vaccine is shown to be satisfactory with respect to safety (*5.2.6*) and efficacy (*5.2.7*) in the species of fish for which it is intended.

The following tests for safety (section 2-2-1) and immunogenicity (section 2-2-2) may be used during the demonstration of safety and efficacy.

2-2-1. **Safety**

2-2-1-1. *Laboratory tests.* Safety is tested using test 2-2-1-1-1, test 2-2-1-1-2, or both, depending on the recommendations for use.

Carry out the test in each species of fish for which the vaccine is intended, using fish of the minimum body mass to be recommended for vaccination. Use a batch of vaccine containing not less than the maximum potency that may be expected in a batch of vaccine. The test is carried out in the conditions to be recommended for use of the vaccine with a water temperature not less than 10 °C.

2-2-1-1-1. *Vaccines intended for administration by injection.* Use not fewer than 50 fish from a population that does not have specific antibodies against *V. salmonicida* and has not been vaccinated against or exposed to cold-water vibriosis. Administer to each fish by the intraperitoneal route a double dose of the vaccine per mass unit. Observe the fish at least daily for 21 days.

The test is invalid if more than 6 per cent of the fish die from causes not attributable to the vaccine. The vaccine complies with the test if no fish shows abnormal local or systemic reactions or dies from causes attributable to the vaccine.

2-2-1-1-2. *Vaccines intended for administration by immersion.* Use not fewer than 50 fish from a population that does not have specific antibodies against *V. salmonicida* and has not been vaccinated against or exposed to cold-water vibriosis. Prepare an immersion bath at twice the concentration to be recommended. Bathe the fish for twice the time to be recommended. Observe the fish at least daily for 21 days.

The test is invalid if more than 6 per cent of the fish die from causes not attributable to the vaccine. The vaccine complies with the test if no fish shows abnormal local or systemic reactions or dies from causes attributable to the vaccine.

2-2-1-2. *Field studies.* Safety is demonstrated in addition in field trials by administering the dose to be recommended to a sufficient number of fish distributed in not fewer than 2 sets of premises.

The vaccine complies with the test if no fish shows abnormal reactions or dies from causes attributable to the vaccine.

2-2-2. **Immunogenicity**. Carry out the test according to a protocol defining limits of body mass for the fish, water source, water flow and temperature limits, and preparation of a standardised challenge. Each test is carried out for each route and method of administration to be recommended. The vaccine administered to each fish is of minimum potency.

Use for the test not fewer than 200 fish. Vaccinate not fewer than 100 fish according to the instructions for use. Perform mock vaccination on a control group of not fewer than 100 fish; mark vaccinated and control fish for identification. Keep all the fish in the same tank or mix equal numbers of controls and vaccinates in each tank if more than one tank is used. Challenge each fish by injection at a fixed interval after vaccination, defined according to the statement regarding development of immunity, with a sufficient quantity of a culture of *V. salmonicida* whose virulence has been verified. Observe the fish at least daily until at least 60 per cent specific mortality is reached in the control group. Plot for both vaccinates and controls a curve of specific mortality against time from challenge and determine by interpolation the time corresponding to 60 per cent specific mortality in controls.

The test is invalid if the specific mortality is less than 60 per cent in the control group 21 days after the first death in the fish. Read from the curve for vaccinates the mortality (*M*) at the time corresponding to 60 per cent mortality in controls. Calculate the relative percentage survival (RPS) using the following expression:

$$\left(1 - \frac{M}{60}\right) \times 100$$

The vaccine complies with the test if the RPS is not less than 60 per cent for vaccines administered by immersion and 90 per cent for vaccines administered by injection.

Vaccines

2-3. *MANUFACTURER'S TESTS*

2-3-1. **Batch potency test**. The potency test (section 3-4) may be carried out for each batch of vaccine, using groups of not fewer than 30 fish of one of the species for which the vaccine is intended. Where the test is not carried out, an alternative validated method based on antibody response may be used, the criteria for acceptance being set with reference to a batch of vaccine that has given satisfactory results in the test described under Potency. The following test may be used.

Use not fewer than 35 fish from a population that does not have specific antibodies against *V. salmonicida* and that are within specified limits for body mass. Carry out the test at a defined temperature. Inject into each of not fewer than 25 fish one dose of vaccine, according to the instructions for use. Perform mock vaccination on a control group of not fewer than 10 fish. Collect blood samples at a defined time after vaccination. Determine for each sample the level of specific antibodies against *V. salmonicida* by a suitable immunochemical method (*2.7.1*). The test is invalid if the control group shows antibodies against *V. salmonicida*. The vaccine complies with the test if the mean level of antibodies in the vaccinates is not significantly lower than that found for a batch that gave satisfactory results in the test described under Potency.

3. BATCH TESTS

3-1. **Identification**. When injected into fish that do not have specific antibodies against *V. salmonicida*, the vaccine stimulates the production of such antibodies.

3-2. **Bacteria and fungi**. The vaccine and, where applicable, the liquid supplied with it comply with the test for sterility prescribed in the monograph *Vaccines for veterinary use (0062)*.

3-3. **Safety**. Use not fewer than 10 fish of one of the species for which the vaccine is intended, having, where possible, the minimum body mass recommended for vaccination; if fish of the minimum body mass are not available, use fish not greater than twice this mass. Use fish from a population that does not have specific antibodies against *V. salmonicida* and that has not been vaccinated against or exposed to cold-water vibriosis. Carry out the test in the conditions recommended for the use of the vaccine with a water temperature not less than 10 °C. For vaccines administered by injection or immersion, administer to each fish by the intraperitoneal route a double dose of the vaccine per mass unit. For vaccines administered by immersion only, use a bath with twice the recommended concentration and bathe the fish for twice the recommended immersion time. Observe the fish at least daily for 21 days.

The test is invalid if more than 10 per cent of the fish die from causes not attributable to the vaccine. The vaccine complies with the test if no fish shows notable signs of disease or dies from causes attributable to the vaccine.

3-4. **Potency**. The vaccine complies with the requirements of the test mentioned under Immunogenicity (section 2-2-2) when administered by a recommended route and method.

4. LABELLING

The label states information on the time needed for development of immunity after vaccination under the range of conditions corresponding to the recommended use.

07/2008:1581

VIBRIOSIS VACCINE (INACTIVATED) FOR SALMONIDS

Vaccinum vibriosidis inactivatum ad salmonidas

1. DEFINITION

Vibriosis vaccine (inactivated) for salmonids is prepared from cultures of one or more suitable strains or serovars of *Vibrio anguillarum*, inactivated while maintaining adequate immunogenic properties; the vaccine may also include *Vibrio ordalii*. This monograph applies to vaccines intended for the active immunisation of salmonids against vibriosis.

2. PRODUCTION

2-1. *PREPARATION OF THE VACCINE*

The strains of *V. anguillarum* and *V. ordalii* are cultured and harvested separately. The harvests are inactivated by a suitable method. They may be purified and concentrated. Whole or disrupted cells may be used and the vaccine may contain extracellular products of the bacterium released into the growth medium.

2-2. *CHOICE OF VACCINE COMPOSITION*

The strains of *V. anguillarum* and *V. ordalii* used are shown to be suitable with respect to production of antigens of assumed immunological importance. The vaccine is shown to be satisfactory with respect to safety (*5.2.6*) and efficacy (*5.2.7*) in the species of fish for which it is intended.

The following tests for safety (section 2-2-1) and immunogenicity (section 2-2-2) may be used during the demonstration of safety and efficacy.

2-2-1. **Safety**

2-2-1-1. *Laboratory tests*. Safety is tested using test 2-2-1-1-1, test 2-2-1-1-2, or both, depending on the recommendations for use.

Carry out the test in each species of fish for which the vaccine is intended, using fish of the minimum body mass to be recommended for vaccination. Use a batch of vaccine containing not less than the maximum potency that may be expected in a batch of vaccine. The test is carried out in the conditions to be recommended for use of the vaccine with a water temperature not less than 10 °C.

2-2-1-1-1. *Vaccines intended for administration by injection*. Use not fewer than 50 fish from a population that does not have specific antibodies against *V. anguillarum* or where applicable *V. ordalii* and has not been vaccinated against or exposed to vibriosis. Administer to each fish by the intraperitoneal route a double dose of the vaccine per mass unit. Observe the fish at least daily for 21 days.

The test is invalid if more than 6 per cent of the fish die from causes not attributable to the vaccine. The vaccine complies with the test if no fish shows abnormal local or systemic reactions or dies from causes attributable to the vaccine.

2-2-1-1-2. *Vaccines intended for administration by immersion*. Use not fewer than 50 fish from a population that does not have antibodies against *V. anguillarum* or where applicable *V. ordalii* and has not been vaccinated against or exposed to vibriosis. Prepare an immersion bath at twice the concentration to be recommended. Bathe the fish for twice the time to be recommended. Observe the fish at least daily for 21 days.

The test is invalid if more than 6 per cent of the fish die from causes not attributable to the vaccine. The vaccine complies with the test if no fish shows abnormal local or systemic reactions or dies from causes attributable to the vaccine.

2-2-1-2. *Field studies*. Safety is demonstrated in addition in field trials by administering the dose to be recommended to a sufficient number of fish distributed in not fewer than 2 sets of premises.

The vaccine complies with the test if no fish shows abnormal reactions or dies from causes attributable to the vaccine.

2-2-2. **Immunogenicity**. Carry out a separate test for each species and each serovar included in the vaccine, according to a protocol defining limits of body mass for the fish, water source, water flow and temperature limits, and preparation of a standardised challenge. Each test is carried out for each route and method of administration to be recommended. The vaccine administered to each fish is of minimum potency.

Use for the test not fewer than 200 fish. Vaccinate not fewer than 100 fish according to the instructions for use. Perform mock vaccination on a control group of not fewer than 100 fish; mark vaccinated and control fish for identification. Keep all the fish in the same tank or mix equal numbers of controls and vaccinates in each tank if more than one tank is used. Challenge each fish by injection at a fixed interval after vaccination, defined according to the statement regarding development of immunity, with a sufficient quantity of cultures of *V. anguillarum* or *V. ordalii* whose virulence has been verified. Observe the fish at least daily until at least 60 per cent specific mortality is reached in the control group. Plot for both vaccinates and controls a curve of specific mortality against time from challenge and determine by interpolation the time corresponding to 60 per cent specific mortality in controls.

The test is invalid if the specific mortality is less than 60 per cent in the control group 21 days after the first death in the fish. Read from the curve for vaccinates the mortality (M) at the time corresponding to 60 per cent mortality in controls. Calculate the relative percentage survival (RPS) using the following expression:

$$\left(1 - \frac{M}{60}\right) \times 100$$

The vaccine complies with the test if the RPS is not less than 60 per cent for vaccines administered by immersion and 75 per cent for vaccines administered by injection.

2-3. *MANUFACTURER'S TESTS*

2-3-1. **Batch potency test**. The potency test (section 3-4) may be carried out for each batch of vaccine, using groups of not fewer than 30 fish of one of the species for which the vaccine is intended. Where the test is not carried out, an alternative validated method based on antibody response may be used, the criteria for acceptance being set with reference to a batch of vaccine that has given satisfactory results in the test described under Potency. The following test may be used.

Use not fewer than 35 fish from a population that does not have specific antibodies against the relevant serovars of *V. anguillarum* included in the vaccine and where applicable against *V. ordalii*, and that are within specified limits for body mass. Carry out the test at a defined temperature. Inject into each of not fewer than 25 fish one dose of vaccine, according to the instructions for use. Perform mock vaccination on a control group of not fewer than 10 fish. Collect blood samples at a defined time after vaccination. Determine for each sample the level of specific antibodies against the different serovars of *V. anguillarum* included in the vaccine and where applicable against *V. ordalii*, by a suitable immunochemical method (*2.7.1*). The test is invalid if the control group shows antibodies against the relevant serovars of *V. anguillarum* or, where applicable, against *V. ordalii*. The vaccine complies with the test if the mean level of antibodies in the vaccinates is not significantly lower than that found for a batch that gave satisfactory results in the test described under Potency.

3. BATCH TESTS

3-1. **Identification**. When injected into fish that do not have specific antibodies against *V. anguillarum* and, where applicable, *V. ordalii*, the vaccine stimulates the production of such antibodies.

3-2. **Bacteria and fungi**. The vaccine and, where applicable, the liquid supplied with it comply with the test for sterility prescribed in the monograph *Vaccines for veterinary use (0062)*.

3-3. **Safety**. Use not fewer than 10 fish of one of the species for which the vaccine is intended, having, where possible, the minimum body mass recommended for vaccination; if fish of the minimum body mass are not available, use fish not greater than twice this mass. Use fish from a population that does not have specific antibodies against the relevant serovars of *V. anguillarum* and where applicable against *V. ordalii*, and which has not been vaccinated against or exposed to vibriosis. Carry out the test in the conditions recommended for the use of the vaccine with a water temperature not less than 10 °C. For vaccines administered by injection or immersion, administer to each fish by the intraperitoneal route a double dose of the vaccine per mass unit. For vaccines administered by immersion only, use a bath with twice the recommended concentration and bathe the fish for twice the recommended immersion time. Observe the fish at least daily for 21 days.

The test is invalid if more than 10 per cent of the fish die from causes not attributable to the vaccine. The vaccine complies with the test if no fish shows notable signs of disease or dies from causes attributable to the vaccine.

3-4. **Potency**. The vaccine complies with the requirements of the test mentioned under Immunogenicity (section 2-2-2) when administered by a recommended route and method.

4. LABELLING

The label states information on the time needed for the development of immunity after vaccination under the range of conditions corresponding to the recommended use.

RADIOPHARMACEUTICAL PREPARATIONS

07/2008:0266

CHROMIUM (^{51}Cr) EDETATE INJECTION

Chromii (^{51}Cr) edetatis solutio iniectabilis

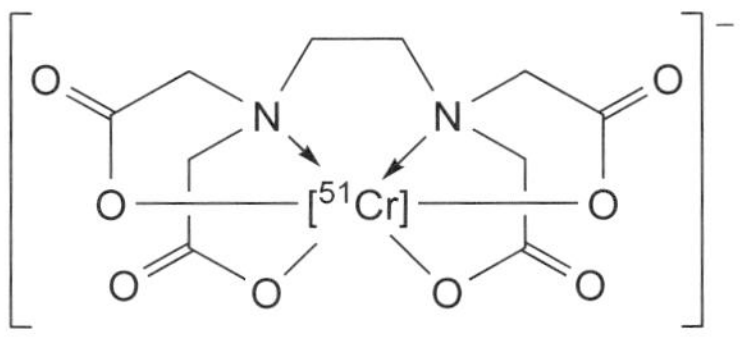

DEFINITION

Sterile solution containing chromium-51 in the form of a complex of chromium(III) with (ethylenedinitrilo)tetraacetic acid, the latter being present in excess. It may be made isotonic by the addition of sodium chloride and may contain a suitable antimicrobial preservative such as benzyl alcohol.

Content:

- *chromium-51*: 90.0 per cent to 110.0 per cent of the declared chromium-51 radioactivity at the date and time stated on the label;
- *chromium*: maximum 1 mg/ml.

PRODUCTION

Chromium-51 is a radioactive isotope of chromium and may be prepared by neutron irradiation of chromium, either of natural isotopic composition or enriched in chromium-50.

CHARACTERS

Appearance: clear, violet solution.

Half-life and nature of radiation of chromium-51: see general chapter *5.7. Table of physical characteristics of radionuclides*.

IDENTIFICATION

A. Radionuclidic purity (see Tests).

B. Examine the chromatograms obtained in the test for radiochemical purity.

Results: the principal peak in the radiochromatogram obtained with the test solution is similar in retardation factor to the principal peak in the chromatogram obtained with the reference solution.

TESTS

pH (*2.2.3*): 3.5 to 6.5.

Chromium. Ultraviolet and visible absorption spectrophotometry (*2.2.25*).

Test solution. The preparation to be examined.

Reference solution: dissolve 0.96 g of *chromic potassium sulphate R* and 2.87 g of *sodium edetate R* in 50 ml of *water R*, boil for 10 min, cool, adjust to pH 3.5-6.5 with *dilute sodium hydroxide solution R* and dilute to 100.0 ml with *water R*.

Measure the absorbance of the test solution and the reference solution at the absorption maximum at 560 nm. The absorbance of the test solution is not greater than that of the reference solution (1 mg/ml).

Sterility. It complies with the test for sterility prescribed in the monograph on *Radiopharmaceutical preparations (0125)*. The injection may be released for use before completion of the test.

RADIONUCLIDIC PURITY

Chromium-51: minimum 99.9 per cent of the total radioactivity.

Gamma-ray spectrometry.

Results: the only gamma photons have an energy of 0.320 MeV.

RADIOCHEMICAL PURITY

[^{51}Cr]Chromium edetate. Descending paper chromatography (*2.2.26*).

Test solution. The preparation to be examined.

Reference solution. Use the reference solution from the test for chromium.

Chromate carrier solution. Dissolve 0.1 g of *potassium chromate R* in 1 ml of *concentrated ammonia R1* and dilute to 100 ml with *water R*.

Paper: *paper for chromatography R*.

Mobile phase: *concentrated ammonia R1, ethanol (96 per cent) R, water R* (1:2:5 *V/V/V*).

Application. Apply a band of a 50 g/l solution of *lead acetate R* to the paper at about 4 cm from the origin and dry in hot air. Apply 10 µl of the chromate carrier solution at the origin, followed by 10 µl of the test solution on the same spot. On a separate sheet, repeat the above procedure, applying 10 µl of the reference solution instead of the test solution.

Development: immediately, over a path of 14 cm.

Drying: in air.

Detection: determine the distribution of radioactivity using a suitable radioactivity detector.

Retardation factors: impurity A = 0; impurity B = 0.2 to 0.4; [^{51}Cr]chromium edetate = 0.8 to 0.9.

System suitability. The band of lead acetate turns yellow due to reaction with the chromate carrier solution.
The retardation factor of the radioactive spot due to [^{51}Cr]chromium edetate in the radiochromatogram obtained with the test solution is similar to that of the violet spot in the chromatogram obtained with the reference solution.

Limit:

- *[^{51}Cr]chromium edetate*: minimum 97.0 per cent of the total radioactivity due to chromium-51.

RADIOACTIVITY

Measure the radioactivity using a calibrated instrument.

IMPURITIES

A. [^{51}Cr]chromium(III) ion,

B. [^{51}Cr]chromate ion.

Radiopharmaceutical preparations

07/2008:1325

FLUDEOXYGLUCOSE (^{18}F) INJECTION

Fludeoxyglucosi (^{18}F) solutio iniectabilis

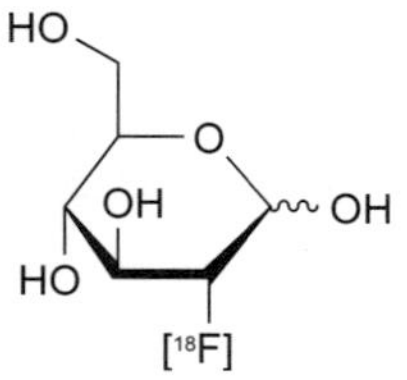

DEFINITION

Sterile solution containing 2-[^{18}F]fluoro-2-deoxy-D-glucopyranose (2-[^{18}F]fluoro-2-deoxy-D-glucose) prepared by nucleophilic substitution. It may also contain 2-[^{18}F]fluoro-2-deoxy-D-mannose.

Content:

- *fluorine-18*: 90 per cent to 110 per cent of the declared fluorine-18 radioactivity at the date and time stated on the label;
- *fluorine-18 in the form of 2-[^{18}F]fluoro-2-deoxy-D-glucose and 2-[^{18}F]fluoro-2-deoxy-D-mannose*: minimum 95 per cent of the total radioactivity;
- *2-[^{18}F]fluoro-2-deoxy-D-mannose*: maximum 10 per cent of the total radioactivity due to 2-[^{18}F]fluoro-2-deoxy-D-glucose and 2-[^{18}F]fluoro-2-deoxy-D-mannose;
- *2-fluoro-2-deoxy-D-glucose*: maximum 0.5 mg per maximum recommended dose, in millilitres.

PRODUCTION

RADIONUCLIDE PRODUCTION

The radionuclide fluorine-18 is most commonly produced by proton irradiation of water enriched in oxygen-18.

RADIOCHEMICAL SYNTHESIS

2-[^{18}F]Fluoro-2-deoxy-D-glucose is mostly prepared by phase transfer catalysed nucleophilic substitution of 1,3,4,6-tetra-*O*-acetyl-2-*O*-trifluoromethanesulphonyl-β-D-mannopyranose (tetraacetylmannose triflate) with [^{18}F]fluoride. Generally, [^{18}F]fluoride is adsorbed on an anion-exchange resin and eluted with a solution of potassium carbonate, which is then evaporated to dryness. Addition of a phase-transfer catalyst, such as an aminopolyether or a tetra-alkyl ammonium salt in dry acetonitrile, may be used to enhance the nucleophilicity of the [^{18}F]fluoride so that it reacts easily with the tetraacetylmannose triflate at elevated temperature. A variation of the method uses solid-phase-catalysed nucleophilic substitution on derivatised anion-exchange resin, for example, derivatised with 4-(4-methylpiperidin-1-yl)pyridine.

Hydrolysis under either alkaline or acidic conditions yields 2-[^{18}F]fluoro-2-deoxy-D-glucose. Depending on the conditions of hydrolysis, variable amounts of 2-chloro-2-deoxy-D-glucose and/or 2-[^{18}F]fluoro-2-deoxy-D-mannose may be formed as a by-product.

The preparation can be purified by serial chromatography on combinations of ion-retardation resin, ion-exchange resin, alumina and octadecylsilyl derivatised silica gel.

CHARACTERS

Appearance: clear, colourless or slightly yellow solution.

Half-life and nature of radiation of fluorine-18: see general chapter *5.7. Table of physical characteristics of radionuclides*.

IDENTIFICATION

A. Test A for radionuclidic purity (see Tests).

B. Determine the approximate half-life by no fewer than 3 measurements of the activity of a sample in the same geometrical conditions within a suitable period of time (for example, 30 min).
Result: 105 to 115 min.

C. Examine the chromatograms obtained in test A for radiochemical purity (see Tests).
Result: the principal peak in the radiochromatogram obtained with the test solution is similar in retention time to the principal peak in the chromatogram obtained with reference solution (a).

TESTS

Particular tests for chemical impurities may be omitted if the substances mentioned are not used or cannot be formed in the production process.

pH (*2.2.3*): 4.5 to 8.5.

2-Fluoro-2-deoxy-D-glucose and impurity A. Liquid chromatography (*2.2.29*).

Test solution. The preparation to be examined.

Reference solution (a). Dissolve 1.0 mg of *2-fluoro-2-deoxy-D-glucose R* in *water R* and dilute to 2.0 ml with the same solvent. Dilute 1.0 ml of the solution to *V* with *water R*, *V* being the maximum recommended dose in millilitres.

Reference solution (b). Dissolve 1.0 mg of *2-chloro-2-deoxy-D-glucose R* (impurity A) in *water R* and dilute to 2.0 ml with the same solvent. Dilute 1.0 ml of the solution to *V* with *water R*, *V* being the maximum recommended dose in millilitres.

Reference solution (c). Dissolve 1.0 mg of *2-fluoro-2-deoxy-D-mannose R* in *water R* and dilute to 2.0 ml with the same solvent. Mix 0.5 ml of this solution with 0.5 ml of reference solution (a).

Column:

- *size*: l = 0.25 m, Ø = 4.0 mm;
- *stationary phase*: *strongly basic anion exchange resin for chromatography R* (10 μm);
- *temperature*: constant, between 20 °C and 25 °C.

Mobile phase: 4 g/l solution of *sodium hydroxide R* in *carbon dioxide-free water R*.

Flow rate: 1 ml/min.

Detection: detector suitable for carbohydrates in the required concentration range, such as pulse amperometric detector and radioactivity detector connected in series.

Injection: 20 μl.

Run time: twice the retention time of 2-fluoro-2-deoxy-D-glucose.

Relative retention with reference to 2-fluoro-2-deoxy-D-glucose (retention time = about 12 min): 2-fluoro-2-deoxy-D-mannose = about 0.9; impurity A = about 1.1.

System suitability: reference solution (c) using the carbohydrate detector:

- *resolution*: minimum 1.5 between the peaks due to 2-fluoro-2-deoxy-D-mannose and 2-fluoro-2-deoxy-D-glucose,
- *signal-to-noise ratio*: minimum 10 for the peak due to 2-fluoro-2-deoxy-D-glucose.

Radiopharmaceutical preparations

Limits: in the chromatogram obtained with the carbohydrate detector:

- *2-fluoro-2-deoxy-D-glucose*: not more than the area of the corresponding peak in the chromatogram obtained with reference solution (a) (0.5 mg/*V*);
- *impurity A*: not more than the area of the corresponding peak in the chromatogram obtained with reference solution (b) (0.5 mg/*V*).

Impurity B. Spot test.

Test solution. The preparation to be examined.

Reference solution (a): *water R.*

Reference solution (b). Dissolve 11.0 mg of *aminopolyether R* (impurity B) in *water R* and dilute to 5.0 ml with the same solvent. Dilute 1 ml of the solution to *V* with *water R, V* being the maximum recommended dose in millilitres.

Plate: *TLC silica gel plate for aminopolyether test R.*

Application: 2.5 μl; in addition, apply 2.5 μl of the test solution and then 2.5 μl of reference solution (b) at the same place.

Detection: visually compare the spots 1 min after application.

System suitability:

- the spot due to the successive application of the test solution and reference solution (b) is similar in appearance to the spot due to reference solution (b), which is characterised by a number of concentric circles; the darker innermost circle (of intensity proportional to the concentration of impurity B) may be surrounded by a bluish-black ring, outside of which is a lighter circle surrounded by a peripheral dark edge;
- the spot due to reference solution (a) has a more diffuse inner circle, which is brownish-pink and without a distinct margin between it and the surrounding lighter zone;
- the spot due to reference solution (b) is clearly different from the spot due to reference solution (a).

Limit:

- the central portion of the spot due to the test solution is less intense than that of the spot due to reference solution (b) (2.2 mg/*V*).

Impurity C. Liquid chromatography (*2.2.29*).

Test solution. The preparation to be examined.

Reference solution (a). Dilute 2.1 ml of a 25.95 g/l solution of *tetrabutylammonium hydroxide R* (impurity C) to 20.0 ml with *water R*. Dilute 1.0 ml of this solution to *V* with *water R, V* being the maximum recommended dose in millilitres.

Reference solution (b). Dilute 1 ml of a 25.95 g/l solution of *tetrabutylammonium hydroxide R* to 10 ml with *water R*. Dilute 1 ml of this solution to 25 ml with *water R*.

Column:

- *size*: *l* = 0.10 m, Ø = 4.6 mm;
- *stationary phase*: *octadecylsilyl silica gel for chromatography R* (3 μm);
- *temperature*: constant, between 20 °C and 25 °C.

Mobile phase: 25 volumes of a 0.95 g/l solution of *toluenesulphonic acid R* and 75 volumes of *acetonitrile R*.

Flow rate: 0.6 ml/min.

Detection: spectrophotometer at 254 nm.

Injection: 20 μl.

Run time: twice the retention time of tetrabutylammonium ions.

Retention time: tetrabutylammonium hydroxide = about 3.3 min.

System suitability: reference solution (b):

- *signal-to-noise ratio*: minimum 10 for the principal peak;
- *symmetry factor*: maximum 1.8 for the principal peak.

Limit:

- *impurity C*: not more than the area of the corresponding peak in the chromatogram obtained with reference solution (a) (2.75 mg/*V*).

Impurity D. Ultraviolet and visible absorption spectrophotometry (*2.2.25*).

Test solution. The preparation to be examined.

Reference solution. Dissolve 20.0 mg of *4-(4-methylpiperidin-1-yl)pyridine R* (impurity D) in *water R* and dilute to 100.0 ml with the same solvent. Dilute 0.1 ml of the solution to *V* with *water R, V* being the maximum recommended dose in millilitres.

Measure the absorbance of the test solution and the reference solution at the absorption maximum of 263 nm.

Limit: the absorbance of the test solution is not greater than that of the reference solution (0.02 mg/*V*).

Residual solvents: limited according to the principles defined in general chapter *5.4*. The preparation may be released for use before completion of the test.

Sterility. It complies with the test for sterility prescribed in the monograph *Radiopharmaceutical preparations (0125)*. The injection may be released for use before completion of the test.

Bacterial endotoxins (*2.6.14*): less than 175/*V* IU/ml, *V* being the maximum recommended dose in millilitres. The injection may be released for use before completion of the test.

RADIONUCLIDIC PURITY

The preparation may be released for use before completion of test B.

A. Gamma-ray spectrometry.

   Results: the only gamma photons have an energy of 0.511 MeV and, depending on the measurement geometry, a sum peak of 1.022 MeV may be observed.

B. Gamma-ray spectrometry.

   Determine the amount of fluorine-18 and radionuclidic impurities with a half-life longer than 2 h. For the detection and quantification of impurities, retain the preparation to be examined for at least 24 h to allow the fluorine-18 to decay to a level that permits the detection of impurities.

   Results: the total radioactivity due to radionuclidic impurities is not more than 0.1 per cent.

RADIOCHEMICAL PURITY

A. Liquid chromatography (*2.2.29*) as described in the test for 2-fluoro-2-deoxy-D-glucose and impurity A. If necessary, dilute the test solution with *water R* to obtain a radioactivity concentration suitable for the radioactivity detector.

   Injection: test solution and reference solutions (a) and (c).

   Relative retention with reference to 2-[^{18}F]fluoro-2-deoxy-D-glucose (retention time = about 12 min): 2-[^{18}F]fluoro-2-deoxy-D-mannose = about 0.9. Partially and fully acetylated derivatives of both compounds hydrolyse under the chromatographic conditions and therefore elute as 2-[^{18}F]fluoro-2-deoxy-D-glucose and 2-[^{18}F]fluoro-2-deoxy-D-mannose.

   Locate the peaks due to 2-[^{18}F]fluoro-2-deoxy-D-glucose and 2-[^{18}F]fluoro-2-deoxy-D-mannose using the chromatograms obtained with the carbohydrate detector and reference solutions (a) and (c).

Radiopharmaceutical preparations

Limits:

– *fluorine-18 in the form of 2-[^{18}F]fluoro-2-deoxy-D-glucose and 2-[^{18}F]fluoro-2-deoxy-D-mannose*: minimum 95 per cent of the total radioactivity;

– *2-[^{18}F]fluoro-2-deoxy-D-mannose*: maximum 10 per cent of the total radioactivity due to 2-[^{18}F]fluoro-2-deoxy-D-glucose and 2-[^{18}F]fluoro-2-deoxy-D-mannose.

B. Thin-layer chromatography (*2.2.27*).

Test solution. The preparation to be examined.

Reference solution: dissolve, with gentle heating, 30 mg of *1,2,3,4-tetra-O-acetyl-β-D-glucopyranose R* and 20 mg of *glucose R* in 1 ml of *water R*.

Plate: *TLC silica gel plate R*.

Mobile phase: *water R, acetonitrile R* (5:95 *V/V*).

Application: about 2 μl.

Development: over a path of 8 cm.

Drying: in air for 15 min.

Detection: determine the distribution of radioactivity using a suitable detector, then immerse the plate in a 75 g/l solution of *sulphuric acid R* in *methanol R* and dry with a heat gun or at 150 °C until the appearance of dark spots in the chromatogram obtained with the reference solution.

Retardation factors: [^{18}F]fluoride = about 0; 2-[^{18}F]fluoro-2-deoxy-D-glucose and 2-[^{18}F]fluoro-2-deoxy-D-mannose = about 0.45; partially or fully acetylated derivatives of 2-[^{18}F]fluoro-2-deoxy-D-glucose and 2-[^{18}F]fluoro-2-deoxy-D-mannose = about 0.8 to 0.95.

System suitability: reference solution:

– the chromatogram shows 2 clearly separated spots.

Limits:

– *fluorine-18 in the form of 2-[^{18}F]fluoro-2-deoxy-D-glucose and 2-[^{18}F]fluoro-2-deoxy-D-mannose*: minimum 95 per cent of the total radioactivity;

– *fluorine-18 in the form of fluoride and partially or fully acetylated derivatives of 2-[^{18}F]fluoro-2-deoxy-D-glucose and 2-[^{18}F]fluoro-2-deoxy-D-mannose*: maximum 5 per cent of the total radioactivity.

RADIOACTIVITY

Measure the radioactivity using a calibrated instrument.

LABELLING

The label states the maximum recommended dose, in millilitres.

IMPURITIES

Specified impurities: *A, B, C, D, E*.

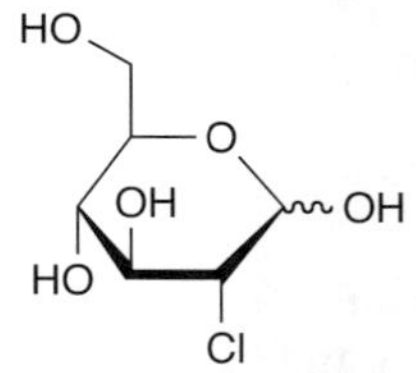

A. 2-chloro-2-deoxy-D-glucopyranose (2-chloro-2-deoxy-D-glucose),

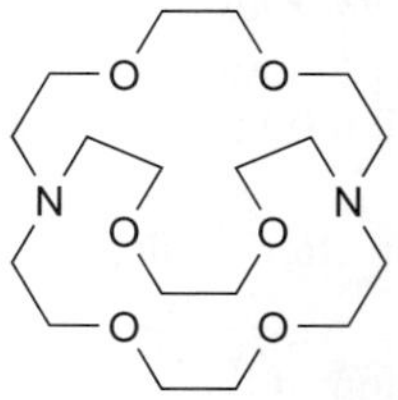

B. 4,7,13,16,21,24-hexaoxa-1,10-diazabicyclo[8.8.8]-hexacosane (aminopolyether),

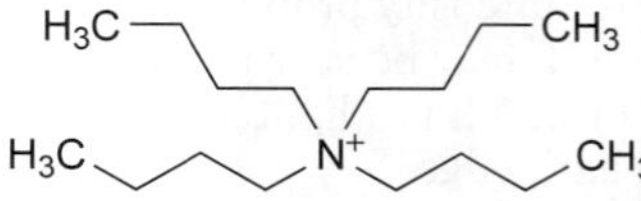

C. *N,N,N*-tributylbutan-1-aminium (tetrabutylammonium),

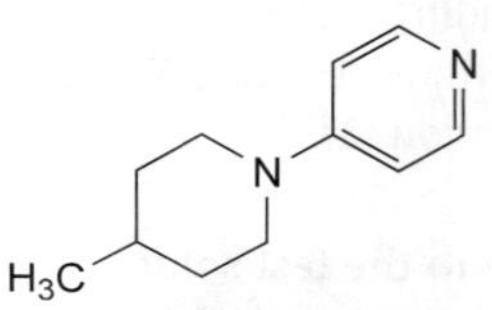

D. 4-(4-methylpiperidin-1-yl)pyridine,

E. [^{18}F]fluoride.

A

07/2008:0307

ACACIA

Acaciae gummi

DEFINITION

Air-hardened, gummy exudate flowing naturally from or obtained by incision of the trunk and branches of *Acacia senegal* L. Willdenow, other species of *Acacia* of African origin and *Acacia seyal Del.*

CHARACTERS

Acacia is almost completely but very slowly soluble, after about 2 h, in twice its mass of water leaving only a very small residue of vegetable particles; the liquid obtained is colourless or yellowish, dense, viscous, adhesive, translucent and weakly acid to blue litmus paper. Acacia is practically insoluble in ethanol (96 per cent).

IDENTIFICATION

A. Acacia occurs as yellowish-white, yellow or pale amber, sometimes with a pinkish tint, friable, opaque, spheroidal, oval or reniform pieces (tears) of a diameter from about 1-3 cm, frequently with a cracked surface, easily broken into irregular, whitish or slightly yellowish angular fragments with conchoidal fracture and a glassy and transparent appearance. In the centre of an unbroken tear there is sometimes a small cavity.

B. Reduce to a powder (355) (*2.9.12*). The powder is white or yellowish-white. Examine under a microscope using a 50 per cent *V/V* solution of *glycerol R*. The powder shows the following diagnostic characters: angular, irregular, colourless, transparent fragments. Only traces of starch or vegetable tissues are visible. No stratified membrane is apparent.

C. Examine the chromatograms obtained in the test for glucose and fructose.

   Results: the chromatogram obtained with the test solution shows 3 zones due to galactose, arabinose and rhamnose. No other important zones are visible, particularly in the upper part of the chromatogram.

D. Dissolve 1 g of the powdered drug (355) (*2.9.12*) in 2 ml of *water R* by stirring frequently for 2 h. Add 2 ml of *ethanol (96 per cent) R*. After shaking, a white, gelatinous mucilage is formed which becomes fluid on adding 10 ml of *water R*.

TESTS

Solution S. Dissolve 3.0 g of the powdered drug (355) (*2.9.12*) in 25 ml of *water R* by stirring for 30 min. Allow to stand for 30 min and dilute to 30 ml with *water R*.

Insoluble matter: maximum 0.5 per cent.

To 5.0 g of the powdered drug (355) (*2.9.12*) add 100 ml of *water R* and 14 ml of *dilute hydrochloric acid R*, boil gently for 15 min, shaking frequently and filter while hot through a tared sintered-glass filter (*2.1.2*). Wash with hot *water R* and dry at 100-105 °C. The residue weighs a maximum of 25 mg.

Glucose and fructose. Thin-layer chromatography (*2.2.27*).

Test solution. To 0.100 g of the powdered drug (355) (*2.9.12*) in a thick-walled centrifuge tube add 2 ml of a 100 g/l solution of *trifluoroacetic acid R*, shake vigorously to dissolve the forming gel, stopper the tube and heat the mixture at 120 °C for 1 h. Centrifuge the hydrolysate, transfer the clear supernatant carefully into a 50 ml flask, add 10 ml of *water R* and evaporate the solution to dryness under reduced pressure. To the resulting clear film add 0.1 ml of *water R* and 0.9 ml of *methanol R*. Centrifuge to separate the amorphous precipitate. Dilute the supernatant, if necessary, to 1 ml with *methanol R*.

Reference solution. Dissolve 10 mg of *arabinose R*, 10 mg of *galactose R*, 10 mg of *glucose R*, 10 mg of *rhamnose R* and 10 mg of *xylose R* in 1 ml of *water R* and dilute to 10 ml with *methanol R*.

Plate: *TLC silica gel plate R.*

Mobile phase: 16 g/l solution of *sodium dihydrogen phosphate R, butanol R, acetone R* (10:40:50 *V/V/V*).

Application: 10 µl as bands.

Developement A: over a path of 10 cm.

Drying A: in a current of warm air for a few minutes.

Development B: over a path of 15 cm using the same mobile phase.

Drying B: at 110 °C for 10 min.

Detection: spray with *anisaldehyde solution R* and heat at 110 °C for 10 min.

Results: the chromatogram obtained with the reference solution shows 5 clearly separated coloured zones due to galactose (greyish-green or green), glucose (grey), arabinose (yellowish-green), xylose (greenish-grey or yellowish-grey) and rhamnose (yellowish-green), in order of increasing R_F value. The chromatogram obtained with the test solution shows no grey zone and no greyish-green zone between the zones corresponding to galactose and arabinose in the chromatogram obtained with the reference solution.

Starch, dextrin and agar. To 10 ml of solution S previously boiled and cooled add 0.1 ml of *0.05 M iodine*. No blue or reddish-brown colour develops.

Sterculia gum

A. Place 0.2 g of the powdered drug (355) (*2.9.12*) in a 10 ml ground-glass-stoppered cylinder graduated in 0.1 ml. Add 10 ml of *ethanol (60 per cent V/V) R* and shake. Any gel formed occupies a maximum of 1.5 ml.

B. To 1.0 g of the powdered drug (355) (*2.9.12*) add 100 ml of *water R* and shake. Add 0.1 ml of *methyl red solution R*. Not more than 5.0 ml of *0.01 M sodium hydroxide* is required to change the colour of the indicator.

Tannins. To 10 ml of solution S add 0.1 ml of *ferric chloride solution R1*. A gelatinous precipitate is formed, but neither the precipitate nor the liquid are dark blue.

Tragacanth. Examine the chromatograms obtained in the test for glucose and fructose.

Results: the chromatogram obtained with the test solution shows no greenish-grey or yellowish-grey zone corresponding to the zone of xylose in the chromatogram obtained with the reference solution.

Loss on drying (*2.2.32*): maximum 15.0 per cent, determined on 1.000 g of the powdered drug (355) (*2.9.12*) by drying in an oven at 105 °C.

Total ash (*2.4.16*): maximum 4.0 per cent.

Microbial contamination. Total viable aerobic count (*2.6.12*) not more than 10^4 micro-organisms per gram, determined by plate count. It complies with the test for *Escherichia coli* (*2.6.13*).

FUNCTIONALITY-RELATED CHARACTERISTICS

This section provides information on characteristics that are recognised as being relevant control parameters for one or more functions of the substance when used as an excipient (see chapter 5.15). This section is a non-mandatory part of the monograph and it is not necessary to verify the characteristics to demonstrate

Monographs A-C

compliance. Control of these characteristics can however contribute to the quality of a medicinal product by improving the consistency of the manufacturing process and the performance of the medicinal product during use. Where control methods are cited, they are recognised as being suitable for the purpose, but other methods can also be used. Wherever results for a particular characteristic are reported, the control method must be indicated.

The following characteristic may be relevant for acacia used as a viscosity-increasing agent and/or suspending agent in aqueous preparations.

Apparent viscosity. Determine the dynamic viscosity using a capillary viscometer (*2.2.9*) or a rotating viscometer (*2.2.10*) on a 100 g/l solution of acacia (dried substance).

07/2008:0308

ACACIA, SPRAY-DRIED

Acaciae gummi dispersione desiccatum

DEFINITION

Spray-dried acacia is obtained from a solution of acacia.

CHARACTERS

It dissolves completely and rapidly, after about 20 min, in twice its mass of water. The liquid obtained is colourless or yellowish, dense, viscous, adhesive, translucent and weakly acid to blue litmus paper. Spray-dried acacia is practically insoluble in ethanol (96 per cent).

IDENTIFICATION

A. Examined under a microscope, in *ethanol (96 per cent) R*, the powder is seen to consist predominantly of spheroidal particles about 4-40 μm in diameter, with a central cavity containing 1 or several air-bubbles; a few minute flat fragments are present. Only traces of starch granules are visible. No vegetable tissue is seen.

B. Examine the chromatograms obtained in the test for glucose and fructose.

   Results: the chromatogram obtained with the test solution shows 3 zones due to galactose, arabinose and rhamnose. No other important zones are visible, particularly in the upper part of the chromatogram.

C. Dissolve 1 g of the drug to be examined in 2 ml of *water R* by stirring frequently for 20 min. Add 2 ml of *ethanol (96 per cent) R*. After shaking a white gelatinous mucilage is formed which becomes fluid on adding 10 ml of *water R*.

TESTS

Solution S. Dissolve 3.0 g of the drug to be examined in 25 ml of *water R* by stirring for 10 min. Allow to stand for 20 min and dilute to 30 ml with *water R*.

Glucose and fructose. Thin-layer chromatography (*2.2.27*).

Test solution. To 0.100 g in a thick-walled centrifuge tube add 2 ml of a 100 g/l solution of *trifluoroacetic acid R*, shake vigorously to dissolve the forming gel, stopper the tube and heat the mixture at 120 °C for 1 h. Centrifuge the hydrolysate, transfer the clear supernatant carefully into a 50 ml flask, add 10 ml of *water R* and evaporate to dryness under reduced pressure. To the resulting clear film add 0.1 ml of *water R* and 0.9 ml of *methanol R*. Centrifuge to separate the amorphous precipitate. Dilute the supernatant, if necessary, to 1 ml with *methanol R*.

Reference solution. Dissolve 10 mg of *arabinose R*, 10 mg of *galactose R*, 10 mg of *glucose R*, 10 mg of *rhamnose R* and 10 mg of *xylose R* in 1 ml of *water R* and dilute to 10 ml with *methanol R*.

Plate: *TLC silica gel plate R*.

Mobile phase: 16 g/l solution of *sodium dihydrogen phosphate R*, *butanol R*, *acetone R* (10:40:50 *V/V/V*).

Application: 10 μl as bands.

Development A: over a path of 10 cm.

Drying A: in a current of warm air for a few minutes.

Development B: over a path of 15 cm using the same mobile phase.

Detection: spray with *anisaldehyde solution R* and heat at 110 °C for 10 min.

Results: the chromatogram obtained with the reference solution shows 5 clearly separated coloured zones due to galactose (greyish-green or green), glucose (grey), arabinose (yellowish-green), xylose (greenish-grey or yellowish-grey) and rhamnose (yellowish-green), in order of increasing R_F value. The chromatogram obtained with the test solution shows no grey zone and no greyish-green zone between the zones corresponding to galactose and arabinose in the chromatogram obtained with the reference solution.

Starch, dextrin and agar. To 10 ml of solution S previously boiled and cooled add 0.1 ml of *0.05 M iodine*. No blue or reddish-brown colour develops.

Sterculia gum

A. Place 0.2 g in a 10 ml ground-glass-stoppered cylinder graduated in 0.1 ml. Add 10 ml of *ethanol (60 per cent V/V) R* and shake. Any gel formed occupies not more than 1.5 ml.

B. To 1.0 g add 100 ml of *water R* and shake. Add 0.1 ml of *methyl red solution R*. Not more than 5.0 ml of *0.01 M sodium hydroxide* is required to change the colour of the indicator.

Tannins. To 10 ml of solution S add 0.1 ml of *ferric chloride solution R1*. A gelatinous precipitate is formed, but neither the precipitate nor the liquid shows a dark blue colour.

Tragacanth. Examine the chromatograms obtained in the test for Glucose and fructose.

Results: the chromatogram obtained with the test solution shows no greenish-grey or yellowish-grey zone corresponding to the zone of xylose in the chromatogram obtained with the reference solution.

Loss on drying (*2.2.32*): maximum 10.0 per cent, determined on 1.000 g by drying in an oven at 105 °C.

Total ash (*2.4.16*).: maximum 4.0 per cent.

Microbial contamination. Total viable aerobic count (*2.6.12*) not more than 10^4 micro-organisms per gram, determined by plate count. It complies with the test for *Escherichia coli* (*2.6.13*).

FUNCTIONALITY-RELATED CHARACTERISTICS

This section provides information on characteristics that are recognised as being relevant control parameters for one or more functions of the substance when used as an excipient (see chapter 5.15). This section is a non-mandatory part of the monograph and it is not necessary to verify the characteristics to demonstrate compliance. Control of these characteristics can however contribute to the quality of a medicinal product by improving the consistency of the manufacturing process and the performance of the medicinal product during use. Where control methods are cited, they are recognised as

Monographs A-C

being suitable for the purpose, but other methods can also be used. Wherever results for a particular characteristic are reported, the control method must be indicated.

The following characteristic may be relevant for spray-dried acacia used as a viscosity-increasing agent and/or suspending agent in aqueous preparations.

Apparent viscosity. Determine the dynamic viscosity using a capillary viscometer (*2.2.9*) or a rotating viscometer (*2.2.10*) on a 100 g/l solution of spray-dried acacia (dried substance).

07/2008:1281

ACECLOFENAC

Aceclofenacum

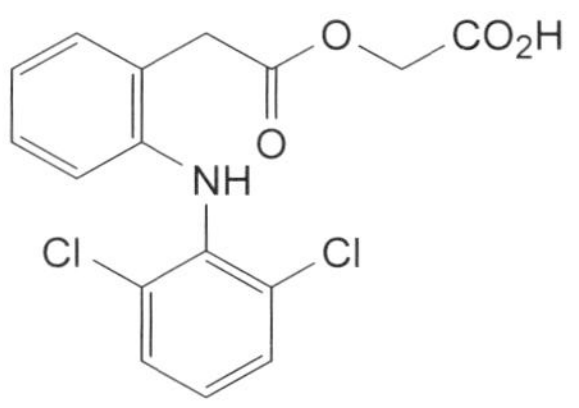

$C_{16}H_{13}Cl_2NO_4$ M_r 354.2
[89796-99-6]

DEFINITION

[[[2-[(2,6-Dichlorophenyl)amino]phenyl]acetyl]oxy]acetic acid.

Content: 99.0 per cent to 101.0 per cent (dried substance).

CHARACTERS

Appearance: white or almost white, crystalline powder.

Solubility: practically insoluble in water, freely soluble in acetone, soluble in ethanol (96 per cent).

IDENTIFICATION

First identification: B.

Second identification: A, C.

A. Dissolve 50.0 mg in *methanol R* and dilute to 100.0 ml with the same solvent. Dilute 2.0 ml of the solution to 50.0 ml with *methanol R*. Examined between 220 nm and 370 nm (*2.2.25*), the solution shows an absorption maximum at 275 nm. The specific absorbance at the absorption maximum is 320 to 350.

B. Infrared absorption spectrophotometry (*2.2.24*).

Comparison: Ph. Eur. reference spectrum of aceclofenac.

C. Dissolve about 10 mg in 10 ml of *ethanol (96 per cent) R*. To 1 ml of the solution, add 0.2 ml of a mixture, prepared immediately before use, of equal volumes of a 6 g/l solution of *potassium ferricyanide R* and a 9 g/l solution of *ferric chloride R*. Allow to stand protected from light for 5 min. Add 3 ml of a 10.0 g/l solution of *hydrochloric acid R*. Allow to stand protected from light for 15 min. A blue colour develops and a precipitate is formed.

TESTS

Related substances. Liquid chromatography (*2.2.29*). *Prepare the solutions immediately before use.*

Test solution. Dissolve 50.0 mg of the substance to be examined in a mixture of 30 volumes of mobile phase A and 70 volumes of mobile phase B and dilute to 25.0 ml with the same mixture of solvents.

Reference solution (a). Dissolve 21.6 mg of *diclofenac sodium CRS* (impurity A) in a mixture of 30 volumes of mobile phase A and 70 volumes of mobile phase B and dilute to 50.0 ml with the same mixture of solvents.

Reference solution (b). Dilute 2.0 ml of the test solution to 10.0 ml with a mixture of 30 volumes of mobile phase A and 70 volumes of mobile phase B.

Reference solution (c). Mix 1.0 ml of reference solution (a) and 1.0 ml of reference solution (b) and dilute to 100.0 ml with a mixture of 30 volumes of mobile phase A and 70 volumes of mobile phase B.

Reference solution (d). Dissolve 4.0 mg of *aceclofenac impurity F CRS* and 2.0 mg of *aceclofenac impurity H CRS* in a mixture of 30 volumes of mobile phase A and 70 volumes of mobile phase B then dilute to 10.0 ml with the same mixture of solvents.

Reference solution (e). Mix 1.0 ml of reference solution (b) and 1.0 ml of reference solution (d) and dilute to 100.0 ml with a mixture of 30 volumes of mobile phase A and 70 volumes of mobile phase B.

Reference solution (f). Dissolve the contents of a vial of *diclofenac impurity A CRS* (aceclofenac impurity I) in 1.0 ml of a mixture of 30 volumes of mobile phase A and 70 volumes of mobile phase B, add 1.5 ml of the same mixture of solvents and mix.

Column:

- *size*: *l* = 0.25 m, Ø = 4.6 mm;
- *stationary phase*: spherical *end-capped octadecylsilyl silica gel for chromatography R* (5 µm) with a pore size of 10 nm and a carbon loading of 19 per cent;
- *temperature*: 40 °C.

Mobile phase:

- *mobile phase A*: 1.12 g/l solution of *phosphoric acid R* adjusted to pH 7.0 using a 42 g/l solution of *sodium hydroxide R*;
- *mobile phase B*: *water R, acetonitrile R* (1:9 *V/V*);

Time (min)	Mobile phase A (per cent *V/V*)	Mobile phase B (per cent *V/V*)
0 - 25	70 → 50	30 → 50
25 - 30	50 → 20	50 → 80
30 - 50	20	80

Flow rate: 1.0 ml/min.

Detection: spectrophotometer at 275 nm.

Injection: 10 µl of the test solution and reference solutions (c), (e) and (f).

Relative retention with reference to aceclofenac (retention time = about 14 min): impurity A = about 0.8; impurity G = about 1.3; impurity H = about 1.5; impurity I = about 2.3; impurity D = about 2.6; impurity B = about 2.7; impurity E = about 2.8; impurity C = about 3.0; impurity F = about 3.2.

System suitability: reference solution (c):

- *resolution*: minimum 5.0 between the peaks due to impurity A and aceclofenac.

Limits:

- *impurity A*: not more than the area of the corresponding peak in the chromatogram obtained with reference solution (c) (0.2 per cent);

Monographs A-C

- *impurities B, C, D, E, G*: for each impurity, not more than the area of the peak due to aceclofenac in the chromatogram obtained with reference solution (e) (0.2 per cent);
- *impurity F*: not more than the area of the corresponding peak in the chromatogram obtained with reference solution (e) (0.2 per cent);
- *impurity H*: not more than the area of the corresponding peak in the chromatogram obtained with reference solution (e) (0.1 per cent);
- *impurity I*: not more than the area of the corresponding peak in the chromatogram obtained with reference solution (f) (0.1 per cent);
- *unspecified impurities*: not more than 0.5 times the area of the peak due to aceclofenac in the chromatogram obtained with reference solution (e) (0.10 per cent);
- *total*: not more than 0.7 per cent;
- *disregard limit*: 0.1 times the area of the peak due to aceclofenac in the chromatogram obtained with reference solution (e) (0.02 per cent).

Heavy metals (*2.4.8*): maximum 10 ppm.

To 2.0 g in a silica crucible, add 2 ml of *sulphuric acid R* to wet the substance. Heat progressively to ignition and continue heating until an almost white or at most a greyish residue is obtained. Carry out the ignition at a temperature not exceeding 800 °C. Allow to cool. Add 3 ml of *hydrochloric acid R* and 1 ml of *nitric acid R*. Heat and evaporate slowly to dryness. Cool and add 1 ml of a 100 g/l solution of *hydrochloric acid R* and 10.0 ml of *distilled water R*. Neutralise with a 1.0 g/l solution of *ammonia R* using 0.1 ml of *phenolphthalein solution R* as indicator. Add 2.0 ml of a 60 g/l solution of *anhydrous acetic acid R* and dilute to 20 ml with *distilled water R*. 12 ml of the solution complies with test A. Prepare the reference solution using *lead standard solution (1 ppm Pb) R*.

Loss on drying (*2.2.32*): maximum 0.5 per cent, determined on 1.000 g by drying in an oven at 105 °C.

Sulphated ash (*2.4.14*): maximum 0.1 per cent, determined on 1.0 g.

ASSAY

Dissolve 0.300 g in 40 ml of *methanol R*. Titrate with *0.1 M sodium hydroxide*, determining the end-point potentiometrically (*2.2.20*).

1 ml of *0.1 M sodium hydroxide* is equivalent to 35.42 mg of $C_{16}H_{13}Cl_2NO_4$.

STORAGE

In an airtight container, protected from light.

IMPURITIES

Specified impurities: A, B, C, D, E, F, G, H, I.

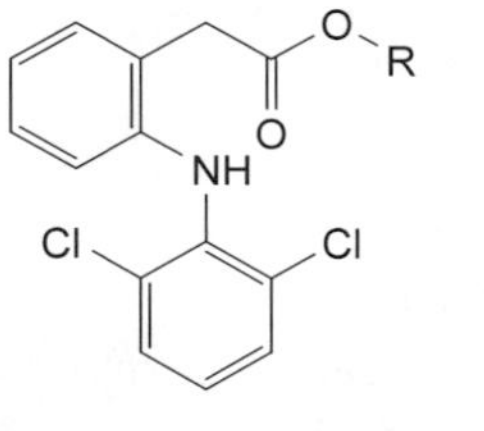

A. R = H: [2-[(2,6-dichlorophenyl)amino]phenyl]acetic acid (diclofenac),

B. R = CH_3: methyl [2-[(2,6-dichlorophenyl)amino]phenyl]-acetate (methyl ester of diclofenac),

C. R = C_2H_5: ethyl [2-[(2,6-dichlorophenyl)amino]phenyl]-acetate (ethyl ester of diclofenac),

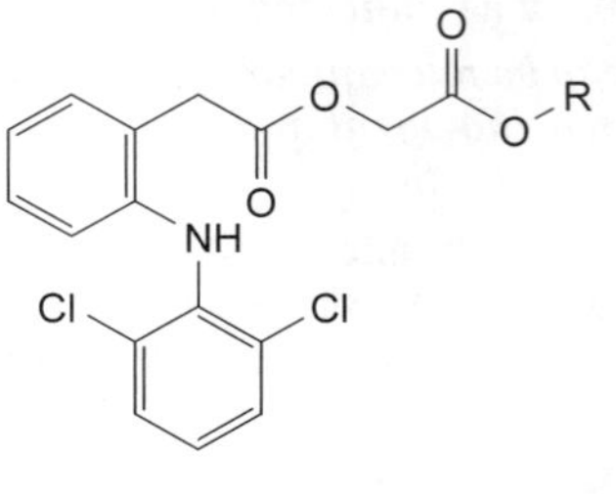

D. R = CH_3: methyl [[[2-[(2,6-dichlorophenyl)-amino]phenyl]acetyl]oxy]acetate (methyl ester of aceclofenac),

E. R = C_2H_5: ethyl [[[2-[(2,6-dichlorophenyl)-amino]phenyl]acetyl]oxy]acetate (ethyl ester of aceclofenac),

F. R = CH_2-C_6H_5: benzyl [[[2-[(2,6-dichlorophenyl)-amino]phenyl]acetyl]oxy]acetate (benzyl ester of aceclofenac),

G. R = CH_2-CO_2H: [[[[[2-[(2,6-dichlorophenyl)-amino]phenyl]acetyl]oxy]acetyl]oxy]acetic acid (acetic aceclofenac),

H. R = CH_2-CO-O-CH_2-CO_2H: [[[[[[[2-[(2,6-dichlorophenyl)-amino]phenyl]acetyl]oxy]acetyl]oxy]acetyl]oxy]acetic acid (diacetic aceclofenac),

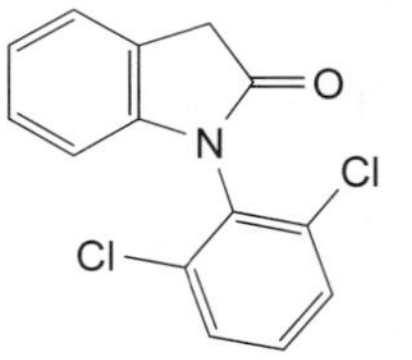

I. 1-(2,6-dichlorophenyl)-1,3-dihydro-2*H*-indol-2-one.

07/2008:2303

ADRENALINE

Adrenalinum

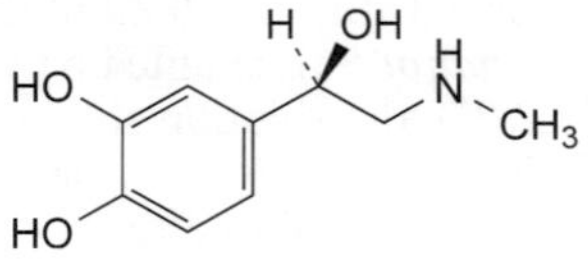

$C_9H_{13}NO_3$ M_r 183.2
[51-43-4]

DEFINITION

4-[(1*R*)-1-Hydroxy-2-(methylamino)ethyl]benzene-1,2-diol.

Synthetic product.

Content: 99.0 per cent to 101.0 per cent (dried substance).

CHARACTERS

Appearance: white or almost white crystalline powder, becoming coloured on exposure to air and light.

Solubility: practically insoluble in water, in ethanol (96 per cent) and in methylene chloride. It dissolves in hydrochloric acid.

IDENTIFICATION

A. Infrared absorption spectrophotometry (*2.2.24*).
Comparison: *adrenaline CRS*.

B. Specific optical rotation (see Tests).

TESTS

Solution S. Dissolve 1.000 g in a 25.75 g/l solution of *hydrochloric acid R* and dilute to 50.0 ml with the same solvent. Examine the solution immediately.

Appearance of solution. Solution S is not more opalescent than reference suspension II (*2.2.1*) and not more intensely coloured than reference solution BY_5 (*2.2.2, Method II*).

Specific optical rotation (*2.2.7*): – 50.0 to – 54.0 (dried substance), determined on solution S.

Related substances. Liquid chromatography (*2.2.29*). *Prepare the solutions protected from light.*

Solvent mixture A. Dissolve 5.0 g of *potassium dihydrogen phosphate R* and 2.6 g of *sodium octanesulphonate R* in *water for chromatography R* and dilute to 1000 ml with the same solvent (it is usually necessary to stir for at least 30 min to achieve complete dissolution). Adjust to pH 2.8 with *phosphoric acid R.*

Solvent mixture B: *acetonitrile R1*, solvent mixture A (13:87 *V/V*).

Test solution. Dissolve 40 mg of the substance to be examined in 5 ml of *0.1 M hydrochloric acid* and dilute to 50.0 ml with solvent mixture B.

Reference solution (a). Dilute 1.0 ml of the test solution to 100.0 ml with solvent mixture B. Dilute 1.0 ml of this solution to 10.0 ml with solvent mixture B.

Reference solution (b). Dissolve 1.5 mg of *noradrenaline tartrate CRS* (impurity B) and 1.5 mg of *adrenalone hydrochloride R* (impurity C) in solvent mixture B, add 1.0 ml of the test solution and dilute to 100 ml with solvent mixture B.

Reference solution (c). Dissolve the contents of a vial of *adrenaline impurity mixture CRS* (containing impurities D and E) in 1.0 ml of the blank solution.

Reference solution (d). Dissolve 4 mg of *adrenaline with impurity F CRS* in 0.5 ml of *0.1 M hydrochloric acid* and dilute to 5 ml with solvent mixture B.

Blank solution: *0.1 M hydrochloric acid,* solvent mixture B (1:9 *V/V*).

Column:

– *size*: *l* = 0.10 m, Ø = 4.6 mm;
– *stationary phase*: *end-capped octadecylsilyl silica gel for chromatography R* (3 µm);
– *temperature*: 50 °C.

Mobile phase:

– *mobile phase A*: *acetonitrile R1*, solvent mixture A (5:95 *V/V*);
– *mobile phase B*: *acetonitrile R1*, solvent mixture A (45:55 *V/V*);

Time (min)	Mobile phase A (per cent *V/V*)	Mobile phase B (per cent *V/V*)
0 - 15	92 → 50	8 → 50
15 - 20	50 → 92	50 → 8
20 - 25	92	8

Flow rate: 2.0 ml/min.

Detection: spectrophotometer at 210 nm.

Injection: 20 µl.

Identification of impurities: use the chromatogram supplied with *adrenaline impurity mixture CRS* and the chromatogram obtained with reference solution (c) to identify the peaks due to impurities D and E; use the chromatogram supplied with *adrenaline with impurity F CRS* and the chromatogram obtained with reference solution (d) to identify the peak due to impurity F.

Relative retention with reference to adrenaline (retention time = about 4 min): impurity F = about 0.2; impurity B = about 0.8; impurity C = about 1.3; impurity D = about 3.3; impurity E = about 3.7.

System suitability: reference solution (b):

– *resolution*: minimum 3.0 between the peaks due to impurity B and adrenaline.

Limits:

– *correction factors*: for the calculation of content, multiply the peak areas of the following impurities by the corresponding correction factor: impurity D = 0.7; impurity E = 0.6;
– *impurities B, C, F*: for each impurity, not more than twice the area of the principal peak in the chromatogram obtained with reference solution (a) (0.2 per cent);
– *impurities D, E*: for each impurity, not more than the area of the principal peak in the chromatogram obtained with reference solution (a) (0.1 per cent);
– *unspecified impurities*: for each impurity, not more than the area of the principal peak in the chromatogram obtained with reference solution (a) (0.10 per cent);
– *total*: not more than 5 times the area of the principal peak in the chromatogram obtained with reference solution (a) (0.5 per cent);
– *disregard limit*: 0.5 times the area of the principal peak in the chromatogram obtained with reference solution (a) (0.05 per cent).

Loss on drying (*2.2.32*): maximum 0.5 per cent, determined on 1.000 g by drying over *diphosphorus pentoxide R* at a pressure not exceeding 0.7 kPa for 18 h.

Sulphated ash (*2.4.14*): maximum 0.1 per cent, determined on 1.0 g.

ASSAY

Dissolve 0.150 g in 50 ml of *anhydrous acetic acid R.* Titrate with *0.1 M perchloric acid,* determining the end-point potentiometrically (*2.2.20*).

1 ml of *0.1 M perchloric acid* is equivalent to 18.32 mg of $C_9H_{13}NO_3$.

STORAGE

Under nitrogen, protected from light.

IMPURITIES

Specified impurities: B, C, D, E, F.

B. noradrenaline,

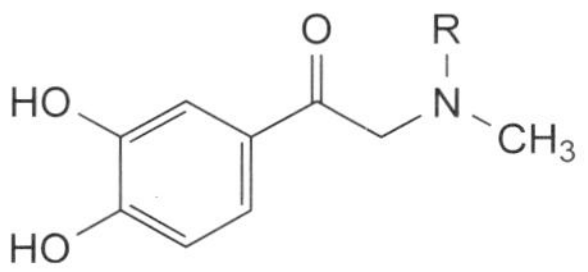

C. R = H: 1-(3,4-dihydroxyphenyl)-2-(methylamino)ethanone (adrenalone),

E. R = CH_2-C_6H_5: 2-(benzylmethylamino)-1-(3,4-dihydroxyphenyl)ethanone,

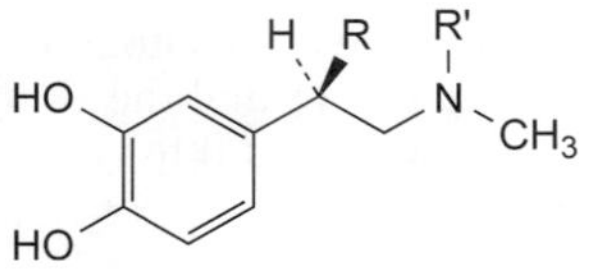

D. R = OH, R′ = CH_2-C_6H_5: 4-[(1*R*)-2-(benzylmethylamino)-1-hydroxyethyl]benzene-1,2-diol,

F. R = SO_3H, R′ = H: (1*R*)-1-(3,4-dihydroxyphenyl)-2-(methylamino)ethanesulphonic acid.

01/2008:0310

AGAR

Agar

DEFINITION

Polysaccharides from various species of Rhodophyceae mainly belonging to the genus *Gelidium*. It is prepared by treating the algae with boiling water; the extract is filtered whilst hot, concentrated and dried.

CHARACTERS

Appearance: powder or crumpled strips 2-5 mm wide or sometimes flakes, colourless or pale yellow, translucent, somewhat tough and difficult to break, becoming more brittle on drying.

Mucilaginous taste.

IDENTIFICATION

A. Examine under a microscope. When mounted in *0.005 M iodine*, the strips or flakes are partly stained brownish-violet. Magnified 100 times, they show the following diagnostic characters: numerous minute, colourless, ovoid or rounded grains on an amorphous background; occasional brown, round or ovoid spores with a reticulated surface, measuring up to 60 µm, may be present. Reduce to a powder, if necessary. The powder is yellowish-white. Examine under a microscope using *0.005 M iodine*. The powder presents angular fragments with numerous grains similar to those seen in the strips and flakes; some of the fragments are stained brownish-violet.

B. Dissolve 0.1 g with heating in 50 ml of *water R*. Cool. To 1 ml of the mucilage carefully add 3 ml of *water R* so as to form 2 separate layers. Add 0.1 ml of *0.05 M iodine*. A dark brownish-violet colour appears at the interface. Mix. The liquid becomes pale yellow.

C. Heat 5 ml of the mucilage prepared for identification test B on a water-bath with 0.5 ml of *hydrochloric acid R* for 30 min. Add 1 ml of *barium chloride solution R1*. A white turbidity develops within 30 min.

D. Heat 0.5 g with 50 ml of *water R* on a water-bath until dissolved. Only a few fragments remain insoluble. During cooling, the solution gels between 35 °C and 30 °C. Heat the gel thus obtained on a water-bath; it does not liquefy below 80 °C.

TESTS

Swelling index (*2.8.4*): minimum 10 and within 10 per cent of the value stated on the label, determined on the powdered drug (355) (*2.9.12*).

Insoluble matter: maximum 1.0 per cent.

To 5.00 g of the powdered drug (355) (*2.9.12*) add 100 ml of *water R* and 14 ml of *dilute hydrochloric acid R*. Boil gently for 15 min with frequent stirring. Filter the hot liquid through a tared, sintered-glass filter (160) (*2.1.2*), rinse the filter with hot *water R* and dry at 100-105 °C. The residue weighs a maximum of 50 mg.

Gelatin. To 1.00 g add 100 ml of *water R* and heat on a water-bath until dissolved. Allow to cool to 50 °C. To 5 ml of this solution add 5 ml of *picric acid solution R*. No turbidity appears within 10 min.

Loss on drying (*2.2.32*): maximum 20.0 per cent, determined on 1.000 g of the powdered drug (355) (*2.9.12*) by drying in an oven at 105 °C.

Total ash (*2.4.16*): maximum 5.0 per cent.

Microbial contamination. Total viable aerobic count (*2.6.12*) not more than 10^3 micro-organisms per gram, determined by plate-count. It complies with the tests for *Escherichia coli* and *Salmonella* (*2.6.13*).

LABELLING

The label states the swelling index.

01/2008:2147
corrected 6.2

AGNUS CASTUS FRUIT

Agni casti fructus

DEFINITION

Whole, ripe, dried fruit of *Vitex agnus-castus* L.

Content: minimum 0.08 per cent of casticin ($C_{19}H_{18}O_8$; M_r 374.3) (dried drug).

IDENTIFICATION

A. Agnus castus fruit is oval to almost globular, with a diameter of up to 5 mm. The persistent calyx is greenish-grey, finely pubescent, ends in 4-5 short teeth and envelops 2/3 to 3/4 of the surface of the fruit. The blackish-brown fruit consists of a pericarp that becomes progressively sclerous up to the endocarp. The style scar is often visible. Some of the fruits may retain a stalk, about 1 mm long. A transverse section of the fruit shows 4 locules, each containing an elongated seed.

B. Reduce to a powder (355) (*2.9.12*). Examine under a microscope using *chloral hydrate solution R*. The powder shows the following diagnostic characters: fragments of the outer epidermis of the calyx composed of polygonal cells densely covered with short, bent or undulate, uni-, bi- or tri-cellular uniseriate covering trichomes; cells of the epicarp with thick walls and well-marked, large pits; isolated glandular trichomes with a unicellular stalk and a uni- or multi-cellular head; layers of parenchyma from the outer part of the mesocarp, some containing brown pigment, others extending into septa; fragments from the inner part of the mesocarp composed of thin-walled, pitted, sclerenchymatous cells and of typical isodiametric sclerous cells with very thick, deeply grooved walls and a narrow, stellate lumen; small brown cells of the endocarp; fragments of the testa containing areas of fairly large, thin-walled lignified cells with reticulate bands of thickening; numerous fragments of the endosperm composed of thin-walled parenchymatous cells containing aleurone grains and oil droplets.

C. Thin-layer chromatography (*2.2.27*).

Test solution. To 1.0 g of the powdered drug (355) (*2.9.12*) add 10 ml of *methanol R*. Heat in a water-bath at 60 °C for 10 min. Allow to cool and filter.

Reference solution. Dissolve 0.5 mg of *aucubin R* and 1 mg of *agnuside R* in *methanol R* and dilute to 1.0 ml with the same solvent.

Monographs A-C

Plate: *TLC silica gel F_{254} plate R* (5-40 µm) [or *TLC silica gel F_{254} plate R* (2-10 µm)].

Mobile phase: *water R, methanol R, ethyl acetate R* (8:15:77 *V/V/V*).

Application: 10 µl [or 8 µl] as bands.

Development: over a path of 8 cm [or 5 cm].

Drying: in air.

Detection: spray with *formic acid R* and heat at 120 °C for 10 min; examine in daylight.

Results: see below the sequence of zones present in the chromatograms obtained with the reference solution and the test solution. Furthermore, other zones may be present in the chromatogram obtained with the test solution.

Top of the plate	
———	———
Agnuside: a blue zone	A blue zone (agnuside)
———	———
Aucubin: a blue zone	A blue zone (aucubin)
Reference solution	**Test solution**

TESTS

Foreign matter (*2.8.2*): maximum 3.0 per cent.

Other species of *Vitex*, in particular *Vitex negundo*. No fruit of other species with a much greater diameter is present.

Total ash (*2.4.16*): maximum 5.0 per cent.

Loss on drying (*2.2.32*): maximum 10.0 per cent, determined on 1.000 g of the powdered drug (355) (*2.9.12*) by drying in an oven at 105 °C for 2 h.

ASSAY

Liquid chromatography (*2.2.29*).

Test solution. Extract 1.000 g of the powdered drug (355) (*2.9.12*) with 40 ml of *methanol R* for 2 min using a suitable-speed homogeniser. Collect the supernatant liquid and filter into a 250 ml flask. Repeat the extraction with a further 40 ml of *methanol R*, collecting the supernatant liquid and filtering as before. Rinse the residue carefully with a small quantity of *methanol R*. Combine the methanol extracts and rinsings and evaporate to dryness *in vacuo* in a water-bath at not more than 30 °C. With the aid of ultrasound, dissolve the residue obtained in *methanol R* and dilute to 20.0 ml with the same solvent. Filter the solution through a membrane filter (0.45 µm). Dilute 1.0 ml to 10.0 ml with *methanol R*.

Reference solution. Dissolve 100.0 mg of *agnus castus fruit standardised dry extract CRS* in 20.0 ml of *methanol R* with the aid of ultrasound for 20 min, then dilute to 25.0 ml with the same solvent. Filter the solution through a membrane filter (0.45 µm).

Column:
- *size*: *l* = 0.125 m, Ø = 3.0 mm;
- *stationary phase*: *octadecylsilyl silica gel for chromatography R* (3 µm);
- *temperature*: 25 °C.

Mobile phase:
- *mobile phase A*: 5.88 g/l solution of *phosphoric acid R*;
- *mobile phase B*: *methanol R*;

Time (min)	Mobile phase A (per cent *V/V*)	Mobile phase B (per cent *V/V*)
0 - 13	50 → 35	50 → 65
13 - 18	35 → 0	65 → 100
18 - 23	0 → 50	100 → 50

Flow rate: 1.0 ml/min.

Detection: spectrophotometer at 348 nm.

Injection: 10 µl.

System suitability: test solution:
- *resolution*: minimum 1.5 between the peaks due to penduletin and casticin (see Figure 2147.-1).

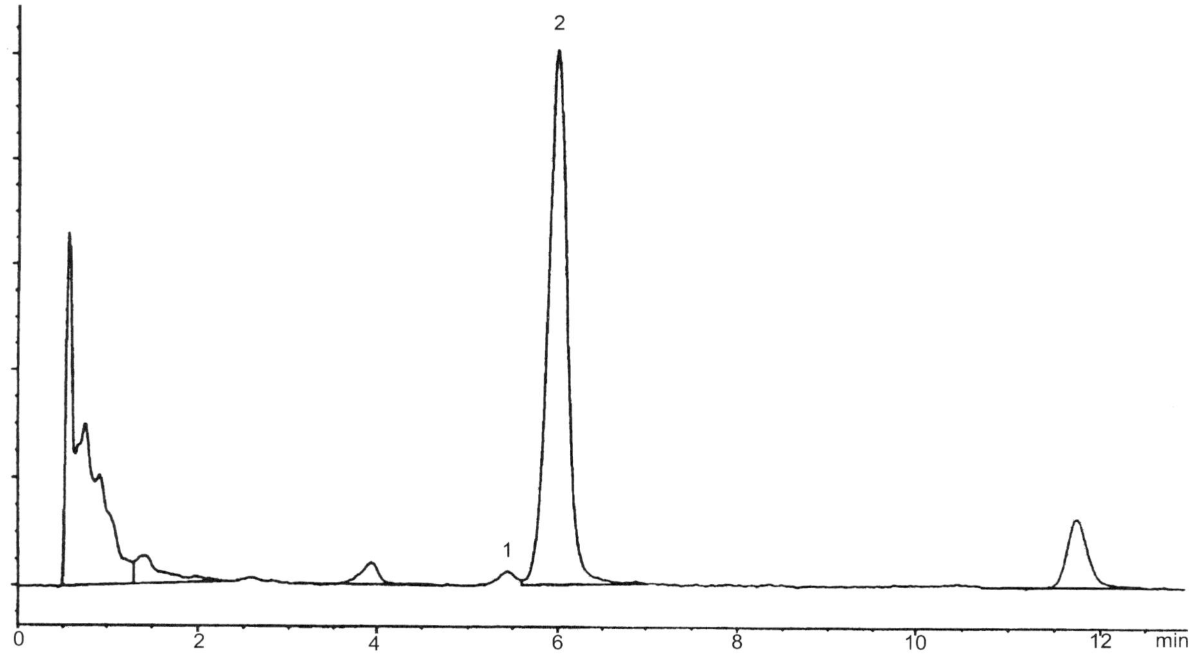

1. penduletin 2. casticin

Figure 2147.-1. – *Chromatogram for the assay of casticin in Agnus castus fruit: test solution*

Monographs A-C

Calculate the percentage content of casticin using the following expression:

$$\frac{F_1 \times m_2 \times p_1 \times 8}{F_2 \times m_1}$$

F_1 = area of the peak due to casticin in the chromatogram obtained with the test solution;

F_2 = area of the peak due to casticin in the chromatogram obtained with the reference solution;

m_1 = mass of the drug used to prepare the test solution, in grams;

m_2 = mass of *agnus castus fruit standardised dry extract CRS* used to prepare the reference solution, in grams;

p_1 = percentage content of casticin in *agnus castus fruit standardised dry extract CRS.*

07/2008:0591

ALGINIC ACID

Acidum alginicum

DEFINITION

Mixture of polyuronic acids [$(C_6H_8O_6)_n$] composed of residues of D-mannuronic and L-guluronic acids, obtained mainly from algae belonging to the Phaeophyceae. A small proportion of the carboxyl groups may be neutralised.

Content: 19.0 per cent to 25.0 per cent of carboxyl groups ($-CO_2H$) (dried substance).

CHARACTERS

Appearance: white or pale yellowish-brown, crystalline or amorphous powder.

Solubility: very slightly soluble or practically insoluble in ethanol (96 per cent), practically insoluble in organic solvents. It swells in water but does not dissolve; it dissolves in solutions of alkali hydroxides.

IDENTIFICATION

A. To 0.2 g add 20 ml of *water R* and 0.5 ml of *sodium carbonate solution R*. Shake and filter. To 5 ml of the filtrate add 1 ml of *calcium chloride solution R*. A voluminous gelatinous mass is formed.

B. To 5 ml of the filtrate obtained in identification test A add 0.5 ml of a 123 g/l solution of *magnesium sulphate R*. No voluminous gelatinous mass is formed.

C. To 5 mg add 5 ml of *water R*, 1 ml of a freshly prepared 10 g/l solution of *1,3-dihydroxynaphthalene R* in *ethanol (96 per cent) R* and 5 ml of *hydrochloric acid R*. Boil gently for 3 min, cool, add 5 ml of *water R*, and shake with 15 ml of *di-isopropyl ether R*. Carry out a blank test. The upper layer obtained with the substance to be examined exhibits a deeper bluish-red colour than that obtained with the blank.

TESTS

Chlorides: maximum 1,0 per cent.

To 2.50 g add 50 ml of *dilute nitric acid R*, shake for 1 h and dilute to 100.0 ml with *dilute nitric acid R*. Filter. To 50.0 ml of the filtrate add 10.0 ml of *0.1 M silver nitrate* and 5 ml of *toluene R*. Titrate with *0.1 M ammonium thiocyanate*, using 2 ml of *ferric ammonium sulphate solution R2* as indicator and shaking vigorously towards the end-point.

1 ml of *0.1 M silver nitrate* is equivalent to 3.545 mg of Cl.

Heavy metals (*2.4.8*): maximum 20 ppm.

1.0 g complies with test F. Prepare the reference solution using 2 ml of *lead standard solution (10 ppm Pb) R*.

Loss on drying (*2.2.32*): maximum 15.0 per cent, determined on 0.1000 g by drying in an oven at 105 °C for 4 h.

Sulphated ash (*2.4.14*): maximum 8.0 per cent (dried substance), determined on 0.100 g.

Microbial contamination. Total viable aerobic count (*2.6.12*) not more than 10^2 micro-organisms per gram, determined by plate-count. It complies with the tests for *Escherichia coli* and *Salmonella* (*2.6.13*).

ASSAY

To 0.2500 g add 25 ml of *water R*, 25.0 ml of *0.1 M sodium hydroxide* and 0.2 ml of *phenolphthalein solution R*. Titrate with *0.1 M hydrochloric acid*.

1 ml of *0.1 M sodium hydroxide* is equivalent to 4.502 mg of carboxyl groups ($-CO_2H$).

FUNCTIONALITY-RELATED CHARACTERISTICS

This section provides information on characteristics that are recognised as being relevant control parameters for one or more functions of the substance when used as an excipient (see chapter 5.15). This section is a non-mandatory part of the monograph and it is not necessary to verify the characteristics to demonstrate compliance. Control of these characteristics can however contribute to the quality of a medicinal product by improving the consistency of the manufacturing process and the performance of the medicinal product during use. Where control methods are cited, they are recognised as being suitable for the purpose, but other methods can also be used. Wherever results for a particular characteristic are reported, the control method must be indicated.

The following characteristics may be relevant for alginic acid used as disintegrant and/or binder.

Particle-size distribution (*2.9.31* or *2.9.38*).

Settling volume. Place 75 ml of *water R* in a 100 ml graduated cylinder and add 1.5 g of the substance to be examined in 0.5 g portions, shaking vigorously after each addition. Dilute to 100.0 ml with *water R* and shake again until the substance is homogeneously distributed. Allow to stand for 4 h and determine the volume of the settled mass.

The following characteristic may be relevant for alginic acid used as gelling agent or viscosity-increasing agent.

Apparent viscosity. Determine the dynamic viscosity using a rotating viscometer (*2.2.10*).

Prepare a 20 g/l suspension of alginic acid (dried substance) and add *0.1 M sodium hydroxide* until a solution is obtained.

01/2008:0259

ALOES DRY EXTRACT, STANDARDISED

Aloes extractum siccum normatum

DEFINITION

Standardised dry extract prepared from Barbados aloes or Cape aloes, or a mixture of both.

Content: 19.0 per cent to 21.0 per cent of hydroxyanthracene derivatives, expressed as barbaloin ($C_{21}H_{22}O_9$; M_r 418.4) adjusted, if necessary (dried extract).

PRODUCTION

The extract is produced from the herbal drug by a suitable procedure using boiling water.

CHARACTERS

Appearance: brown or yellowish-brown powder.

Solubility: sparingly soluble in boiling water.

IDENTIFICATION

A. Thin-layer chromatography (*2.2.27*).

Test solution. To 0.25 g of the extract to be examined add 20 ml of *methanol R* and heat to boiling in a water-bath. Shake for a few minutes and decant the solution. Store at about 4 °C and use within 24 h.

Reference solution. Dissolve 25 mg of *barbaloin R* in *methanol R* and dilute to 10 ml with the same solvent.

Plate: *TLC silica gel G plate R.*

Mobile phase: *water R, methanol R, ethyl acetate R* (13:17:100 *V/V/V*).

Application: 10 µl as bands of 20 mm by not more than 3 mm.

Development: over a path of 10 cm.

Drying: in air.

Detection: spray with a 100 g/l solution of *potassium hydroxide R* in *methanol R* and examine in ultraviolet light at 365 nm.

Results: the chromatogram obtained with the test solution shows, in the central part, a zone of yellow fluorescence (barbaloin) similar in position to the zone due to barbaloin in the chromatogram obtained with the reference solution and in the lower part, a zone of light blue fluorescence (aloesine). In the lower part of the chromatogram obtained with the test solution 2 zones of yellow fluorescence (aloinosides A and B) (Cape aloes) and a zone of violet fluorescence just below the zone due to barbaloin (Barbados aloes) may be present.

B. Shake 1 g with 100 ml of boiling *water R*. Cool, add 1 g of *talc R* and filter. To 10 ml of the filtrate add 0.25 g of *disodium tetraborate R* and heat to dissolve. Pour 2 ml of this solution into 20 ml of *water R*. A yellowish-green fluorescence appears which is particularly marked in ultraviolet light at 365 nm.

TESTS

Loss on drying (*2.8.17*): maximum 4.0 per cent *m/m*.

Total ash (*2.4.16*): maximum 2.0 per cent.

ASSAY

Carry out the assay protected from bright light.

Introduce 0.400 g into a 250 ml conical flask. Moisten with 2 ml of *methanol R*, add 5 ml of *water R* warmed to about 60 °C, mix, add a further 75 ml of *water R* at about 60 °C and shake for 30 min. Cool, filter into a volumetric flask, rinse the conical flask and the filter with 20 ml of *water R*, add the rinsings to the volumetric flask and dilute to 1000.0 ml with *water R*. Transfer 10.0 ml of this solution to a 100 ml round-bottomed flask containing 1 ml of a 600 g/l solution of *ferric chloride R* and 6 ml of *hydrochloric acid R*. Heat in a water-bath under a reflux condenser for 4 h, with the water level above that of the liquid in the flask. Allow to cool, transfer the solution to a separating funnel, rinse the flask successively with 4 ml of *water R*, 4 ml of *1 M sodium hydroxide* and 4 ml of *water R*, and add the rinsings to the separating funnel. Shake the contents of the separating funnel with 3 quantities, each of 20 ml, of *ether R*. Wash the combined ether layers with 2 quantities, each of 10 ml, of *water R*. Discard the washings and dilute the organic layer to 100.0 ml with *ether R*. Evaporate 20.0 ml carefully to dryness on a water-bath and dissolve the residue in 10.0 ml of a 5 g/l solution of *magnesium acetate R* in *methanol R*. Measure the absorbance (*2.2.25*) at 512 nm using *methanol R* as the compensation liquid.

Calculate the percentage content of hydroxyanthracene derivatives, expressed as barbaloin, using the following expression:

$$\frac{A \times 19.6}{m}$$

i.e. taking the specific absorbance of barbaloin to be 255.

A = absorbance at 512 nm;

m = mass of the substance to be examined, in grams.

07/2008:2185

ALTIZIDE

Altizidum

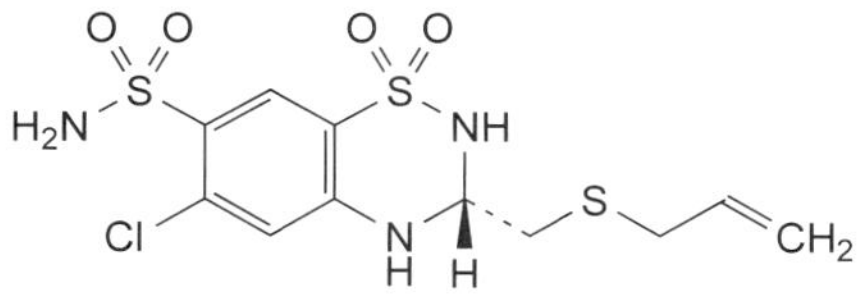

and enantiomer

$C_{11}H_{14}ClN_3O_4S_3$ M_r 383.9

[5588-16-9]

DEFINITION

(3*RS*)-6-Chloro-3-[(prop-2-enylsulphanyl)methyl]-3,4-dihydro-2*H*-1,2,4-benzothiadiazine-7-sulphonamide 1,1-dioxide.

Content: 97.5 per cent to 102.0 per cent (anhydrous substance).

CHARACTERS

Appearance: white or almost white powder.

Solubility: practically insoluble in water, soluble in methanol, practically insoluble in dichloromethane.

It shows polymorphism (*5.9*).

IDENTIFICATION

Infrared absorption spectrophotometry (*2.2.24*).

Comparison: *altizide CRS.*

If the spectra obtained show differences, dissolve 50 mg of the substance to be examined and 50 mg of the reference substance separately in 2 ml of *acetone R* and evaporate the solvent. Precipitate by adding 1 ml of *methylene chloride R*. Evaporate to dryness and record new spectra using the residues.

TESTS

Impurity B. Thin-layer chromatography (*2.2.27*).

Test solution. Dissolve 0.200 g of the substance to be examined in *acetone R* and dilute to 2.0 ml with the same solvent.

Reference solution (a). Dissolve 10.0 mg of *altizide impurity B CRS* in *acetone R* and dilute to 25.0 ml with the same solvent.

Reference solution (b). To 1.0 ml of reference solution (a) add 1.0 ml of the test solution.

Reference solution (c). Dilute 5.0 ml of reference solution (a) to 10.0 ml with *acetone R*.

Plate: *TLC silica gel F_{254} plate R.*

Monographs A-C

Mobile phase: *acetone R, methylene chloride R* (25:75 *V/V*).

Application: 10 µl of the test solution and reference solutions (b) and (c).

Development: over 2/3 of the plate.

Drying: in air.

Detection: spray with a mixture of equal volumes of a 10 g/l solution of *potassium permanganate R* and a 50 g/l solution of *sodium carbonate R*, prepared immediately before use. Allow to stand for 30 min and examine in daylight.

System suitability: reference solution (b):

– the chromatogram shows 2 clearly separated spots.

Limit: any spot due to impurity B is not more intense than the principal spot in the chromatogram obtained with reference solution (c) (0.2 per cent).

Related substances. Liquid chromatography (*2.2.29*). *Prepare the solutions immediately before use, except reference solution (b).*

Test solution. Dissolve 50 mg of the substance to be examined in 5 ml of *acetonitrile R* and dilute to 25 ml with the mobile phase.

Reference solution (a). Dilute 1.0 ml of the test solution to 100.0 ml with the mobile phase. Dilute 1.0 ml of this solution to 10.0 ml with the mobile phase.

Reference solution (b). In order to produce impurity A *in situ*, dissolve 50 mg of the substance to be examined in 5 ml of *acetonitrile R* and dilute to 25 ml with *water R*. Allow to stand for 30 min.

Reference solution (c). Dissolve 4 mg of *furosemide CRS* in 2 ml of *acetonitrile R*, add 2 ml of the test solution and dilute to 100 ml with the mobile phase.

Column:

– *size*: l = 0.15 m, Ø = 3.9 mm;
– *stationary phase*: *end-capped octadecylsilyl silica gel for chromatography R* (5 µm);
– *temperature*: 30 °C.

Mobile phase: *acetonitrile R, water R* previously adjusted to pH 2.0 with *perchloric acid R* (25:75 *V/V*).

Flow rate: 0.7 ml/min.

Detection: spectrophotometer at 270 nm.

Injection: 5 µl.

Run time: twice the retention time of altizide.

Relative retention with reference to altizide (retention time = about 25 min): impurity A = about 0.15; furosemide = about 1.05.

System suitability: reference solution (c):

– *resolution*: minimum 1.0 between the peaks due to altizide and furosemide.

Limits:

– *impurity A*: not more than 3 times the area of the principal peak in the chromatogram obtained with reference solution (a) (0.3 per cent);
– *unspecified impurities*: for each impurity, not more than the area of the principal peak in the chromatogram obtained with reference solution (a) (0.10 per cent);
– *total*: not more than 5 times the area of the principal peak in the chromatogram obtained with reference solution (a) (0.5 per cent);
– *disregard limit*: 0.5 times the area of the principal peak in the chromatogram obtained with reference solution (a) (0.05 per cent).

Water (*2.5.32*): maximum 0.5 per cent, determined on 50.0 mg.

Sulphated ash (*2.4.14*): maximum 0.1 per cent, determined on 1.0 g.

ASSAY

Liquid chromatography (*2.2.29*) as described in the test for related substances, with the following modifications.

Test solution. Dissolve 25.0 mg of the substance to be examined in 2 ml of *acetonitrile R* and dilute to 25.0 ml with the mobile phase.

Reference solution. Dissolve 25.0 mg of *altizide CRS* in 2 ml of *acetonitrile R* and dilute to 25.0 ml with the mobile phase.

Calculate the percentage content of $C_{11}H_{14}ClN_3O_4S_3$ from the declared content of *altizide CRS*.

IMPURITIES

Specified impurities: *A, B*.

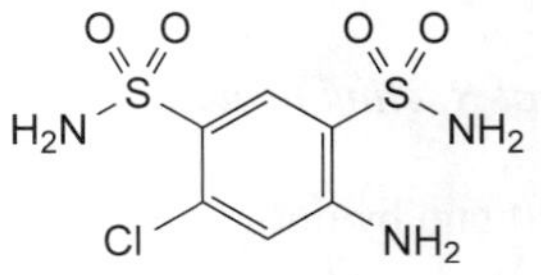

A. 4-amino-6-chlorobenzene-1,3-disulphonamide,

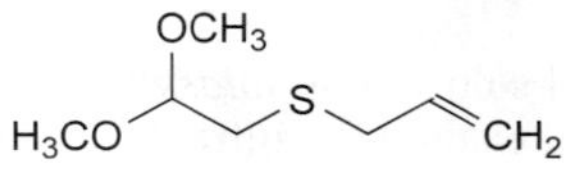

B. 3-[(2,2-dimethoxyethyl)sulphanyl]prop-1-ene.

01/2008:0579
corrected 6.2

APROTININ CONCENTRATED SOLUTION

Aprotinini solutio concentrata

DEFINITION

Aprotinin concentrated solution is a solution of aprotinin, a polypeptide consisting of a chain of 58 amino acids, which inhibits stoichiometrically the activity of several proteolytic enzymes such as chymotrypsin, kallikrein, plasmin and trypsin. It contains not less than 15.0 Ph. Eur. U. of aprotinin activity per millilitre.

PRODUCTION

The animals from which aprotinin is derived must fulfil the requirements for the health of animals suitable for human consumption to the satisfaction of the competent authority.

The manufacturing process is validated to demonstrate suitable inactivation or removal of any contamination by viruses or other infectious agents.

The method of manufacture is validated to demonstrate that the product, if tested, would comply with the following tests.

Abnormal toxicity (*2.6.9*). Inject into each mouse a quantity of the preparation to be examined containing 2 Ph. Eur. U. diluted with a sufficient quantity of *water for injections R* to give a volume of 0.5 ml.

Histamine (*2.6.10*): maximum 0.2 µg of histamine base per 3 Ph. Eur. U.

CHARACTERS

Appearance: clear, colourless liquid.

IDENTIFICATION

A. Thin-layer chromatography (*2.2.27*).

Test solution. Solution S (see Tests).

Reference solution. Aprotinin solution BRP.

Plate: *TLC silica gel G plate R.*

Mobile phase: *water R, glacial acetic acid R* (80:100 *V/V*) containing 100 g/l of *sodium acetate R*).

Application: 10 μl.

Development: over a path of 12 cm.

Drying: in air.

Detection: spray with a solution of 0.1 g of *ninhydrin R* in a mixture of 6 ml of a 10 g/l solution of *cupric chloride R*, 21 ml of *glacial acetic acid R* and 70 ml of *anhydrous ethanol R*. Dry the plate at 60 °C.

Results: the principal spot in the chromatogram obtained with the test solution is similar in position, colour and size to the principal spot in the chromatogram obtained with the reference solution.

B. Determine the ability of the preparation to be examined to inhibit trypsin activity using the method described below.

Test solution. Dilute 1 ml of solution S to 50 ml with *buffer solution pH 7.2 R.*

Trypsin solution. Dissolve 10 mg of *trypsin BRP* in *0.002 M hydrochloric acid* and dilute to 100 ml with the same acid.

Casein solution. Dissolve 0.2 g of *casein R* in *buffer solution pH 7.2 R* and dilute to 100 ml with the same buffer solution.

Precipitating solution. Mix 1 volume of *glacial acetic acid R*, 49 volumes of *water R* and 50 volumes of *anhydrous ethanol R.*

Mix 1 ml of the test solution with 1 ml of the trypsin solution. Allow to stand for 10 min and add 1 ml of the casein solution. Incubate at 35 °C for 30 min. Cool in iced water and add 0.5 ml of the precipitating solution. Shake and allow to stand at room temperature for 15 min. The solution is cloudy. Carry out a blank test under the same conditions using *buffer solution pH 7.2 R* instead of the test solution. The solution is not cloudy.

TESTS

Solution S. Prepare a solution containing 15 Ph. Eur. U./ml, if necessary by dilution on the basis of the activity stated on the label.

Appearance of solution. Solution S is clear (*2.2.1*).

Absorbance (*2.2.25*): maximum 0.80 by measuring at the absorption maximum at 277 nm.

Prepare from the concentrated solution a dilution containing 3.0 Ph. Eur. U./ml.

Protein impurities of higher molecular mass. Size-exclusion chromatography (*2.2.30*).

Freeze-dry the preparation to be examined using a pressure of 2.7 Pa and a temperature of − 30 °C; the operation, including freeze-drying and a period of drying at 15-25 °C, takes 6-12 h.

Use *cross-linked dextran for chromatography R2*. Use a 180 g/l solution of *anhydrous acetic acid R* to swell the gel and as the eluent. Prepare a column of gel 0.8 m to 1.0 m long and 25 mm in diameter, taking care to avoid the introduction of air bubbles. Place at the top of the column a quantity of the preparation to be examined containing 300 Ph. Eur. U. dissolved in 1 ml of a 180 g/l solution of *anhydrous acetic acid R* and allow to elute. Collect the eluate in fractions of 2 ml. Measure the absorbance (*2.2.25*) of each fraction at the absorption maximum at 277 nm and plot the values on a graph. The chromatogram obtained does not present an absorption maximum before the elution of the aprotinin.

Specific activity of the dry residue: minimum 3.0 Ph. Eur. U. of aprotinin activity per milligram of dry residue.

Evaporate 25.0 ml to dryness in a water-bath, dry the residue at 110 °C for 15 h and weigh. From the mass of the residue and the activity determined as described below, calculate the number of European Pharmacopoeia Units per milligram of dry residue.

Bacterial endotoxins (*2.6.14*): less than 0.14 IU per European Pharmacopoeia Unit of aprotinin, if intended for use in the manufacture of parenteral preparations without a further appropriate procedure for the removal of bacterial endotoxins.

ASSAY

The activity of aprotinin is determined by measuring its inhibitory action on a solution of trypsin of known activity. The inhibiting activity of the aprotinin is calculated from the difference between the initial activity and the residual activity of the trypsin.

The inhibiting activity of aprotinin is expressed in European Pharmacopoeia Units. 1 Ph. Eur. U. inhibits 50 per cent of the enzymatic activity of 2 microkatals of trypsin.

Use a reaction vessel with a capacity of about 30 ml and provided with:

– a device that will maintain a temperature of 25 ± 0.1 °C;
– a stirring device, such as a magnetic stirrer;
– a lid with 5 holes for accommodating the electrodes, the tip of a burette, a tube for the admission of nitrogen and the introduction of the reagents.

An automatic or manual titration apparatus may be used. In the latter case the burette is graduated in 0.05 ml and the pH-meter is provided with a wide reading scale and glass and calomel electrodes.

Test solution. With *0.0015 M borate buffer solution pH 8.0 R* prepare an appropriate dilution (*D*) of the concentrated solution expected on the basis of the stated potency to contain 1.67 Ph. Eur. U./ml.

Trypsin solution. Prepare a solution of *trypsin BRP* containing about 0.8 microkatals per millilitre (about 1 mg/ml), using *0.001 M hydrochloric acid* as the solvent. Use a freshly prepared solution and keep in iced water.

Trypsin and aprotinin solution. To 4.0 ml of the trypsin solution add 1.0 ml of the test solution. Dilute immediately to 40.0 ml with *0.0015 M borate buffer solution pH 8.0 R.* Allow to stand at room temperature for 10 min and then keep in iced water. Use within 6 h of preparation.

Dilute trypsin solution. Dilute 0.5 ml of the trypsin solution to 10.0 ml with *0.0015 M borate buffer solution pH 8.0 R.* Allow to stand at room temperature for 10 min and then keep in iced water.

Maintain an atmosphere of nitrogen in the reaction flask and stir continuously; introduce 9.0 ml of *0.0015 M borate buffer solution pH 8.0 R* and 1.0 ml of a freshly prepared 6.9 g/l solution of *benzoylarginine ethyl ester hydrochloride R.* Adjust to pH 8.0 with *0.1 M sodium hydroxide.* When the temperature has reached equilibrium at 25 ± 0.1 °C, add 1.0 ml of the trypsin and aprotinin solution and start a timer. Maintain at pH 8.0 by the addition of *0.1 M sodium hydroxide* and note the volume added every 30 s. Continue the reaction for 6 min. Determine the number of millilitres of *0.1 M sodium hydroxide* used per second (n_1 ml). Carry out, under the same conditions, a titration using 1.0 ml of the dilute trypsin solution. Determine the number of millilitres of *0.1 M sodium hydroxide* used per second (n_2 ml).

Calculate the aprotinin activity in European Pharmacopoeia Units per millilitre using the following expression:

$$4000\,(2n_2 - n_1) \times D$$

D = dilution factor of the aprotinin concentrated solution to be examined in order to obtain a solution containing 1.67 Ph. Eur. U./ml.

The estimated activity is not less than 90 per cent and not more than 110 per cent of the activity stated on the label.

STORAGE

In an airtight, tamper-proof container, protected from light.

LABELLING

The label states the number of European Pharmacopoeia Units of aprotinin activity per millilitre.

01/2008:1171
corrected 6.2

ARACHIS OIL, HYDROGENATED

Arachidis oleum hydrogenatum

DEFINITION

Oil obtained by refining, bleaching, hydrogenating and deodorising oil obtained from the shelled seeds of *Arachis hypogaea* L. Each type of hydrogenated arachis oil is characterised by its nominal drop point.

CHARACTERS

Appearance: white or faintly yellowish, soft mass which melts to a clear, pale yellow liquid when heated.

Solubility: practically insoluble in water, freely soluble in methylene chloride and in light petroleum (bp: 65-70 °C), very slightly soluble in ethanol (96 per cent).

IDENTIFICATION

First identification: A, B.

Second identification: A, C.

A. Drop point (see Tests).

B. Identification of fatty oils by thin-layer chromatography (*2.3.2*).

   Results: the chromatogram obtained is similar to the typical chromatogram for arachis oil.

C. Composition of fatty acids (see Tests).

TESTS

Drop point (*2.2.17*): 32 °C to 43 °C, and within 3 °C of the nominal value.

Acid value (*2.5.1*): maximum 0.5.

Dissolve 10.0 g in 50 ml of the prescribed solvent by heating on a water-bath.

Peroxide value (*2.5.5, Method A*): maximum 5.0.

Dissolve 5.0 g in 30 ml of the prescribed solvent by heating on a water-bath.

Unsaponifiable matter (*2.5.7*): maximum 1.0 per cent.

Alkaline impurities in fatty oils (*2.4.19*). It complies with the test.

Composition of fatty acids (*2.4.22, Method A*). Use the mixture of calibrating substances in Table 2.4.22.-3.

Column:

- *material*: fused silica;
- *size*: *l* = 25 m, Ø = 0.25 mm;
- *stationary phase*: *poly(cyanopropyl)siloxane R* (film thickness 0.2 μm).

Carrier gas: *helium for chromatography R.*

Flow rate: 0.7 ml/min.

Split ratio: 1:100.

Temperature:

- *column*: 180 °C for 20 min;
- *injection port and detector*: 250 °C.

Detection: flame ionisation.

Composition of the fatty-acid fraction of the oil:

- *saturated fatty acids of chain length less than C_{14}*: maximum 0.5 per cent;
- *myristic acid*: maximum 0.5 per cent;
- *palmitic acid*: 7.0 per cent to 16.0 per cent;
- *stearic acid*: 3.0 per cent to 19.0 per cent;
- *oleic acid and isomers*: 54.0 per cent to 78.0 per cent;
- *linoleic acid and isomers*: maximum 10.0 per cent;
- *arachidic acid*: 1.0 per cent to 3.0 per cent;
- *eicosenoic acids*: maximum 2.1 per cent;
- *behenic acid*: 1.0 per cent to 5.0 per cent;
- *erucic acid and isomers*: maximum 0.5 per cent;
- *lignoceric acid*: 0.5 per cent to 3.0 per cent.

Nickel: maximum 1.0 ppm.

Atomic absorption spectrometry (*2.2.23, Method II*).

Test solution. Into a platinum or silica crucible previously tared after ignition introduce 5.0 g. Cautiously heat and introduce into the substance a wick formed from twisted ashless filter paper. Ignite the wick. When the substance has ignited stop heating. After combustion, ignite in a muffle furnace at about 600 ± 50 °C. Continue ignition until white ash is obtained. After cooling, take up the residue with 2 quantities, each of 2 ml, of *dilute hydrochloric acid R* and transfer into a 25 ml graduated flask. Add 0.3 ml of *nitric acid R* and dilute to 25.0 ml with *water R.*

Reference solutions. Prepare 3 reference solutions by adding 1.0 ml, 2.0 ml and 4.0 ml of *nickel standard solution (0.2 ppm Ni) R* to 2.0 ml of the test solution and diluting to 10.0 ml with *water R.*

Source: nickel hollow-cathode lamp.

Wavelength: 232 nm.

Atomisation device: graphite furnace.

Carrier gas: *argon R.*

Water (*2.5.12*): maximum 0.3 per cent, determined on 1.000 g.

STORAGE

Protected from light.

LABELLING

The label states the nominal drop point.

B

Monographs
A-C

01/2008:1294

BELLADONNA LEAF DRY EXTRACT, STANDARDISED

Belladonnae folii extractum siccum normatum

DEFINITION

Standardised dry extract obtained from *Belladonna leaf (0221)*.

Content: 0.95 per cent to 1.05 per cent of total alkaloids, expressed as hyoscyamine ($C_{17}H_{23}NO_3$; M_r 289.4) (dried extract).

PRODUCTION

The extract is produced from the herbal drug by a suitable procedure using ethanol (70 per cent *V/V*).

CHARACTERS

Appearance: brown or greenish, hygroscopic powder.

IDENTIFICATION

A. Thin-layer chromatography (*2.2.27*).

Test solution. To 1 g of the extract to be examined add 5.0 ml of *methanol R*. Shake for 2 min and filter.

Reference solution. Dissolve 1.0 mg of *chlorogenic acid R* and 2.5 mg of *rutin R* in 10 ml of *methanol R*.

Plate: *TLC silica gel plate R*.

Mobile phase: *anhydrous formic acid R, water R, methyl ethyl ketone R, ethyl acetate R* (10:10:30:50 *V/V/V/V*).

Application: 20 µl as bands.

Development: over a path of 15 cm.

Drying: at 100-105 °C.

Detection: spray the warm plate with a 10 g/l solution of *diphenylboric acid aminoethyl ester R* in *methanol R*, then spray with a 50 g/l solution of *macrogol 400 R* in *methanol R*; allow to dry in air for 30 min and examine in ultraviolet light at 365 nm.

Results: the chromatograms obtained with the reference solution and the test solution show in the central part a light blue fluorescent zone (chlorogenic acid) and in the lower part a yellowish-brown fluorescent zone (rutin); furthermore, the chromatogram obtained with the test solution shows a little above the start a yellowish-brown fluorescent zone and directly above that a yellow fluorescent zone, and a yellow or yellowish-brown fluorescent zone between the zone due to rutin and the zone due to chlorogenic acid. Further zones may be present.

B. Examine the chromatograms obtained in the test for atropine.

Results: the principal zones in the chromatogram obtained with the test solution are similar in position and colour to the principal zones in the chromatogram obtained with the reference solution.

TESTS

Atropine. Thin-layer chromatography (*2.2.27*).

Test solution. To 0.20 g of the extract to be examined add 10.0 ml of *0.05 M sulphuric acid*, shake for 2 min and filter. Add 1.0 ml of *concentrated ammonia R* and shake with 2 quantities, each of 10 ml, of *peroxide-free ether R*. If necessary, separate by centrifugation. Dry the combined ether layers over about 2 g of *anhydrous sodium sulphate R*, filter and evaporate to dryness on a water-bath. Dissolve the residue in 0.5 ml of *methanol R*.

Reference solution. Dissolve 50 mg of *hyoscyamine sulphate R* in 9 ml of *methanol R*. Dissolve 15 mg of *hyoscine hydrobromide R* in 10 ml of *methanol R*. Mix 1.8 ml of the hyoscine hydrobromide solution and 8 ml of the hyoscyamine sulphate solution.

Plate: *TLC silica gel plate R*.

Mobile phase: *concentrated ammonia R, water R, acetone R* (3:7:90 *V/V/V*).

Application: 20 µl as bands.

Development: over a path of 10 cm.

Drying: at 100-105 °C for 15 min; allow to cool.

Detection A: spray with *potassium iodobismuthate solution R2*, until orange or brown zones become visible against a yellow background.

Results A: the zones in the chromatogram obtained with the test solution are similar in position (hyoscyamine in the lower third, hyoscine in the upper third) and colour to those in the chromatogram obtained with the reference solution. Other faint zones may be present in the chromatogram obtained with the test solution.

Detection B: spray with *sodium nitrite solution R* until the coating is transparent and examine after 15 min.

Results B: the zones due to hyoscyamine in the chromatograms obtained with the test solution and the reference solution change from orange or brown to reddish-brown but not to greyish-blue (atropine).

Loss on drying (*2.8.17*): maximum 5.0 per cent.

Microbial contamination. Total viable aerobic count (*2.6.12*) not more than 10^4 micro-organisms per gram of which not more than 10^2 fungi per gram, determined by plate count. It complies with the tests for *Escherichia coli* and for *Salmonella* (*2.6.13*).

ASSAY

At each extraction stage it is necessary to check that the alkaloids have been completely extracted. If the extraction is into the organic phase this is done by evaporating to dryness a few millilitres of the last organic layer, dissolving the residue in *0.25 M sulphuric acid* and verifying the absence of alkaloids using *potassium tetraiodomercurate solution R*. If the extraction is into the acid aqueous phase, this is done by taking a few millilitres of the last acid aqueous phase and verifying the absence of alkaloids using *potassium tetraiodomercurate solution R*.

Disperse 3.00 g in a mixture of 5 ml of *ammonia R* and 15 ml of *water R*. Shake with no fewer than 3 quantities, each of 40 ml, of a mixture of 1 volume of *methylene chloride R* and 3 volumes of *peroxide-free ether R* until the alkaloids are completely extracted. Concentrate the combined organic layers to about 50 ml by distilling on a water-bath and transfer the resulting liquid to a separating funnel, rinsing with *peroxide-free ether R*. Add a quantity of *peroxide-free ether R* equal to at least 2.1 times the volume of the liquid to produce a layer having a density well below that of water. Shake the resulting solution with no fewer than 3 quantities, each of 20 ml, of *0.25 M sulphuric acid* until the alkaloids are completely extracted. Separate the layers by centrifugation, if necessary, and transfer the acid layers to a 2nd separating funnel. Make the combined acid layers alkaline with *ammonia R* and shake with no fewer than 3 quantities, each of 30 ml, of *methylene chloride R* until the alkaloids are completely extracted. Combine the organic layers, add 4 g of *anhydrous sodium sulphate R* and allow to stand for 30 min with occasional shaking. Decant

Monographs A-C

the methylene chloride and wash the sodium sulphate with 3 quantities, each of 10 ml, of *methylene chloride R*. Combine the organic extracts and evaporate to dryness on a water-bath. Heat the residue in an oven at 100-105 °C for 15 min. Dissolve the residue in a few millilitres of *methylene chloride R*, evaporate to dryness on a water-bath and again heat the residue in an oven at 100-105 °C for 15 min. Dissolve the residue in a few millilitres of *methylene chloride R*, add 20.0 ml of *0.01 M sulphuric acid* and remove the methylene chloride by evaporation on a water-bath. Titrate the excess of acid with *0.02 M sodium hydroxide* using *methyl red mixed solution R* as indicator.

Calculate the percentage content of total alkaloids, expressed as hyoscyamine, using the following expression:

$$\frac{57.88 \times (20 - n)}{100 \times m}$$

n = volume of *0.02 M sodium hydroxide* used, in millilitres;

m = mass of drug used, in grams.

01/2008:0222

BELLADONNA, PREPARED

Belladonnae pulvis normatus

DEFINITION

Belladonna leaf powder (180) (*2.9.12*) adjusted, if necessary, by adding powdered lactose or belladonna leaf powder with a lower alkaloidal content.

Content: 0.28 per cent to 0.32 per cent of total alkaloids, expressed as hyoscyamine (M_r 289.4) (dried drug).

CHARACTERS

Slightly nauseous odour.

IDENTIFICATION

A. The powder is dark green. Examine under a microscope, using *chloral hydrate solution R*. The powder shows the following diagnostic characters: fragments of leaf lamina showing sinuous-walled epidermal cells, a striated cuticle and numerous stomata predominantly present on the lower epidermis (anisocytic and also some anomocytic) (*2.8.3*); multicellular uniseriate covering trichomes with smooth cuticle, glandular trichomes with unicellular heads and multicellular, uniseriate stalks or with multicellular heads and unicellular stalks; parenchyma cells including rounded cells containing microsphenoidal crystals of calcium oxalate; annular and spirally thickened vessels. The powdered drug may also show the following: fibres and reticulately thickened vessels from the stems; subspherical pollen grains, 40-50 µm in diameter, with 3 germinal pores, 3 furrows and an extensively pitted exine; fragments of the corolla, with a papillose epidermis or bearing numerous covering or glandular trichomes of the types previously described; brownish-yellow seed fragments containing irregularly sclerified and pitted cells of the testa. Examined in *glycerol (85 per cent) R*, the powder may be seen to contain lactose crystals.

B. Shake 1 g with 10 ml of *0.05 M sulphuric acid* for 2 min. Filter and add to the filtrate 1 ml of *concentrated ammonia R* and 5 ml of *water R*. Shake cautiously with 15 ml of *ether R*, avoiding formation of an emulsion. Separate the ether layer and dry over *anhydrous sodium sulphate R*. Filter and evaporate the ether in a porcelain dish. Add 0.5 ml of *fuming nitric acid R* and evaporate to dryness on a water-bath. Add 10 ml of *acetone R* and, dropwise, a 30 g/l solution of *potassium hydroxide R* in *ethanol (96 per cent) R*. A deep violet colour develops.

C. Examine the chromatograms obtained in the test Chromatography.

Results: the principal zones in the chromatograms obtained with the test solution are similar in position, colour and size to the principal zones in the chromatogram obtained with the same volume of the reference solution.

TESTS

Chromatography. Thin-layer chromatography (*2.2.27*).

Test solution. To 0.6 g of the drug to be examined add 15 ml of *0.05 M sulphuric acid*, shake for 15 min and filter. Wash the filter with *0.05 M sulphuric acid* until 20 ml of filtrate is obtained. To the filtrate add 1 ml of *concentrated ammonia R* and shake with 2 quantities, each of 10 ml, of *peroxide-free ether R*. If necessary, separate by centrifugation. Dry the combined ether layers over *anhydrous sodium sulphate R*, filter, and evaporate to dryness on a water-bath. Dissolve the residue in 0.5 ml of *methanol R*.

Reference solution. Dissolve 50 mg of *hyoscyamine sulphate R* in 9 ml of *methanol R*. Dissolve 15 mg of *hyoscine hydrobromide R* in 10 ml of *methanol R*. Mix 1.8 ml of the hyoscine hydrobromide solution and 8 ml of the hyoscyamine sulphate solution.

Plate: *TLC silica gel G plate R*.

Mobile phase: *concentrated ammonia R, water R, acetone R* (3:7:90 *V/V/V*).

Application: 10 µl and 20 µl of each solution, as bands of 20 mm by 3 mm, leaving 1 cm between each band.

Development: over a path of 10 cm.

Drying: at 100-105 °C for 15 min; allow to cool.

Detection A: spray with *potassium iodobismuthate solution R2*, using about 10 ml for a plate 200 mm square, until orange or brown zones become visible against a yellow background.

Results A: the zones in the chromatograms obtained with the test solution are similar in position (hyoscyamine in the lower third, hyoscine in the upper third) and colour to those in the chromatograms obtained with the reference solution; the zones in the chromatograms obtained with the test solution are at least equal in size to the corresponding zones in the chromatogram obtained with the same volume of the reference solution; faint secondary zones may appear, particularly in the middle of the chromatogram obtained with 20 µl of the test solution or near the starting-point in the chromatogram obtained with 10 µl of the test solution.

Detection B: spray with *sodium nitrite solution R* until the coating is transparent and examine after 15 min.

Results B: the zones due to hyoscyamine in the chromatograms obtained with the test solution and the reference solution change from brown to reddish-brown but not to greyish-blue (atropine), and any secondary zones disappear.

Loss on drying (*2.2.32*): maximum 5.0 per cent, determined on 1.000 g by drying in an oven at 105 °C.

Total ash (*2.4.16*): maximum 16.0 per cent.

Ash insoluble in hydrochloric acid (*2.8.1*): maximum 4.0 per cent.

Monographs A-C

ASSAY

a) Determine the loss on drying (*2.2.32*) on 2.000 g by drying in an oven at 105 °C.

b) Moisten 10.00 g with a mixture of 5 ml of *ammonia R*, 10 ml of *ethanol (96 per cent) R* and 30 ml of *peroxide-free ether R* and mix thoroughly. Transfer the mixture to a suitable percolator, if necessary with the aid of the extracting mixture. Allow to macerate for 4 h and percolate with a mixture of 1 volume of *chloroform R* and 3 volumes of *peroxide-free ether R* until the alkaloids are completely extracted. Evaporate to dryness a few millilitres of the liquid flowing from the percolator, dissolve the residue in *0.25 M sulphuric acid* and verify the absence of alkaloids using *potassium tetraiodomercurate solution R*. Concentrate the percolate to about 50 ml by distilling on a water-bath and transfer it to a separating funnel, rinsing with *peroxide-free ether R*. Add a quantity of *peroxide-free ether R* equal to at least 2.1 times the volume of the percolate to produce a liquid of a density well below that of water. Shake the solution with no fewer than 3 quantities, each of 20 ml, of *0.25 M sulphuric acid*, separate the 2 layers by centrifugation if necessary and transfer the acid layers to a 2nd separating funnel. Make the acid layer alkaline with *ammonia R* and shake with 3 quantities, each of 30 ml, of *chloroform R*. Combine the chloroform layers, add 4 g of *anhydrous sodium sulphate R* and allow to stand for 30 min with occasional shaking. Decant the chloroform and wash the sodium sulphate with 3 quantities, each of 10 ml, of *chloroform R*. Add the washings to the chloroform extract, evaporate to dryness on a water-bath and heat in an oven at 100-105 °C for 15 min. Dissolve the residue in a few millilitres of *chloroform R*, add 20.0 ml of *0.01 M sulphuric acid* and remove the chloroform by evaporation on a water-bath. Titrate the excess of acid with *0.02 M sodium hydroxide* using *methyl red mixed solution R* as indicator.

Calculate the percentage content of total alkaloids, expressed as hyoscyamine, using the following expression:

$$\frac{57.88 \times (20 - n)}{(100 - d) \times m}$$

d = loss on drying as a percentage;

n = volume of *0.02 M sodium hydroxide* used, in millilitres;

m = mass of drug used, in grams.

STORAGE

In an airtight container.

07/2008:1174

BIRCH LEAF

Betulae folium

DEFINITION

Whole or fragmented dried leaves of *Betula pendula* Roth and/or *Betula pubescens* Ehrh. as well as hybrids of both species.

Content: minimum 1.5 per cent of flavonoids, expressed as hyperoside ($C_{21}H_{20}O_{12}$; M_r 464.4) (dried drug).

IDENTIFICATION

A. The leaves of both species are dark green on the adaxial surface and lighter greenish-grey on the abaxial surface; they show a characteristic dense reticulate venation. The veins are light brown or almost white.

The leaves of *Betula pendula* are glabrous and show closely spaced glandular pits on both surfaces. The leaves of *Betula pendula* are 3-7 cm long and 2-5 cm wide; the petiole is long and the doubly dentate lamina is triangular or rhomboid and broadly cuneate or truncate at the base. The angle on each side is unrounded or slightly rounded, and the apex is long and acuminate.

The leaves of *Betula pubescens* show few glandular trichomes and are slightly pubescent on both surfaces. The abaxial surface shows small bundles of yellowish-grey trichomes at the branch points of the veins. The leaves of *Betula pubescens* are slightly smaller, oval or rhomboid and more rounded. They are more roughly and more regularly dentate. The apex is neither long nor acuminate.

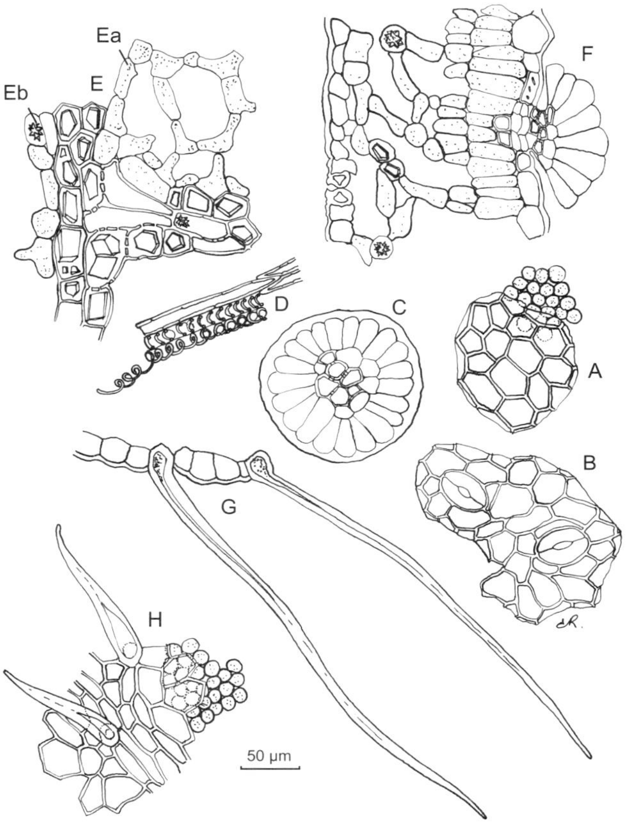

A. Upper epidermis of the lamina accompanied by palisade parenchyma	E. Crystal sheaths containing prisms of calcium oxalate, spongy parenchyma (Ea) and cells containing cluster crystals of calcium oxalate (Eb)
B. Lower epidermis of the lamina with anomocytic stomata	F. Transverse section of the lamina, showing a peltate gland in side view
C. Peltate gland, in surface view	G. Covering trichomes on the margin of the lamina (*B. pubescens*)
D. Xylem vessels accompanied by sclerenchyma fibres	H. Covering trichomes on the upper epidermis of the lamina (*B. pubescens*)

Figure 1174.-1. – *Illustration of powdered herbal drug of birch leaf (see Identification B)*

B. Reduce to a powder (355) (*2.9.12*). The powder is greenish-grey. Examine under a microscope using *chloral hydrate solution R*. The powder shows the following diagnostic characters: numerous fragments of lamina with straight-walled epidermal cells and cells of the lower epidermis surrounding anomocytic stomata (*2.8.3*). Peltate large glands usually measuring 100-120 µm are found on the upper and lower epidermises. The mesophyll

Monographs A-C

fragments contain calcium oxalate crystals. Fragments of radial vascular bundles and sclerenchyma fibres are accompanied by crystal sheaths. If *Betula pubescens* is present, the powder also contains unicellular covering trichomes with very thick walls, about 80-600 µm long, usually 100-200 µm.

C. Thin-layer chromatography (*2.2.27*).

Test solution. To 1 g of the powdered drug (355) (*2.9.12*) add 10 ml of *methanol R*. Heat in a water-bath at 60 °C for 5 min. Cool and filter the solution.

Reference solution. Dissolve 1 mg of *caffeic acid R* and 1 mg of *chlorogenic acid R*, 2.5 mg of *hyperoside R* and 2.5 mg of *rutin R* in 10 ml of *methanol R*.

Plate: *TLC silica gel plate R*.

Mobile phase: *anhydrous formic acid R, water R, methyl ethyl ketone R, ethyl acetate R* (10:10:30:50 *V/V/V/V*).

Application: 10 µl, as bands.

Development: over a path of 10 cm.

Drying: in a current of warm air.

Detection: spray with a 10 g/l solution of *diphenylboric acid aminoethyl ester R* in *methanol R*; subsequently spray with a 50 g/l solution of *macrogol 400 R* in *methanol R*; allow to dry in air for 30 min and examine in ultraviolet light at 365 nm.

Results: the chromatogram obtained with the reference solution shows 3 zones in its lower half: in increasing order of R_F a yellowish-brown fluorescent zone (rutin), a light blue fluorescent zone (chlorogenic acid) and a yellowish-brown fluorescent zone (hyperoside), and in its upper third, a light blue fluorescent zone (caffeic acid). The chromatogram obtained with the test solution shows 3 zones similar in position and fluorescence to the zones due to rutin, chlorogenic acid and hyperoside in the chromatogram obtained with the reference solution. The zone due to rutin is very faint and the zone due to hyperoside is intense. It also shows other yellowish-brown faint fluorescence zones between the zones due to caffeic acid and chlorogenic acid in the chromatogram obtained with the reference solution. Near the solvent front, the red fluorescent zone due to chlorophylls is visible. In the chromatogram obtained with the test solution, between this zone and the zone due to caffeic acid in the chromatogram obtained with the reference solution, there is a brownish-yellow zone due to quercetin.

TESTS

Foreign matter (*2.8.2*): maximum 3 per cent of fragments of female catkins and maximum 3 per cent of other foreign matter.

Loss on drying (*2.2.32*): maximum 10.0 per cent, determined on 1.000 g of powered drug (355) by drying in an oven at 105 °C for 2 h.

Total ash (*2.4.16*): maximum 5.0 per cent.

ASSAY

Stock solution. In a 100 ml round-bottomed flask introduce 0.200 g of the powdered drug (355) (*2.9.12*), 1 ml of a 5 g/l solution of *hexamethylenetetramine R*, 20 ml of *acetone R* and 2 ml of *hydrochloric acid R1*. Boil the mixture under a reflux condenser for 30 min. Filter the liquid through a plug of absorbent cotton in a 100 ml flask. Add the absorbent cotton to the residue in the round-bottomed flask and extract with 2 quantities, each of 20 ml, of *acetone R*, each time boiling under a reflux condenser for 10 min. Allow to cool to room temperature, filter the liquid through a plug of absorbent cotton then through a filter-paper in the volumetric flask, and dilute to 100.0 ml with *acetone R* by rinsing of the flask and filter. Introduce 20.0 ml of the solution into a separating funnel, add 20 ml of *water R* and extract the mixture with 1 quantity of 15 ml and then 3 quantities, each of 10 ml, of *ethyl acetate R*. Combine the ethyl acetate extracts in a separating funnel, rinse with 2 quantities, each of 50 ml, of *water R*, and filter the extract over 10 g of *anhydrous sodium sulphate R* into a 50 ml volumetric flask and dilute to 50.0 ml with *ethyl acetate R*.

Test solution. To 10.0 ml of the stock solution add 1 ml of *aluminium chloride reagent R* and dilute to 25.0 ml with a 5 per cent *V/V* solution of *glacial acetic acid R* in *methanol R*.

Compensation liquid. Dilute 10.0 ml of the stock solution to 25.0 ml with a 5 per cent *V/V* solution of *glacial acetic acid R* in *methanol R*.

Measure the absorbance (*2.2.25*) of the test solution after 30 min, by comparison with the compensation liquid at 425 nm.

Calculate the percentage content of flavonoids, expressed as hyperoside, using the following expression:

$$\frac{A \times 1.25}{m}$$

i.e. taking the specific absorbance of hyperoside to be 500.

A = absorbance at 425 nm;

m = mass of the substance to be examined, in grams.

C

07/2008:0014

CALCIUM CARBONATE

Calcii carbonas

$CaCO_3$ M_r 100.1
[471-34-1]

DEFINITION

Content: 98.5 per cent to 100.5 per cent (dried substance).

CHARACTERS

Appearance: white or almost white powder.

Solubility: practically insoluble in water.

IDENTIFICATION

A. It gives the reaction of carbonates (*2.3.1*).

B. 0.2 ml of solution S (see Tests) gives the reactions of calcium (*2.3.1*).

TESTS

Solution S. Dissolve 5.0 g in 80 ml of *dilute acetic acid R*. When the effervescence ceases, boil for 2 min. Allow to cool, dilute to 100 ml with *dilute acetic acid R* and filter, if necessary, through a sintered-glass filter (*2.1.2*).

Substances insoluble in acetic acid: maximum 0.2 per cent.

Wash any residue obtained during the preparation of solution S with 4 quantities, each of 5 ml, of hot *water R* and dry at 100-105 °C for 1 h. The residue weighs a maximum of 10 mg.

Chlorides (*2.4.4*): maximum 330 ppm.

Dilute 3 ml of solution S to 15 ml with *water R*.

Sulphates (*2.4.13*): maximum 0.25 per cent.

Dilute 1.2 ml of solution S to 15 ml with *distilled water R*.

Arsenic (*2.4.2, Method A*): maximum 4 ppm, determined on 5 ml of solution S.

Barium. To 10 ml of solution S add 10 ml of *calcium sulphate solution R*. After at least 15 min, any opalescence in the solution is not more intense than that in a mixture of 10 ml of solution S and 10 ml of *distilled water R*.

Iron (*2.4.9*): maximum 200 ppm.

Dissolve 50 mg in 5 ml of *dilute hydrochloric acid R* and dilute to 10 ml with *water R*.

Magnesium and alkali metals: maximum 1.5 per cent.

Dissolve 1.0 g in 12 ml of *dilute hydrochloric acid R*. Boil the solution for about 2 min and add 20 ml of *water R*, 1 g of *ammonium chloride R* and 0.1 ml of *methyl red solution R*. Add *dilute ammonia R1* until the colour of the indicator changes and then add 2 ml in excess. Heat to boiling and add 50 ml of hot *ammonium oxalate solution R*. Allow to stand for 4 h, dilute to 100 ml with *water R* and filter through a suitable filter. To 50 ml of the filtrate add 0.25 ml of *sulphuric acid R*. Evaporate to dryness on a water-bath and ignite to constant mass at 600 ± 50 °C. The residue weighs a maximum of 7.5 mg.

Heavy metals (*2.4.8*): maximum 20 ppm.

12 ml of solution S complies with test A. Prepare the reference solution using *lead standard solution (1 ppm Pb) R*.

Loss on drying (*2.2.32*): maximum 2.0 per cent, determined on 1.000 g by drying in an oven at 200 ± 10 °C.

ASSAY

Dissolve 0.150 g in a mixture of 3 ml of *dilute hydrochloric acid R* and 20 ml of *water R*. Boil for 2 min, allow to cool and dilute to 50 ml with *water R*. Carry out the complexometric titration of calcium (*2.5.11*).

1 ml of *0.1 M sodium edetate* is equivalent to 10.01 mg of $CaCO_3$.

FUNCTIONALITY-RELATED CHARACTERISTICS

This section provides information on characteristics that are recognised as being relevant control parameters for one or more functions of the substance when used as an excipient (see chapter 5.15). This section is a non-mandatory part of the monograph and it is not necessary to verify the characteristics to demonstrate compliance. Control of these characteristics can however contribute to the quality of a medicinal product by improving the consistency of the manufacturing process and the performance of the medicinal product during use. Where control methods are cited, they are recognised as being suitable for the purpose, but other methods can also be used. Wherever results for a particular characteristic are reported, the control method must be indicated.

The following characteristics may be relevant for calcium carbonate used as filler in tablets and capsules.

Particle-size distribution (*2.9.31* or *2.9.38*).

Powder flow (*2.9.36*).

07/2008:1183

CALCIUM DOBESILATE MONOHYDRATE

Calcii dobesilas monohydricus

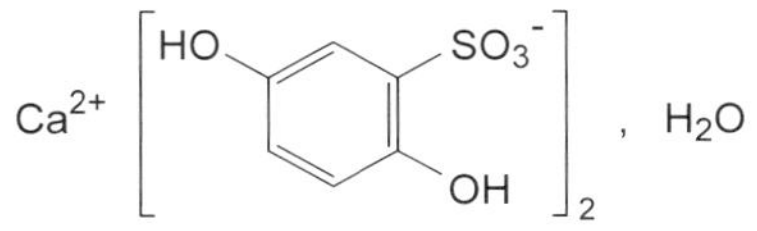

$C_{12}H_{10}CaO_{10}S_2,H_2O$ M_r 436.4

DEFINITION

Calcium di(2,5-dihydroxybenzenesulphonate) monohydrate.

Content: 99.0 per cent to 101.0 per cent (anhydrous substance).

CHARACTERS

Appearance: white or almost white, hygroscopic powder.

Solubility: very soluble in water, freely soluble in anhydrous ethanol, very slightly soluble in 2-propanol, practically insoluble in methylene chloride.

IDENTIFICATION

A. Ultraviolet and visible absorption spectrophotometry (*2.2.25*).

Test solution. Dissolve 0.100 g in *water R* and dilute to 200.0 ml with the same solvent. Dilute 5.0 ml of this solution to 100.0 ml with *water R*.

Spectral range: 210-350 nm.

Absorption maxima: at 221 nm and 301 nm.

Specific absorbance at the absorption maximum at 301 nm: 174 to 181.

Monographs A-C

B. Mix 1 ml of *ferric chloride solution R2*, 1 ml of a freshly prepared 10 g/l solution of *potassium ferricyanide R* and 0.1 ml of *nitric acid R*. To this mixture add 5 ml of freshly prepared solution S (see Tests): a blue colour and a precipitate are immediately produced.

C. 2 ml of freshly prepared solution S gives reaction (b) of calcium (*2.3.1*).

TESTS

Solution S. Dissolve 10.0 g in *carbon dioxide-free water R* and dilute to 100 ml with the same solvent.

Appearance of solution. Solution S, when freshly prepared, is clear (*2.2.1*) and colourless (*2.2.2, Method II*).

pH (*2.2.3*): 4.5 to 6.0 for solution S.

Related substances. Liquid chromatography (*2.2.29*). *Keep all solutions at 2-8 °C.*

Buffer solution. Dissolve 1.2 g of *anhydrous sodium dihydrogen phosphate R* in 900 ml of *water for chromatography R*, adjust to pH 6.5 with *disodium hydrogen phosphate solution R* and dilute to 1000 ml with *water for chromatography R*.

Test solution. Dissolve 0.100 g of the substance to be examined in *water R* and dilute to 10.0 ml with the same solvent.

Reference solution (a). Dilute 1.0 ml of the test solution to 100.0 ml with *water R*. Dilute 1.0 ml of this solution to 10.0 ml with *water R*.

Reference solution (b). Dissolve 10 mg of the substance to be examined and 10 mg of *hydroquinone R* (impurity A) in *water R* and dilute to 10 ml with the same solvent. Dilute 1 ml of this solution to 100 ml with *water R*.

Column:

- *size*: *l* = 0.25 m, Ø = 4.6 mm;
- *stationary phase*: spherical *end-capped octadecylsilyl silica gel for chromatography R* (5 µm).

Mobile phase: *acetonitrile R1*, buffer solution (10:90 *V/V*).

Flow rate: 0.8 ml/min.

Detection: spectrophotometer at 220 nm.

Injection: 10 µl.

Run time: 2.5 times the retention time of dobesilate.

Relative retention with reference to dobesilate (retention time = about 6 min): impurity A = about 1.7.

System suitability: reference solution (b):

- *resolution*: minimum 8.0 between the peaks due to dobesilate and impurity A.

Limits:

- *correction factor*: for the calculation of content, multiply the peak area of impurity A by 0.6;
- *impurity A*: not more than the area of the principal peak in the chromatogram obtained with reference solution (a) (0.1 per cent);
- *unspecified impurities*: for each impurity, not more than the area of the principal peak in the chromatogram obtained with reference solution (a) (0.10 per cent);
- *total*: not more than twice the area of the principal peak in the chromatogram obtained with reference solution (a) (0.2 per cent);
- *disregard limit*: 0.5 times the area of the principal peak in the chromatogram obtained with reference solution (a) (0.05 per cent).

Heavy metals (*2.4.8*): maximum 15 ppm.

1.0 g complies with test C. Prepare the reference solution using 1.5 ml of *lead standard solution (10 ppm Pb) R*.

Iron (*2.4.9*): maximum 10 ppm, determined on 10 ml of solution S.

Water (*2.5.12*): 4.0 per cent to 6.0 per cent, determined on 0.500 g.

ASSAY

Dissolve 0.200 g in a mixture of 10 ml of *water R* and 40 ml of *dilute sulphuric acid R*. Titrate with *0.1 M cerium sulphate*, determining the end-point potentiometrically (*2.2.20*).

1 ml of *0.1 M cerium sulphate* is equivalent to 10.45 mg of $C_{12}H_{10}CaO_{10}S_2$.

STORAGE

In an airtight container, protected from light.

IMPURITIES

Specified impurities: A.

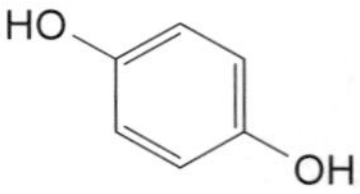

A. benzene-1,4-diol (hydroquinone).

07/2008:1859

CAPSICUM

Capsici fructus

DEFINITION

Dried ripe fruits of *Capsicum annuum* L. var. *minimum* (Miller) Heiser and small-fruited varieties of *Capsicum frutescens* L.

Content: minimum 0.4 per cent of total capsaicinoids, expressed as capsaicin ($C_{18}H_{27}NO_3$; M_r 305.4) (dried drug).

CHARACTERS

Extremely pungent taste.

IDENTIFICATION

A. The fruit is yellowish-orange or reddish-brown, oblong conical with an obtuse apex, about 1-3 cm long and up to 1 cm in diameter at the widest part, occasionally attached to a 5-toothed inferior calyx and a straight pedicel. Pericarp somewhat shrivelled, glabrous, enclosing about 10-20 flat, reniform seeds 3-4 mm long, either loose or attached to a reddish dissepiment.

B. Reduce to a powder (355) (*2.9.12*). The powder is orange. Examine under a microscope using *chloral hydrate solution R*. The powder shows the following diagnostic characters: fragments of the pericarp having an outer epicarp with cells often arranged in rows of 5 to 7, cuticle uniformly striated, parenchymatous cells frequently containing droplets of red oil, occasionally containing microsphenoidal crystals of calcium oxalate, endocarp with characteristic island groups of sclerenchymatous cells, the groups being separated by thin-walled parenchymatous cells; fragments of the seeds having an episperm composed of large, greenish-yellow, sinuous-walled sclereids with thin outer walls and strongly and unevenly thickened radial and inner walls which are conspicuously pitted, endosperm parenchymatous cells with drops of fixed oil and aleurone grains 3-6 µm in diameter; occasional fragments from the calyx having an outer epidermis with anisocytic stomata (*2.8.3*), inner epidermis with many trichomes but no stomata, trichomes glandular, with uniseriate stalks and multicellular heads, mesophyll with many idioblasts containing microsphenoidal crystals of calcium oxalate.

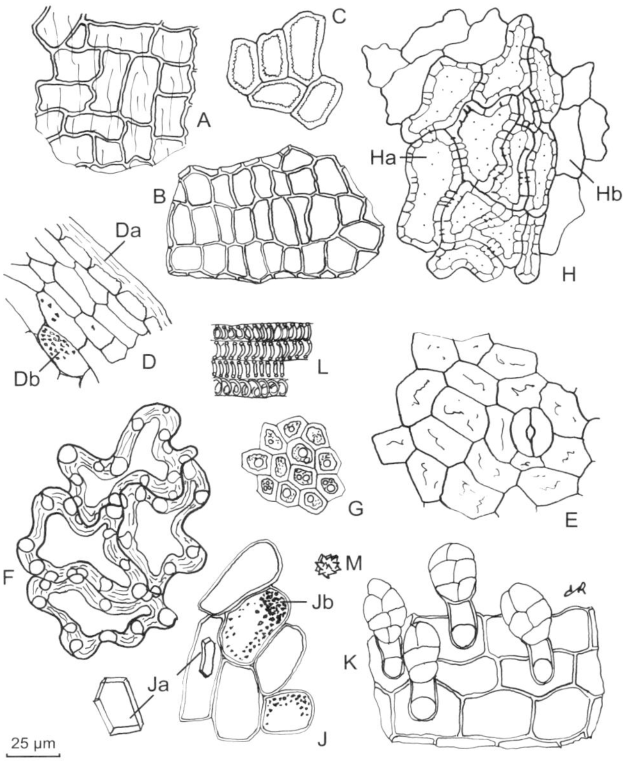

A, B, C. Epicarp: cells with striated cuticle (A); cells arranged in rows (B) and cells close to the peduncle (C)

D. Epicarp in transverse section showing cuticle (Da), accompanied by parenchyma containing microcrystals of calcium oxalate (Db)

E. Outer epidermis of the calyx with anisocytic stoma

F. Episperm

G. Endosperm with aleurone grains

H. Fragment of endocarp in transverse section with sclerenchymatous cells (Ha) and thin-walled parenchymatous cells (Hb)

J. Mesophyll of the calyx with prisms (Ja), microcrystals (Jb) and cluster crystals of calcium oxalate

K. Inner epidermis of the calyx with glandular trichomes

L. Vessels

M. Calcium oxalate cluster

Figure 1859.-1. – *Illustration of powdered herbal drug of capsicum (see identification B)*

C. Thin-layer chromatography (*2.2.27*).

Test solution. To 0.50 g of the powdered drug (500) (*2.9.12*) add 5.0 ml of *ether R*, shake for 5 min and filter.

Reference solution. Dissolve 2 mg of *capsaicin R* and 2 mg of *dihydrocapsaicin R* in 5.0 ml of *ether R*.

Plate: *TLC octadecylsilyl silica gel plate R*.

Mobile phase: *water R*, *methanol R* (20:80 *V/V*).

Application: 20 µl as bands.

Development: over a path of 12 cm.

Drying: in air.

Detection: spray with a 5 g/l solution of *dichloroquinonechlorimide R* in *methanol R*. Expose to ammonia vapour until blue zones appear. Examine in daylight.

Results: see below the sequence of zones present in the chromatograms obtained with the reference solution and the test solution. Furthermore, other zones may be present in the chromatogram obtained with the test solution.

Top of the plate	
_______	_______
Capsaicin: a blue zone	A blue zone (capsaicin)
Dihydrocapsaicin: a blue zone	A blue zone (dihydrocapsaicin)
_______	_______
Reference solution	**Test solution**

TESTS

Nonivamide. Liquid chromatography (*2.2.29*).

Test solution. To 2.5 g of the powdered drug (500) (*2.9.12*) add 100 ml of *methanol R*. Allow to macerate for 30 min. Place in an ultrasonic bath for 15 min. Filter into a 100 ml volumetric flask, rinse the flask and filter with *methanol R*, then dilute to 100.0 ml with the same solvent.

Reference solution. Dissolve 20.0 mg of *capsaicin CRS* and 4.0 mg of *nonivamide CRS* in *methanol R* and dilute to 100.0 ml with the same solvent.

Column:

- *size*: *l* = 0.25 m, Ø = 4.6 mm;
- *stationary phase*: *phenylsilyl silica gel for chromatography R* (5 µm);
- *temperature*: 30 °C.

Mobile phase: mix 40 volumes of *acetonitrile R* and 60 volumes of a 1 g/l solution of *phosphoric acid R*.

Flow rate: 1.0 ml/min.

Detection: spectrophotometer at 225 nm.

Injection: 10 µl.

Elution order: nordihydrocapsaicin, nonivamide, capsaicin, dihydrocapsaicin.

System suitability: reference solution:

- *resolution*: minimum 1.5 between the peaks due to nonivamide and capsaicin.

Calculate the percentage content of nonivamide using the following expression:

$$\frac{F_1 \times m_2 \times p_1}{F_2 \times m_1}$$

F_1 = area of the peak corresponding to nonivamide in the chromatogram obtained with the test solution;

F_2 = area of the peak corresponding to nonivamide in the chromatogram obtained with the reference solution;

m_1 = mass of the drug to be examined, in grams;

m_2 = mass of *nonivamide CRS* used to prepare the reference solution, in grams;

p_1 = percentage content of nonivamide in *nonivamide CRS*.

Limit:

- *nonivamide*: maximum 5.0 per cent of the total capsaicinoid content.

Foreign matter (*2.8.2*). Fruits of *C. annuum* L. var. *longum* (Sendtn.) are absent.

Loss on drying (*2.2.32*): maximum 11.0 per cent, determined on 1.000 g of the powdered drug (500) (*2.9.12*) by drying in an oven at 105 °C for 2 h.

Total ash (*2.4.16*): maximum 10.0 per cent.

ASSAY

Liquid chromatography (*2.2.29*) as described in the test for nonivamide.

Calculate the percentage content of total capsaicinoids, expressed as capsaicin, using the following expression:

$$\frac{(F_3 + F_5 + F_6) \times m_4 \times p_2}{F_4 \times m_3}$$

F_3 = area of the peak corresponding to capsaicin in the chromatogram obtained with the test solution;

F_4 = area of the peak corresponding to capsaicin in the chromatogram obtained with the reference solution;

F_5 = area of the peak corresponding to dihydrocapsaicin in the chromatogram obtained with the test solution;

F_6 = area of the peak corresponding to nordihydrocapsaicin in the chromatogram obtained with the test solution;

m_3 = mass of the drug to be examined, in grams;

m_4 = mass of *capsaicin CRS* used to prepare the reference solution, in grams;

p_2 = percentage content of capsaicin in *capsaicin CRS*.

07/2008:2201

CARPROFEN FOR VETERINARY USE

Carprofenum ad usum veterinarium

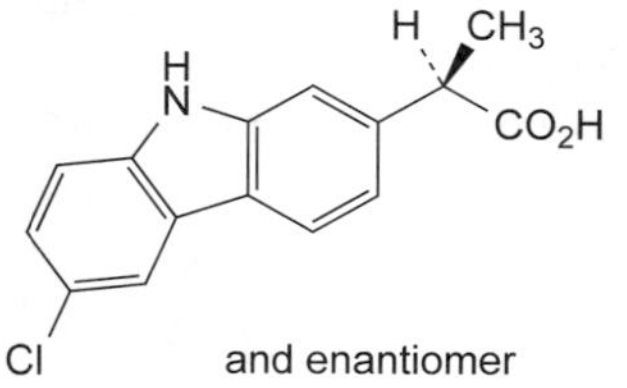

$C_{15}H_{12}ClNO_2$ M_r 273.7
[53716-49-7]

DEFINITION

(2*RS*)-2-(6-Chloro-9*H*-carbazol-2-yl)propanoic acid.

Content: 98.5 per cent to 101.5 per cent (dried substance).

CHARACTERS

Appearance: white or almost white, crystalline powder.

Solubility: practically insoluble in water, freely soluble in acetone, soluble in methanol, slightly soluble in 2-propanol.

It shows polymorphism (*5.9*).

IDENTIFICATION

Infrared absorption spectrophotometry (*2.2.24*).

Comparison: *carprofen CRS*.

If the spectra obtained in the solid state show differences, dissolve the substance to be examined and the reference substance separately in *acetone R*, evaporate to dryness and record new spectra using the residues.

TESTS

Appearance of solution. The solution is clear and not more intensely coloured than reference solution BY_3 (*2.2.2, Method II*).

Dissolve 1.0 g in *methanol R* and dilute to 25 ml with the same solvent.

Related substances. Liquid chromatography (*2.2.29*). *Carry out the test protected from light.*

Test solution. Dissolve 50 mg of the substance to be examined in the mobile phase and dilute to 100.0 ml with the mobile phase.

Reference solution (a). Dissolve 2.5 mg of *carprofen for system suitability CRS* (containing impurity C) in the mobile phase and dilute to 5.0 ml with the mobile phase.

Reference solution (b). Dilute 1.0 ml of the test solution to 100.0 ml with the mobile phase. Dilute 1.0 ml of this solution to 10.0 ml with the mobile phase.

Column:

- *size*: *l* = 0.25 m, Ø = 4.6 mm;
- *stationary phase*: *end-capped polar-embedded octadecylsilyl amorphous organosilica polymer R* (5 μm).

Mobile phase: mix 30 volumes of a 1.36 g/l solution of *potassium dihydrogen phosphate R* adjusted to pH 3.0 with *phosphoric acid R* and 70 volumes of *methanol R2*.

Flow rate: 1.3 ml/min.

Detection: spectrophotometer at 235 nm.

Injection: 20 μl.

Run time: 4 times the retention time of carprofen.

Retention time: carprofen = about 10 min.

System suitability: reference solution (a):

- *resolution*: minimum 1.5 between the peaks due to impurity C and carprofen.

Limits:

- *unspecified impurities*: for each impurity, not more than twice the area of the principal peak in the chromatogram obtained with reference solution (b) (0.2 per cent);
- *total*: not more than 5 times the area of the principal peak in the chromatogram obtained with reference solution (b) (0.5 per cent);
- *disregard limit*: the area of the principal peak in the chromatogram obtained with reference solution (b) (0.1 per cent).

Heavy metals (*2.4.8*): maximum 20 ppm.

Dissolve 2.0 g in *ethanol (96 per cent) R* and dilute to 20 ml with the same solvent. 12 ml of the solution complies with test B. Prepare the reference solution using *lead standard solution (2 ppm Pb) R*.

Loss on drying (*2.2.32*): maximum 0.5 per cent, determined on 1.000 g by drying in an oven at 105 °C for 2 h.

Sulphated ash (*2.4.14*): maximum 0.1 per cent, determined on 1.0 g.

ASSAY

Dissolve 0.200 g in 50 ml of *ethanol (96 per cent) R*. Add 1.0 ml of *0.1 M hydrochloric acid*. Titrate with *0.1 M sodium hydroxide*, determining the end-point potentiometrically (*2.2.20*). Read the volume added between the 2 points of inflexion.

1 ml of *0.1 M sodium hydroxide* is equivalent to 27.37 mg of $C_{15}H_{12}ClNO_2$.

STORAGE

Protected from light.

IMPURITIES

Other detectable impurities (the following substances would, if present at a sufficient level, be detected by one or other of the tests in the monograph. They are limited by the general acceptance criterion for other/unspecified impurities and/or by the general monograph *Substances for pharmaceutical use (2034)*. It is therefore not necessary to identify these impurities for demonstration of compliance. See also *5.10. Control of impurities in substances for pharmaceutical use*): *A, B, C, D, E, F, G, H.*

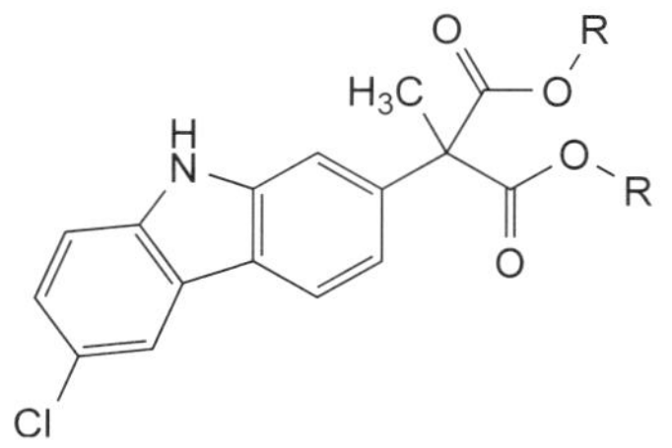

A. R = H: 2-(6-chloro-9*H*-carbazol-2-yl)-2-methylpropanedioic acid,

F. R = C_2H_5: diethyl 2-(6-chloro-9*H*-carbazol-2-yl)-2-methylpropanedioate,

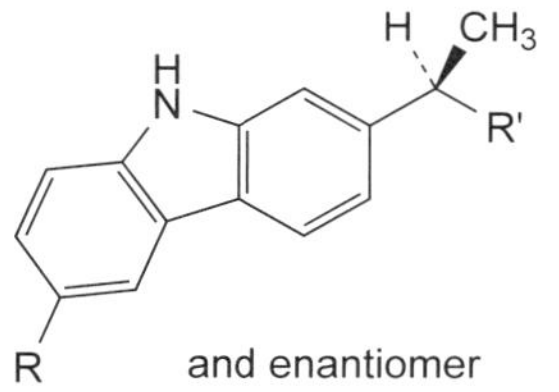

and enantiomer

B. R = H, R′ = CO_2H: (2*RS*)-2-(9*H*-carbazol-2-yl)propanoic acid,

C. R = Cl, R′ = OH: (1*RS*)-1-(6-chloro-9*H*-carbazol-2-yl)ethanol,

G. R = Cl, R′ = CO-O-C_2H_5: ethyl (2*RS*)-2-(6-chloro-9*H*-carbazol-2-yl)propanoate,

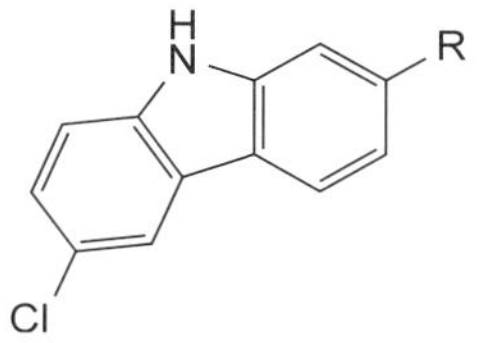

D. R = CO-CH_3: 1-(6-chloro-9*H*-carbazol-2-yl)ethanone,

E. R = H: 3-chloro-9*H*-carbazole,

H. R = C_2H_5: 6-chloro-2-ethyl-9*H*-carbazole.

01/2008:1496

CASSIA OIL

Cinnamomi cassiae aetheroleum

DEFINITION

Essential oil obtained by steam distillation of the leaves and young branches of *Cinnamomum cassia* Blume (*C. aromaticum* Nees).

CHARACTERS

Appearance: clear, mobile, yellow or reddish-brown liquid.

Characteristic odour reminiscent of cinnamic aldehyde.

IDENTIFICATION

First identification: B.

Second identification: A.

A. Thin-layer chromatography (*2.2.27*).

Test solution. Dissolve 0.5 ml of the oil to be examined in *acetone R* and dilute to 10 ml with the same solvent.

Reference solution. Dissolve 50 µl of *trans-cinnamic aldehyde R*, 10 µl of *eugenol R* and 50 mg of *coumarin R* in *acetone R* and dilute to 10 ml with the same solvent.

Plate: *TLC silica gel plate R*.

Mobile phase: *methanol R, toluene R* (10:90 *V/V*).

Application: 10 µl as bands.

Development: over a path of 15 cm.

Drying: in air.

Detection A: examine in ultraviolet light at 365 nm.

Results A: the zone of blue fluorescence in the chromatogram obtained with the test solution is similar in position and colour to the zone in the chromatogram obtained with the reference solution (coumarin).

Detection B: spray with *anisaldehyde solution R*; examine in daylight while heating at 100-105 °C for 5-10 min.

Results B: the chromatogram obtained with the reference solution shows in its upper part a violet zone (eugenol) and above this zone a greenish-blue zone (*trans*-cinnamic aldehyde). The chromatogram obtained with the test solution shows a zone similar in position and colour to the zone due to *trans*-cinnamic aldehyde in the chromatogram obtained with the reference solution and may show a very faint zone due to eugenol. Other faint zones are present.

B. Examine the chromatograms obtained in the test for chromatographic profile.

Results: the principal peaks in the chromatogram obtained with the test solution are similar in retention time to those in the chromatogram obtained with the reference solution. Eugenol may be absent from the chromatogram obtained with the test solution.

TESTS

Relative density (*2.2.5*): 1.052 to 1.070.

Refractive index (*2.2.6*): 1.600 to 1.614.

Optical rotation (*2.2.7*): – 1° to + 1°.

Chromatographic profile. Gas chromatography (*2.2.28*): use the normalisation procedure.

Test solution. The oil to be examined.

Reference solution. Dissolve 100 µl of *trans-cinnamic aldehyde R,* 10 µl of *cinnamyl acetate R,* 10 µl of *eugenol R,* 10 µl of *trans-2-methoxycinnamaldehyde R* and 20 mg of *coumarin R* in 1 ml of *acetone R.*

Column:

– *material*: fused silica;

– *size*: l = 60 m, Ø = about 0.25 mm;

– *stationary phase*: bonded *macrogol 20 000 R.*

Carrier gas: *helium for chromatography R.*

Flow rate: 1.5 ml/min.

Split ratio: 1:100.

Temperature:

	Time (min)	Temperature (°C)
Column	0 - 10	60
	10 - 75	60 → 190
	75 - 160	190
Injection port		200
Detector		240

Detection: flame ionisation.

Injection: 0.2 µl.

Elution order: order indicated in the composition of the reference solution, depending on the operating conditions and the state of the column, coumarin may elute before or after *trans*-2-methoxycinnamaldehyde; record the retention times of these substances.

System suitability: reference solution:

– *resolution*: minimum 1.5 between the peaks due to *trans*-2-methoxycinnamaldehyde and coumarin.

Identification of components: using the retention times determined from the chromatogram obtained with the reference solution, locate the components of the reference solution in the chromatogram obtained with the test solution.

Determine the percentage content of each of these components. The percentages are within the following ranges:

– *trans-cinnamic aldehyde*: 70 per cent to 90 per cent;

– *cinnamyl acetate*: 1.0 per cent to 6.0 per cent;

– *eugenol*: less than 0.5 per cent;

– *trans-2-methoxycinnamaldehyde*: 3.0 per cent to 15 per cent;

– *coumarin*: 1.5 per cent to 4.0 per cent.

STORAGE

Protected from heat.

07/2008:0316

CELLULOSE, MICROCRYSTALLINE

Cellulosum microcristallinum

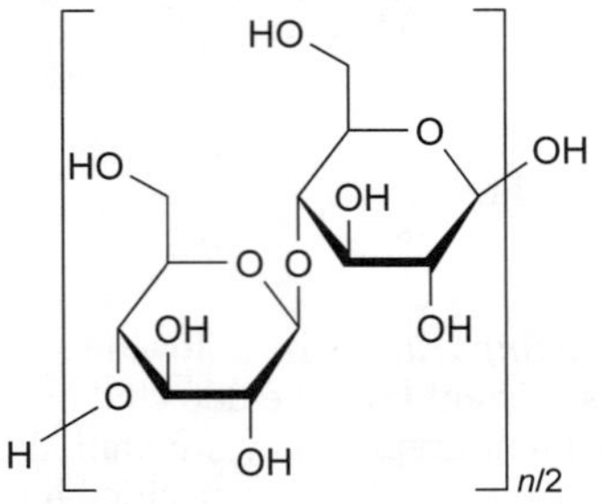

$C_{6n}H_{10n+2}O_{5n+1}$

DEFINITION

Purified, partly depolymerised cellulose prepared by treating alpha-cellulose, obtained as a pulp from fibrous plant material, with mineral acids.

CHARACTERS

Appearance: white or almost white, fine or granular powder.

Solubility: practically insoluble in water, in acetone, in anhydrous ethanol, in toluene, in dilute acids and in a 50 g/l solution of sodium hydroxide.

IDENTIFICATION

A. Place about 10 mg on a watch-glass and disperse in 2 ml of *iodinated zinc chloride solution R.* The substance becomes violet-blue.

B. The degree of polymerisation is not more than 350.

Transfer 1.300 g to a 125 ml conical flask. Add 25.0 ml of *water R* and 25.0 ml of *cupriethylenediamine hydroxide solution R.* Immediately purge the solution with *nitrogen R,* insert the stopper and shake until completely dissolved. Transfer an appropriate volume of the solution to a suitable capillary viscometer (*2.2.9*). Equilibrate the solution at 25 ± 0.1 °C for at least 5 min. Record the flow time (t_1) in seconds between the 2 marks on the viscometer. Calculate the kinematic viscosity (ν_1) of the solution using the following expression:

$$t_1\,(k_1)$$

where k_1 is the viscometer constant.

Dilute a suitable volume of *cupriethylenediamine hydroxide solution R* with an equal volume of *water R* and measure the flow time (t_2) using a suitable capillary viscometer. Calculate the kinematic viscosity (ν_2) of the solvent using the following expression:

$$t_2\,(k_2)$$

where k_2 is the viscometer constant.

Determine the relative viscosity (η_{rel}) of the substance to be examined using the following expression:

$$\nu_1/\nu_2$$

Determine the intrinsic viscosity ($[\eta]_c$) by interpolation, using the intrinsic viscosity table (Table 0316.-1).

Calculate the degree of polymerisation (*P*) using the following expression:

$$\frac{95\,[\eta]_c}{m\,[(100-b)/100]}$$

where *m* is the mass in grams of the substance to be examined and *b* is the loss on drying as a percentage.

TESTS

Solubility. Dissolve 50 mg in 10 ml of *ammoniacal solution of copper tetrammine R*. It dissolves completely, leaving no residue.

pH (*2.2.3*): 5.0 to 7.5 for the supernatant liquid.

Shake 5 g with 40 ml of *carbon dioxide-free water R* for 20 min and centrifuge.

Conductivity (*2.2.38*). The conductivity of the test solution does not exceed the conductivity of the water by more than 75 μS·cm^{-1}.

Use as test solution the supernatant liquid obtained in the test for pH. Measure the conductivity of the supernatant liquid after a stable reading has been obtained and measure the conductivity of the water used to prepare the test solution.

Ether-soluble substances: maximum 0.05 per cent (5 mg) for the difference between the weight of the residue and the weight obtained from a blank determination.

Place 10.0 g in a chromatography column about 20 mm in internal diameter and pass 50 ml of *peroxide-free ether R* through the column. Evaporate the eluate to dryness. Dry the residue at 105 °C for 30 min, allow to cool in a dessicator and weigh. Carry out a blank determination.

Water-soluble substances: maximum 0.25 per cent (12.5 mg) for the difference between the mass of the residue and the mass obtained from a blank determination.

Shake 5.0 g with 80 ml of *water R* for 10 min. Filter through a filter paper with the aid of vacuum into a tared flask. Evaporate to dryness on a water-bath avoiding charring. Dry at 105 °C for 1 h and weigh. Carry out a blank determination.

Heavy metals (*2.4.8*): maximum 10 ppm.

2.0 g complies with test C. Prepare the reference solution using 2 ml of *lead standard solution (10 ppm Pb) R*.

Loss on drying (*2.2.32*): maximum 7.0 per cent, determined on 1.000 g by drying in an oven at 105 °C for 3 h.

Sulphated ash (*2.4.14*): maximum 0.1 per cent, determined on 1.0 g.

Microbial contamination. Total viable aerobic count (*2.6.12*) not more than 10^3 micro-organisms per gram and with a limit for fungi of 10^2 per gram, determined by plate count. It complies with the tests for *Escherichia coli*, for *Pseudomonas aeruginosa*, for *Staphylococcus aureus* and for *Salmonella* (*2.6.13*).

Table 0316.-1. – *Intrinsic viscosity table*

Intrinsic viscosity $[\eta]_c$ at different values of relative viscosity η_{rel}										
					$[\eta]_c$					
η_{rel}	0.00	0.01	0.02	0.03	0.04	0.05	0.06	0.07	0.08	0.09
1.1	0.098	0.106	0.115	0.125	0.134	0.143	0.152	0.161	0.170	0.180
1.2	0.189	0.198	0.207	0.216	0.225	0.233	0.242	0.250	0.259	0.268
1.3	0.276	0.285	0.293	0.302	0.310	0.318	0.326	0.334	0.342	0.350
1.4	0.358	0.367	0.375	0.383	0.391	0.399	0.407	0.414	0.422	0.430
1.5	0.437	0.445	0.453	0.460	0.468	0.476	0.484	0.491	0.499	0.507
1.6	0.515	0.522	0.529	0.536	0.544	0.551	0.558	0.566	0.573	0.580
1.7	0.587	0.595	0.602	0.608	0.615	0.622	0.629	0.636	0.642	0.649
1.8	0.656	0.663	0.670	0.677	0.683	0.690	0.697	0.704	0.710	0.717
1.9	0.723	0.730	0.736	0.743	0.749	0.756	0.762	0.769	0.775	0.782
2.0	0.788	0.795	0.802	0.809	0.815	0.821	0.827	0.833	0.840	0.846
2.1	0.852	0.858	0.864	0.870	0.876	0.882	0.888	0.894	0.900	0.906
2.2	0.912	0.918	0.924	0.929	0.935	0.941	0.948	0.953	0.959	0.965
2.3	0.971	0.976	0.983	0.988	0.994	1.000	1.006	1.011	1.017	1.022
2.4	1.028	1.033	1.039	1.044	1.050	1.056	1.061	1.067	1.072	1.078
2.5	1.083	1.089	1.094	1.100	1.105	1.111	1.116	1.121	1.126	1.131
2.6	1.137	1.142	1.147	1.153	1.158	1.163	1.169	1.174	1.179	1.184
2.7	1.190	1.195	1.200	1.205	1.210	1.215	1.220	1.225	1.230	1.235
2.8	1.240	1.245	1.250	1.255	1.260	1.265	1.270	1.275	1.280	1.285
2.9	1.290	1.295	1.300	1.305	1.310	1.314	1.319	1.324	1.329	1.333
3.0	1.338	1.343	1.348	1.352	1.357	1.362	1.367	1.371	1.376	1.381

Intrinsic viscosity $[\eta]_c$ at different values of relative viscosity η_{rel}

	$[\eta]_c$									
η_{rel}	0.00	0.01	0.02	0.03	0.04	0.05	0.06	0.07	0.08	0.09
3.1	1.386	1.390	1.395	1.400	1.405	1.409	1.414	1.418	1.423	1.427
3.2	1.432	1.436	1.441	1.446	1.450	1.455	1.459	1.464	1.468	1.473
3.3	1.477	1.482	1.486	1.491	1.496	1.500	1.504	1.508	1.513	1.517
3.4	1.521	1.525	1.529	1.533	1.537	1.542	1.546	1.550	1.554	1.558
3.5	1.562	1.566	1.570	1.575	1.579	1.583	1.587	1.591	1.595	1.600
3.6	1.604	1.608	1.612	1.617	1.621	1.625	1.629	1.633	1.637	1.642
3.7	1.646	1.650	1.654	1.658	1.662	1.666	1.671	1.675	1.679	1.683
3.8	1.687	1.691	1.695	1.700	1.704	1.708	1.712	1.715	1.719	1.723
3.9	1.727	1.731	1.735	1.739	1.742	1.746	1.750	1.754	1.758	1.762
4.0	1.765	1.769	1.773	1.777	1.781	1.785	1.789	1.792	1.796	1.800
4.1	1.804	1.808	1.811	1.815	1.819	1.822	1.826	1.830	1.833	1.837
4.2	1.841	1.845	1.848	1.852	1.856	1.859	1.863	1.867	1.870	1.874
4.3	1.878	1.882	1.885	1.889	1.893	1.896	1.900	1.904	1.907	1.911
4.4	1.914	1.918	1.921	1.925	1.929	1.932	1.936	1.939	1.943	1.946
4.5	1.950	1.954	1.957	1.961	1.964	1.968	1.971	1.975	1.979	1.982
4.6	1.986	1.989	1.993	1.996	2.000	2.003	2.007	2.010	2.013	2.017
4.7	2.020	2.023	2.027	2.030	2.033	2.037	2.040	2.043	2.047	2.050
4.8	2.053	2.057	2.060	2.063	2.067	2.070	2.073	2.077	2.080	2.083
4.9	2.087	2.090	2.093	2.097	2.100	2.103	2.107	2.110	2.113	2.116
5.0	2.119	2.122	2.125	2.129	2.132	2.135	2.139	2.142	2.145	2.148
5.1	2.151	2.154	2.158	2.160	2.164	2.167	2.170	2.173	2.176	2.180
5.2	2.183	2.186	2.190	2.192	2.195	2.197	2.200	2.203	2.206	2.209
5.3	2.212	2.215	2.218	2.221	2.224	2.227	2.230	2.233	2.236	2.240
5.4	2.243	2.246	2.249	2.252	2.255	2.258	2.261	2.264	2.267	2.270
5.5	2.273	2.276	2.279	2.282	2.285	2.288	2.291	2.294	2.297	2.300
5.6	2.303	2.306	2.309	2.312	2.315	2.318	2.320	2.324	2.326	2.329
5.7	2.332	2.335	2.338	2.341	2.344	2.347	2.350	2.353	2.355	2.358
5.8	2.361	2.364	2.367	2.370	2.373	2.376	2.379	2.382	2.384	2.387
5.9	2.390	2.393	2.396	2.400	2.403	2.405	2.408	2.411	2.414	2.417
6.0	2.419	2.422	2.425	2.428	2.431	2.433	2.436	2.439	2.442	2.444
6.1	2.447	2.450	2.453	2.456	2.458	2.461	2.464	2.467	2.470	2.472
6.2	2.475	2.478	2.481	2.483	2.486	2.489	2.492	2.494	2.497	2.500
6.3	2.503	2.505	2.508	2.511	2.513	2.516	2.518	2.521	2.524	2.526
6.4	2.529	2.532	2.534	2.537	2.540	2.542	2.545	2.547	2.550	2.553
6.5	2.555	2.558	2.561	2.563	2.566	2.568	2.571	2.574	2.576	2.579
6.6	2.581	2.584	2.587	2.590	2.592	2.595	2.597	2.600	2.603	2.605
6.7	2.608	2.610	2.613	2.615	2.618	2.620	2.623	2.625	2.627	2.630
6.8	2.633	2.635	2.637	2.640	2.643	2.645	2.648	2.650	2.653	2.655
6.9	2.658	2.660	2.663	2.665	2.668	2.670	2.673	2.675	2.678	2.680
7.0	2.683	2.685	2.687	2.690	2.693	2.695	2.698	2.700	2.702	2.705
7.1	2.707	2.710	2.712	2.714	2.717	2.719	2.721	2.724	2.726	2.729

Intrinsic viscosity $[\eta]_c$ at different values of relative viscosity η_{rel}

η_{rel}	$[\eta]_c$ 0.00	0.01	0.02	0.03	0.04	0.05	0.06	0.07	0.08	0.09
7.2	2.731	2.733	2.736	2.738	2.740	2.743	2.745	2.748	2.750	2.752
7.3	2.755	2.757	2.760	2.762	2.764	2.767	2.769	2.771	2.774	2.776
7.4	2.779	2.781	2.783	2.786	2.788	2.790	2.793	2.795	2.798	2.800
7.5	2.802	2.805	2.807	2.809	2.812	2.814	2.816	2.819	2.821	2.823
7.6	2.826	2.828	2.830	2.833	2.835	2.837	2.840	2.842	2.844	2.847
7.7	2.849	2.851	2.854	2.856	2.858	2.860	2.863	2.865	2.868	2.870
7.8	2.873	2.875	2.877	2.879	2.881	2.884	2.887	2.889	2.891	2.893
7.9	2.895	2.898	2.900	2.902	2.905	2.907	2.909	2.911	2.913	2.915
8.0	2.918	2.920	2.922	2.924	2.926	2.928	2.931	2.933	2.935	2.937
8.1	2.939	2.942	2.944	2.946	2.948	2.950	2.952	2.955	2.957	2.959
8.2	2.961	2.963	2.966	2.968	2.970	2.972	2.974	2.976	2.979	2.981
8.3	2.983	2.985	2.987	2.990	2.992	2.994	2.996	2.998	3.000	3.002
8.4	3.004	3.006	3.008	3.010	3.012	3.015	3.017	3.019	3.021	3.023
8.5	3.025	3.027	3.029	3.031	3.033	3.035	3.037	3.040	3.042	3.044
8.6	3.046	3.048	3.050	3.052	3.054	3.056	3.058	3.060	3.062	3.064
8.7	3.067	3.069	3.071	3.073	3.075	3.077	3.079	3.081	3.083	3.085
8.8	3.087	3.089	3.092	3.094	3.096	3.098	3.100	3.102	3.104	3.106
8.9	3.108	3.110	3.112	3.114	3.116	3.118	3.120	3.122	3.124	3.126
9.0	3.128	3.130	3.132	3.134	3.136	3.138	3.140	3.142	3.144	3.146
9.1	3.148	3.150	3.152	3.154	3.156	3.158	3.160	3.162	3.164	3.166
9.2	3.168	3.170	3.172	3.174	3.176	3.178	3.180	3.182	3.184	3.186
9.3	3.188	3.190	3.192	3.194	3.196	3.198	3.200	3.202	3.204	3.206
9.4	3.208	3.210	3.212	3.214	3.215	3.217	3.219	3.221	3.223	3.225
9.5	3.227	3.229	3.231	3.233	3.235	3.237	3.239	3.241	3.242	3.244
9.6	3.246	3.248	3.250	3.252	3.254	3.256	3.258	3.260	3.262	3.264
9.7	3.266	3.268	3.269	3.271	3.273	3.275	3.277	3.279	3.281	3.283
9.8	3.285	3.287	3.289	3.291	3.293	3.295	3.297	3.298	3.300	3.302
9.9	3.304	3.305	3.307	3.309	3.311	3.313	3.316	3.318	3.320	3.321

Intrinsic viscosity $[\eta]_c$ at different values of relative viscosity η_{rel}

η_{rel}	$[\eta]_c$ 0.0	0.1	0.2	0.3	0.4	0.5	0.6	0.7	0.8	0.9
10	3.32	3.34	3.36	3.37	3.39	3.41	3.43	3.45	3.46	3.48
11	3.50	3.52	3.53	3.55	3.56	3.58	3.60	3.61	3.63	3.64
12	3.66	3.68	3.69	3.71	3.72	3.74	3.76	3.77	3.79	3.80
13	3.80	3.83	3.85	3.86	3.88	3.89	3.90	3.92	3.93	3.95
14	3.96	3.97	3.99	4.00	4.02	4.03	4.04	4.06	4.07	4.09
15	4.10	4.11	4.13	4.14	4.15	4.17	4.18	4.19	4.20	4.22
16	4.23	4.24	4.25	4.27	4.28	4.29	4.30	4.31	4.33	4.34
17	4.35	4.36	4.37	4.38	4.39	4.41	4.42	4.43	4.44	4.45
18	4.46	4.47	4.48	4.49	4.50	4.52	4.53	4.54	4.55	4.56
19	4.57	4.58	4.59	4.60	4.61	4.62	4.63	4.64	4.65	4.66

FUNCTIONALITY-RELATED CHARACTERISTICS

This section provides information on characteristics that are recognised as being relevant control parameters for one or more functions of the substance when used as an excipient. This section is a non-mandatory part of the monograph and it is not necessary to verify the characteristics to demonstrate compliance. Control of these characteristics can however contribute to the quality of a medicinal product by improving the consistency of the manufacturing process and the performance of the medicinal product during use. Where control methods are cited, they are recognised as being suitable for the purpose, but other methods can also be used. Wherever results for a particular characteristic are reported, the control method must be indicated.

The following characteristics may be relevant for microcrystalline cellulose used as binder, diluent or disintegrant.

Particle-size distribution (*2.9.31* or *2.9.38*).

Powder flow (*2.9.36*).

07/2008:0315

CELLULOSE, POWDERED

Cellulosi pulvis

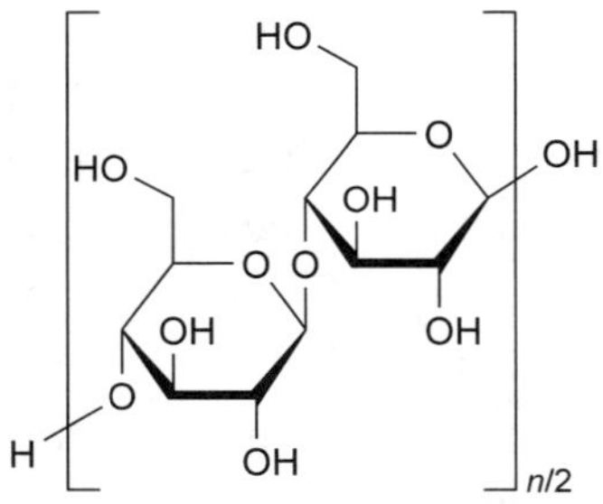

$C_{6n}H_{10n+2}O_{5n+1}$

DEFINITION

Purified, mechanically disintegrated cellulose prepared by processing alpha-cellulose obtained as a pulp from fibrous plant material.

CHARACTERS

Appearance: white or almost white, fine or granular powder.

Solubility: practically insoluble in water, slightly soluble in a 50 g/l solution of sodium hydroxide, practically insoluble in acetone, in anhydrous ethanol, in toluene, in dilute acids and in most organic solvents.

IDENTIFICATION

A. Place about 10 mg on a watch-glass and disperse in 2 ml of *iodinated zinc chloride solution R*. The substance becomes violet-blue.

B. The degree of polymerisation is greater than 440.

Transfer 0.250 g to a 125 ml conical flask. Add 25.0 ml of *water R* and 25.0 ml of *cupriethylenediamine hydroxide solution R*. Immediately purge the solution with *nitrogen R*, insert the stopper and shake until completely dissolved. Transfer an appropriate volume of the solution to a suitable capillary viscometer (*2.2.9*). Equilibrate the solution at 25 ± 0.1 °C for at least 5 min. Record the flow time (t_1) in seconds between the 2 marks on the viscometer. Calculate the kinematic viscosity (ν_1) of the solution using the following expression:

$$t_1\,(k_1)$$

where k_1 is the viscometer constant.

Dilute a suitable volume of *cupriethylenediamine hydroxide solution R* with an equal volume of *water R* and measure the flow time (t_2) using a suitable capillary viscometer. Calculate the kinematic viscosity (ν_2) of the solvent using the following expression:

$$t_2\,(k_2)$$

where k_2 is the viscometer constant.

Determine the relative viscosity (η_{rel}) of the substance to be examined using the following expression:

$$\nu_1/\nu_2$$

Determine the intrinsic viscosity ($[\eta]_c$) by interpolation, using the intrinsic viscosity table (Table 0315.-1).

Calculate the degree of polymerisation (*P*) using the following expression:

$$\frac{95\,[\eta]_c}{m\,[(100-b)/100]}$$

where *m* is the mass in grams of the substance to be examined and *b* is the loss on drying as a percentage.

TESTS

Solubility. Dissolve 50 mg in 10 ml of *ammoniacal solution of copper tetrammine R*. It dissolves completely, leaving no residue.

pH (*2.2.3*): 5.0 to 7.5 for the supernatant liquid.

Mix 10 g with 90 ml of *carbon dioxide-free water R* and allow to stand with occasional stirring for 1 h.

Ether-soluble substances: maximum 0.15 per cent (15 mg) for the difference between the mass of the residue and the mass obtained from a blank determination.

Place 10.0 g in a chromatography column about 20 mm in internal diameter and pass 50 ml of *peroxide-free ether R* through the column. Evaporate the eluate to dryness in a previously dried and tared evaporating dish, with the aid of a current of air in a fume hood. After all the ether has evaporated, dry the residue at 105 °C for 30 min, allow to cool in a dessiccator and weigh. Carry out a blank determination.

Water-soluble substances: maximum 1.5 per cent (15.0 mg) for the difference between the mass of the residue and the mass obtained from a blank determination.

Shake 6.0 g with 90 ml of *carbon dioxide-free water R* for 10 min. Filter with the aid of vacuum into a tared flask. Discard the first 10 ml of the filtrate and pass the filtrate through the same filter a second time, if necessary, to obtain a clear filtrate. Evaporate a 15.0 ml portion of the filtrate to dryness in a tared evaporating dish without charring. Dry at 105 °C for 1 h, allow to cool in a desiccator and weigh. Carry out a blank determination.

Heavy metals (*2.4.8*): maximum 10 ppm.

2.0 g complies with test C. Prepare the reference solution using 2 ml of *lead standard solution (10 ppm Pb) R.*

Loss on drying (*2.2.32*): maximum 6.5 per cent, determined on 1.000 g by drying in an oven at 105 °C for 3 h.

Sulphated ash (*2.4.14*): maximum 0.3 per cent, determined on 1.0 g (dried substance).

Microbial contamination. Total viable aerobic count (*2.6.12*) not more than 10^3 micro-organisms per gram and with a limit for fungi of 10^2 per gram, determined by plate count. It complies with the tests for *Escherichia coli*, for *Pseudomonas aeruginosa*, for *Staphylococcus aureus* and for *Salmonella* (*2.6.13*).

Table 0315.-1. – *Intrinsic viscosity table*

Intrinsic viscosity $[\eta]_c$ at different values of relative viscosity η_{rel}										
					$[\eta]_c$					
η_{rel}	0.00	0.01	0.02	0.03	0.04	0.05	0.06	0.07	0.08	0.09
1.1	0.098	0.106	0.115	0.125	0.134	0.143	0.152	0.161	0.170	0.180
1.2	0.189	0.198	0.207	0.216	0.225	0.233	0.242	0.250	0.259	0.268
1.3	0.276	0.285	0.293	0.302	0.310	0.318	0.326	0.334	0.342	0.350
1.4	0.358	0.367	0.375	0.383	0.391	0.399	0.407	0.414	0.422	0.430
1.5	0.437	0.445	0.453	0.460	0.468	0.476	0.484	0.491	0.499	0.507
1.6	0.515	0.522	0.529	0.536	0.544	0.551	0.558	0.566	0.573	0.580
1.7	0.587	0.595	0.602	0.608	0.615	0.622	0.629	0.636	0.642	0.649
1.8	0.656	0.663	0.670	0.677	0.683	0.690	0.697	0.704	0.710	0.717
1.9	0.723	0.730	0.736	0.743	0.749	0.756	0.762	0.769	0.775	0.782
2.0	0.788	0.795	0.802	0.809	0.815	0.821	0.827	0.833	0.840	0.846
2.1	0.852	0.858	0.864	0.870	0.876	0.882	0.888	0.894	0.900	0.906
2.2	0.912	0.918	0.924	0.929	0.935	0.941	0.948	0.953	0.959	0.965
2.3	0.971	0.976	0.983	0.988	0.994	1.000	1.006	1.011	1.017	1.022
2.4	1.028	1.033	1.039	1.044	1.050	1.056	1.061	1.067	1.072	1.078
2.5	1.083	1.089	1.094	1.100	1.105	1.111	1.116	1.121	1.126	1.131
2.6	1.137	1.142	1.147	1.153	1.158	1.163	1.169	1.174	1.179	1.184
2.7	1.190	1.195	1.200	1.205	1.210	1.215	1.220	1.225	1.230	1.235
2.8	1.240	1.245	1.250	1.255	1.260	1.265	1.270	1.275	1.280	1.285
2.9	1.290	1.295	1.300	1.305	1.310	1.314	1.319	1.324	1.329	1.333
3.0	1.338	1.343	1.348	1.352	1.357	1.362	1.367	1.371	1.376	1.381
3.1	1.386	1.390	1.395	1.400	1.405	1.409	1.414	1.418	1.423	1.427
3.2	1.432	1.436	1.441	1.446	1.450	1.455	1.459	1.464	1.468	1.473
3.3	1.477	1.482	1.486	1.491	1.496	1.500	1.504	1.508	1.513	1.517
3.4	1.521	1.525	1.529	1.533	1.537	1.542	1.546	1.550	1.554	1.558
3.5	1.562	1.566	1.570	1.575	1.579	1.583	1.587	1.591	1.595	1.600
3.6	1.604	1.608	1.612	1.617	1.621	1.625	1.629	1.633	1.637	1.642
3.7	1.646	1.650	1.654	1.658	1.662	1.666	1.671	1.675	1.679	1.683
3.8	1.687	1.691	1.695	1.700	1.704	1.708	1.712	1.715	1.719	1.723
3.9	1.727	1.731	1.735	1.739	1.742	1.746	1.750	1.754	1.758	1.762
4.0	1.765	1.769	1.773	1.777	1.781	1.785	1.789	1.792	1.796	1.800
4.1	1.804	1.808	1.811	1.815	1.819	1.822	1.826	1.830	1.833	1.837
4.2	1.841	1.845	1.848	1.852	1.856	1.859	1.863	1.867	1.870	1.874
4.3	1.878	1.882	1.885	1.889	1.893	1.896	1.900	1.904	1.907	1.911
4.4	1.914	1.918	1.921	1.925	1.929	1.932	1.936	1.939	1.943	1.946

Intrinsic viscosity $[\eta]_c$ at different values of relative viscosity η_{rel}

	$[\eta]_c$									
η_{rel}	0.00	0.01	0.02	0.03	0.04	0.05	0.06	0.07	0.08	0.09
4.5	1.950	1.954	1.957	1.961	1.964	1.968	1.971	1.975	1.979	1.982
4.6	1.986	1.989	1.993	1.996	2.000	2.003	2.007	2.010	2.013	2.017
4.7	2.020	2.023	2.027	2.030	2.033	2.037	2.040	2.043	2.047	2.050
4.8	2.053	2.057	2.060	2.063	2.067	2.070	2.073	2.077	2.080	2.083
4.9	2.087	2.090	2.093	2.097	2.100	2.103	2.107	2.110	2.113	2.116
5.0	2.119	2.122	2.125	2.129	2.132	2.135	2.139	2.142	2.145	2.148
5.1	2.151	2.154	2.158	2.160	2.164	2.167	2.170	2.173	2.176	2.180
5.2	2.183	2.186	2.190	2.192	2.195	2.197	2.200	2.203	2.206	2.209
5.3	2.212	2.215	2.218	2.221	2.224	2.227	2.230	2.233	2.236	2.240
5.4	2.243	2.246	2.249	2.252	2.255	2.258	2.261	2.264	2.267	2.270
5.5	2.273	2.276	2.279	2.282	2.285	2.288	2.291	2.294	2.297	2.300
5.6	2.303	2.306	2.309	2.312	2.315	2.318	2.320	2.324	2.326	2.329
5.7	2.332	2.335	2.338	2.341	2.344	2.347	2.350	2.353	2.355	2.358
5.8	2.361	2.364	2.367	2.370	2.373	2.376	2.379	2.382	2.384	2.387
5.9	2.390	2.393	2.396	2.400	2.403	2.405	2.408	2.411	2.414	2.417
6.0	2.419	2.422	2.425	2.428	2.431	2.433	2.436	2.439	2.442	2.444
6.1	2.447	2.450	2.453	2.456	2.458	2.461	2.464	2.467	2.470	2.472
6.2	2.475	2.478	2.481	2.483	2.486	2.489	2.492	2.494	2.497	2.500
6.3	2.503	2.505	2.508	2.511	2.513	2.516	2.518	2.521	2.524	2.526
6.4	2.529	2.532	2.534	2.537	2.540	2.542	2.545	2.547	2.550	2.553
6.5	2.555	2.558	2.561	2.563	2.566	2.568	2.571	2.574	2.576	2.579
6.6	2.581	2.584	2.587	2.590	2.592	2.595	2.597	2.600	2.603	2.605
6.7	2.608	2.610	2.613	2.615	2.618	2.620	2.623	2.625	2.627	2.630
6.8	2.633	2.635	2.637	2.640	2.643	2.645	2.648	2.650	2.653	2.655
6.9	2.658	2.660	2.663	2.665	2.668	2.670	2.673	2.675	2.678	2.680
7.0	2.683	2.685	2.687	2.690	2.693	2.695	2.698	2.700	2.702	2.705
7.1	2.707	2.710	2.712	2.714	2.717	2.719	2.721	2.724	2.726	2.729
7.2	2.731	2.733	2.736	2.738	2.740	2.743	2.745	2.748	2.750	2.752
7.3	2.755	2.757	2.760	2.762	2.764	2.767	2.769	2.771	2.774	2.776
7.4	2.779	2.781	2.783	2.786	2.788	2.790	2.793	2.795	2.798	2.800
7.5	2.802	2.805	2.807	2.809	2.812	2.814	2.816	2.819	2.821	2.823
7.6	2.826	2.828	2.830	2.833	2.835	2.837	2.840	2.842	2.844	2.847
7.7	2.849	2.851	2.854	2.856	2.858	2.860	2.863	2.865	2.868	2.870
7.8	2.873	2.875	2.877	2.879	2.881	2.884	2.887	2.889	2.891	2.893
7.9	2.895	2.898	2.900	2.902	2.905	2.907	2.909	2.911	2.913	2.915
8.0	2.918	2.920	2.922	2.924	2.926	2.928	2.931	2.933	2.935	2.937
8.1	2.939	2.942	2.944	2.946	2.948	2.950	2.952	2.955	2.957	2.959
8.2	2.961	2.963	2.966	2.968	2.970	2.972	2.974	2.976	2.979	2.981
8.3	2.983	2.985	2.987	2.990	2.992	2.994	2.996	2.998	3.000	3.002
8.4	3.004	3.006	3.008	3.010	3.012	3.015	3.017	3.019	3.021	3.023
8.5	3.025	3.027	3.029	3.031	3.033	3.035	3.037	3.040	3.042	3.044

Intrinsic viscosity $[\eta]_c$ at different values of relative viscosity η_{rel}

	$[\eta]_c$									
η_{rel}	0.00	0.01	0.02	0.03	0.04	0.05	0.06	0.07	0.08	0.09
8.6	3.046	3.048	3.050	3.052	3.054	3.056	3.058	3.060	3.062	3.064
8.7	3.067	3.069	3.071	3.073	3.075	3.077	3.079	3.081	3.083	3.085
8.8	3.087	3.089	3.092	3.094	3.096	3.098	3.100	3.102	3.104	3.106
8.9	3.108	3.110	3.112	3.114	3.116	3.118	3.120	3.122	3.124	3.126
9.0	3.128	3.130	3.132	3.134	3.136	3.138	3.140	3.142	3.144	3.146
9.1	3.148	3.150	3.152	3.154	3.156	3.158	3.160	3.162	3.164	3.166
9.2	3.168	3.170	3.172	3.174	3.176	3.178	3.180	3.182	3.184	3.186
9.3	3.188	3.190	3.192	3.194	3.196	3.198	3.200	3.202	3.204	3.206
9.4	3.208	3.210	3.212	3.214	3.215	3.217	3.219	3.221	3.223	3.225
9.5	3.227	3.229	3.231	3.233	3.235	3.237	3.239	3.241	3.242	3.244
9.6	3.246	3.248	3.250	3.252	3.254	3.256	3.258	3.260	3.262	3.264
9.7	3.266	3.268	3.269	3.271	3.273	3.275	3.277	3.279	3.281	3.283
9.8	3.285	3.287	3.289	3.291	3.293	3.295	3.297	3.298	3.300	3.302
9.9	3.304	3.305	3.307	3.309	3.311	3.313	3.316	3.318	3.320	3.321

Intrinsic viscosity $[\eta]_c$ at different values of relative viscosity η_{rel}

	$[\eta]_c$									
η_{rel}	0.0	0.1	0.2	0.3	0.4	0.5	0.6	0.7	0.8	0.9
10	3.32	3.34	3.36	3.37	3.39	3.41	3.43	3.45	3.46	3.48
11	3.50	3.52	3.53	3.55	3.56	3.58	3.60	3.61	3.63	3.64
12	3.66	3.68	3.69	3.71	3.72	3.74	3.76	3.77	3.79	3.80
13	3.80	3.83	3.85	3.86	3.88	3.89	3.90	3.92	3.93	3.95
14	3.96	3.97	3.99	4.00	4.02	4.03	4.04	4.06	4.07	4.09
15	4.10	4.11	4.13	4.14	4.15	4.17	4.18	4.19	4.20	4.22
16	4.23	4.24	4.25	4.27	4.28	4.29	4.30	4.31	4.33	4.34
17	4.35	4.36	4.37	4.38	4.39	4.41	4.42	4.43	4.44	4.45
18	4.46	4.47	4.48	4.49	4.50	4.52	4.53	4.54	4.55	4.56
19	4.57	4.58	4.59	4.60	4.61	4.62	4.63	4.64	4.65	4.66

FUNCTIONALITY-RELATED CHARACTERISTICS

This section provides information on characteristics that are recognised as being relevant control parameters for one or more functions of the substance when used as an excipient. This section is a non-mandatory part of the monograph and it is not necessary to verify the characteristics to demonstrate compliance. Control of these characteristics can however contribute to the quality of a medicinal product by improving the consistency of the manufacturing process and the performance of the medicinal product during use. Where control methods are cited they are recognised as being suitable for the purpose but other methods can also be used. Wherever results for a particular characteristic are reported, the control method must be indicated.

The following characteristics may be relevant for powdered cellulose used as diluent or disintegrant.

Particle-size distribution (*2.9.31* or *2.9.38*).

Powder flow (*2.9.36*).

01/2008:1084
corrected 6.2

CETIRIZINE DIHYDROCHLORIDE

Cetirizini dihydrochloridum

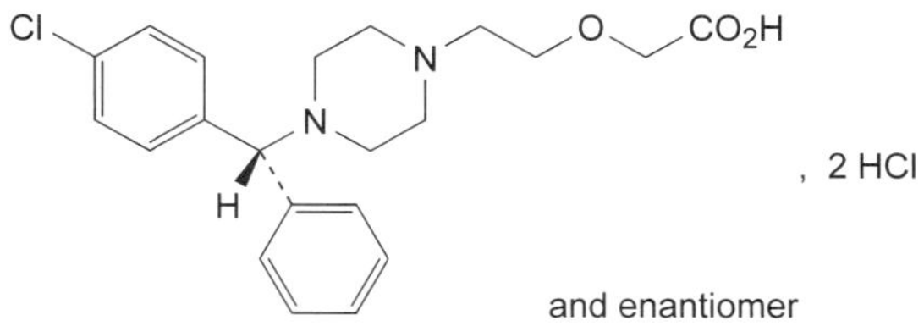

and enantiomer

$C_{21}H_{27}Cl_3N_2O_3$ M_r 461.8
[83881-52-1]

DEFINITION

(*RS*)-2-[2-[4-[(4-Chlorophenyl)phenylmethyl]piperazin-1-yl]ethoxy]acetic acid dihydrochloride.

Content: 99.0 per cent to 100.5 per cent (dried substance).

CHARACTERS

Appearance: white or almost white powder.

Solubility: freely soluble in water, practically insoluble in acetone and in methylene chloride.

IDENTIFICATION

First identification: B, D.

Second identification: A, C, D.

A. Ultraviolet and visible absorption spectrophotometry (*2.2.25*).

Test solution. Dissolve 20.0 mg in 50 ml of a 10.3 g/l solution of *hydrochloric acid R* and dilute to 100.0 ml with the same acid. Dilute 10.0 ml of this solution to 100.0 ml with a 10.3 g/l solution of *hydrochloric acid R.*

Spectral range: 210-350 nm.

Absorption maximum: at 231 nm.

Specific absorbance at the absorption maximum: 359 to 381.

B. Infrared absorption spectrophotometry (*2.2.24*).

Comparison: *cetirizine dihydrochloride CRS.*

C. Thin-layer chromatography (*2.2.27*).

Test solution. Dissolve 10 mg of the substance to be examined in *water R* and dilute to 5 ml with the same solvent.

Reference solution (a). Dissolve 10 mg of *cetirizine dihydrochloride CRS* in *water R* and dilute to 5 ml with the same solvent.

Reference solution (b). Dissolve 10 mg of *chlorphenamine maleate CRS* in *water R* and dilute to 5 ml with the same solvent. To 1 ml of the solution add 1 ml of reference solution (a).

Plate: *TLC silica gel GF_{254} plate R.*

Mobile phase: *ammonia R, methanol R, methylene chloride R* (1:10:90 *V/V/V*).

Application: 5 µl.

Development: over 2/3 of the plate.

Drying: in a current of cold air.

Detection: examine in ultraviolet light at 254 nm.

System suitability: reference solution (b):

- the chromatogram obtained shows 2 clearly separated spots.

Results: the principal spot in the chromatogram obtained with the test solution is similar in position and size to the principal spot in the chromatogram obtained with reference solution (a).

D. It gives reaction (a) of chlorides (*2.3.1*).

TESTS

Solution S. Dissolve 1.0 g in *carbon dioxide-free water R* and dilute to 20 ml with the same solvent.

Appearance of solution. Solution S is clear (*2.2.1*) and not more intensely coloured than reference solution BY_7 (*2.2.2, Method II*).

pH (*2.2.3*): 1.2 to 1.8 for solution S.

Related substances. Liquid chromatography (*2.2.29*).

Test solution. Dissolve 20.0 mg of the substance to be examined in the mobile phase and dilute to 100.0 ml with the mobile phase.

Reference solution (a). Dissolve 2 mg of *cetirizine dihydrochloride CRS* and 2 mg of *cetirizine impurity A CRS* in the mobile phase and dilute to 10.0 ml with the mobile phase. Dilute 1.0 ml of the solution to 100.0 ml with the mobile phase.

Reference solution (b). Dilute 2.0 ml of the test solution to 50.0 ml with the mobile phase. Dilute 5.0 ml of this solution to 100.0 ml with the mobile phase.

Column:

- *size*: *l* = 0.25 m, Ø = 4.6 mm;
- *stationary phase*: *silica gel for chromatography R* (5 µm).

Mobile phase: *dilute sulphuric acid R, water R, acetonitrile R* (0.4:6.6:93 *V/V/V*).

Flow rate: 1 ml/min.

Detection: spectrophotometer at 230 nm.

Injection: 20 µl.

Run time: 3 times the retention time of cetirizine.

System suitability: reference solution (a):

- *resolution*: minimum 3 between the peaks due to cetirizine and impurity A;
- *symmetry factors*: maximum 2.0.

Limits:

- *impurities A, B, C, D, E, F*: for each impurity, not more than 0.5 times the area of the principal peak in the chromatogram obtained with reference solution (b) (0.1 per cent);
- *unspecified impurities*: for each impurity, not more than 0.5 times the area of the principal peak in the chromatogram obtained with reference solution (b) (0.1 per cent);
- *total*: not more than 1.5 times the area of the principal peak in the chromatogram obtained with reference solution (b) (0.3 per cent);
- *disregard limit*: 0.1 times the area of the principal peak in the chromatogram obtained with reference solution (b) (0.02 per cent).

Loss on drying (*2.2.32*): maximum 0.5 per cent, determined on 1.000 g by drying in an oven at 105 °C.

Sulphated ash (*2.4.14*): maximum 0.2 per cent, determined on 1.0 g.

ASSAY

Dissolve 0.100 g in 70 ml of a mixture of 30 volumes of *water R* and 70 volumes of *acetone R.* Titrate with *0.1 M sodium hydroxide* to the 2nd point of inflexion. Determine the end-point potentiometrically (*2.2.20*). Carry out a blank titration.

1 ml of *0.1 M sodium hydroxide* is equivalent to 15.39 mg of $C_{21}H_{27}Cl_3N_2O_3$.

STORAGE

Protected from light.

IMPURITIES

Specified impurities: A, B, C, D, E, F.

Other detectable impurities (the following substances would, if present at a sufficient level, be detected by one or other of the tests in the monograph. They are limited by the general acceptance criterion for other/unspecified impurities and/or by the general monograph *Substances for pharmaceutical use (2034).* It is therefore not necessary to

Monographs A-C

identify these impurities for demonstration of compliance. See also *5.10. Control of impurities in substances for pharmaceutical use*): *G*.

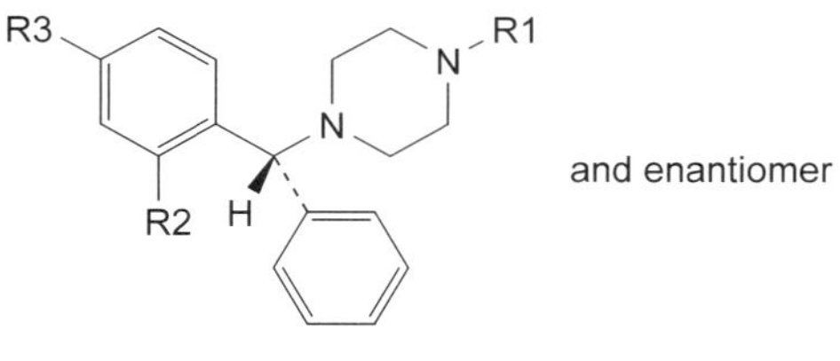

A. R1 = R2 = H, R3 = Cl: (*RS*)-1-[(4-chlorophenyl)phenylmethyl]piperazine,

B. R1 = CH_2-CO_2H, R2 = H, R3 = Cl: (*RS*)-2-[4-[(4-chlorophenyl)phenylmethyl]piperazin-1-yl]acetic acid,

C. R1 = CH_2-CH_2-O-CH_2-CO_2H, R2 = Cl, R3 = H: (*RS*)-2-[2-[4-[(2-chlorophenyl)phenylmethyl]piperazin-1-yl]ethoxy]acetic acid,

E. R1 = CH_2-[CH_2-O-CH_2]$_2$-CO_2H, R2 = H, R3 = Cl: (*RS*)-2-[2-[2-[4-[(4-chlorophenyl)phenylmethyl]piperazin-1-yl]ethoxy]ethoxy]acetic acid (ethoxycetirizine),

F. R1 = CH_2-CH_2-O-CH_2-CO_2H, R2 = R3 = H: [2-[4-(diphenylmethyl)piperazin-1-yl]ethoxy]acetic acid,

G. R1 = CH_2-CH_2-OH, R2 = H, R3 = Cl: 2-[4-[(*RS*)-(4-chlorophenyl)phenylmethyl]piperazin-1-yl]ethanol,

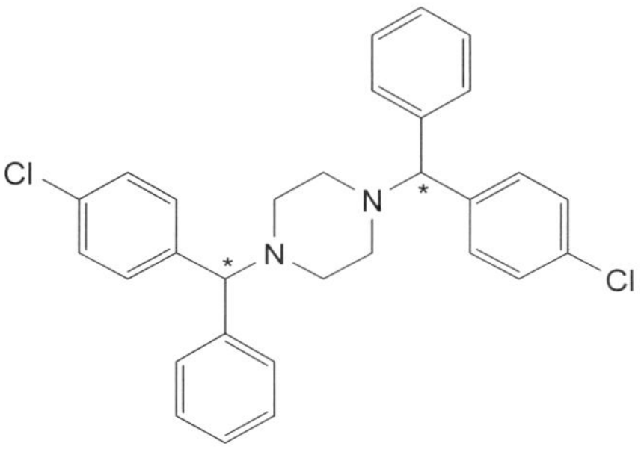

D. 1,4-bis[(4-chlorophenyl)phenylmethyl]piperazine.

07/2008:0801
corrected 6.2

CETOSTEARYL ALCOHOL (TYPE A), EMULSIFYING

Alcohol cetylicus et stearylicus emulsificans A

DEFINITION

Mixture of cetostearyl alcohol and sodium cetostearyl sulphate. A suitable buffer may be added.

Content:

– *cetostearyl alcohol*: minimum 80.0 per cent (anhydrous substance);
– *sodium cetostearyl sulphate*: minimum 7.0 per cent (anhydrous substance).

CHARACTERS

Appearance: white or pale yellow, waxy mass, plates, flakes or granules.

Solubility: soluble in hot water giving an opalescent solution, practically insoluble in cold water, slightly soluble in ethanol (96 per cent).

IDENTIFICATION

First identification: B, C, D.

Second identification: A, C.

A. Thin-layer chromatography (*2.2.27*).

Test solution (a). Dissolve 0.1 g of the substance to be examined in 10 ml of *trimethylpentane R*, heating on a water-bath. Shake with 2 ml of *ethanol (70 per cent V/V) R* and allow to separate. Use the lower layer as test solution (b). Dilute 1 ml of the upper layer to 8 ml with *trimethylpentane R*.

Test solution (b). Use the lower layer obtained in the preparation of test solution (a).

Reference solution (a). Dissolve 24 mg of *cetyl alcohol CRS* and 16 mg of *stearyl alcohol CRS* in 10 ml of *trimethylpentane R*.

Reference solution (b). Dissolve 20 mg of *sodium cetostearyl sulphate R* in 10 ml of *ethanol (70 per cent V/V) R*, heating on a water-bath.

Plate: *TLC silanised silica gel plate R*.

Mobile phase: *water R, acetone R, methanol R* (20:40:40 *V/V/V*).

Application: 2 µl.

Development: over a path of 12 cm.

Drying: in air.

Detection: spray with a 50 g/l solution of *phosphomolybdic acid R* in *ethanol (96 per cent) R*; heat at 120 °C until spots appear (about 3 h).

Results:

– the 2 principal spots in the chromatogram obtained with test solution (a) are similar in position and colour to the principal spots in the chromatogram obtained with reference solution (a);
– 2 of the spots in the chromatogram obtained with test solution (b) are similar in position and colour to the principal spots in the chromatogram obtained with reference solution (b).

B. Examine the chromatograms obtained in the assay.

Results: the 2 principal peaks in the chromatogram obtained with test solution (b) are similar in retention time to the 2 principal peaks in the chromatogram obtained with the reference solution.

C. It gives a yellow colour to a non-luminous flame.

D. To 0.3 g add 20 ml of *anhydrous ethanol R* and heat to boiling on a water-bath with shaking. Filter the mixture immediately, evaporate to dryness and take up the residue in 7 ml of *water R*. To 1 ml of the solution add 0.1 ml of a 1 g/l solution of *methylene blue R*, 2 ml of *dilute sulphuric acid R* and 2 ml of *methylene chloride R* and shake. A blue colour develops in the lower layer.

TESTS

Acid value (*2.5.1*): maximum 2.0.

Iodine value (*2.5.4, Method A*): maximum 3.0.

Dissolve 2.00 g in 25 ml of *methylene chloride R*.

Saponification value (*2.5.6*): maximum 2.0.

Water (*2.5.12*): maximum 3.0 per cent, determined on 2.50 g.

ASSAY

Cetostearyl alcohol. Gas chromatography (*2.2.28*).

Internal standard solution. Dissolve 0.60 g of *heptadecanol CRS* in *anhydrous ethanol R* and dilute to 150 ml with the same solvent.

Test solution (a). Dissolve 0.300 g of the substance to be examined in 50 ml of the internal standard solution, add 50 ml of *water R* and shake with 4 quantities, each of 25 ml, of *pentane R*, adding *sodium chloride R*, if necessary, to facilitate the separation of the layers. Combine the organic layers. Wash with 2 quantities, each of 30 ml, of *water R*, dry over *anhydrous sodium sulphate R* and filter.

Test solution (b). Dissolve 0.300 g of the substance to be examined in 50 ml of *anhydrous ethanol R*, add 50 ml of *water R* and shake with 4 quantities, each of 25 ml, of *pentane R*, adding *sodium chloride R*, if necessary, to facilitate the separation of the layers. Combine the organic layers. Wash with 2 quantities, each of 30 ml, of *water R*, dry over *anhydrous sodium sulphate R* and filter.

Reference solution. Dissolve 50 mg of *cetyl alcohol CRS* and 50 mg of *stearyl alcohol CRS* in *anhydrous ethanol R* and dilute to 10 ml with the same solvent.

Column:

- *material*: fused silica;
- *size*: l = 25 m, Ø = 0.25 mm;
- *stationary phase*: *poly(dimethyl)siloxane R.*

Carrier gas: *nitrogen for chromatography R.*

Flow rate: 1 ml/min.

Split ratio: 1:100.

Temperature:

	Time (min)	Temperature (°C)
Column	0 - 20	150 → 250
Injection port		250
Detector		250

Detection: flame ionisation.

Elution order: cetyl alcohol, heptadecanol, stearyl alcohol.

Inject 1 µl of test solution (a) and 1 µl of test solution (b). If the chromatogram obtained with test solution (b) shows a peak with the same retention time as the peak due to the internal standard in the chromatogram obtained with test solution (a), calculate the ratio r using the following expression:

$$\frac{S_{ci}}{S_i}$$

S_{ci} = area of the peak due to cetyl alcohol in the chromatogram obtained with test solution (b);

S_i = area of the peak with the same retention time as the peak due to the internal standard in the chromatogram obtained with test solution (a).

If r is less than 300, calculate the corrected area $S_{Ha(corr)}$ of the peak due to the internal standard in the chromatogram obtained with test solution (a) using the following expression:

$$S'_{Ha} - \frac{S_i \times S_c}{S_{ci}}$$

S'_{Ha} = area of the peak due to the internal standard in the chromatogram obtained with test solution (a);

S_c = area of the peak due to cetyl alcohol in the chromatogram obtained with test solution (a).

Inject, under the same conditions, equal volumes of the reference solution and of test solution (a). Identify the peaks in the chromatogram obtained with test solution (a) by comparing their retention times with those of the peaks in the chromatogram obtained with the reference solution and determine the area of each peak.

Calculate the percentage content of cetyl alcohol using the following expression:

$$S_A \frac{100 \times m_H}{S_{Ha(corr)} \times m}$$

S_A = area of the peak due to cetyl alcohol in the chromatogram obtained with test solution (a);

m_H = mass of the internal standard in test solution (a), in milligrams;

$S_{Ha(corr)}$ = corrected area of the peak due to the internal standard in the chromatogram obtained with test solution (a);

m = mass of the substance to be examined in test solution (a), in milligrams.

Calculate the percentage content of stearyl alcohol using the following expression:

$$S_B \frac{100 \times m_H}{S_{Ha(corr)} \times m}$$

S_B = area of the peak due to stearyl alcohol in the chromatogram obtained with test solution (a).

The percentage content of cetostearyl alcohol corresponds to the sum of the percentage content of cetyl alcohol and of stearyl alcohol.

Sodium cetostearyl sulphate. Disperse 0.300 g in 25 ml of *methylene chloride R.* Add 50 ml of *water R* and 10 ml of *dimidium bromide-sulphan blue mixed solution R.* Titrate with *0.004 M benzethonium chloride*, using sonication, heating and allowing the layers to separate before each addition, until the colour of the lower layer changes from pink to grey.

1 ml of *0.004 M benzethonium chloride* is equivalent to 1.434 mg of sodium cetostearyl sulphate.

LABELLING

The label states, where applicable, the name and concentration of any added buffer.

07/2008:0802
corrected 6.2

CETOSTEARYL ALCOHOL (TYPE B), EMULSIFYING

Alcohol cetylicus et stearylicus emulsificans B

DEFINITION

Mixture of cetostearyl alcohol and sodium laurilsulfate. A suitable buffer may be added.

Content:

- *cetostearyl alcohol*: minimum 80.0 per cent (anhydrous substance);
- *sodium laurilsulfate*: minimum 7.0 per cent (anhydrous substance).

CHARACTERS

Appearance: white or pale yellow, waxy mass, plates, flakes or granules.

Solubility: soluble in hot water giving an opalescent solution, practically insoluble in cold water, slightly soluble in ethanol (96 per cent).

IDENTIFICATION

First identification: B, C, D.

Second identification: A, C.

A. Thin-layer chromatography (*2.2.27*).

Test solution (a). Dissolve 0.1 g of the substance to be examined in 10 ml of *trimethylpentane R,* heating on a water-bath. Shake with 2 ml of *ethanol (70 per cent V/V) R* and allow to separate. Use the lower layer as test solution (b). Dilute 1 ml of the upper layer to 8 ml with *trimethylpentane R.*

Test solution (b). Use the lower layer obtained in the preparation of test solution (a).

Reference solution (a). Dissolve 24 mg of *cetyl alcohol CRS* and 16 mg of *stearyl alcohol CRS* in 10 ml of *trimethylpentane R.*

Reference solution (b). Dissolve 20 mg of *sodium laurilsulfate CRS* in 10 ml of *ethanol (70 per cent V/V) R,* heating on a water-bath.

Plate: *TLC silanised silica gel plate R.*

Mobile phase: *water R, acetone R, methanol R* (20:40:40 *V/V/V*).

Application: 2 µl.

Development: over a path of 12 cm.

Drying: in air.

Detection: spray with a 50 g/l solution of *phosphomolybdic acid R* in *ethanol (96 per cent) R*; heat at 120 °C until spots appear (about 3 h).

Results:

- the 2 principal spots in the chromatogram obtained with test solution (a) are similar in position and colour to the principal spots in the chromatogram obtained with reference solution (a);
- 1 of the spots in the chromatogram obtained with test solution (b) is similar in position and colour to the principal spot in the chromatogram obtained with reference solution (b).

B. Examine the chromatograms obtained in the assay.

Results: the 2 principal peaks in the chromatogram obtained with test solution (b) are similar in retention time to the 2 principal peaks in the chromatogram obtained with the reference solution.

C. It gives a yellow colour to a non-luminous flame.

D. To 0.3 g add 20 ml of *anhydrous ethanol R* and heat to boiling on a water-bath with shaking. Filter the mixture immediately, evaporate to dryness and take up the residue in 7 ml of *water R.* To 1 ml of the solution add 0.1 ml of a 1 g/l solution of *methylene blue R,* 2 ml of *dilute sulphuric acid R* and 2 ml of *methylene chloride R* and shake. A blue colour develops in the lower layer.

TESTS

Acid value (*2.5.1*): maximum 2.0.

Iodine value (*2.5.4, Method A*): maximum 3.0.

Dissolve 2.00 g in 25 ml of *methylene chloride R.*

Saponification value (*2.5.6*): maximum 2.0.

Water (*2.5.12*): maximum 3.0 per cent, determined on 2.50 g.

ASSAY

Cetostearyl alcohol. Gas chromatography (*2.2.28*).

Internal standard solution. Dissolve 0.60 g of *heptadecanol CRS* in *anhydrous ethanol R* and dilute to 150 ml with the same solvent.

Test solution (a). Dissolve 0.300 g of the substance to be examined in 50 ml of the internal standard solution, add 50 ml of *water R* and shake with 4 quantities, each of 25 ml, of *pentane R,* adding *sodium chloride R,* if necessary, to facilitate the separation of the layers. Combine the organic layers. Wash with 2 quantities, each of 30 ml, of *water R,* dry over *anhydrous sodium sulphate R* and filter.

Test solution (b). Dissolve 0.300 g of the substance to be examined in 50 ml of *anhydrous ethanol R,* add 50 ml of *water R* and shake with 4 quantities, each of 25 ml, of *pentane R,* adding *sodium chloride R,* if necessary, to facilitate the separation of the layers. Combine the organic layers. Wash with 2 quantities, each of 30 ml, of *water R,* dry over *anhydrous sodium sulphate R* and filter.

Reference solution. Dissolve 50 mg of *cetyl alcohol CRS* and 50 mg of *stearyl alcohol CRS* in *anhydrous ethanol R* and dilute to 10 ml with the same solvent.

Column:

- *material*: fused silica;
- *size*: l = 25 m, Ø = 0.25 mm;
- *stationary phase*: *poly(dimethyl)siloxane R.*

Carrier gas: *nitrogen for chromatography R.*

Flow rate: 1 ml/min.

Split ratio: 1:100.

Temperature:

	Time (min)	Temperature (°C)
Column	0 - 20	150 → 250
Injection port		250
Detector		250

Detection: flame ionisation.

Elution order: cetyl alcohol, heptadecanol, stearyl alcohol.

Inject 1 µl of test solution (a) and 1 µl of test solution (b). If the chromatogram obtained with test solution (b) shows a peak with the same retention time as the peak due to the internal standard in the chromatogram obtained with test solution (a), calculate the ratio r using the following expression:

$$\frac{S_{ci}}{S_i}$$

S_{ci} = area of the peak due to cetyl alcohol in the chromatogram obtained with test solution (b);

S_i = area of the peak with the same retention time as the peak due to the internal standard in the chromatogram obtained with test solution (a).

If r is less than 300, calculate the corrected area $S_{Ha(corr)}$ of the peak due to the internal standard in the chromatogram obtained with test solution (a) using the following expression:

$$S'_{Ha} - \frac{S_i \times S_c}{S_{ci}}$$

S'_{Ha} = area of the peak due to the internal standard in the chromatogram obtained with test solution (a);

S_c = area of the peak due to cetyl alcohol in the chromatogram obtained with test solution (a).

Inject, under the same conditions, equal volumes of the reference solution and of test solution (a). Identify the peaks in the chromatogram obtained with test solution (a) by comparing their retention times with those of the peaks in the chromatogram obtained with the reference solution and determine the area of each peak.

Calculate the percentage content of cetyl alcohol using the following expression:

$$S_A \frac{100 \times m_H}{S_{Ha(corr)} \times m}$$

S_A = area of the peak due to cetyl alcohol in the chromatogram obtained with test solution (a);

m_H = mass of the internal standard in test solution (a), in milligrams;

$S_{Ha(corr)}$ = corrected area of the peak due to the internal standard in the chromatogram obtained with test solution (a);

m = mass of the substance to be examined in test solution (a), in milligrams.

Calculate the percentage content of stearyl alcohol using the following expression:

$$S_B \frac{100 \times m_H}{S_{Ha(corr)} \times m}$$

S_B = area of the peak due to stearyl alcohol in the chromatogram obtained with test solution (a).

The percentage content of cetostearyl alcohol corresponds to the sum of the percentage content of cetyl alcohol and of stearyl alcohol.

Sodium laurilsulfate. Disperse 0.300 g in 25 ml of *methylene chloride R*. Add 50 ml of *water R* and 10 ml of *dimidium bromide-sulphan blue mixed solution R*. Titrate with *0.004 M benzethonium chloride*, using sonication, heating, and allowing the layers to separate before each addition, until the colour of the lower layer changes from pink to grey. 1 ml of *0.004 M benzethonium chloride* is equivalent to 1.154 mg of sodium laurilsulfate.

LABELLING

The label states, where applicable, the name and concentration of any added buffer.

07/2008:0174

CINCHONA BARK

Cinchonae cortex

DEFINITION

Whole or cut, dried bark of *Cinchona pubescens* Vahl (*Cinchona succirubra* Pav.), of *Cinchona calisaya* Wedd., of *Cinchona ledgeriana* Moens ex Trimen or of their varieties or hybrids.

Content: minimum 6.5 per cent of total alkaloids, of which 30 per cent to 60 per cent consists of quinine-type alkaloids (dried drug).

CHARACTERS

Intense bitter, somewhat astringent taste.

IDENTIFICATION

A. The stem and branch bark is supplied in quilled or curved pieces 2-6 mm thick. The outer surface is dull brownish-grey or grey and frequently bears lichens; it is usually rough, marked with transverse fissures and longitudinally furrowed or wrinkled; exfoliation of the outer surface occurs in some varieties. The inner surface is striated and deep reddish-brown; the fracture is short in the outer part and fibrous in the inner part.

B. Reduce to a powder (355) (*2.9.12*). The powder is reddish-brown. Examine under a microscope using *chloral hydrate solution R*. The powder shows the following diagnostic characters: thin-walled cork cells filled with reddish-brown contents; yellow, spindle-shaped striated phloem fibres up to 90 μm in diameter and up to 1300 μm in length, very thick-walled with an uneven lumen and with conspicuous, funnel-shaped pits; parenchymatous idioblasts filled with microprisms of calcium oxalate; clusters of thin-walled phloem parenchyma cells. Examine under a microscope using a 50 per cent *V/V* solution of *glycerol R*. The powder shows a few starch granules 6-10 μm in diameter; mostly simple but occasionally with 2 or 3 components.

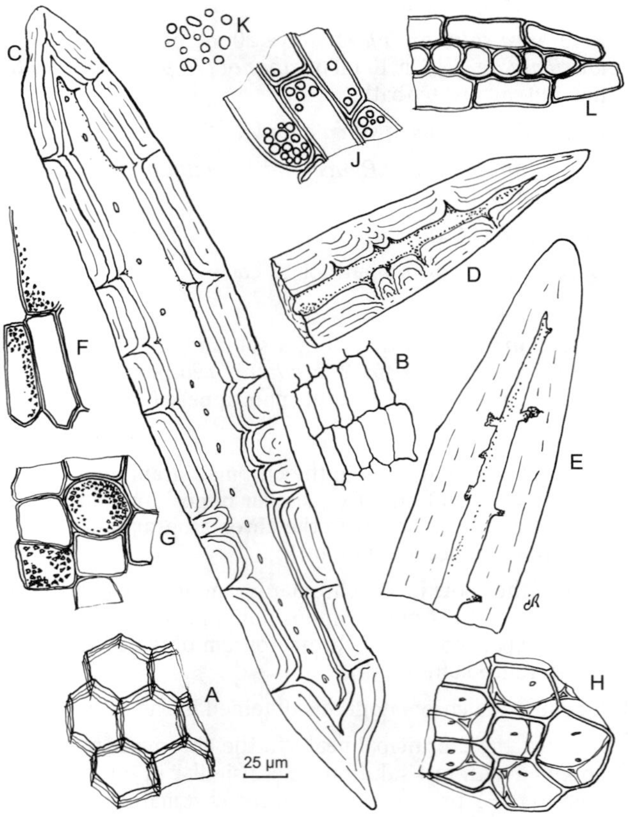

A, B. Cork cells in surface view (A) and in transverse section (B)

C, D, E. Phloem fibres

F, G. Parenchymatous idioblasts filled with microprisms of calcium oxalate

H. Parenchymatous cells

J. Parenchymatous cells containing starch granules

K. Starch granules

L. Phloem parenchyma with medullary ray in tangential section

Figure 0174.-1. – *Illustration of powdered herbal drug of cinchona bark (see Identification B)*

C. Thin-layer chromatography (*2.2.27*).

Test solution. To 0.10 g of the powdered drug (180) (*2.9.12*) in a test-tube add 0.1 ml of *concentrated ammonia R* and 5 ml of *methylene chloride R*. Shake vigorously occasionally during 30 min and filter. Evaporate the filtrate to dryness on a water-bath and dissolve the residue in 1 ml of *anhydrous ethanol R*.

Reference solution. Dissolve 17.5 mg of *quinine R*, 2.5 mg of *quinidine R*, 10 mg of *cinchonine R* and 10 mg of *cinchonidine R* in 5 ml of *anhydrous ethanol R*.

Plate: *TLC silica gel plate R*.

Mobile phase: *diethylamine R, ethyl acetate R, toluene R* (10:20:70 *V/V/V*).

Application: 10 µl, as bands.

Development: twice over a path of 15 cm.

Drying: at 100-105 °C, then allow to cool.

Detection A: spray with *anhydrous formic acid R* and allow to dry in air; examine in ultraviolet light at 365 nm.

Results A: see below the sequence of zones present in the chromatograms obtained with the reference solution and the test solution. Furthermore, other fluorescent zones are present in the chromatogram obtained with the test solution.

Top of the plate	
_______	_______
Quinidine: a distinct blue fluorescent zone	A distinct blue fluorescent zone (quinidine)
_______	_______
Quinine: a distinct blue fluorescent zone	A distinct blue fluorescent zone (quinine)
Reference solution	**Test solution**

Detection B: spray with *iodoplatinate reagent R*.

Results B: see below the sequence of zones present in the chromatograms obtained with the reference solution and the test solution. Furthermore, other zones are present in the chromatogram obtained with the test solution.

Top of the plate	
_______	_______
Cinchonine: a violet zone that becomes violet-grey	A violet zone that becomes violet-grey (cinchonine)
Quinidine: a violet zone that becomes violet-grey	A violet zone that becomes violet-grey (quinidine)
Cinchonidine: an intense dark blue zone	An intense dark blue zone (cinchonidine)
_______	_______
Quinine: a violet zone that becomes violet-grey	A violet zone that becomes violet-grey (quinine)
Reference solution	**Test solution**

TESTS

Total ash (*2.4.16*): maximum 6.0 per cent.

Loss on drying (*2.2.32*): maximum 10 per cent, determined on 1.000 g of the powdered drug (355) (*2.9.12*) by drying in an oven at 105 °C for 2 h.

ASSAY

Test solution. In a 250 ml conical flask mix 1.000 g of the powdered drug (180) (*2.9.12*) with 10 ml of *water R* and 7 ml of *dilute hydrochloric acid R*. Heat in a water-bath for 30 min, allow to cool and add 25 ml of *methylene chloride R*, 50 ml of *ether R* and 5 ml of a 200 g/l solution of *sodium hydroxide R*. Shake the mixture repeatedly for 30 min, add 3 g of powdered *tragacanth R* and shake until the mixture becomes clear. Filter through a plug of absorbent cotton and rinse the flask and the cotton with 5 quantities, each of 20 ml, of a mixture of 1 volume of *methylene chloride R* and 2 volumes of *ether R*. Combine the filtrate and washings, evaporate to dryness and dissolve the residue in 10.0 ml of *anhydrous ethanol R*. Evaporate 5.0 ml of this solution to dryness, dissolve the residue in *0.1 M hydrochloric acid* and dilute to 1000.0 ml with the same acid.

Reference solutions. Dissolve separately 30.0 mg of *quinine R* and 30.0 mg of *cinchonine R* in *0.1 M hydrochloric acid* and dilute each solution to 1000.0 ml with the same acid.

Measure the absorbances (*2.2.25*) of the 3 solutions at 316 nm and 348 nm using *0.1 M hydrochloric acid* as the compensation liquid.

Calculate the percentage content of alkaloids using the following equations:

$$x = \frac{[A_{316} \times A_{348c}] - [A_{316c} \times A_{348}]}{[A_{316q} \times A_{348c}] - [A_{316c} \times A_{348q}]} \times \frac{100}{m} \times \frac{2}{1000}$$

$$y = \frac{[A_{316} \times A_{348q}] - [A_{316q} \times A_{348}]}{[A_{316c} \times A_{348q}] - [A_{316q} \times A_{348c}]} \times \frac{100}{m} \times \frac{2}{1000}$$

m = mass of the drug used, in grams;

x = percentage content of quinine-type alkaloids;

y = percentage content of cinchonine-type alkaloids;

A_{316} = absorbance of the test solution at 316 nm;

A_{348} = absorbance of the test solution at 348 nm;

A_{316c} = absorbance of the reference solution containing cinchonine at 316 nm, corrected to a concentration of 1 mg/1000 ml;

A_{316q} = absorbance of the reference solution containing quinine at 316 nm, corrected to a concentration of 1 mg/1000 ml;

A_{348c} = absorbance of the reference solution containing cinchonine at 348 nm, corrected to a concentration of 1 mg/1000 ml;

A_{348q} = absorbance of the reference solution containing quinine at 348 nm, corrected to a concentration of 1 mg/1000 ml.

Calculate the content of total alkaloids ($x + y$), and calculate the relative content of quinine-type alkaloids using the following expression:

$$\frac{100x}{x + y}$$

01/2008:1501

CINNAMON BARK OIL, CEYLON

Cinnamomi zeylanicii corticis aetheroleum

DEFINITION

Essential oil obtained by steam distillation of the bark of the shoots of *Cinnamomum zeylanicum* Nees (*C. Verum* J.S. Presl.).

CHARACTERS

Appearance: clear, mobile, light yellow liquid becoming reddish over time.

It has a characteristic odour reminiscent of cinnamic aldehyde.

Monographs A-C

IDENTIFICATION

First identification: B.

Second identification: A.

A. Thin-layer chromatography (*2.2.27*).

Test solution. Dissolve 1 ml of the essential oil to be examined in *acetone R* and dilute to 10 ml with the same solvent.

Reference solution. Dissolve 50 µl of *trans-cinnamic aldehyde R,* 10 µl of *eugenol R,* 10 µl of *linalol R* and 10 µl of *β-caryophyllene R* in *ethanol (96 per cent) R* and dilute to 10 ml with the same solvent.

Plate: *TLC silica gel plate R.*

Mobile phase: *methanol R, toluene R* (10:90 *V/V*).

Application: 10 µl as bands.

Development: over a path of 15 cm.

Drying: in air.

Detection: spray with *anisaldehyde solution R*; examine in daylight while heating at 100-105 °C for 5-10 min.

Results: the zones in the chromatogram obtained with the test solution are similar in position and colour to those in the chromatogram obtained with the reference solution.

B. Examine the chromatograms obtained in the test for chromatographic profile.

Results: the principal peaks in the chromatogram obtained with the test solution are similar in retention time to those in the chromatogram obtained with the reference solution. Safrole, coumarin and cineole may be absent from the chromatogram obtained with the test solution.

TESTS

Relative density (*2.2.5*): 1.000 to 1.030.

Refractive index (*2.2.6*): 1.572 to 1.591.

Optical rotation (*2.2.7*): − 2° to + 1°.

Chromatographic profile. Gas chromatography (*2.2.28*): use the normalisation procedure.

Test solution. The essential oil to be examined.

Reference solution. Dissolve 10 µl of *cineole R,* 10 µl of *linalol R,* 10 µl of *β-caryophyllene R,* 10 µl of *safrole R,* 100 µl of *trans-cinnamic aldehyde R,* 10 µl of *eugenol R,* 20 mg of *coumarin R,* 10 µl of *trans-2-methoxycinnamaldehyde R* and 10 µl of *benzyl benzoate R* in 1 ml of *acetone R.*

Column:
- *material*: fused silica;
- *size*: *l* = 60 m, Ø = 0.25 mm;
- *stationary phase*: bonded *macrogol 20 000 R.*

Carrier gas: *helium for chromatography R.*

Flow rate: 1.5 ml/min.

Split ratio: 1:100.

Temperature:

	Time (min)	Temperature (°C)
Column	0 - 10	60
	10 - 75	60 → 190
	75 - 200	190
Injection port		200
Detector		240

Detection: flame ionisation.

Injection: 0.2 µl.

Elution order: order indicated in the composition of the reference solution; depending on the operating conditions and the state of the column, coumarin may elute before or after *trans*-2-methoxycinnamaldehyde; record the retention times of these substances.

System suitability: reference solution:
- *resolution*: minimum 1.5 between the peaks due to linalol and β-caryophyllene.

Identification of components: using the retention times determined from the chromatogram obtained with the reference solution, locate the components of the reference solution in the chromatogram obtained with the test solution.

Determine the percentage content of each of these components. The percentages are within the following ranges:
- *cineole*: less than 3.0 per cent;
- *linalol*: 1.0 per cent to 6.0 per cent;
- *β-caryophyllene*: 1.0 per cent to 4.0 per cent;
- *safrole*: less than 0.5 per cent;
- *trans-cinnamic aldehyde*: 55 per cent to 75 per cent;
- *eugenol*: less than 7.5 per cent;
- *coumarin*: less than 0.5 per cent;
- *trans-2-methoxycinnamaldehyde*: 0.1 per cent to 1.0 per cent;
- *benzyl benzoate*: less than 1.0 per cent.

STORAGE

Protected from heat.

07/2008:1777

CLODRONATE DISODIUM TETRAHYDRATE

Dinatrii clodronas tetrahydricus

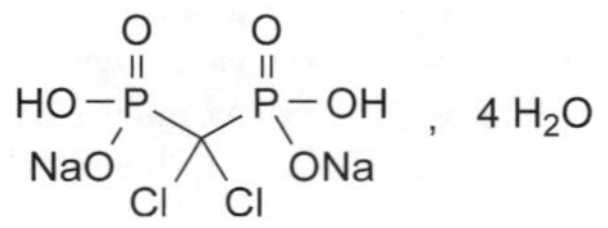

$CH_2Cl_2Na_2O_6P_2,4H_2O$ M_r 360.9

DEFINITION

Disodium (dichloromethylene)bis(hydrogen phosphonate) tetrahydrate.

Content: 99.0 per cent to 101.0 per cent (anhydrous substance).

CHARACTERS

Appearance: white or almost white, crystalline powder.

Solubility: freely soluble in water, practically insoluble in ethanol (96 per cent), slightly soluble in methanol.

IDENTIFICATION

A. Infrared absorption spectrophotometry (*2.2.24*).

Comparison: *clodronate disodium tetrahydrate CRS.*

B. Dissolve 0.5 g in 10 ml of *water R.* The solution gives reaction (a) of sodium (*2.3.1*).

TESTS

Solution S. Dissolve 1.0 g in *carbon dioxide-free water R* and dilute to 20 ml with the same solvent.

Appearance of solution. Solution S is clear (*2.2.1*) and colourless (*2.2.2, Method II*).

pH (*2.2.3*): 3.0 to 4.5, for solution S.

Related substances. Liquid chromatography (*2.2.29*).

Test solution. Dissolve 0.125 g of the substance to be examined in 30 ml of *water R*, sonicate for 10 min and dilute to 50.0 ml with *water R* (*test stock solution*). Dilute 10.0 ml of the test stock solution to 20.0 ml of *water R*.

Reference solution (a). Dilute 1.0 ml of the test solution to 10.0 ml with *water R*. Dilute 1.0 ml of this solution to 50.0 ml with *water R*.

Reference solution (b). Dissolve 1 mg of *clodronate impurity D CRS* in 10 ml of *water R*, sonicate for 10 min and dilute to 20.0 ml with *water R*. Mix 2.0 ml of this solution with 10.0 ml of the test stock solution and dilute to 20.0 ml with *water R*.

Reference solution (c). Dilute 1.0 ml of a 0.3 g/l solution of *phosphoric acid R* (impurity B) to 100.0 ml with *water R*.

Precolumn:
- *size*: l = 0.05 m, Ø = 4 mm;
- *stationary phase*: *anion exchange resin R*;
- *particle size*: 9 μm.

Column:
- *size*: l = 0.25 m, Ø = 4 mm;
- *stationary phase*: *anion exchange resin R*;
- *particle size*: 9 μm.

Mobile phase:
- *mobile phase A*: 0.21 g/l solution of *sodium hydroxide R* in *carbon dioxide-free water R*; close immediately, mix and use under helium pressure;
- *mobile phase B*: 4.2 g/l solution of *sodium hydroxide R* in *carbon dioxide-free water R*; close immediately, mix and use under helium pressure;

Time (min)	Mobile phase A (per cent *V/V*)	Mobile phase B (per cent *V/V*)
0 - 10	90 → 60	10 → 40
10 - 22	60 → 50	40 → 50
22 - 23	50 → 20	50 → 80
23 - 25	20	80

Flow rate: 1 ml/min.

Detection: conductivity detector. Use a self-regenerating anion suppressor.

Injection: 20 μl.

Identification of impurities: use the chromatogram obtained with reference solution (c) to identify the peak due to impurity B.

Relative retention with reference to clodronate (retention time = about 13 min): impurities A and B = about 0.7; impurity D = about 1.1.

System suitability: reference solution (b):
- *peak-to-valley ratio*: minimum 3, where H_p = height above the baseline of the peak due to impurity D and H_v = height above the baseline of the lowest point of the curve separating this peak from the peak due to clodronate.

Limits:
- *sum of impurities A and B*: not more than the area of the principal peak in the chromatogram obtained with reference solution (a) (0.2 per cent);
- *unspecified impurities*: for each impurity, not more than 0.5 times the area of the principal peak in the chromatogram obtained with reference solution (a) (0.10 per cent);
- *total*: not more than 1.5 times the area of the principal peak in the chromatogram obtained with reference solution (a) (0.3 per cent);
- *disregard limit*: 0.25 times the area of the principal peak in the chromatogram obtained with reference solution (a) (0.05 per cent).

Heavy metals (*2.4.8*): maximum 20 ppm.

0.5 g complies with test G. Prepare the reference solution using 1 ml of *lead standard solution (10 ppm Pb) R*.

Water (*2.5.12*): 18.5 per cent to 21.0 per cent, determined on 0.100 g.

ASSAY

Dissolve 0.140 g in 10 ml of *water R*. Add 10 ml of *concentrated sodium hydroxide solution R* and some glass beads. Boil until the solution is completely decolourised (about 10 min). Cool in an ice-bath and add 30 ml of *water R* and 10 ml of *nitric acid R*. Titrate with *0.1 M silver nitrate*, determining the end-point potentiometrically (*2.2.20*).

1 ml of *0.1 M silver nitrate* is equivalent to 14.44 mg of $CH_2Cl_2Na_2O_6P_2$.

IMPURITIES

Specified impurities: *A, B.*

Other detectable impurities (the following substances would, if present at a sufficient level, be detected by one or other of the tests in the monograph. They are limited by the general acceptance criterion for other/unspecified impurities and/or by the general monograph *Substances for pharmaceutical use (2034)*. It is therefore not necessary to identify these impurities for demonstration of compliance. See also *5.10. Control of impurities in substances for pharmaceutical use*): *D*.

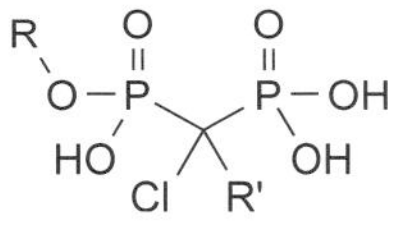

A. R = $CH(CH_3)_2$, R' = Cl: [dichloro[hydroxy(1-methylethoxy)phosphinoyl]methyl]phosphonic acid,

D. R = R' = H: (chloromethylene)bis(phosphonic acid),

B. phosphoric acid.

01/2008:1410

COCONUT OIL, REFINED

Cocois oleum raffinatum

[8001-31-8]

DEFINITION

Fatty oil obtained from the dried, solid part of the endosperm of *Cocos nucifera* L., then refined.

CHARACTERS

Appearance: white or almost white, unctuous mass.

Solubility: practically insoluble in water, freely soluble in methylene chloride and in light petroleum (bp: 65-70 °C), very slightly soluble in ethanol (96 per cent).

Refractive index: about 1.449, determined at 40 °C.

IDENTIFICATION

A. Melting point (see Tests).

B. Composition of fatty acids (see Tests).

TESTS

Melting point (*2.2.14*): 23 °C to 26 °C.

Acid value (*2.5.1*): maximum 0.5, determined on 20.0 g.

Peroxide value (*2.5.5, Method A*): maximum 5.0.

Unsaponifiable matter (*2.5.7*): maximum 1.0 per cent, determined on 5.0 g.

Alkaline impurities in fatty oils (*2.4.19*). It complies with the test.

Composition of fatty acids (*2.4.22, Method B*). Refined coconut oil is melted under gentle heating to a homogeneous liquid prior to sampling.

Reference solution. Dissolve 15.0 mg of *tricaproin CRS,* 80.0 mg of *tristearin CRS,* 0.150 g of *tricaprin CRS,* 0.200 g of *tricaprylin CRS,* 0.450 g of *trimyristin CRS* and 1.25 g of *trilaurin CRS* in a mixture of 2 volumes of *methylene chloride R* and 8 volumes of *heptane R,* then dilute to 50 ml with the same mixture of solvents heating at 45-50 °C. Transfer 2 ml of this mixture to a 10 ml centrifuge tube with a screw cap and evaporate the solvent in a current of *nitrogen R.* Dissolve with 1 ml of *heptane R* and 1 ml of *dimethyl carbonate R* and mix vigorously under gentle heating (50-60 °C). Add, while still warm, 1 ml of a 12 g/l solution of *sodium R* in *anhydrous methanol R,* prepared with the necessary precautions, and mix vigorously for about 5 min. Add 3 ml of *distilled water R* and mix vigorously for about 30 s. Centrifuge for 15 min at 1500 *g*. Inject 1 µl of the organic phase.

Calculate the percentage content of each fatty acid using the following expression:

$$\frac{A_{x,s,c}}{\sum A_{x,s,c}} \times 100 \text{ per cent } m/m$$

$A_{x,s,c}$ is the corrected peak area of each fatty acid in the test solution:

$$A_{x,s,c} = A_{x,s} \times R_c$$

R_c is the relative correction factor:

$$R_c = \frac{m_{x,r} \times A_{1,r}}{A_{x,r} \times m_{1,r}}$$

for the peaks due to caproic, caprylic, capric, lauric and myristic acid methyl esters.

$m_{x,r}$ = mass of tricaproin, tricaprylin, tricaprin, trilaurin or trimyristin in the reference solution, in milligrams;

$m_{1,r}$ = mass of tristearin in the reference solution, in milligrams:

$A_{x,r}$ = area of the peaks due to caproic, caprylic, capric, lauric and myristic acid methyl esters in the reference solution;

$A_{1,r}$ = area of the peak due to stearic acid methyl ester in the reference solution;

$A_{x,s}$ = area of the peaks due to any specified or unspecified fatty acid methyl esters;

R_c = 1 for the peaks due to each of the remaining specified fatty acid methyl esters or any unspecified fatty acid methyl ester.

Composition of the fatty-acid fraction of the oil:

- *caproic acid (R_{Rt} 0.11)*: maximum 1.5 per cent;
- *caprylic acid (R_{Rt} 0.23)*: 5.0 per cent to 11.0 per cent;
- *capric acid (R_{Rt} 0.56)*: 4.0 per cent to 9.0 per cent;
- *lauric acid (R_{Rt} 0.75)*: 40.0 per cent to 50.0 per cent;
- *myristic acid (R_{Rt} 0.85)*: 15.0 per cent to 20.0 per cent;
- *palmitic acid (R_{Rt} 0.93)*: 7.0 per cent to 12.0 per cent;
- *stearic acid (R_{Rt} 1.00)*: 1.5 per cent to 5.0 per cent;
- *oleic acid and isomers (R_{Rt} 1.01)*: 4.0 per cent to 10.0 per cent;
- *linoleic acid (R_{Rt} 1.03)*: 1.0 per cent to 3.0 per cent;
- *linolenic acid (R_{Rt} 1.06)*: maximum 0.2 per cent;
- *arachidic acid (R_{Rt} 1.10)*: maximum 0.2 per cent;
- *eicosenoic acid (R_{Rt} 1.11)*: maximum 0.2 per cent.

STORAGE

In a well-filled container, protected from light.

01/2008:1305
corrected 6.2

COTTONSEED OIL, HYDROGENATED

Gossypii oleum hydrogenatum

DEFINITION

Product obtained by refining and hydrogenation of oil obtained from seeds of cultivated plants of various varieties of *Gossypium hirsutum* L. or of other species of *Gossypium*. The product consists mainly of triglycerides of palmitic and stearic acids.

CHARACTERS

Appearance: white or almost white mass or powder which melts to a clear, pale yellow liquid when heated.

Solubility: practically insoluble in water, freely soluble in methylene chloride and in toluene, very slightly soluble in ethanol (96 per cent).

IDENTIFICATION

A. Melting point (see Tests).

B. Composition of fatty acids (see Tests).

TESTS

Melting point (*2.2.14*): 57 °C to 70 °C.

Acid value (*2.5.1*): maximum 0.5.

Dissolve 10.0 g in 50 ml of a hot mixture of equal volumes of *ethanol (96 per cent) R* and *toluene R,* previously neutralised with *0.1 M potassium hydroxide* using 0.5 ml of *phenolphthalein solution R1* as indicator. Titrate the solution immediately while still hot.

Peroxide value (*2.5.5, Method A*): maximum 5.0.

Unsaponifiable matter (*2.5.7*): maximum 1.0 per cent, determined on 5.0 g.

Alkaline impurities. Dissolve by gentle heating 2.0 g in a mixture of 1.5 ml of *ethanol (96 per cent) R* and 3 ml of *toluene R.* Add 0.05 ml of a 0.4 g/l solution of *bromophenol blue R* in *ethanol (96 per cent) R.* Not more than 0.4 ml of *0.01 M hydrochloric acid* is required to change the colour to yellow.

Composition of fatty acids (*2.4.22, Method A*). Use the mixture of calibrating substances in Table 2.4.22.-3.

Column:

- *material*: fused silica;
- *size*: *l* = 25 m, Ø = 0.25 mm;
- *stationary phase*: *poly(cyanopropyl)siloxane R* (film thickness 0.2 µm).

Monographs A-C

Carrier gas: *helium for chromatography R*.

Flow rate: 0.65 ml/min.

Split ratio: 1:100.

Temperature:

- *column*: 180 °C for 35 min;
- *injection port and detector*: 250 °C.

Detection: flame ionisation.

Composition of the fatty-acid fraction of the oil:

- *saturated fatty acids of chain length less than* C_{14}: maximum 0.2 per cent;
- *myristic acid*: maximum 1.0 per cent;
- *palmitic acid*: 19.0 per cent to 26.0 per cent;
- *stearic acid*: 68.0 per cent to 80.0 per cent;
- *oleic acid and isomers*: maximum 4.0 per cent;
- *linoleic acid and isomers*: maximum 1.0 per cent;
- *arachidic acid*: maximum 1.0 per cent;
- *behenic acid*: maximum 1.0 per cent;
- *lignoceric acid*: maximum 0.5 per cent.

Nickel: maximum 1.0 ppm.

Atomic absorption spectrometry (*2.2.23, Method II*).

Test solution. Introduce 5.0 g into a platinum or silica crucible tared after ignition. Cautiously heat and introduce into the substance a wick formed from twisted ashless filter paper. Ignite the wick. When the substance ignites, stop heating. After combustion, ignite in a muffle furnace at about 600 ± 50 °C. Continue the incineration until white ash is obtained. After cooling, take up the residue with 2 quantities, each of 2 ml, of *dilute hydrochloric acid R* and transfer into a 25 ml graduated flask. Add 0.3 ml of *nitric acid R* and dilute to 25.0 ml with *distilled water R*.

Reference solutions. Prepare 3 reference solutions by adding 1.0 ml, 2.0 ml and 4.0 ml of *nickel standard solution (0.2 ppm Ni) R* to 2.0 ml portions of the test solution, diluting to 10.0 ml with *distilled water R*.

Source: nickel hollow-cathode lamp.

Wavelength: 232 nm.

Atomisation device: graphite furnace.

Carrier gas: *argon R*.

STORAGE

Protected from light.

07/2008:1092

CYCLIZINE HYDROCHLORIDE

Cyclizini hydrochloridum

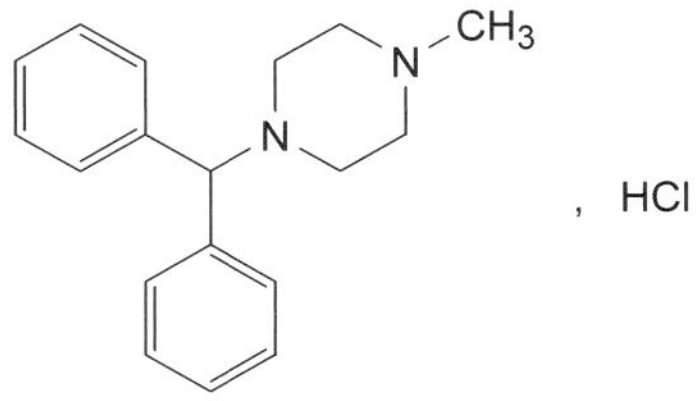

$C_{18}H_{23}ClN_2$ M_r 302.8

[305-25-3]

DEFINITION

1-(Diphenylmethyl)-4-methylpiperazine hydrochloride.

Content: 98.5 per cent to 101.0 per cent (dried substance).

CHARACTERS

Appearance: white or almost white, crystalline powder.

Solubility: slightly soluble in water and in ethanol (96 per cent).

IDENTIFICATION

First identification: B, E.

Second identification: A, C, D, E.

A. Ultraviolet and visible absorption spectrophotometry (*2.2.25*).

Test solution (a). Dissolve 20.0 mg in a 5 g/l solution of *sulphuric acid R* and dilute to 100.0 ml with the same acid solution.

Test solution (b). Dilute 10.0 ml of test solution (a) to 100.0 ml with a 5 g/l solution of *sulphuric acid R*.

Spectral range: 240-350 nm for test solution (a); 210-240 nm for test solution (b).

Resolution (*2.2.25*): minimum 1.7.

Absorption maxima: at 258 nm and 262 nm for test solution (a); at 225 nm for test solution (b).

Absorbance ratio: A_{262}/A_{258} = 1.0 to 1.1.

Specific absorbance at the absorption maximum at 225 nm: 370 to 410 for test solution (b).

B. Infrared absorption spectrophotometry (*2.2.24*).

Comparison: *cyclizine hydrochloride CRS.*

C. Thin-layer chromatography (*2.2.27*).

Test solution. Dissolve 10 mg of the substance to be examined in *methanol R* and dilute to 10 ml with the same solvent.

Reference solution. Dissolve 10 mg of *cyclizine hydrochloride CRS* in *methanol R* and dilute to 10 ml with the same solvent.

Plate: *TLC silica gel* GF_{254} *plate R*.

Mobile phase: *concentrated ammonia R, methanol R, methylene chloride R* (2:13:85 *V/V/V*).

Application: 20 µl.

Development: over 2/3 of the plate.

Drying: in air for 30 min.

Detection: expose to iodine vapour for 10 min.

Results: the principal spot in the chromatogram obtained with the test solution is similar in position, colour and size to the principal spot in the chromatogram obtained with the reference solution.

D. Dissolve 0.5 g in 10 ml of *ethanol (60 per cent) R*, heating if necessary. Cool in iced water. Add 1 ml of *dilute sodium hydroxide solution R* and 10 ml of *water R*. Filter, wash the precipitate with *water R* and dry at 60 °C at a pressure not exceeding 0.7 kPa for 2 h. The melting point (*2.2.14*) is 105 °C to 108 °C.

E. It gives reaction (a) of chlorides (*2.3.1*).

TESTS

pH (*2.2.3*): 4.5 to 5.5.

Dissolve 0.5 g in a mixture of 40 volumes of *ethanol (96 per cent) R* and 60 volumes of *carbon dioxide-free water R* and dilute to 25 ml with the same mixture of solvents.

Related substances. Gas chromatography (*2.2.28*). *Prepare the solutions immediately before use.*

Test solution. Dissolve 0.250 g of the substance to be examined in 4.0 ml of *methanol R* and dilute to 5.0 ml with *1 M sodium hydroxide.*

Monographs A-C

Reference solution (a). Dissolve 25 mg of the substance to be examined in 10.0 ml of *methanol R*. Dilute 1.0 ml of this solution to 50.0 ml with *methanol R*.

Reference solution (b). Dissolve 5 mg of the substance to be examined, 5.0 mg of *cyclizine impurity A CRS* and 5.0 mg of *cyclizine impurity B CRS* in *methanol R* and dilute to 20.0 ml with the same solvent.

Column:

- *material*: fused silica;
- *size*: l = 25 m, Ø = 0.33 mm;
- *stationary phase*: *poly(dimethyl)(diphenyl)siloxane R* (film thickness 0.50 μm).

Carrier gas: *helium for chromatography R*.

Flow rate: 1.0 ml/min.

Split ratio: 1:25.

Temperature:

	Time (min)	Temperature (°C)
Column	0 - 14	100 → 240
	14 - 16	240 → 270
	16 - 30	270
Injection port		250
Detector		290

Detection: flame ionisation.

Injection: 1 μl.

Relative retention with reference to cyclizine (retention time = about 15 min): impurity A = about 0.2; impurity B = about 0.7.

System suitability: reference solution (b):

- *peak-to-valley ratio*: minimum 50, where H_p = height above the baseline of the peak due to impurity A and H_v = height above the baseline of the lowest point of the curve separating this peak from the peak due to methanol.

Limits:

- *impurities A, B*: for each impurity, not more than the area of the corresponding peak in the chromatogram obtained with reference solution (b) (0.5 per cent);
- *unspecified impurities*: for each impurity, not more than the area of the principal peak in the chromatogram obtained with reference solution (a) (0.10 per cent);
- *total*: not more than 10 times the area of the principal peak in the chromatogram obtained with reference solution (a) (1.0 per cent);
- *disregard limit*: 0.5 times the area of the principal peak in the chromatogram obtained with reference solution (a) (0.05 per cent).

Loss on drying (*2.2.32*): maximum 1.0 per cent, determined on 1.000 g by drying in an oven at 130 °C.

Sulphated ash (*2.4.14*): maximum 0.1 per cent, determined on 1.0 g.

ASSAY

In order to avoid overheating in the reaction medium, mix thoroughly throughout and stop the titration immediately after the end-point has been reached.

Dissolve 0.120 g in 15 ml of *anhydrous formic acid R* and add 40 ml of *acetic anhydride R*. Titrate with *0.1 M perchloric acid*, determining the end-point potentiometrically (*2.2.20*).

1 ml of *0.1 M perchloric acid* is equivalent to 15.14 mg of $C_{18}H_{23}ClN_2$.

STORAGE

Protected from light.

IMPURITIES

Specified impurities: A, B.

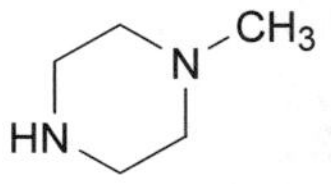

A. 1-methylpiperazine,

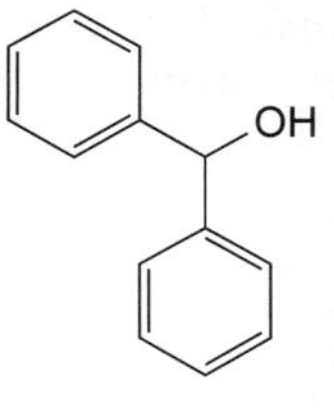

B. diphenylmethanol (benzhydrol).

D

07/2008:1095

DEVIL'S CLAW ROOT

Harpagophyti radix

DEFINITION

Devil's claw root consists of the cut and dried, tuberous secondary roots of *Harpagophytum procumbens* DC. and/or *Harpagophytum zeyheri* Decne.

Content: minimum 1.2 per cent of harpagoside ($C_{24}H_{30}O_{11}$; M_r 494.5) (dried drug).

CHARACTERS

Devil's claw root is greyish-brown to dark brown.

IDENTIFICATION

A. It consists of thick, fan-shaped or rounded slices or of roughly crushed discs. The darker outer surface is traversed by tortuous longitudinal wrinkles. The paler cut surface shows a dark cambial zone and xylem bundles distinctly aligned in radial rows. The central cylinder shows fine concentric striations. Seen under a lens, the cut surface presents yellow to brownish-red granules.

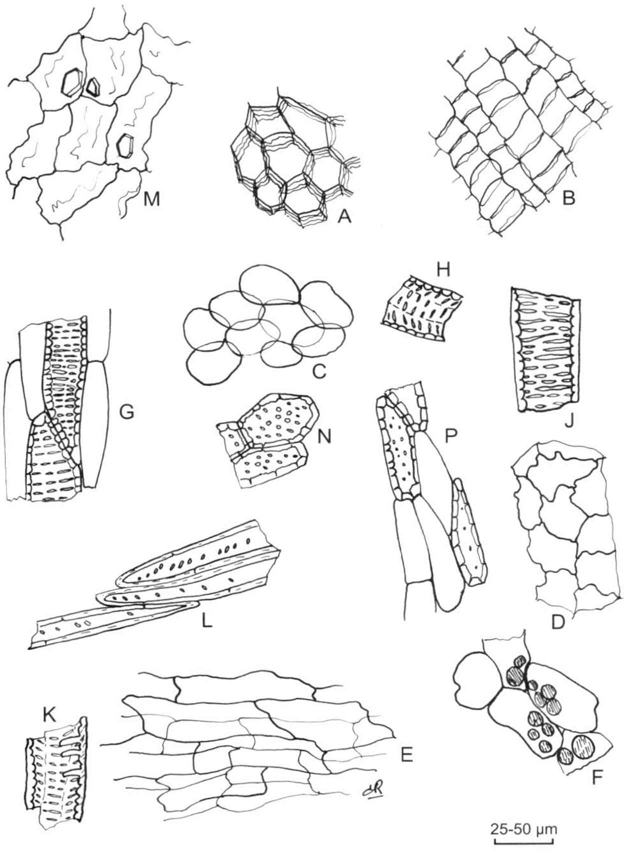

A, B. Fragments of cork layer in surface view (A) and in transverse section (B)

C, D, E, F. Fragments of cortical parenchyma; fragment containing yellow droplets (F)

G, H, J, K. Vessels with reticulate or pitted thickenings

L. Lignified parenchyma from the central cylinder

M. Parenchyma containing prisms of calcium oxalate

N, P. Rectangular or polygonal sclereids

Figure 1095.-1. – *Illustration of powdered herbal drug of devil's claw root (see identification B)*

B. Reduce to a powder (355) (*2.9.12*). The powder is brownish-yellow. Examine under a microscope using *chloral hydrate solution R*. The powder shows the following diagnostic characters: fragments of cork layer consisting of yellowish-brown, thin-walled cells; fragments of cortical parenchyma consisting of large, thin-walled cells, sometimes containing reddish-brown granular inclusions and isolated yellow droplets; fragments of reticulately thickened or pitted vessels and fragments of lignified parenchyma, sometimes associated with vessels from the central cylinder; prism crystals and rare small needles of calcium oxalate in the parenchyma. The powder may show rectangular or polygonal sclereids with dark reddish-brown contents. With a solution of phloroglucinol in hydrochloric acid, the parenchyma turns green.

C. Thin-layer chromatography (*2.2.27*).

Test solution. Heat 1.0 g of the powdered drug (355) (*2.9.12*) with 10 ml of *methanol R* on a water-bath at 60 °C for 10 min. Filter and reduce the filtrate to about 2 ml under reduced pressure at a temperature not exceeding 40 °C.

Reference solution. Dissolve 1 mg of *harpagoside R* and 2.5 mg of *fructose R* in 1 ml of *methanol R*.

Plate: *TLC silica gel plate R* (5-40 µm) [or *TLC silica gel plate R* (2-10 µm)].

Mobile phase: *water R, methanol R, ethyl acetate R* (8:15:77 *V/V/V*).

Application: 20 µl [or 5 µl], as bands.

Development: over a path of 10 cm [or 7.5 cm].

Drying: in a current of warm air.

Detection A: examine in ultraviolet light at 254 nm.

Results A: see below the sequence of zones present in the chromatograms obtained with the reference solution and the test solution. The chromatogram obtained with the test solution shows other distinct zones, mainly above the zone due to harpagoside. Furthermore, other faint zones may be present in the chromatogram obtained with the test solution.

Top of the plate	
_______	_______
Harpagoside: a quenching zone	A quenching zone: harpagoside
_______	_______
Reference solution	**Test solution**

Detection B: spray with a 10 g/l solution of *phloroglucinol R* in *ethanol (96 per cent) R* and then with *hydrochloric acid R*; heat at 80 °C for 5-10 min and examine in daylight.

Results B: see below the sequence of zones present in the chromatograms obtained with the reference solution and the test solution. The chromatogram obtained with the test solution also shows several yellow to brown zones above the zone due to harpagoside. Furthermore, other faint zones may be present in the chromatogram obtained with the test solution.

Top of the plate	
_______	_______
Harpagoside: a green zone	A green zone (harpagoside)
_______	_______
	A yellow zone
	A light green zone
Fructose: a yellowish-grey zone	A yellowish-grey zone may be present (fructose)
	A brown zone
Reference solution	**Test solution**

TESTS

Starch. Examine the powdered drug (355) (*2.9.12*) under a microscope using *water R*. Add *iodine solution R1*. No blue colour develops.

Loss on drying (*2.2.32*): maximum 12.0 per cent, determined on 1.000 g of the powdered drug (355) (*2.9.12*) by drying in an oven at 105 °C.

Total ash (*2.4.16*): maximum 10.0 per cent.

ASSAY

Liquid chromatography (*2.2.29*).

Test solution. To 0.500 g of the powdered drug (355) (*2.9.12*) add 100.0 ml of *methanol R*. Shake for 4 h and filter through a membrane filter (nominal pore size: 0.45 μm).

Reference solution. Dissolve the contents of a vial of *harpagoside CRS* in *methanol R* and dilute to 10.0 ml with the same solvent.

Column:

- *size*: l = 0.10 m, Ø = 4.0 mm;
- *stationary phase*: *octadecylsilyl silica gel for chromatography R* (5 μm).

Mobile phase: *methanol R, water R* (50:50 *V/V*).

Flow rate: 1.5 ml/min.

Detection: spectrophotometer at 278 nm.

Injection: 10 μl.

Run time: 3 times the retention time of harpagoside.

Retention time: harpagoside = about 7 min.

Calculate the percentage content of harpagoside using the following expression:

$$\frac{m_2 \times A_1 \times 1000}{A_2 \times m_1}$$

A_1 = area of the peak due to harpagoside in the chromatogram obtained with the test solution;

A_2 = area of the peak due to harpagoside in the chromatogram obtained with the reference solution;

m_1 = mass of the drug to be examined used to prepare the test solution, in grams;

m_2 = mass of *harpagoside CRS* in the reference solution, in grams.

07/2008:0485

DIHYDROSTREPTOMYCIN SULPHATE FOR VETERINARY USE

Dihydrostreptomycini sulfas ad usum veterinarium

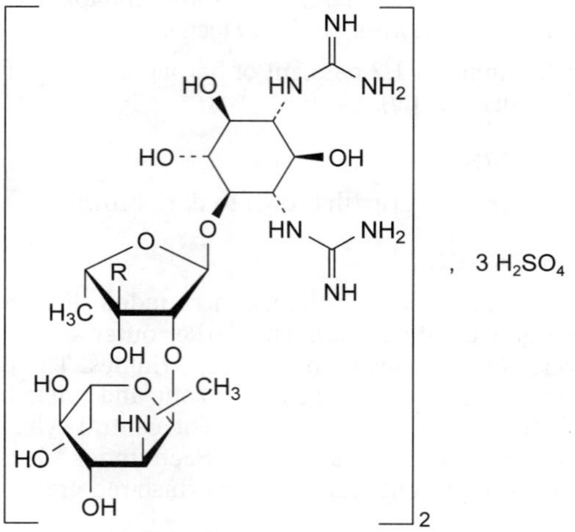

Compound	R	Molec. Formula	M_r
dihydrostreptomycin sulphate	CH_2OH	$C_{42}H_{88}N_{14}O_{36}S_3$	1461
streptomycin sulphate	CHO	$C_{42}H_{84}N_{14}O_{36}S_3$	1457

[5490-27-7]

DEFINITION

Main compound: bis[*N*,*N*'''-[(1*R*,2*R*,3*S*,4*R*,5*R*,6*S*)-4-[[5-deoxy-2-*O*-[2-deoxy-2-(methylamino)-α-L-glucopyranosyl]-3-*C*-(hydroxymethyl)-α-L-lyxofuranosyl]oxy]-2,5,6-trihydroxycyclohexane-1,3-diyl]diguanidine] trisulphate.

Sulphate of a substance obtained by catalytic hydrogenation of streptomycin or by any other means.

Semi-synthetic product derived from a fermentation product.

Stabilisers may be added.

Content:

- *sum of dihydrostreptomycin sulphate and streptomycin sulphate*: 95.0 per cent to 102.0 per cent (dried substance);
- *streptomycin sulphate*: maximum 2.0 per cent (dried substance).

PRODUCTION

The method of manufacture is validated to demonstrate that the product, if tested, would comply with the following test.

Abnormal toxicity (*2.6.9*). Inject into each mouse 1 mg dissolved in 0.5 ml of *water for injections R*.

CHARACTERS

Appearance: white or almost white, hygroscopic powder.

Solubility: freely soluble in water, practically insoluble in acetone, in ethanol (96 per cent) and in methanol.

IDENTIFICATION

First identification: *A, E*.

Second identification: *B, C, D, E*.

A. Examine the chromatograms obtained in the assay.

Results: the principal peak in the chromatogram obtained with the test solution is similar in retention time and size to the principal peak in the chromatogram obtained with reference solution (a).

B. Thin-layer chromatography (*2.2.27*).

Test solution. Dissolve 10 mg of the substance to be examined in *water R* and dilute to 10 ml with the same solvent.

Reference solution (a). Dissolve the contents of a vial of *dihydrostreptomycin sulphate CRS* in 5.0 ml of *water R*. Dilute 1.0 ml of this solution to 5.0 ml with *water R*.

Reference solution (b). Dissolve the contents of a vial of *dihydrostreptomycin sulphate CRS* in 5.0 ml of *water R*.

Reference solution (c). Dissolve 10 mg of *kanamycin monosulphate CRS* and 10 mg of *neomycin sulphate CRS* in *water R*, add 2.0 ml of reference solution (b), mix thoroughly and dilute to 10 ml with *water R*.

Plate: *TLC silica gel plate R*.

Mobile phase: 70 g/l solution of *potassium dihydrogen phosphate R*.

Application: 10 µl.

Development: over 2/3 of the plate.

Drying: in a current of warm air.

Detection: spray with a mixture of equal volumes of a 2 g/l solution of *1,3-dihydroxynaphthalene R* in *ethanol (96 per cent) R* and a 460 g/l solution of *sulphuric acid R*; heat at 150 °C for 5-10 min.

System suitability: reference solution (c):

– the chromatogram shows 3 clearly separated spots.

Results: the principal spot in the chromatogram obtained with the test solution is similar in position, colour and size to the principal spot in the chromatogram obtained with reference solution (a).

C. Dissolve 0.1 g in 2 ml of *water R* and add 1 ml of *α-naphthol solution R* and 2 ml of a mixture of equal volumes of *strong sodium hypochlorite solution R* and *water R*. A red colour develops.

D. Dissolve 10 mg in 5 ml of *water R* and add 1 ml of *1 M hydrochloric acid*. Heat in a water-bath for 2 min. Add 2 ml of a 5 g/l solution of *α-naphthol R* in *1 M sodium hydroxide* and heat in a water-bath for 1 min. A violet-pink colour is produced.

E. It gives reaction (a) of sulphates (*2.3.1*).

TESTS

Solution S. Dissolve 2.5 g in *carbon dioxide-free water R* and dilute to 10 ml with the same solvent.

Appearance of solution. Solution S is not more intensely coloured than intensity 5 of the range of reference solutions of the most appropriate colour (*2.2.2, Method II*). Allow to stand protected from light at about 20 °C for 24 h; solution S is not more opalescent than reference suspension II (*2.2.1*).

pH (*2.2.3*): 5.0 to 7.0 for solution S.

Specific optical rotation (*2.2.7*): – 83.0 to – 91.0 (dried substance).

Dissolve 0.200 g in *water R* and dilute to 10.0 ml with the same solvent.

Related substances. Liquid chromatography (*2.2.29*).

Test solution. Dissolve 50.0 mg of the substance to be examined in *water R* and dilute to 10.0 ml with the same solvent.

Reference solution (a). Dissolve the contents of a vial of *dihydrostreptomycin sulphate CRS* (containing impurities A, B and C) in 5.0 ml of *water R*.

Reference solution (b). Dilute 1.0 ml of the test solution to 100.0 ml with *water R*.

Reference solution (c). Dilute 5.0 ml of reference solution (b) to 50.0 ml with *water R*.

Reference solution (d). Dissolve 10 mg of *streptomycin sulphate CRS* in *water R* and dilute to 20 ml with the same solvent. Mix 0.1 ml of this solution with 1.0 ml of reference solution (a).

Column:

– *size*: l = 0.25 m, Ø = 4.6 mm;
– *stationary phase*: *octadecylsilyl silica gel for chromatography R* (5 µm);
– *temperature*: 45 °C.

Mobile phase: solution in *water R* containing 4.6 g/l of *anhydrous sodium sulphate R*, 1.5 g/l of *sodium octanesulphonate R*, 120 ml/l of *acetonitrile R1* and 50 ml/l of a 27.2 g/l solution of *potassium dihydrogen phosphate R* adjusted to pH 3.0 with a 22.5 g/l solution of *phosphoric acid R*.

Flow rate: 1.0 ml/min.

Detection: spectrophotometer at 205 nm.

Injection: 20 µl.

Run time: 1.5 times the retention time of dihydrostreptomycin.

Identification of impurities: use the chromatogram supplied with *dihydrostreptomycin sulphate CRS* and the chromatogram obtained with reference solution (a) to identify the peaks due to streptomycin and impurities A, B and C.

Relative retention with reference to dihydrostreptomycin (retention time = about 57 min): impurity A = about 0.2; impurity B = about 0.8; streptomycin = about 0.9; impurity C = about 0.95.

System suitability:

– peak-to-valley ratio (a): minimum 1.1, where H_p = height above the baseline of the peak due to streptomycin and H_v = height above the baseline of the lowest point of the curve separating this peak from the peak due to impurity C in the chromatogram obtained with reference solution (d);
– peak-to-valley ratio (b): minimum 5, where H_p = height above the baseline of the peak due to impurity C and H_v = height above the baseline of the lowest point of the curve separating this peak from the peak due to dihydrostreptomycin in the chromatogram obtained with reference solution (d);
– the chromatogram obtained with reference solution (a) is similar to the chromatogram supplied with *dihydrostreptomycin sulphate CRS*.

Limits:

– *correction factor*: for the calculation of content, multiply the peak area of impurity A by 0.5;
– *impurities A, B*: for each impurity, not more than the area of the principal peak in the chromatogram obtained with reference solution (b) (1.0 per cent);
– *impurity C*: not more than twice the area of the principal peak in the chromatogram obtained with reference solution (b) (2.0 per cent);
– *any other impurity*: for each impurity, not more than the area of the principal peak in the chromatogram obtained with reference solution (b) (1.0 per cent);

– *total*: not more than 5 times the area of the principal peak in the chromatogram obtained with reference solution (b) (5.0 per cent);
– *disregard limit*: the area of the principal peak in the chromatogram obtained with reference solution (c) (0.1 per cent); disregard the peak due to streptomycin.

Heavy metals (*2.4.8*): 20 ppm.

1.0 g complies with test C. Prepare the reference solution using 2 ml of *lead standard solution (10 ppm Pb) R*.

Loss on drying (*2.2.32*): maximum 5.0 per cent, determined on 1.000 g by drying under high vacuum at 60 °C for 4 h.

Sulphated ash (*2.4.14*): maximum 1.0 per cent, determined on 1.0 g.

Bacterial endotoxins (*2.6.14*): less than 0.50 IU/mg, if intended for use in the manufacture of parenteral dosage forms without a further appropriate procedure for removal of bacterial endotoxins.

ASSAY

Liquid chromatography (*2.2.29*) as described in the test for related substances with the following modification.

Injection: test solution and reference solution (a).

Calculate the percentage content of $C_{42}H_{88}N_{14}O_{36}S_3$ and of $C_{42}H_{84}N_{14}O_{36}S_3$ using the chromatogram obtained with reference solution (a) and the declared contents of *dihydrostreptomycin sulphate CRS*. Calculate the sum of these percentage contents.

STORAGE

In an airtight container, protected from light. If the substance is sterile, store in a sterile, airtight, tamper-proof container.

IMPURITIES

Specified impurities: A, B, C.

Other detectable impurities (the following substances would, if present at a sufficient level, be detected by one or other of the tests in the monograph. They are limited by the general acceptance criterion for other/unspecified impurities and/or by the general monograph *Substances for pharmaceutical use (2034)*. It is therefore not necessary to identify these impurities for demonstration of compliance. See also *5.10. Control of impurities in substances for pharmaceutical use*): *D*.

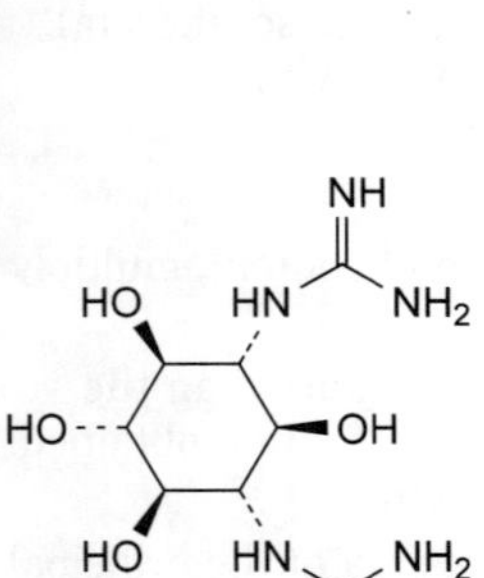

A. *N,N'''*-[(1*R*,2*s*,3*S*,4*R*,5*r*,6*S*)-2,4,5,6-tetrahydroxycyclohexane-1,3-diyl]diguanidine (streptidine),

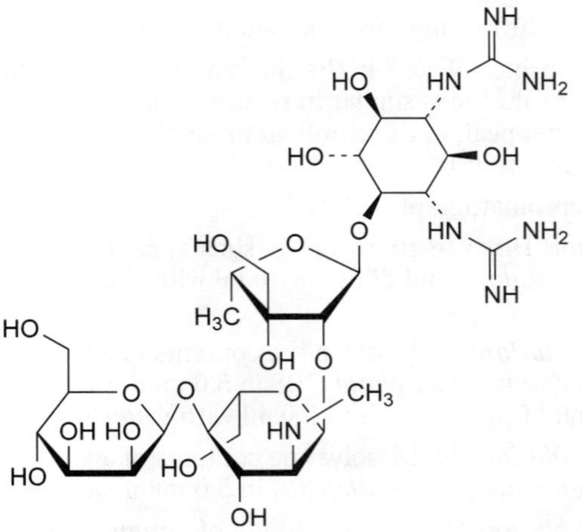

B. *N,N'''*-[(1*S*,2*R*,3*R*,4*S*,5*R*,6*R*)-2,4,5-trihydroxy-6-[[β-D-mannopyranosyl-(1→4)-2-deoxy-2-(methylamino)-α-L-glucopyranosyl-(1→2)-5-deoxy-3-*C*-(hydroxymethyl)-α-L-lyxofuranosyl]oxy]cyclohexane-1,3-diyl]diguanidine (dihydrostreptomycin B),

C. unknown structure,

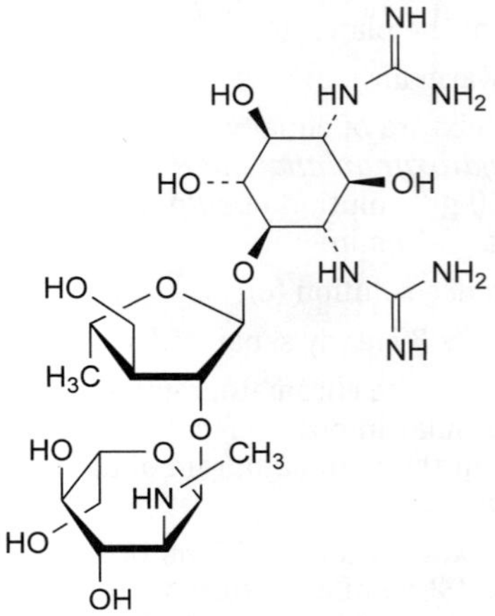

D. *N,N'''*-[(1*R*,2*R*,3*S*,4*R*,5*R*,6*S*)-4-[[3,5-dideoxy-2-*O*-[2-deoxy-2-(methylamino)-α-L-glucopyranosyl]-3-(hydroxymethyl)-α-L-arabinofuranosyl]oxy]-2,5,6-trihydroxycyclohexane-1,3-diyl]diguanidine (deoxydihydrostreptomycin).

01/2008:0138
corrected 6.2

DIMETICONE

Dimeticonum

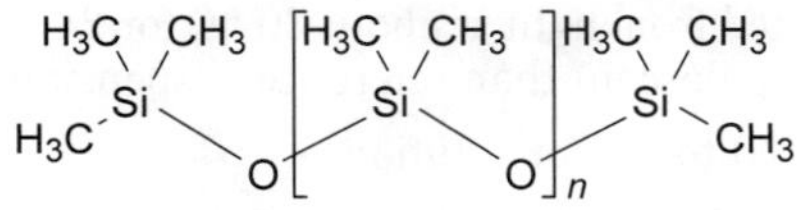

[9006-65-9]

DEFINITION

Poly(dimethylsiloxane) obtained by hydrolysis and polycondensation of dichlorodimethylsilane and chlorotrimethylsilane. Different grades of dimeticone exist which are distinguished by a number indicating the nominal kinematic viscosity placed after the name.

Their degree of polymerisation (*n* = 20 to 400) is such that their kinematic viscosities are nominally between 20 $mm^2 \cdot s^{-1}$ and 1300 $mm^2 \cdot s^{-1}$.

Dimeticones with a nominal viscosity of 50 $mm^2 \cdot s^{-1}$ or lower are intended for external use only.

CHARACTERS

Appearance: clear, colourless liquid of various viscosities.

Solubility: practically insoluble in water, very slightly soluble or practically insoluble in anhydrous ethanol, miscible with ethyl acetate, with methyl ethyl ketone and with toluene.

IDENTIFICATION

A. It is identified by its kinematic viscosity at 25 °C (see Tests).

B. Infrared absorption spectrophotometry (*2.2.24*).

Comparison: *dimeticone CRS.*

The region of the spectrum from 850 cm^{-1} to 750 cm^{-1} is not taken into account.

C. Heat 0.5 g in a test-tube over a small flame until white fumes begin to appear. Invert the tube over a 2nd tube containing 1 ml of a 1 g/l solution of *chromotropic acid, sodium salt R* in *sulphuric acid R* so that the fumes reach the solution. Shake the 2nd tube for about 10 s and heat on a water-bath for 5 min. The solution is violet.

D. In a platinum crucible, prepare the sulphated ash (*2.4.14*) using 50 mg. The residue is a white powder that gives the reaction of silicates (*2.3.1*).

TESTS

Acidity. To 2.0 g add 25 ml of a mixture of equal volumes of *anhydrous ethanol R* and *ether R*, previously neutralised to 0.2 ml of *bromothymol blue solution R1* and shake. Not more than 0.15 ml of *0.01 M sodium hydroxide* is required to change the colour of the solution to blue.

Viscosity (*2.2.9*): 90 per cent to 110 per cent of the nominal kinematic viscosity stated on the label, determined at 25 °C.

Mineral oils. Place 2 g in a test-tube and examine in ultraviolet light at 365 nm. The fluorescence is not more intense than that of a solution containing 0.1 ppm of *quinine sulphate R* in *0.005 M sulphuric acid* examined in the same conditions.

Phenylated compounds. Dissolve 5.0 g with shaking in 10 ml of *cyclohexane R*. At wavelengths from 250 nm to 270 nm, the absorbance (*2.2.25*) of the solution is not greater than 0.2.

Heavy metals: maximum 5 ppm.

Mix 1.0 g with *methylene chloride R* and dilute to 20 ml with the same solvent. Add 1.0 ml of a freshly prepared 0.02 g/l solution of *dithizone R* in *methylene chloride R*, 0.5 ml of *water R* and 0.5 ml of a mixture of 1 volume of *dilute ammonia R2* and 9 volumes of a 2 g/l solution of *hydroxylamine hydrochloride R*. At the same time, prepare a reference solution as follows: to 20 ml of *methylene chloride R* add 1.0 ml of a freshly prepared 0.02 g/l solution of *dithizone R* in *methylene chloride R*, 0.5 ml of *lead standard solution (10 ppm Pb) R* and 0.5 ml of a mixture of 1 volume of *dilute ammonia R2* and 9 volumes of a 2 g/l solution of *hydroxylamine hydrochloride R*. Immediately shake each solution vigorously for 1 min. Any red colour in the test solution is not more intense than that in the reference solution.

Volatile matter: maximum 0.3 per cent, for dimeticones with a nominal viscosity greater than 50 $mm^2 \cdot s^{-1}$, determined on 1.00 g by heating in an oven at 150 °C for 2 h. Carry out the test using a dish 60 mm in diameter and 10 mm deep.

LABELLING

The label states:

- the nominal kinematic viscosity by a number placed after the name of the product,
- where applicable, that the product is intended for external use.

Monographs D-K

E

07/2008:1204

ETAMSYLATE

Etamsylatum

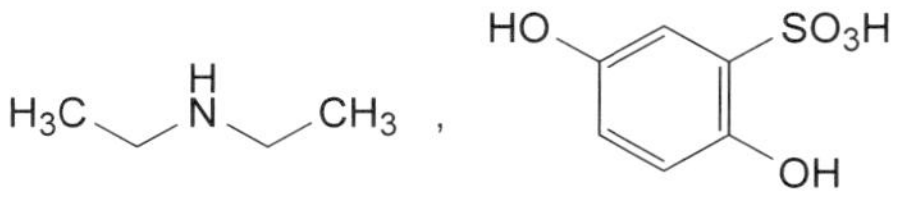

$C_{10}H_{17}NO_5S$ M_r 263.3

[2624-44-4]

DEFINITION

N-Ethylethanamine 2,5-dihydroxybenzenesulphonate.

Content: 99.0 per cent to 101.0 per cent (dried substance).

CHARACTERS

Appearance: white or almost white, crystalline powder.

Solubility: very soluble in water, freely soluble in methanol, soluble in anhydrous ethanol, practically insoluble in methylene chloride.

It shows polymorphism (*5.9*).

IDENTIFICATION

First identification: B.

Second identification: A, C, D.

A. Melting point (*2.2.14*): 127 °C to 134 °C.

B. Infrared absorption spectrophotometry (*2.2.24*).

Comparison: *etamsylate CRS.*

C. Ultraviolet and visible absorption spectrophotometry (*2.2.25*).

Test solution. Dissolve 0.100 g in *water R* and dilute to 200.0 ml with the same solvent. Dilute 5.0 ml of this solution to 100.0 ml with *water R*. Examine immediately.

Spectral range: 210-350 nm.

Absorption maxima: at 221 nm and 301 nm.

Specific absorbance at the absorption maximum at 301 nm: 145 to 151.

D. Into a test-tube, introduce 2 ml of freshly prepared solution S (see Tests) and 0.5 g of *sodium hydroxide R*. Warm the mixture and place a wet strip of *red litmus paper R* near the open end of the tube. The colour of the paper becomes blue.

TESTS

Solution S. Dissolve 10.0 g in *carbon dioxide-free water R* and dilute to 100 ml with the same solvent.

Appearance of solution. Solution S, when freshly prepared, is clear (*2.2.1*) and colourless (*2.2.2, Method II*).

pH (*2.2.3*): 4.5 to 5.6 for solution S.

Related substances. Liquid chromatography (*2.2.29*). *Keep all solutions at 2-8 °C.*

Buffer solution. Dissolve 1.2 g of *anhydrous sodium dihydrogen phosphate R* in 900 ml of *water for chromatography R*. Adjust to pH 6.5 with *disodium hydrogen phosphate solution R* and dilute to 1000 ml with *water for chromatography R*.

Test solution. Dissolve 0.100 g of the substance to be examined in *water R* and dilute to 10.0 ml with the same solvent.

Reference solution (a). Dilute 1.0 ml of the test solution to 100.0 ml with *water R*. Dilute 1.0 ml of this solution to 10.0 ml with *water R*.

Reference solution (b). Dissolve 10 mg of the substance to be examined and 10 mg of *hydroquinone R* (impurity A) in *water R* and dilute to 10 ml with the same solvent. Dilute 1 ml of this solution to 100 ml with *water R*.

Column:

– *size*: *l* = 0.25 m, Ø = 4.6 mm;
– *stationary phase:* spherical *end-capped octadecylsilyl silica gel for chromatography R* (5 µm).

Mobile phase: *acetonitrile R1*, buffer solution (10:90 *V/V*).

Flow rate: 0.8 ml/min.

Detection: spectrophotometer at 220 nm.

Injection: 10 µl.

Run time: 2.5 times the retention time of etamsylate.

Relative retention with reference to etamsylate (retention time = about 6 min): impurity A = about 1.7.

System suitability: reference solution (b):

– *resolution*: minimum 8.0 between the peaks due to etamsylate and impurity A.

Limits:

– *correction factor*: for the calculation of content, multiply the peak area of impurity A by 0.5;
– *impurity A*: not more than the area of the principal peak in the chromatogram obtained with reference solution (a) (0.1 per cent);
– *unspecified impurities*: for each impurity, not more than the area of the principal peak in the chromatogram obtained with reference solution (a) (0.10 per cent);
– *total*: not more than twice the area of principal peak in the chromatogram obtained with reference solution (a) (0.2 per cent);
– *disregard limit*: 0.5 times the area of the principal peak in the chromatogram obtained with reference solution (a) (0.05 per cent).

Iron (*2.4.9*): maximum 10 ppm, determined on solution S.

Heavy metals (*2.4.8*): maximum 15 ppm.

1.0 g complies with test C. Prepare the reference solution using 1.5 ml of *lead standard solution (10 ppm Pb) R.*

Loss on drying (*2.2.32*): maximum 0.5 per cent, determined on 1.000 g by drying *in vacuo* in an oven at 60 °C.

Sulphated ash (*2.4.14*): maximum 0.1 per cent, determined on 1.0 g.

ASSAY

Dissolve 0.200 g in a mixture of 10 ml of *water R* and 40 ml of *dilute sulphuric acid R*. Titrate with *0.1 M cerium sulphate*, determining the end-point potentiometrically (*2.2.20*).

1 ml of *0.1 M cerium sulphate* is equivalent to 13.16 mg of $C_{10}H_{17}NO_5S$.

STORAGE

In an airtight container, protected from light.

IMPURITIES

Specified impurities: A.

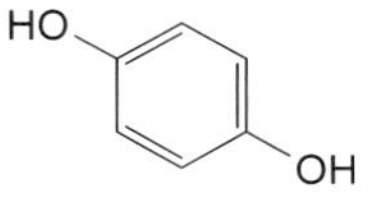

A. benzene-1,4-diol (hydroquinone).

Monographs D-K

01/2008:0390

EUCALYPTUS OIL

Eucalypti aetheroleum

DEFINITION

Essential oil obtained by steam distillation and rectification from the fresh leaves or the fresh terminal branchlets of various species of *Eucalyptus* rich in 1,8-cineole. The species mainly used are *Eucalyptus globulus* Labill., *Eucalyptus polybractea* R.T. Baker and *Eucalyptus smithii* R.T. Baker.

CHARACTERS

Appearance: colourless or pale yellow liquid.

Aromatic and camphoraceous odour, pungent and camphoraceous taste.

IDENTIFICATION

First identification: B.

Second identification: A.

A. Thin-layer chromatography (*2.2.27*).

Test solution. Dissolve 0.1 g of the substance to be examined in *toluene R* and dilute to 10 ml with the same solvent.

Reference solution. Dissolve 50 µl of *cineole R* in *toluene R* and dilute to 5 ml with the same solvent.

Plate: *TLC silica gel plate R.*

Mobile phase: *ethyl acetate R, toluene R* (10:90 *V/V*).

Application: 10 µl as bands.

Development: over a path of 15 cm.

Drying: in air.

Detection: spray with *anisaldehyde solution R* and examine in daylight while heating at 100-105 °C for 5-10 min.

Results: the chromatogram obtained with the reference solution shows in the middle part a zone due to cineole; the chromatogram obtained with the test solution shows a main zone similar in position and colour to the zone due to cineole in the chromatogram obtained with the reference solution. Other weaker zones may be present.

B. Examine the chromatograms obtained in the test for chromatographic profile.

Results: the chromatogram obtained with the test solution shows 5 principal peaks similar in retention time to the 5 principal peaks in the chromatogram obtained with the reference solution.

TESTS

Relative density (*2.2.5*): 0.906 to 0.927.

Refractive index (*2.2.6*): 1.458 to 1.470.

Optical rotation (*2.2.7*): 0° to + 10°.

Solubility in alcohol (*2.8.10*). It is soluble in 5 volumes of *ethanol (70 per cent V/V) R*.

Aldehydes. To 10 ml in a ground-glass-stoppered tube 25 mm in diameter and 150 mm long, add 5 ml of *toluene R* and 4 ml of *alcoholic hydroxylamine solution R*. Shake vigorously and titrate immediately with *0.5 M potassium hydroxide in alcohol (60 per cent V/V)* until the red colour changes to yellow. Continue the titration with shaking; the end-point is reached when the pure yellow colour of the indicator is permanent in the lower layer after shaking vigorously for 2 min and allowing separation to take place. The reaction is complete in about 15 min. Repeat the titration using a further 10 ml of the substance to be examined and, as a reference solution for the end-point, the titrated liquid from the 1st determination to which has been added 0.5 ml of *0.5 M potassium hydroxide in alcohol (60 per cent V/V)*. Not more than 2.0 ml of *0.5 M potassium hydroxide in alcohol (60 per cent V/V)* is required in the 2nd titration.

Chromatographic profile. Gas chromatography (*2.2.28*): use the normalisation procedure.

Test solution. The substance to be examined.

Reference solution. Dissolve 80 µl of *α-pinene R*, 10 µl of *β-pinene R*, 10 µl of *sabinene R*, 10 µl of *α-phellandrene R*, 10 µl of *limonene R*, 0.8 ml of *cineole R* and 10 mg of *camphor R* in 10 ml of *acetone R*.

Column:

- *material*: fused silica;
- *size*: l = 60 m, Ø = about 0.25 mm;
- *stationary phase*: bonded *macrogol 20 000 R*.

Carrier gas: *helium for chromatography R*.

Flow rate: 1.5 ml/min.

Split ratio: 1:100.

Temperature:

	Time (min)	Temperature (°C)
Column	0 - 5	60
	5 - 33	60 → 200
	33 - 38	200
Injection port		220
Detector		220

Detection: flame ionisation.

Injection: 0.5 µl.

Elution order: order indicated in the composition of the reference solution. Record the retention times of these substances.

System suitability: reference solution:

- *resolution*: minimum 1.5 between the peaks due to limonene and cineole;
- *number of theoretical plates*: minimum 30 000, calculated for the peak due to limonene at 110 °C.

Identification of components: using the retention times determined from the chromatogram obtained with the reference solution, locate the components of the reference solution in the chromatogram obtained with the test solution.

Determine the percentage content of each of these components. The percentages are within the following ranges:

- *α-pinene*: traces to 9.0 per cent;
- *β-pinene*: less than 1.5 per cent;
- *sabinene*: less than 0.3 per cent;
- *α-phellandrene*: less than 1.5 per cent;
- *limonene*: traces to 12.0 per cent;
- *1,8-cineole*: minimum 70.0 per cent;
- *camphor*: less than 0.1 per cent.

STORAGE

At a temperature not exceeding 25 °C.

Monographs D-K

F

Monographs
D-K

07/2008:2346

FLUCLOXACILLIN MAGNESIUM OCTAHYDRATE

Flucloxacillinum magnesicum octahydricum

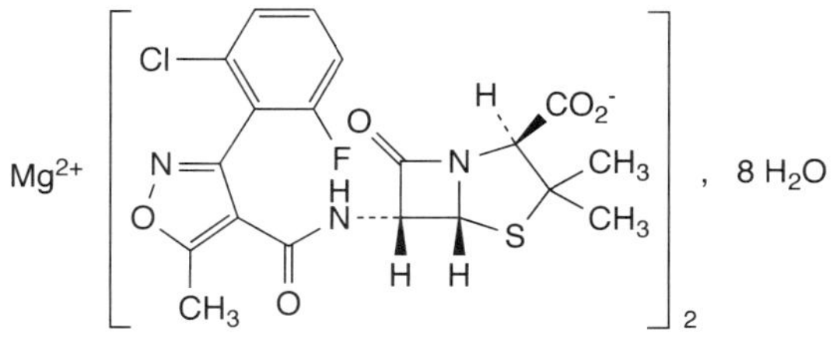

$C_{38}H_{32}Cl_2F_2MgN_6O_{10}S_2,8H_2O$ M_r 1074
[58486-36-5]

DEFINITION

Magnesium bis[(2*S*,5*R*,6*R*)-6-[[[3-(2-chloro-6-fluorophenyl)-5-methylisoxazol-4-yl]carbonyl]amino]-3,3-dimethyl-7-oxo-4-thia-1-azabicyclo[3.2.0]heptane-2-carboxylate] octahydrate.

Semi-synthetic product derived from a fermentation product.

Content: 95.0 per cent to 102.0 per cent (anhydrous substance).

CHARACTERS

Appearance: white or almost white, crystalline powder.

Solubility: slightly soluble in water, freely soluble in methanol.

IDENTIFICATION

First identification: A, C.

Second identification: B, C.

A. Infrared absorption spectrophotometry (*2.2.24*).

Comparison: *flucloxacillin magnesium octahydrate CRS.*

B. Thin-layer chromatography (*2.2.27*).

Test solution. Dissolve 25 mg of the substance to be examined in 5 ml of *water R.*

Reference solution (a). Dissolve 25 mg of *flucloxacillin sodium CRS* in 5 ml of *water R.*

Reference solution (b). Dissolve 25 mg of *cloxacillin sodium CRS*, 25 mg of *dicloxacillin sodium CRS* and 25 mg of *flucloxacillin sodium CRS* in 5 ml of *water R.*

Plate: *TLC silanised silica gel plate R.*

Mobile phase: mix 30 volumes of *acetone R* and 70 volumes of a 154 g/l solution of *ammonium acetate R* previously adjusted to pH 5.0 with *glacial acetic acid R.*

Application: 1 μl.

Development: over 2/3 of the plate.

Drying: in air.

Detection: expose the plate to iodine vapour until the spots appear.

System suitability: reference solution (b):

– the chromatogram shows 3 clearly separated spots.

Results: the principal spot in the chromatogram obtained with the test solution is similar in position, colour and size to the principal spot in the chromatogram obtained with reference solution (a).

C. It gives the reaction of magnesium (*2.3.1*).

TESTS

pH (*2.2.3*): 4.5 to 6.5.

Dissolve 0.25 g in *carbon dioxide-free water R* and dilute to 50 ml with the same solvent.

Specific optical rotation (*2.2.7*): + 163 to + 175 (anhydrous substance).

Dissolve 0.250 g in *water R* and dilute to 50.0 ml with the same solvent.

Related substances. Liquid chromatography (*2.2.29*). *Prepare the solutions immediately before use.*

Test solution (a). Dissolve 50.0 mg of the substance to be examined in the mobile phase and dilute to 50.0 ml with the mobile phase.

Test solution (b). Dilute 5.0 ml of test solution (a) to 50.0 ml with the mobile phase.

Reference solution (a). Dissolve 50.0 mg of *flucloxacillin sodium CRS* in the mobile phase and dilute to 50.0 ml with the mobile phase. Dilute 5.0 ml of this solution to 50.0 ml with the mobile phase.

Reference solution (b). Dilute 5.0 ml of test solution (b) to 50.0 ml with the mobile phase.

Reference solution (c). In order to prepare impurity A *in situ*, add 1 ml of *sodium carbonate solution R* to 10 mg of the substance to be examined, dilute to 25 ml with *water R* and place in an oven at 70 °C for 20 min.

Reference solution (d). Dilute 1 ml of reference solution (c) to 10 ml with a 27 g/l solution of *dipotassium hydrogen phosphate R* previously adjusted to pH 3.5 with *dilute phosphoric acid R.*

Reference solution (e). In order to prepare impurity B *in situ*, add 5 ml of *dilute hydrochloric acid R* to 10 ml of reference solution (c), dilute to 25 ml with *water R* and place in an oven at 70 °C for 1 h. Dilute 1 ml of this solution to 5 ml with a 27 g/l solution of *dipotassium hydrogen phosphate R* previously adjusted to pH 7.0 with *phosphoric acid R.*

Reference solution (f). Dilute 2 ml of reference solution (a) to 10 ml with reference solution (e).

Reference solution (g). Dissolve 1.5 mg of *flucloxacillin impurity C CRS* in 1 ml of the mobile phase and dilute to 50 ml with the mobile phase.

Reference solution (h). Dissolve 1 mg of *flucloxacillin impurity D CRS* in 100 ml of the mobile phase.

Reference solution (i). Dissolve 1 mg of *flucloxacillin impurity E CRS* in 100 ml of the mobile phase.

Column:

– *size*: *l* = 0.25 m, Ø = 4 mm;

– *stationary phase*: *octadecylsilyl silica gel for chromatography R* (5 μm);

– *temperature*: 40 °C.

Mobile phase: mix 25 volumes of *acetonitrile R1* and 75 volumes of a 2.7 g/l solution of *potassium dihydrogen phosphate R* previously adjusted to pH 5.0 with *dilute sodium hydroxide solution R.*

Flow rate: 1 ml/min.

Detection: spectrophotometer at 225 nm.

Injection: 20 μl of test solution (a) and reference solutions (b), (d), (e), (f), (g), (h) and (i).

Run time: 7 times the retention time of flucloxacillin.

Identification of impurities: use the chromatograms obtained with reference solutions (d), (e), (g), (h) and (i) to identify the peaks due to impurities A, B, C, D and E respectively.

Relative retention with reference to flucloxacillin (retention time = about 8 min): impurity C = about 0.2; impurity A (isomer 1) = about 0.3; impurity A (isomer 2) = about 0.5; impurity D = about 0.6; impurity B (isomer 1) = about 0.8; impurity B (isomer 2) = about 0.9; impurity E = about 6.

System suitability: reference solution (f):

– *resolution*: minimum 2.0 between the 2nd peak due to impurity B (isomer 2) and the peak due to flucloxacillin.

Limits:

– *correction factor*: for the calculation of content, multiply the peak area of impurity C by 3.3;
– *impurity A* (sum of the 2 isomers): the sum of the areas of the 2 peaks is not more than twice the area of the principal peak in the chromatogram obtained with reference solution (b) (2.0 per cent);
– *impurity B* (sum of the 2 isomers): the sum of the areas of the 2 peaks is not more than the area of the principal peak in the chromatogram obtained with reference solution (b) (1.0 per cent);
– *impurity C*: not more than the area of the principal peak in the chromatogram obtained with reference solution (b) (1.0 per cent);
– *impurities D, E*: for each impurity, not more than 0.3 times the area of the principal peak in the chromatogram obtained with reference solution (b) (0.3 per cent);
– *any other impurity*: for each impurity, not more than 0.3 times the area of the principal peak in the chromatogram obtained with reference solution (b) (0.3 per cent);
– *total*: not more than 3 times the area of the principal peak in the chromatogram obtained with reference solution (b) (3.0 per cent);
– *disregard limit*: 0.05 times the area of the principal peak in the chromatogram obtained with reference solution (b) (0.05 per cent).

2-Ethylhexanoic acid (*2.4.28*): maximum 0.8 per cent *m/m*.

Water (*2.5.12*): 12.0 per cent to 15.0 per cent, determined on 0.100 g.

ASSAY

Liquid chromatography (*2.2.29*) as described in the test for related substances with the following modifications.

Injection: test solution (b) and reference solution (a).

Calculate the percentage content of $C_{38}H_{32}Cl_2F_2MgN_6O_{10}S_2$ from the declared content of *flucloxacillin sodium CRS*, multiplying by 0.9773.

IMPURITIES

Specified impurities: A, B, C, D, E.

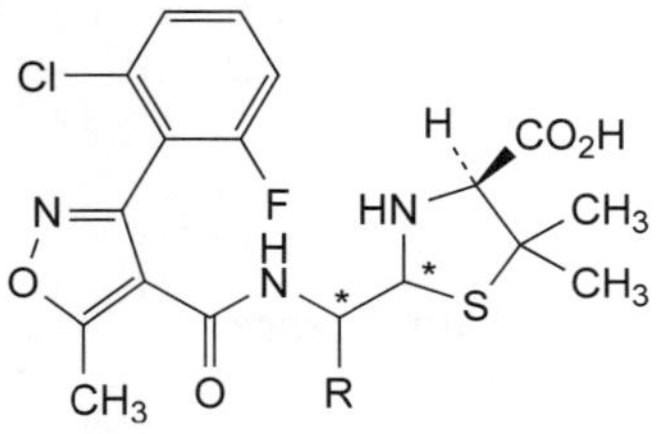

A. R = CO_2H: (4*S*)-2-[carboxy[[[3-(2-chloro-6-fluorophenyl)-5-methylisoxazol-4-yl]carbonyl]amino]methyl]-5,5-dimethylthiazolidine-4-carboxylic acid (penicilloic acids of flucloxacillin),

B. R = H: (2*RS*,4*S*)-2-[[[[3-(2-chloro-6-fluorophenyl)-5-methylisoxazol-4-yl]carbonyl]amino]methyl]-5,5-dimethylthiazolidine-4-carboxylic acid (penilloic acids of flucloxacillin),

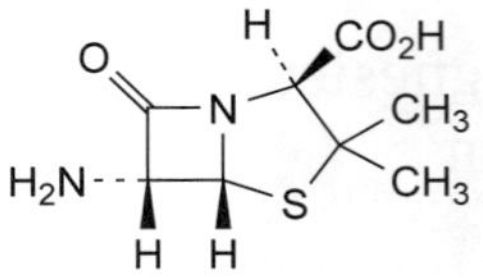

C. (2*S*,5*R*,6*R*)-6-amino-3,3-dimethyl-7-oxo-4-thia-1-azabicyclo[3.2.0]heptane-2-carboxylic acid (6-aminopenicillanic acid),

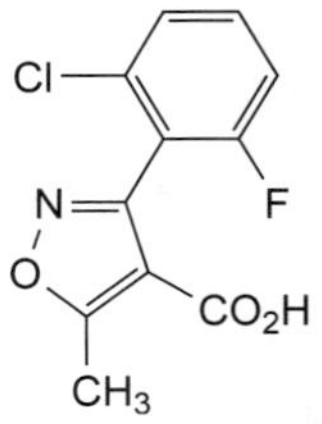

D. 3-(2-chloro-6-fluorophenyl)-5-methylisoxazole-4-carboxylic acid,

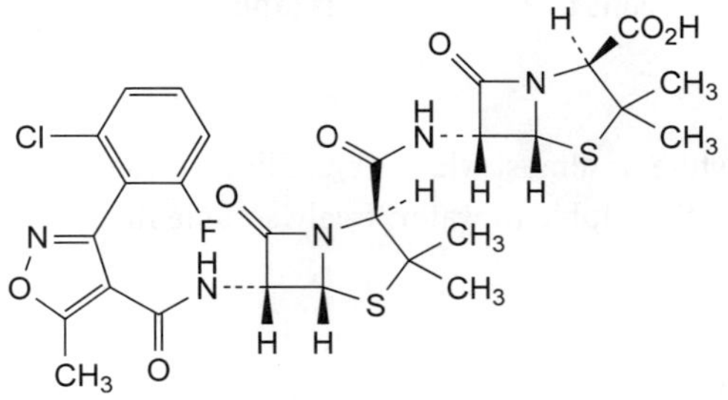

E. (2*S*,5*R*,6*R*)-6-[[[(2*S*,5*R*,6*R*)-6-[[[3-(2-chloro-6-fluorophenyl)-5-methylisoxazol-4-yl]carbonyl]amino]-3,3-dimethyl-7-oxo-4-thia-1-azabicyclo[3.2.0]hept-2-yl]carbonyl]amino]-3,3-dimethyl-7-oxo-4-thia-1-azabicyclo[3.2.0]heptane-2-carboxylic acid (6-APA flucloxacillin amide).

07/2008:1977

FLUVOXAMINE MALEATE

Fluvoxamini maleas

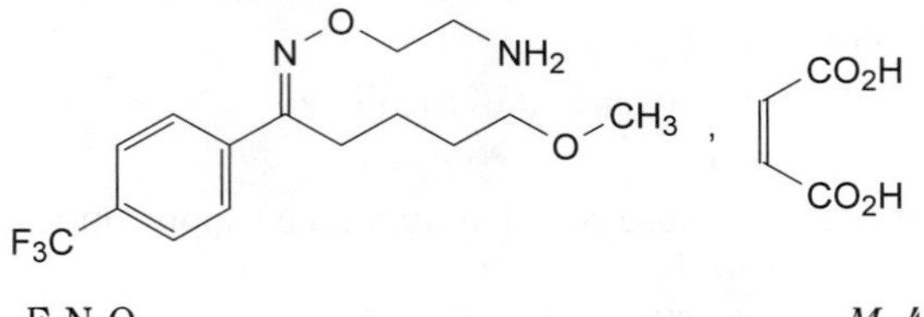

$C_{19}H_{25}F_3N_2O_6$ M_r 434.4
[61718-82-9]

DEFINITION

2-[[[(1*E*)-5-Methoxy-1-[4-(trifluoromethyl)phenyl]pentylidene]amino]oxy]ethanamine (*Z*)-butenedioate.

Content: 99.0 per cent to 101.0 per cent (dried substance).

PRODUCTION

The production method must be evaluated to determine the potential for formation of aziridine. Where necessary, a validated test for the substance is carried out or the production method is validated to demonstrate acceptable clearance.

CHARACTERS

Appearance: white or almost white, crystalline powder.

Solubility: sparingly soluble in water, freely soluble in ethanol (96 per cent) and in methanol.

IDENTIFICATION

Infrared absorption spectrophotometry (*2.2.24*).

Comparison: *fluvoxamine maleate CRS*.

TESTS

Related substances. Liquid chromatography (*2.2.29*). *Prepare the test solution immediately before use.*

Test solution. Dissolve 50 mg of the substance to be examined in the mobile phase and dilute to 25 ml with the mobile phase.

Reference solution (a). Dilute 1.0 ml of the test solution to 10.0 ml with the mobile phase. Dilute 1.0 ml of this solution to 100.0 ml with the mobile phase.

Reference solution (b). Dissolve the contents of a vial of *fluvoxamine for system suitability CRS* (containing impurities A, B, C and F) in the mobile phase and dilute to 5 ml with the mobile phase.

Reference solution (c). Dissolve 3.0 mg of *fluvoxamine impurity D CRS* in 5 ml of the mobile phase and dilute to 10.0 ml with the mobile phase. Dilute 1.0 ml of this solution to 100.0 ml with the mobile phase.

Column:

- *size*: l = 0.25 m, Ø = 4.6 mm;
- *stationary phase*: *octylsilyl silica gel for chromatography R* (5 μm).

Mobile phase: mix 370 volumes of *acetonitrile R1* and 630 volumes of a buffer solution containing 1.1 g/l of *potassium dihydrogen phosphate R* and 1.9 g/l of *sodium pentanesulphonate R* in *water R*, previously adjusted to pH 3.0 with *phosphoric acid R*.

Flow rate: 1.2 ml/min.

Detection: spectrophotometer at 234 nm.

Injection: 20 μl.

Run time: 6 times the retention time of fluvoxamine.

Identification of impurities: use the chromatogram supplied with *fluvoxamine for system suitability CRS* and the chromatogram obtained with reference solution (b) to identify the peaks due to impurities A, B, C and F.

Relative retention with reference to fluvoxamine (retention time = about 15 min): maleic acid = about 0.15; impurities F and G = about 0.5; impurity C = about 0.6; impurity B = about 0.8; impurity A = about 2.5; impurity D = about 5.4.

System suitability: reference solution (b):

- *resolution*: minimum 1.5 between the peaks due to impurities F and C.

Limits:

- *impurity B*: not more than 5 times the area of the principal peak in the chromatogram obtained with reference solution (a) (0.5 per cent);
- *impurity C*: not more than 3 times the area of the principal peak in the chromatogram obtained with reference solution (a) (0.3 per cent);
- *impurity A*: not more than twice the area of the principal peak in the chromatogram obtained with reference solution (a) (0.2 per cent);
- *impurity D*: not more than the area of the corresponding peak in the chromatogram obtained with reference solution (c) (0.15 per cent);
- *sum of impurities F and G*: not more than 3 times the area of the principal peak in the chromatogram obtained with reference solution (a) (0.3 per cent);
- *unspecified impurities*: for each impurity, not more than the area of the principal peak in the chromatogram obtained with reference solution (a) (0.10 per cent);
- *total*: not more than 10 times the area of the principal peak in the chromatogram obtained with reference solution (a) (1.0 per cent);
- *disregard limit*: 0.5 times the area of the principal peak in the chromatogram obtained with reference solution (a) (0.05 per cent); disregard the peak due to maleic acid.

Heavy metals (*2.4.8*): maximum 20 ppm.

1.0 g complies with test B. Prepare the reference solution using 2 ml of *lead standard solution (10 ppm Pb) R*.

Loss on drying (*2.2.32*): maximum 0.5 per cent, determined on 1.000 g by drying *in vacuo* at 80 °C for 2 h.

Sulphated ash (*2.4.14*): maximum 0.1 per cent, determined on 1.0 g in a platinum crucible.

ASSAY

Dissolve 0.350 g in 50 ml of *anhydrous acetic acid R*. Titrate with *0.1 M perchloric acid*, determining the end-point potentiometrically (*2.2.20*).

1 ml of *0.1 M perchloric acid* is equivalent to 43.44 mg of $C_{19}H_{25}F_3N_2O_6$.

IMPURITIES

Specified impurities: A, B, C, D, F, G.

Other detectable impurities (the following substances would, if present at a sufficient level, be detected by one or other of the tests in the monograph. They are limited by the general acceptance criterion for other/unspecified impurities and/or by the general monograph *Substances for pharmaceutical use (2034)*. It is therefore not necessary to identify these impurities for demonstration of compliance. See also *5.10. Control of impurities in substances for pharmaceutical use*): *E, I, J.*

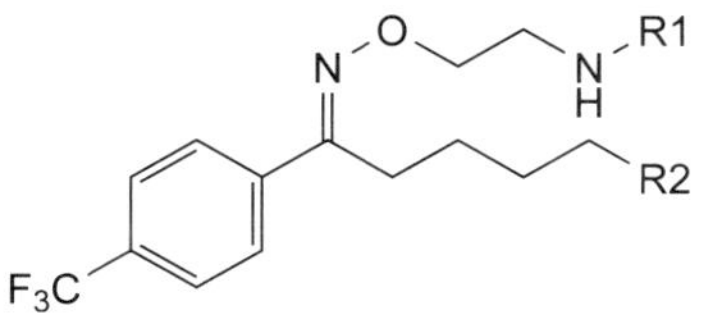

A. R1 = R2 = H: 2-[[[(1*E*)-1-[4-(trifluoromethyl)phenyl]pentylidene]amino]oxy]ethanamine,

F. R1 = CH_2-CH_2-NH_2, R2 = OCH_3: *N*-[2-[[[(1*E*)-5-methoxy-1-[4-(trifluoromethyl)phenyl]pentylidene]amino]oxy]ethyl]-ethane-1,2-diamine,

G. R1 = H, R2 = OH: (5*E*)-5-[(2-aminoethoxy)imino]-5-[4-(trifluoromethyl)phenyl]pentan-1-ol,

Monographs D-K

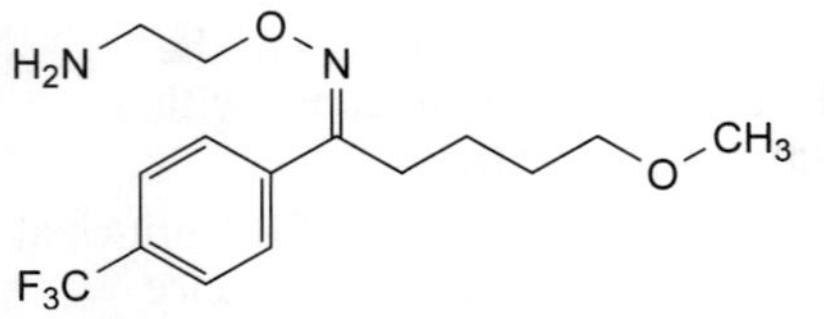

B. 2-[[[(1*Z*)-5-methoxy-1-[4-(trifluoromethyl)phenyl]pentylidene]amino]oxy]ethanamine,

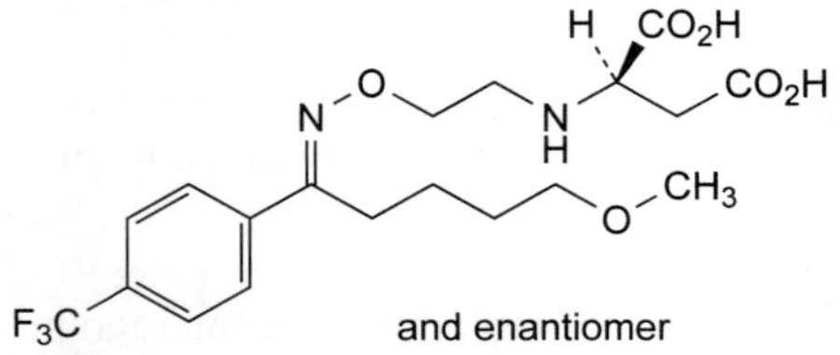

C. (2*RS*)-2-[[2-[[[(1*E*)-5-methoxy-1-[4-(trifluoromethyl)-phenyl]pentylidene]amino]oxy]ethyl]amino]butanedioic acid,

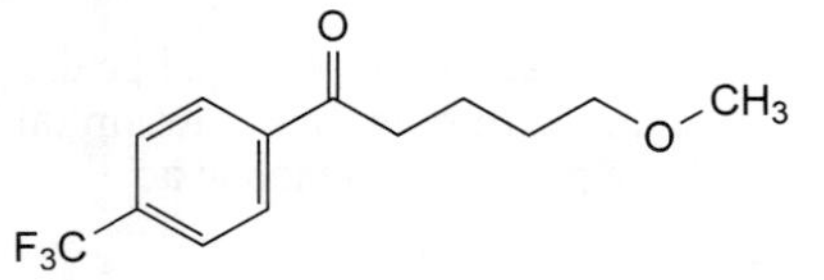

D. 5-methoxy-1-[4-(trifluoromethyl)phenyl]pentan-1-one,

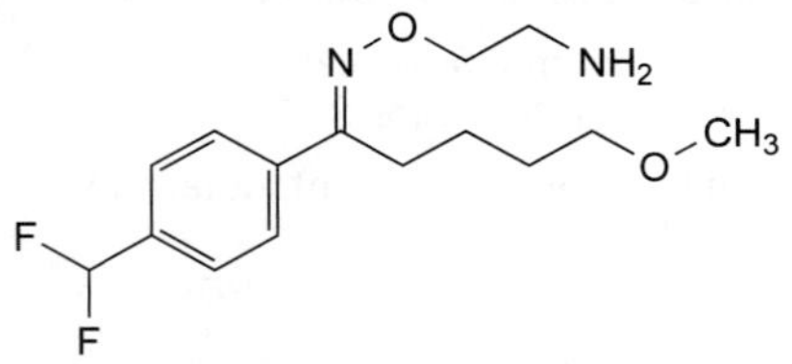

E. 2-[[[(1*E*)-1-[4-(difluoromethyl)phenyl]-5-methoxypentylidene]amino]oxy]ethanamine,

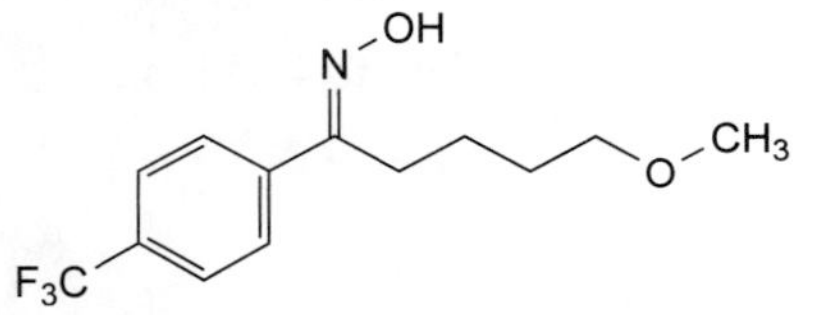

I. (*E*)-*N*-[5-methoxy-1-[4-(trifluoromethyl)phenyl]pentylidene]hydroxylamine,

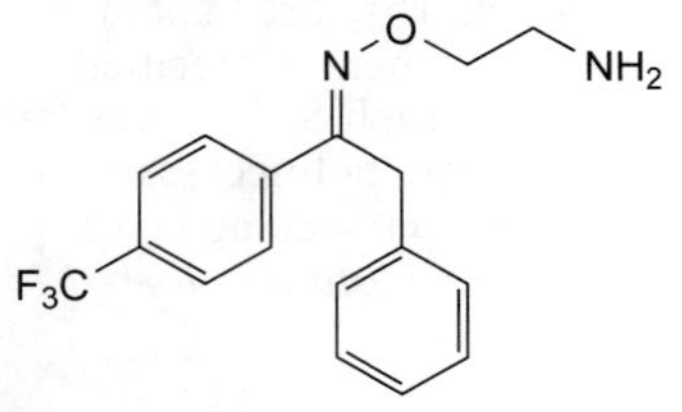

J. 2-[[[(1*E*)-2-phenyl-1-[4-(trifluoromethyl)phenyl]-ethylidene]amino]oxy]ethanamine.

01/2008:1214

FRANGULA BARK DRY EXTRACT, STANDARDISED

Frangulae corticis extractum siccum normatum

DEFINITION

Standardised dry extract obtained from *Frangula bark (0025)*.

Content: 15.0 per cent to 30.0 per cent of glucofrangulins, expressed as glucofrangulin A ($C_{27}H_{30}O_{14}$; M_r 578.5) (dried extract); the measured content does not deviate from that stated on the label by more than ± 10 per cent.

PRODUCTION

The extract is produced from the herbal drug by a suitable procedure using ethanol (50-80 per cent *V/V*).

CHARACTERS

Appearance: yellowish-brown, fine powder.

IDENTIFICATION

A. Thin-layer chromatography (*2.2.27*).

Test solution. To 0.05 g of the extract to be examined add 5 ml of *ethanol (70 per cent V/V) R* and heat to boiling. Cool and centrifuge. Decant the supernatant solution immediately and use within 30 min.

Reference solution. Dissolve 20 mg of *barbaloin R* in *ethanol (70 per cent V/V) R* and dilute to 10 ml with the same solvent.

Plate: *TLC silica gel plate R.*

Mobile phase: *water R, methanol R, ethyl acetate R* (13:17:100 *V/V/V*).

Application: 10 µl as bands.

Development: over a path of 10 cm.

Drying: in air for 5 min.

Detection: spray with a 50 g/l solution of *potassium hydroxide R* in *ethanol (50 per cent V/V) R* and heat at 100-105 °C for 15 min; examine immediately after heating.

Results: the chromatogram obtained with the reference solution shows in the median third a reddish-brown zone due to barbaloin. The chromatogram obtained with the test solution shows 2 orange-brown zones (glucofrangulins) in the lower third and 2-4 red zones (frangulins, not always clearly separated, and above them frangula-emodin) in the upper third.

B. To about 25 mg add 25 ml of *dilute hydrochloric acid R* and heat the mixture on a water-bath for 15 min. Allow to cool, shake with 20 ml of *ether R* and discard the aqueous layer. Shake the ether layer with 10 ml of *dilute ammonia R1*. The aqueous layer becomes reddish-violet.

TESTS

Loss on drying (*2.8.17*): maximum 5.0 per cent.

Microbial contamination. Total viable aerobic count (*2.6.12*) not more than 10^4 per gram of which not more than 10^2 fungi per gram, determined by plate count. It complies with the test for *Escherichia coli* and *Salmonella* (*2.6.13*).

ASSAY

Carry out the assay protected from bright light.

In a tared round-bottomed flask with a ground-glass neck, weigh 0.100 g. Add 25.0 ml of a 70 per cent *V/V* solution of *methanol R*, mix and weigh again. Heat the flask in a water-bath under a reflux condenser at 70 °C for 15 min. Allow to cool, weigh and adjust to the original mass with a 70 per cent *V/V* solution of *methanol R*. Filter and transfer 5.0 ml of the filtrate to a separating funnel. Add 50 ml of *water R* and 0.1 ml of *hydrochloric acid R*. Shake with 5 quantities, each of 20 ml, of *light petroleum R1*. Allow the layers to separate and transfer the aqueous layer to a 100 ml volumetric flask. Combine the light petroleum layers and wash with 2 quantities, each of 15 ml, of *water R*. Use this water for washing the separating funnel and add it to the aqueous solution in the volumetric flask. Add 5 ml of a 50 g/l solution of *sodium carbonate R* and dilute to 100.0 ml with *water R*. Discard the light petroleum layer. Transfer 40.0 ml of the aqueous solution to a 200 ml round-bottomed flask with a ground-glass neck. Add 20 ml of a 200 g/l solution of *ferric chloride R* and heat under a reflux condenser for 20 min in a water-bath with the water level above that of the liquid in the flask. Add 2 ml of *hydrochloric acid R* and continue heating for 20 min, shaking frequently, until the precipitate is dissolved. Allow to cool, transfer the mixture to a separating funnel and shake with 3 quantities, each of 25 ml, of *ether R*, previously used to rinse the flask. Combine the ether extracts and wash with 2 quantities, each of 15 ml, of *water R*. Transfer the ether layer to a volumetric flask and dilute to 100.0 ml with *ether R*. Evaporate 20.0 ml carefully to dryness and dissolve the residue in 10.0 ml of a 5 g/l solution of *magnesium acetate R* in *methanol R*. Measure the absorbance (*2.2.25*) at 515 nm using *methanol R* as the compensation liquid.

Calculate the percentage content of glucofrangulins, expressed as glucofrangulin A, using the following expression:

$$\frac{A \times 3.06}{m}$$

i.e. taking the specific absorbance of glucofrangulin A to be 204, calculated on the basis of the specific absorbance of barbaloin.

A = absorbance at 515 nm;

m = mass of the preparation to be examined, in grams.

LABELLING

The label states the content of glucofrangulins.

07/2008:2394

FRESH BILBERRY FRUIT DRY EXTRACT, REFINED AND STANDARDISED

Myrtilli fructus recentis extractum siccum raffinatum et normatum

DEFINITION

Refined and standardised dry extract produced from *Bilberry fruit, fresh (1602).*

Content: 32.4 per cent to 39.6 per cent of anthocyanins, expressed as cyanidin 3-*O*-glucoside chloride [chrysanthemin ($C_{21}H_{21}ClO_{11}$; M_r 484.8)] (dried extract).

PRODUCTION

The extract is produced from the herbal drug by a suitable procedure using ethanol (96 per cent *V/V*) or methanol (100 per cent). Refinement may be performed by ion-exchange chromatography.

CHARACTERS

Appearance: dark reddish-violet, amorphous, hygroscopic powder.

IDENTIFICATION

First identification: B.

Second identification: A.

A. Thin-layer chromatography (*2.2.27*).

Test solution. Dissolve 0.10 g of the extract to be examined in 25 ml of *methanol R*. Stir for 15 min and filter.

Reference solution. Dissolve 2 mg of *chrysanthemin R* and 2 mg of *myrtillin R* in 5 ml of *methanol R*.

Plate: TLC plate coated with *cellulose for chromatography R* (5-40 μm) [or TLC plate coated with *cellulose for chromatography R* (2-10 μm)].

Mobile phase:

– *mobile phase A*: *hydrochloric acid R, acetic acid R, water R* (3:15:82 *V/V/V*);

– *mobile phase B*: *water R, acetic acid R* (40:60 *V/V*).

Application: 10 μl [or 2 μl] as bands of 10 mm [or 6 mm].

Development A: over a path of 10 cm [or 6 cm] with mobile phase A.

Drying A: in warm air.

Development B: over a path of 10 cm [or 6 cm] with mobile phase B.

Drying B: in air.

Detection: examine in daylight.

Results: see below the sequence of zones present in the chromatograms obtained with the reference solution and the test solution. Furthermore, other faint zones may be present in the chromatogram obtained with the test solution.

Top of the plate	
_______	_______
	A violet-red zone
Chrysanthemin: a violet-red zone	A violet-red zone (chrysanthemin)
Myrtillin: a violet-red zone	A violet-red zone (myrtillin)
_______	_______
Reference solution	**Test solution**

B. Liquid chromatography (*2.2.29*) as described in the test for total anthocyanidins.

The characteristic anthocyanin peaks (peaks 1-8, 10-15 and 17) in the chromatogram obtained with the test solution are similar in their retention times to those in the chromatogram obtained with reference solution (b).

TESTS

Loss on drying (*2.8.17*): maximum 4.5 per cent.

Total ash (*2.4.16*): maximum 2.0 per cent.

Total anthocyanidins. Liquid chromatography (*2.2.29*). *Maintain the solutions at 4 °C.*

Solvent mixture: *hydrochloric acid R, methanol R* (2:98 *V/V*).

Test solution. Dissolve 125.0 mg of the extract to be examined in the solvent mixture and dilute to 25.0 ml with the solvent mixture. Dilute 5.0 ml of this solution to 20.0 ml with *dilute phosphoric acid R.*

Reference solution (a). Dissolve 10.0 mg of *cyanidin chloride CRS* in the solvent mixture and dilute to 25.0 ml with the solvent mixture. Dilute 2.0 ml of this solution to 100.0 ml with *dilute phosphoric acid R.*

Reference solution (b). Dissolve 125.0 mg of *bilberry dry extract CRS* in the solvent mixture and dilute to 25.0 ml with the solvent mixture. Dilute 5.0 ml of this solution to 20.0 ml with *dilute phosphoric acid R.*

Monographs D-K

Column:

- *size*: l = 0.250 m, Ø = 4.6 mm;
- *stationary phase*: *octadecylsilyl silica gel for chromatography R* (5 µm);
- *temperature*: 30 °C.

Mobile phase:

- *mobile phase A*: *anhydrous formic acid R, water R* (8.5:91.5 *V/V*);
- *mobile phase B*: *anhydrous formic acid R, acetonitrile R, methanol R, water R,* (8.5:22.5:22.5:41.5 *V/V/V/V*);

Time (min)	Mobile phase A (per cent *V/V*)	Mobile phase B (per cent *V/V*)
0 - 35	93 → 75	7 → 25
35 - 45	75 → 35	25 → 65
45 - 46	35 → 0	65 → 100
46 - 50	0	100

Flow rate: 1.0 ml/min.

Detection: spectrophotometer at 535 nm.

Injection: 10 µl.

Identification of peaks: use the chromatogram supplied with *bilberry dry extract CRS* and the chromatograms obtained with reference solutions (a) and (b) to identify the peaks due to the anthocyanins and the anthocyanidins.

Retention times: the retention times and the elution order of the peaks are similar to those shown in the chromatogram (Figure 2394.-1).

System suitability: reference solution (b):

- *peak-to-valley ratio*: minimum 2.0, where H_p = height above the baseline of the peak due to cyanidin 3-*O*-galactoside (peak 3) and H_v = height above the baseline of the lowest point of the curve separating this peak from the peak due to delphinidin 3-*O*-arabinoside (peak 4).

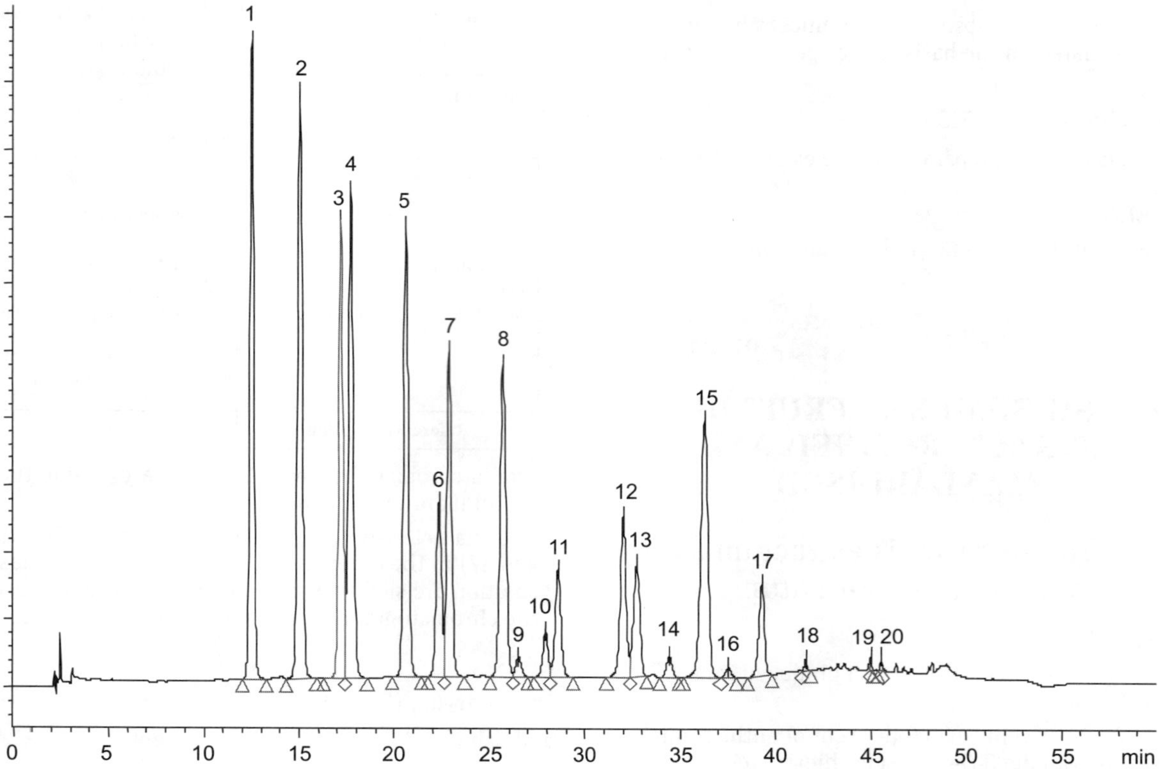

1. delphinidin 3-*O*-galactoside chloride
2. myrtillin (delphinidin 3-*O*-glucoside chloride)
3. cyanidin 3-*O*-galactoside chloride
4. delphinidin 3-*O*-arabinoside chloride
5. chrysanthemin (cyanidin 3-*O*-glucoside chloride)
6. petunidin 3-*O*-galactoside chloride
7. cyanidin 3-*O*-arabinoside chloride
8. petunidin 3-*O*-glucoside chloride
9. delphinidin chloride
10. peonidin 3-*O*-galactoside chloride
11. petunidin 3-*O*-arabinoside chloride
12. peonidin 3-*O*-glucoside chloride
13. malvidin 3-*O*-galactoside chloride
14. peonidin 3-*O*-arabinoside chloride
15. malvidin 3-*O*-glucoside chloride
16. cyanidin chloride
17. malvidin 3-*O*-arabinoside chloride
18. petunidin chloride
19. peonidin chloride
20. malvidin chloride

Figure 2394.-1. – *Chromatogram for the assay of refined and standardised fresh bilberry fruit dry extract*

Monographs D-K

Calculate the percentage content of total anthocyanidins, expressed as cyanidin chloride, using the following expression:

$$\frac{A_1 \times m_2 \times 100 \times p}{m_1 \times A_2 \times 1250}$$

A_1 = sum of the areas of the peaks due to the anthocyanidins (peaks 9, 16, 18-20) in the chromatogram obtained with the test solution;

A_2 = area of the peak due to cyanidin chloride (peak 16) in the chromatogram obtained with reference solution (a);

m_1 = mass of the extract to be examined used to prepare the test solution, in grams;

m_2 = mass of *cyanidin chloride CRS* used to prepare reference solution (a), in grams;

p = percentage content of cyanidin chloride in *cyanidin chloride CRS*.

Limits: not more than 1.0 per cent of total anthocyanidins, expressed as cyanidin chloride.

ASSAY

Liquid chromatography (*2.2.29*) as described in the test for total anthocyanidins with the following modification.

Injection: test solution and reference solution (b).

Calculate the percentage content of total anthocyanins expressed as cyanidin 3-*O*-glucoside chloride, using the following expression:

$$\frac{A_1 \times m_2 \times p}{m_1 \times A_2}$$

A_1 = sum of the areas of the peaks due to the anthocyanins (peaks 1-8, 10-15 and 17) in the chromatogram obtained with the test solution;

A_2 = area of the peak due to cyanidin 3-*O*-glucoside chloride (peak 5) in the chromatogram obtained with reference solution (b);

m_1 = mass of the extract to be examined used to prepare the test solution, in grams;

m_2 = mass of *bilberry dry extract CRS* used to prepare reference solution (b), in grams;

p = percentage content of cyanidin 3-*O*-glucoside chloride in *bilberry dry extract CRS*.

G

07/2008:1522

GINGER

Zingiberis rhizoma

DEFINITION

Dried, whole or cut rhizome of *Zingiber officinale* Roscoe, with the cork removed, either completely or from the wide flat surfaces only.

Content: minimum 15 ml/kg of essential oil (anhydrous drug).

CHARACTERS

Characteristic aromatic odour.

Spicy and burning taste.

IDENTIFICATION

A. The rhizome is laterally compressed, bearing short, flattened, obovate oblique branches on the upper side, each sometimes having a depressed scar at the apex; the whole rhizomes are about 5-10 cm long, 1.5-3 cm or 4 cm wide and 1-1.5 cm thick, sometimes split longitudinally. The scraped rhizome with a light-brown external surface shows longitudinal striations and occasional loose fibres; the outer surface of the unscraped rhizome varies from pale to dark brown and is more or less covered with cork which shows conspicuous, narrow, longitudinal and transverse ridges; the cork readily exfoliates from the lateral surfaces but persists between the branches. The fracture is short and starchy with projecting fibres. The smoothed transversely cut surface exhibits a narrow cortex separated by an endodermis from a much wider stele; it shows numerous, scattered, fibrovascular bundles and abundant scattered oleoresin cells with yellow contents. The unscraped rhizome shows, in addition, an outer layer of dark brown cork.

B. Reduce to a powder (355) (*2.9.12*). The powder is pale yellow or brownish. Examine under a microscope using *chloral hydrate solution R*. The powder shows the following diagnostic characters: groups of large, thin-walled, septate fibres, with one wall frequently dentate; fairly large vessels with reticulate thickening and often accompanied by narrow, thin-walled cells containing brown pigment; abundant thin-walled parenchyma of the ground tissue, some cells containing brown oleoresin; fragments of brown cork, usually seen in surface view. Examine under a microscope using a 50 per cent *V/V* solution of *glycerol R*. The powder shows abundant starch granules, simple, flattened, oblong or oval or irregular, up to about 50 µm long and 25 µm wide, with a small point hilum situated at the narrower end; occasional granules show faint, transverse striations.

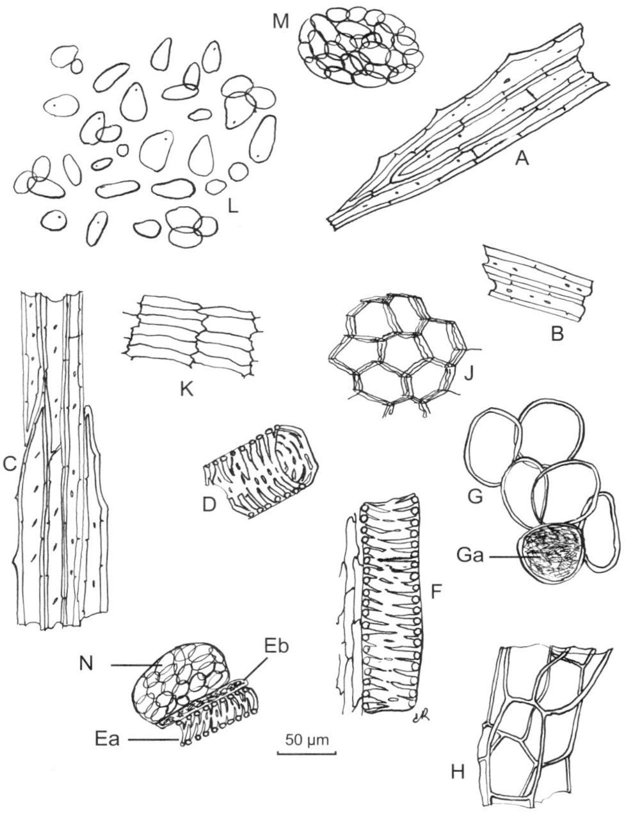

A, B, C. Groups of septate fibres, sometimes with dentate walls

D, E, F. Vessels with reticulate thickening (Ea), sometimes accompanied by cells with brown contents (Eb)

G, H. Parenchyma with cells containing oleoresin (Ga)

J, K. Fragments of cork, in surface view (J) and in transverse section (K)

L, M, N. Starch granules, free (L) and in parenchymatous cells (M, N)

Figure 1522.-1. – *Illustration of powdered herbal drug of ginger (see Identification B)*

C. Thin-layer chromatography (*2.2.27*).

Test solution. To 1.0 g of the powdered drug (710) (*2.9.12*) add 5 ml of *methanol R*. Shake for 15 min and filter.

Reference solution. Dissolve 10 µl of *citral R* and 10 mg of *resorcinol R* in 10 ml of *methanol R*. Prepare the solution immediately before use.

Plate: *TLC silica gel plate R.*

Mobile phase: *hexane R, ether R* (40:60 *V/V*).

Application: 20 µl, as bands.

Development: in an unsaturated tank, over a path of 15 cm.

Drying: in air.

Detection: spray with a 10 g/l solution of *vanillin R* in *sulphuric acid R* and examine in daylight while heating at 100-105 °C for 10 min.

Results: the chromatogram obtained with the reference solution shows in the lower half an intense red zone (resorcinol) and in the upper half 2 violet zones (citral). The chromatogram obtained with the test solution shows below the zone due to resorcinol in the chromatogram obtained with the reference solution 2 intense violet zones (gingerols) and in the middle, between the zones due to resorcinol and citral in the chromatogram obtained with the reference solution, 2 other less intense violet zones (shogaols). Other zones may be present.

Monographs D-K

TESTS

Water (*2.2.13*): maximum 100 ml/kg, determined by distillation on 20.0 g of the powdered drug (710) (*2.9.12*).

Total ash (*2.4.16*): maximum 6.0 per cent.

ASSAY

Carry out the determination of essential oils in herbal drugs (*2.8.12*). Use 20.0 g of the freshly, coarsely powdered drug, a 1000 ml round-bottomed flask, 10 drops of *liquid paraffin R* or other antifoam, 500 ml of *water R* as distillation liquid and 0.5 ml of *xylene R* in the graduated tube. Distil at a rate of 2-3 ml/min for 4 h.

07/2008:1330

GLUCOSE, LIQUID

Glucosum liquidum

DEFINITION

Aqueous solution containing a mixture of glucose, oligosaccharides and polysaccharides obtained by hydrolysis of starch.

It contains a minimum of 70.0 per cent dry matter.

The degree of hydrolysis, expressed as dextrose equivalent (DE), is not less than 20 (nominal value).

CHARACTERS

Appearance: clear, colourless or brown, viscous liquid.

Solubility: miscible with water.

It may partly or totally solidify at room temperature and liquefies again when heated to 50 °C.

IDENTIFICATION

A. Dissolve 0.1 g in 2.5 ml of *water R* and heat with 2.5 ml of *cupri-tartaric solution R*. A red precipitate is formed.

B. Dip, for 1 s, a suitable stick with a reactive pad containing glucose-oxidase, peroxidase and a hydrogen-donating substance, such as tetramethylbenzidine, in a 5 g/l solution of the substance to be examined. Observe the colour of the reactive pad; within 60 s the colour changes from yellow to green or blue.

C. It is a clear, colourless or brown, viscous liquid, miscible with water. The substance may partly or totally solidify at room temperature and liquefies again when heated to 50 °C.

D. Dextrose equivalent (see Tests).

TESTS

Solution S. Dissolve 25.0 g in *carbon dioxide-free water R* and dilute to 50.0 ml with the same solvent.

pH (*2.2.3*): 4.0 to 6.0.

Mix 1 ml of a 223.6 g/l solution of *potassium chloride R* and 30 ml of solution S.

Sulphur dioxide (*2.5.29*): maximum 20 ppm; maximum 400 ppm if intended for the production of lozenges or pastilles obtained by high boiling techniques, provided that the final product contains maximum 50 ppm of sulphur dioxide.

Heavy metals (*2.4.8*): maximum 10 ppm.

Dilute 2 ml of solution S to 30 ml with *water R*. The solution complies with test E. Prepare the reference solution using 10 ml of *lead standard solution (1 ppm Pb) R*.

Loss on drying (*2.2.32*): maximum 30.0 per cent, determined on 1.000 g. Triturate the sample with 3.000 g of *kieselguhr G R*, previously dried at 80 °C under high vacuum for 2 h, and dry at 80 °C under high vacuum for 2 h.

Sulphated ash (*2.4.14*): maximum 0.5 per cent, determined on 1.0 g.

Dextrose equivalent (DE): within 10 per cent of the nominal value.

Weigh an amount of the substance to be examined equivalent to 2.85-3.15 g of reducing carbohydrates, calculated as dextrose equivalent, into a 500 ml volumetric flask. Dissolve in *water R* and dilute to 500.0 ml with the same solvent. Transfer the solution to a 50 ml burette.

Pipette 25.0 ml of *cupri-tartaric solution R* into a 250 ml flask and add 18.5 ml of the test solution from the burette, mix and add a few glass beads. Place the flask on a hot plate, previously adjusted so that the solution begins to boil after 2 min ± 15 s. Allow to boil for exactly 120 s, add 1 ml of a 1 g/l solution of *methylene blue R* and titrate with the test solution (V_1) until the blue colour disappears. Maintain the solution at boiling throughout the titration.

Standardise the cupri-tartaric solution using a 6.00 g/l solution of *glucose R* (V_0).

Calculate the dextrose equivalent using the following expression:

$$\frac{300 \times V_0 \times 100}{V_1 \times M \times D}$$

V_0 = total volume of glucose standard solution, in millilitres,

V_1 = total volume of test solution, in millilitres,

M = mass of the sample, in grams,

D = percentage content of dry matter in the substance.

LABELLING

The label states the dextrose equivalent (DE) (= nominal value).

01/2008:1218

GUAR

Cyamopsidis seminis pulvis

DEFINITION

Guar is obtained by grinding the endosperms of seeds of *Cyamopsis tetragonolobus* (L.) Taub. It consists mainly of guar galactomannan.

CHARACTERS

Appearance: white or almost white powder.

Solubility: it yields a mucilage of variable viscosity when dissolved in water, practically insoluble in ethanol (96 per cent).

IDENTIFICATION

A. Examined under a microscope in *glycerol R*, the substance to be examined (125) (*2.9.12*) shows pyriform or ovoid cells, usually isolated, having very thick walls around a central somewhat elongated lumen with granular contents, and smaller polyhedral cells, isolated or in clusters, with thinner walls.

B. In a conical flask place 2 g, add rapidly 45 ml of *water R* and stir vigorously for 30 s. After 5-10 min a stiff gel forms which does not flow when the flask is inverted.

Monographs D-K

C. Mix a suspension of 0.1 g in 10 ml of *water R* with 1 ml of a 10 g/l solution of *disodium tetraborate R*; the mixture soon gels.

D. Thin-layer chromatography (*2.2.27*).

Test solution. To 10 mg in a thick-walled centrifuge test tube add 2 ml of a 100 g/l solution of *trifluoroacetic acid R*, shake vigorously to dissolve the forming gel, stopper the test tube and heat the mixture at 120 °C for 1 h. Centrifuge the hydrolysate, transfer the clear supernatant liquid carefully into a 50 ml flask, add 10 ml of *water R* and evaporate the solution to dryness under reduced pressure. To the resulting clear film add 0.1 ml of *water R* and 0.9 ml of *methanol R*. Centrifuge to separate the amorphous precipitate. Dilute the supernatant liquid, if necessary, to 1 ml with *methanol R*.

Reference solution. Dissolve 10 mg of *galactose R* and 10 mg of *mannose R* in 2 ml of *water R*, then dilute to 20 ml with *methanol R*.

Plate: *TLC silica gel plate R*.

Mobile phase: *water R, acetonitrile R* (15:85 *V/V*).

Application: 5 µl, as bands.

Development: over a path of 15 cm.

Detection: spray with *aminohippuric acid reagent R* and dry at 120 °C for 5 min.

Results: the chromatogram obtained with the reference solution shows, in the lower part 2 clearly separated brownish zones due to galactose and mannose in order of increasing R_F value. The chromatogram obtained with the test solution shows 2 zones due to galactose and mannose.

TESTS

Tragacanth, sterculia gum, agar, alginates, carrageenan. To a small amount of the substance to be examined add 0.2 ml of freshly prepared *ruthenium red solution R*. Examined under a microscope the cell walls do not stain red.

Protein: maximum 8.0 per cent.

Carry out the determination of nitrogen by the method of sulphuric acid digestion (*2.5.9*) using 0.170 g. Multiply the result by 6.25.

Apparent viscosity (*2.2.10*): 85 per cent to 115 per cent of the value stated on the label.

Moisten a quantity equivalent to 1.00 g of the dried substance with 2.5 ml of *2-propanol R*. While stirring, dilute to 100.0 ml with *water R*. After 1 h, determine the viscosity at 20 °C using a rotating viscometer and a shear rate of 100 s^{-1}.

Loss on drying (*2.2.32*): maximum 15.0 per cent, determined on 1.000 g by drying in an oven at 105 °C for 5 h.

Total ash (*2.4.16*): maximum 1.8 per cent.

Microbial contamination. Total viable aerobic count (*2.6.12*) not more than 10^4 micro-organisms per gram, determined by plate-count. It complies with the tests *Escherichia coli* and for *Salmonella* (*2.6.13*).

LABELLING

The label states the apparent viscosity in millipascal seconds for a 10 g/l solution.

01/2008:0908

GUAR GALACTOMANNAN

Guar galactomannanum

DEFINITION

Guar galactomannan is obtained from the seeds of *Cyamopsis tetragonolobus* (L.) Taub. by grinding of the endosperms and subsequent partial hydrolysis. The main components are polysaccharides composed of D-galactose and D-mannose at molecular ratios of 1:1.4 to 1:2. The molecules consist of a linear main chain of β-(1→4)-glycosidically linked mannopyranoses and single α-(1→6)-glycosidically linked galactopyranoses.

CHARACTERS

Appearance: yellowish-white powder.

Solubility: soluble in cold water and in hot water, practically insoluble in organic solvents.

IDENTIFICATION

A. Mix 5 g of solution S (see Tests) with 0.5 ml of a 10 g/l solution of *disodium tetraborate R*. A gel forms within a short time.

B. Heat 20 g of solution S in a water-bath for 10 min. Allow to cool and adjust to the original mass with *water R*. The solution does not gel.

C. Thin-layer chromatography (*2.2.27*).

Test solution. To 10 mg of the substance to be examined in a thick-walled centrifuge tube add 2 ml of a 230 g/l solution of *trifluoroacetic acid R*, shake vigorously to dissolve the forming gel, stopper the tube and heat the mixture at 120 °C for 1 h. Centrifuge the hydrolysate, transfer the clear supernatant liquid carefully into a 50 ml flask, add 10 ml of *water R* and evaporate the solution to dryness under reduced pressure. Take up the residue in 10 ml of *water R* and evaporate again to dryness under reduced pressure. To the resulting clear film, which has no odour of acetic acid, add 0.1 ml of *water R* and 1 ml of *methanol R*. Centrifuge to separate the amorphous precipitate. Dilute the supernatant liquid, if necessary, to 1 ml with *methanol R*.

Reference solution. Dissolve 10 mg of *galactose R* and 10 mg of *mannose R* in 2 ml of *water R* and dilute to 10 ml with *methanol R*.

Plate: *TLC silica gel G plate R*.

Mobile phase: *water R, acetonitrile R* (15:85 *V/V*).

Application: 5 µl, as bands of 20 mm by 3 mm.

Development: over a path of 15 cm.

Detection: spray with *aminohippuric acid reagent R* and heat at 120 °C for 5 min.

Results: the chromatogram obtained with the reference solution shows in the lower part 2 clearly separated brownish zones (galactose and mannose in order of increasing R_F value). The chromatogram obtained with the test solution shows 2 zones due to galactose and mannose.

TESTS

Solution S. Moisten 1.0 g with 2 ml of *2-propanol R*. While stirring, dilute to 100 g with *water R* and stir until the substance is uniformly dispersed. Allow to stand for at least 1 h. If the apparent viscosity is below 200 mPa·s, use 3.0 g of substance instead of 1.0 g.

pH (*2.2.3*): 5.5 to 7.5 for solution S.

Apparent viscosity (*2.2.10*): 75 per cent to 140 per cent of the value stated on the label.

Moisten a quantity of the substance to be examined equivalent to 2.00 g of the dried substance with 2.5 ml of *2-propanol R* and, while stirring, dilute to 100.0 ml with *water R*. After 1 h, determine the viscosity at 20 °C using a rotating viscometer and a shear rate of 100 s^{-1}.

Insoluble matter: maximum 7.0 per cent.

In a 250 ml flask disperse, while stirring, 1.50 g in a mixture of 1.6 ml of *sulphuric acid R* and 150 ml of *water R* and weigh. Immerse the flask in a water-bath and heat under a reflux condenser for 6 h. Adjust to the original mass with *water R*. Filter the hot solution through a tared, sintered-glass filter (160) (*2.1.2*). Rinse the filter with hot *water R* and dry at 100-105 °C. The residue weighs a maximum of 105 mg.

Protein: maximum 5.0 per cent.

Carry out the determination of nitrogen by sulphuric acid digestion (*2.5.9*), using 0.400 g. Multiply the result by 6.25.

Tragacanth, sterculia gum, agar, alginates and carrageenan. To a small amount of the substance to be examined, add 0.2 ml of freshly prepared *ruthenium red solution R*. Examined under a microscope, none of the structures are red.

Loss on drying (*2.2.32*): maximum 15.0 per cent, determined on 1.000 g by drying in an oven at 105 °C for 5 h.

Total ash (*2.4.16*): maximum 1.8 per cent, determined on 1.00 g after wetting with 10 ml of *water R*.

Microbial contamination. Total viable aerobic count (*2.6.12*) not more than 10^3 micro-organisms per gram, determined by plate count. It complies with the tests for *Escherichia coli* and for *Salmonella* (*2.6.13*).

LABELLING

The label states the apparent viscosity in millipascal seconds for a 20 g/l solution.

H

Monographs D-K

07/2008:0557

HUMAN ANTI-D IMMUNOGLOBULIN

Immunoglobulinum humanum anti-D

DEFINITION

Human anti-D immunoglobulin is a liquid or freeze-dried preparation containing immunoglobulins, mainly immunoglobulin G. The preparation is intended for intramuscular administration. It contains specific antibodies against erythrocyte D-antigen and may also contain small quantities of other blood-group antibodies. *Human normal immunoglobulin (0338)* and/or *Human albumin solution (0255)* may be added.

It complies with the monograph *Human normal immunoglobulin (0338)*, except for the minimum number of donors and the minimum total protein content.

The test for anti-D antibodies (*2.6.26*) prescribed in the monograph *Human normal immunoglobulin (0338)* is not carried out, since it is replaced by the assay of human anti-D immunoglobulin (*2.7.13*) as prescribed below under Potency.

For products prepared by a method that eliminates immunoglobulins with specificities other than anti-D, where authorised, the test for antibodies to hepatitis B surface antigen is not required.

PRODUCTION

Human anti-D immunoglobulin is preferably obtained from the plasma of donors with a sufficient titre of previously acquired anti-D antibodies. Where necessary, in order to ensure an adequate supply of human anti-D immunoglobulin, it is obtained from plasma derived from donors immunised with D-positive erythrocytes that are compatible in relevant blood group systems in order to avoid formation of undesirable antibodies.

ERYTHROCYTE DONORS

Erythrocyte donors comply with the requirements for donors prescribed in the monograph *Human plasma for fractionation (0853)*.

IMMUNISATION

Immunisation of the plasma donor is carried out under proper medical supervision. Recommendations concerning donor immunisation, including testing of erythrocyte donors, have been formulated by the World Health Organisation (*Requirements for the collection, processing and quality control of blood, blood components and plasma derivatives*, WHO Technical Report Series, No. 840, 1994 or subsequent revision).

POOLED PLASMA

To limit the potential B19 virus burden in plasma pools used for the manufacture of anti-D immunoglobulin, the plasma pool is tested for B19 virus using validated nucleic acid amplification techniques (*2.6.21*).

B19 virus DNA: maximum 10.0 IU/μl.

A positive control with 10.0 IU of B19 virus DNA per microlitre and, to test for inhibitors, an internal control prepared by addition of a suitable marker to a sample of the plasma pool are included in the test. The test is invalid if the positive control is non-reactive or if the result obtained with the internal control indicates the presence of inhibitors.

B19 virus DNA for NAT testing BRP is suitable for use as a positive control.

If *Human normal immunoglobulin (0338)* and/or *Human albumin solution (0255)* are added to the preparation, the plasma pool or pools from which they are derived comply with the above requirement for B19 virus DNA.

POTENCY

Carry out the assay of human anti-D immunoglobulin (*2.7.13, Method A*). The estimated potency is not less than 90 per cent of the stated potency. The confidence limits (P = 0.95) are not less than 80 per cent and not more than 120 per cent of the estimated potency.

Method B or C (*2.7.13*) may be used for potency determination if a satisfactory correlation with the results obtained by Method A has been established for the particular product.

STORAGE

See *Human normal immunoglobulin (0338)*.

LABELLING

See *Human normal immunoglobulin (0338)*.

The label states the number of International Units per container.

07/2008:0338

HUMAN NORMAL IMMUNOGLOBULIN

Immunoglobulinum humanum normale

DEFINITION

Human normal immunoglobulin is a liquid or freeze-dried preparation containing immunoglobulins, mainly immunoglobulin G (IgG). Other proteins may be present. Human normal immunoglobulin contains the IgG antibodies of normal subjects. It is intended for intramuscular or subcutaneous administration.

Human normal immunoglobulin is obtained from plasma that complies with the requirements of the monograph on *Human plasma for fractionation (0853)*. No antibiotic is added to the plasma used.

PRODUCTION

The method of preparation includes a step or steps that have been shown to remove or to inactivate known agents of infection; if substances are used for inactivation of viruses, it shall have been shown that any residues present in the final product have no adverse effects on the patients treated with the immunoglobulin.

The product shall have been shown, by suitable tests in animals and evaluation during clinical trials, to be well tolerated when administered intramuscularly or subcutaneously.

Human normal immunoglobulin is prepared from pooled material from at least 1000 donors by a method that has been shown to yield a product that:

- does not transmit infection;
- at a protein concentration of 160 g/l, contains antibodies for at least 2 of which (1 viral and 1 bacterial) an International Standard or Reference Preparation is available, the concentration of such antibodies being at least 10 times that in the initial pooled material.

If the human normal immunoglobulin is intended for subcutaneous administration, the production method shall have been shown to consistently yield products that comply with the test for Fc function of immunoglobulin (*2.7.9*).

Human normal immunoglobulin is prepared as a stabilised solution, for example in a 9 g/l solution of sodium chloride, a 22.5 g/l solution of glycine or, if the preparation is to be freeze-dried, a 60 g/l solution of glycine. Multidose preparations contain an antimicrobial preservative. Single-dose preparations do not contain an antimicrobial preservative. Any antimicrobial preservative or stabilising agent used shall have been shown to have no deleterious effect on the final product in the amount present. The solution is passed through a bacteria-retentive filter. The preparation may subsequently be freeze-dried and the containers closed under vacuum or under an inert gas.

The stability of the preparation is demonstrated by suitable tests carried out during development studies.

CHARACTERS

The liquid preparation is clear and pale-yellow or light-brown; during storage it may show formation of slight turbidity or a small amount of particulate matter. The freeze-dried preparation is a hygroscopic, white or slightly yellow powder or solid, friable mass.

For the freeze-dried preparation, reconstitute as stated on the label immediately before carrying out the identification and the tests, except those for solubility and water.

IDENTIFICATION

Examine by a suitable immunoelectrophoresis technique. Using antiserum to normal human serum, compare normal human serum and the preparation to be examined, both diluted to a protein concentration of 10 g/l. The main component of the preparation to be examined corresponds to the IgG component of normal human serum. The solution may show the presence of small quantities of other plasma proteins.

TESTS

Solubility. For the freeze-dried preparation, add the volume of the liquid stated on the label. The preparation dissolves completely within 20 min at 20-25 °C.

pH (*2.2.3*): 5.0 to 7.2.

Dilute the preparation to be examined with a 9 g/l solution of *sodium chloride R* to a protein concentration of 10 g/l.

Total protein. Dilute the preparation to be examined with a 9 g/l solution of *sodium chloride R* to obtain a solution containing about 15 mg of protein in 2 ml. To 2.0 ml of this solution in a round-bottomed centrifuge tube add 2 ml of a 75 g/l solution of *sodium molybdate R* and 2 ml of a mixture of 1 volume of *nitrogen-free sulphuric acid R* and 30 volumes of *water R*. Shake, centrifuge for 5 min, decant the supernatant liquid and allow the inverted tube to drain on filter paper. Determine the nitrogen in the residue by the method of sulphuric acid digestion (*2.5.9*) and calculate the content of protein by multiplying the result by 6.25. The preparation has a protein concentration of not less than 100 g/l and not more than 180 g/l and contains not less than 90 per cent and not more than 110 per cent of the quantity of protein stated on the label.

Protein composition. Examine by zone electrophoresis (*2.2.31*).

Use strips of suitable cellulose acetate gel or suitable agarose gel as the supporting medium and *barbital buffer solution pH 8.6 R1* as the electrolyte solution.

If cellulose acetate is the supporting material, the method described below can be used. If agarose gels are used, and because they are normally part of an automated system, the manufacturer's instructions are followed instead.

Test solution. Dilute the preparation to be examined with a 9 g/l solution of *sodium chloride R* to a protein concentration of 50 g/l.

Reference solution. Reconstitute *human immunoglobulin for electrophoresis BRP* and dilute with a 9 g/l solution of *sodium chloride R* to a protein concentration of 50 g/l.

To a strip apply 2.5 µl of the test solution as a 10 mm band or apply 0.25 µl per millimetre if a narrower strip is used. To another strip apply in the same manner the same volume of the reference solution. Apply a suitable electric field such that the albumin band of normal human serum applied on a control strip migrates at least 30 mm. Stain the strip with *amido black 10B solution R* for 5 min. Decolourise with a mixture of 10 volumes of *glacial acetic acid R* and 90 volumes of *methanol R* so that the background is just free of colour. Develop the transparency of the strips with a mixture of 19 volumes of *glacial acetic acid R* and 81 volumes of *methanol R*. Measure the absorbance of the bands at 600 nm in an instrument having a linear response over the range of measurement. Calculate the result as the mean of 3 measurements of each strip.

System suitability: in the electropherogram obtained with the reference solution on cellulose acetate or on agarose gels, the proportion of protein in the principal band is within the limits stated in the leaflet accompanying the reference preparation.

Results: in the electropherogram obtained with the test solution on cellulose acetate or on agarose gels, not more than 10 per cent of protein has a mobility different from that of the principal band.

Distribution of molecular size. Liquid chromatography (*2.2.29*).

Test solution. Dilute the preparation to be examined with a 9 g/l solution of *sodium chloride R* to a concentration suitable for the chromatographic system used. A concentration in the range of 4-12 g/l and injection of 50-600 µg of protein are usually suitable.

Reference solution. Dilute *human immunoglobulin (molecular size) BRP* with a 9 g/l solution of *sodium chloride R* to the same protein concentration as the test solution.

Column:

- *size*: l = 0.6 m, Ø = 7.5 mm [or l = 0.3 m, Ø = 7.8 mm];
- *stationary phase*: *hydrophilic silica gel for chromatography R*, of a grade suitable for fractionation of globular proteins with relative molecular masses in the range 10 000 to 500 000.

Mobile phase: dissolve 4.873 g of *disodium hydrogen phosphate dihydrate R*, 1.741 g of *sodium dihydrogen phosphate monohydrate R*, 11.688 g of *sodium chloride R* and 50 mg of *sodium azide R* in 1 litre of *water R*.

Flow rate: 0.5 ml/min.

Detection: spectrophotometer at 280 nm.

In the chromatogram obtained with the reference solution, the principal peak corresponds to the IgG monomer and there is a peak corresponding to the dimer with a relative retention to the principal peak of about 0.85. Identify the peaks in the chromatogram obtained with the test solution by comparison with the chromatogram obtained with the reference solution; any peak with a retention time shorter than that of the dimer corresponds to polymers

Monographs D-K

and aggregates. The preparation to be examined complies with the test if, in the chromatogram obtained with the test solution:

- *relative retention*: for the monomer and for the dimer, the relative retention to the corresponding peak in the chromatogram obtained with the reference solution is 1 ± 0.02;
- *peak area*: the sum of the peak areas of the monomer and the dimer represent not less than 85 per cent of the total area of the chromatogram and the sum of the peak areas of polymers and aggregates represents not more than 10 per cent of the total area of the chromatogram.

Anti-A and anti-B haemagglutinins (*2.6.20*). If human normal immunoglobulin is intended for subcutaneous administration, carry out the tests for anti-A and anti-B haemagglutinins. Dilute the preparation to be examined to an immunoglobulin concentration of 30 g/l before preparing the dilutions to be used in the test. The 64-fold dilutions do not show agglutination.

Anti-D antibodies (*2.6.26*). If human normal immunoglobulin is intended for subcutaneous administration, it complies with the test for anti-D antibodies in human immunoglobulin for intravenous administration.

Antibody to hepatitis B surface antigen. Not less than 0.5 IU/g of immunoglobulin, determined by a suitable immunochemical method (*2.7.1*).

Antibody to hepatitis A virus. If intended for use in the prophylaxis of hepatitis A, it complies with the following additional requirement. Determine the antibody content by comparison with a reference preparation calibrated in International Units, using an immunoassay of suitable sensitivity and specificity (*2.7.1*).

The International Unit is the activity contained in a stated amount of the International Standard for anti-hepatitis A immunoglobulin. The equivalence in International Units of the International Standard is stated by the World Health Organisation.

Human hepatitis A immunoglobulin BRP is calibrated in International Units by comparison with the International Standard.

The stated potency is not less than 100 IU/ml. The estimated potency is not less than the stated potency. The confidence limits (P = 0.95) of the estimated potency are not less than 80 per cent and not more than 125 per cent.

Water. Determined by a suitable method, such as the semi-micro determination of water (*2.5.12*), loss on drying (*2.2.32*) or near infrared spectrophotometry (*2.2.40*), the water content is within the limits approved by the competent authority.

Sterility (*2.6.1*). It complies with the test for sterility.

Pyrogens (*2.6.8*). It complies with the test for pyrogens. Inject 1 ml per kilogram of the rabbit's mass.

STORAGE

For the liquid preparation, in a colourless glass container, protected from light. For the freeze-dried preparation, in an airtight colourless glass container, protected from light.

LABELLING

The label states:

- for liquid preparations, the volume of the preparation in the container and the protein content expressed in grams per litre;
- for freeze-dried preparations, the quantity of protein in the container;
- the route of administration;
- for freeze-dried preparations, the name or composition and the volume of the reconstituting liquid to be added;
- where applicable, that the preparation is suitable for use in the prophylaxis of hepatitis A infection;
- where applicable, the anti-hepatitis A virus activity in International Units per millilitre;
- where applicable, the name and amount of antimicrobial preservative in the preparation.

07/2008:0853

HUMAN PLASMA FOR FRACTIONATION

Plasma humanum ad separationem

DEFINITION

Human plasma for fractionation is the liquid part of human blood remaining after separation of the cellular elements from blood collected in a receptacle containing an anticoagulant, or separated by continuous filtration or centrifugation of anticoagulated blood in an apheresis procedure; it is intended for the manufacture of plasma-derived products.

PRODUCTION

DONORS

Only a carefully selected, healthy donor who, as far as can be ascertained after medical examination, laboratory blood tests and a study of the donor's medical history, is free from detectable agents of infection transmissible by plasma-derived products may be used. Recommendations in this field are made by the Council of Europe [*Recommendation No. R (95) 15 on the preparation, use and quality assurance of blood components*, or subsequent revision]; a directive of the European Union also deals with the matter: *Commission Directive 2004/33/EC of 22 March 2004 implementing Directive 2002/98/EC of the European Parliament and of the Council as regards certain technical requirements for blood and blood components*.

Immunisation of donors. Immunisation of donors to obtain immunoglobulins with specific activities may be carried out when sufficient supplies of material of suitable quality cannot be obtained from naturally immunised donors. Recommendations for such immunisations are formulated by the World Health Organisation (*Requirements for the collection, processing and quality control of blood, blood components and plasma derivatives*, WHO Technical Report Series, No. 840, 1994 or subsequent revision).

Records. Records of donors and donations made are kept in such a way that, while maintaining the required degree of confidentiality concerning the donor's identity, the origin of each donation in a plasma pool and the results of the corresponding acceptance procedures and laboratory tests can be traced.

Laboratory tests. Laboratory tests are carried out for each donation to detect the following viral markers:

1. antibodies against human immunodeficiency virus 1 (anti-HIV-1);
2. antibodies against human immunodeficiency virus 2 (anti-HIV-2);
3. hepatitis B surface antigen (HBsAg);
4. antibodies against hepatitis C virus (anti-HCV).

The test methods used are of suitable sensitivity and specificity and comply with the regulations in force. If a repeat-reactive result is found in any of these tests, the donation is not accepted.

INDIVIDUAL PLASMA UNITS

The plasma is prepared by a method that removes cells and cell debris as completely as possible. Whether prepared from whole blood or by plasmapheresis, the plasma is separated from the cells by a method designed to prevent the introduction of micro-organisms. No antibacterial or antifungal agent is added to the plasma. The containers comply with the requirements for glass containers (*3.2.1*) or for plastic containers for blood and blood components (*3.2.3*). The containers are closed so as to prevent any possibility of contamination.

If 2 or more units are pooled prior to freezing, the operations are carried out using sterile connecting devices or under aseptic conditions and using containers that have not previously been used.

When obtained by plasmapheresis or from whole blood (after separation from cellular elements), plasma intended for the recovery of proteins that are labile in plasma is frozen within 24 h of collection by cooling rapidly in conditions validated to ensure that a temperature of – 25 °C or below is attained at the core of each plasma unit within 12 h of placing in the freezing apparatus.

When obtained by plasmapheresis, plasma intended solely for the recovery of proteins that are not labile in plasma is frozen by cooling rapidly in a chamber at – 20 °C or below as soon as possible and at the latest within 24 h of collection.

When obtained from whole blood, plasma intended solely for the recovery of proteins that are not labile in plasma is separated from cellular elements and frozen in a chamber at – 20 °C or below as soon as possible and at the latest within 72 h of collection.

It is not intended that the determination of total protein and factor VIII shown below be carried out on each unit of plasma. They are rather given as guidelines for good manufacturing practice, the test for factor VIII being relevant for plasma intended for use in the preparation of concentrates of labile proteins.

The total protein content of a unit of plasma depends on the serum protein content of the donor and the degree of dilution inherent in the donation procedure. When plasma is obtained from a suitable donor and using the intended proportion of anticoagulant solution, a total protein content complying with the limit of 50 g/l is obtained. If a volume of blood or plasma smaller than intended is collected into the anticoagulant solution, the resulting plasma is not necessarily unsuitable for pooling for fractionation. The aim of good manufacturing practice must be to achieve the prescribed limit for all normal donations.

Preservation of factor VIII in the donation depends on the collection procedure and the subsequent handling of the blood and plasma. With good practice, 0.7 IU/ml can usually be achieved, but units of plasma with a lower activity may still be suitable for use in the production of coagulation factor concentrates. The aim of good manufacturing practice is to conserve labile proteins as much as possible.

Total protein. Carry out the test using a pool of not fewer than 10 units. Dilute the pool with a 9 g/l solution of *sodium chloride R* to obtain a solution containing about 15 mg of protein in 2 ml. To 2.0 ml of this solution in a round-bottomed centrifuge tube add 2 ml of a 75 g/l solution of *sodium molybdate R* and 2 ml of a mixture of 1 volume of *nitrogen-free sulphuric acid R* and 30 volumes of *water R*. Shake, centrifuge for 5 min, decant the supernatant liquid and allow the inverted tube to drain on filter paper. Determine the nitrogen in the residue by the method of sulphuric acid digestion (*2.5.9*) and calculate the protein content by multiplying the quantity of nitrogen by 6.25. The total protein content is not less than 50 g/l.

Factor VIII. Carry out the test using a pool of not fewer than 10 units. Thaw the samples to be examined, if necessary, at 37 °C. Carry out the assay of factor VIII (*2.7.4*), using a reference plasma calibrated against the International Standard for human coagulation factor VIII in plasma. The activity is not less than 0.7 IU/ml.

STORAGE AND TRANSPORT

Frozen plasma is stored and transported in conditions designed to maintain the temperature at or below – 20 °C; for accidental reasons, the storage temperature may rise above – 20 °C on one or more occasions during storage and transport but the plasma is nevertheless considered suitable for fractionation if all the following conditions are fulfilled:

– the total period of time during which the temperature exceeds – 20 °C does not exceed 72 h;
– the temperature does not exceed – 15 °C on more than one occasion;
– the temperature at no time exceeds – 5 °C.

POOLED PLASMA

During the manufacture of plasma products, the first homogeneous pool of plasma (for example, after removal of cryoprecipitate) is tested for HBsAg and for HIV antibodies using test methods of suitable sensitivity and specificity; the pool must give negative results in these tests.

The plasma pool is also tested for hepatitis C virus RNA using a validated nucleic acid amplification technique (*2.6.21*). A positive control with 100 IU/ml of hepatitis C virus RNA and, to test for inhibitors, an internal control prepared by addition of a suitable marker to a sample of the plasma pool are included in the test. The test is invalid if the positive control is non-reactive or if the result obtained with the internal control indicates the presence of inhibitors. The plasma pool complies with the test if it is found non-reactive for hepatitis C virus RNA.

Hepatitis C virus RNA for NAT testing BRP is suitable for use as a positive control.

CHARACTERS

Before freezing, a clear to slightly turbid liquid without visible signs of haemolysis; it may vary in colour from light yellow to green.

LABELLING

The label enables each individual unit to be traced to a specific donor.

07/2008:1646

HUMAN PLASMA (POOLED AND TREATED FOR VIRUS INACTIVATION)

Plasma humanum coagmentatum conditumque ad exstinguendum virum

DEFINITION

Human plasma (pooled and treated for virus inactivation) is a frozen or freeze-dried, sterile, non-pyrogenic preparation obtained from human plasma derived from donors belonging to the same ABO blood group. The preparation is thawed or reconstituted before use to give a solution for infusion.

The human plasma used complies with the monograph on *Human plasma for fractionation (0853)*.

PRODUCTION

The units of plasma to be used are cooled to – 30 °C or lower within 6 h of separation of cells and always within 24 h of collection.

The pool is prepared by mixing units of plasma belonging to the same ABO blood group.

The pool of plasma is tested for hepatitis B surface antigen (HBsAg) and for HIV antibodies using test methods of suitable sensitivity and specificity; the pool must give negative results in these tests.

Hepatitis C virus RNA. The plasma pool is tested using a validated nucleic acid amplification technique (*2.6.21*). A positive control with 100 IU of hepatitis C virus RNA per millilitre and, to test for inhibitors, an internal control prepared by addition of a suitable marker to a sample of the plasma pool are included in the test. The test is invalid if the positive control is non-reactive or if the result obtained with the internal control indicates the presence of inhibitors. The pool complies with the test if it is found non-reactive for hepatitis C virus RNA.

Hepatitis C virus RNA for NAT testing BRP is suitable for use as a positive control.

To limit the potential burden of B19 virus in plasma pools, the plasma pool is also tested for B19 virus using a validated nucleic acid amplification technique (*2.6.21*).

B19 virus DNA. The plasma pool contains not more than 10.0 IU/μl.

A positive control with 10.0 IU of B19 virus DNA per microlitre and, to test for inhibitors, an internal control prepared by addition of a suitable marker to a sample of the plasma pool are included in the test. The test is invalid if the positive control is non-reactive or if the result obtained with the internal control indicates the presence of inhibitors.

B19 virus DNA for NAT testing BRP is suitable for use as a positive control.

The method of preparation is designed to minimise activation of any coagulation factor (to minimise potential thrombogenicity) and includes a step or steps that have been shown to inactivate known agents of infection; if substances are used for the inactivation of viruses during production, the subsequent purification procedure must be validated to demonstrate that the concentration of these substances is reduced to a suitable level and that any residues are such as not to compromise the safety of the preparation for patients.

Inactivation process. The solvent-detergent process, which is one of the methods used to inactivate enveloped viruses, uses treatment with a combination of tributyl phosphate and octoxinol 10; these reagents are subsequently removed by oil extraction or by solid phase extraction so that the amount in the final product is less than 2 μg/ml for tributyl phosphate and less than 5 μg/ml for octoxinol 10.

No antimicrobial preservative is added.

The solution is passed through a bacteria-retentive filter, distributed aseptically into the final containers and immediately frozen; it may subsequently be freeze-dried.

Plastic containers comply with the requirements for sterile plastic containers for human blood and blood components (*3.2.3*).

Glass containers comply with the requirements for glass containers for pharmaceutical use (*3.2.1*).

CHARACTERS

The frozen preparation, after thawing, is a clear or slightly opalescent liquid free from solid and gelatinous particles. The freeze-dried preparation is an almost white or slightly yellow powder or friable solid.

Thaw or reconstitute the preparation to be examined as stated on the label immediately before carrying out the identification, tests and assay.

IDENTIFICATION

A. Examine by electrophoresis (*2.2.31*) comparing with normal human plasma. The electropherograms show the same bands.

B. It complies with the test for anti-A and anti-B haemagglutinins (see Tests).

TESTS

pH (*2.2.3*): 6.5 to 7.6.

Osmolality (*2.2.35*): minimum 240 mosmol/kg.

Total protein: minimum 45 g/l.

Dilute with a 9 g/l solution of *sodium chloride R* to obtain a solution containing about 15 mg of protein in 2 ml. Place 2.0 ml of this solution in a round-bottomed centrifuge tube and add 2 ml of a 75 g/l solution of *sodium molybdate R* and 2 ml of a mixture of 1 volume of *nitrogen-free sulphuric acid R* and 30 volumes of *water R*. Shake, centrifuge for 5 min, decant the supernatant and allow the inverted tube to drain on filter paper. Determine the nitrogen in the residue by the method of sulphuric acid digestion (*2.5.9*) and calculate the quantity of protein by multiplying the result by 6.25.

Activated coagulation factors (*2.6.22*). It complies with the test for activated coagulation factors. Carry out the test with 0.1 ml of the preparation to be examined instead of 10-fold and 100-fold dilutions. The coagulation time for the preparation to be examined is not less than 150 s.

Anti-A and anti-B haemagglutinins (*2.6.20*). The presence of haemagglutinins (anti-A or anti-B) corresponds to the blood group stated on the label.

Hepatitis A virus antibodies: minimum 2 IU/ml, determined by a suitable immunochemical method (*2.7.1*).

Human hepatitis A immunoglobulin BRP is suitable for use as a reference preparation.

Irregular erythrocyte antibodies. The preparation to be examined does not show the presence of irregular erythrocyte antibodies when examined without dilution by an indirect antiglobulin test.

Citrate. Liquid chromatography (*2.2.29*).

Test solution. Dilute the preparation to be examined with an equal volume of a 9 g/l solution of *sodium chloride R*. Filter the solution using a filter with 0.45 μm pores.

Reference solution. Dissolve 0.300 g of *sodium citrate R* in *water R* and dilute to 100.0 ml with the same solvent.

Column:

– *size*: l = 0.3 m, Ø = 7.8 mm;

– *stationary phase*: *cation exchange resin R* (9 μm).

Mobile phase: 0.51 g/l solution of *sulphuric acid R*.

Flow rate: 0.5 ml/min.

Detection: spectrophotometer at 215 nm.

Equilibration: 15 min.

Injection: 10 μl.

Retention time: citrate = about 10 min.

Limit:

– *citrate*: maximum 25 mmol/l.

Calcium: maximum 5.0 mmol/l.

Atomic absorption spectrometry (*2.2.23, Method I*).

Source: calcium hollow-cathode lamp using a transmission band preferably of 0.5 nm.

Wavelength: 622 nm.

Atomisation device: air-acetylene or acetylene-propane flame.

Potassium: maximum 5.0 mmol/l.

Atomic emission spectrometry (*2.2.22, Method I*).

Wavelength: 766.5 nm.

Sodium: maximum 2.00×10^2 mmol/l.

Atomic emission spectrometry (*2.2.22, Method I*).

Wavelength: 589 nm.

Water: determined by a suitable method, such as the semi-micro determination of water (*2.5.12*), loss on drying (*2.2.32*) or near-infrared spectrometry (*2.2.40*), the water content is within the limits approved by the competent authority (freeze-dried product).

Sterility (*2.6.1*). It complies with the test for sterility.

Pyrogens (*2.6.8*). It complies with the test for pyrogens. Inject 3 ml per kilogram of the rabbit's mass.

ASSAY

Factor VIII. Carry out the assay of human coagulation factor VIII (*2.7.4*) using a reference plasma calibrated against the International Standard for blood coagulation factor VIII in plasma.

The estimated potency is not less than 0.5 IU/ml. The confidence limits ($P = 0.95$) are not less than 80 per cent and not more than 120 per cent of the estimated potency.

Factor V. Carry out the assay of human coagulation factor V described below using a reference plasma calibrated against the International Standard for blood coagulation factor V in plasma.

Using *imidazole buffer solution pH 7.3 R*, prepare at least 3 two-fold dilutions of the preparation to be examined, preferably in duplicate, from 1 in 10 to 1 in 40. Test each dilution as follows: mix 1 volume of *plasma substrate deficient in factor V R*, 1 volume of the dilution to be examined, 1 volume of *thromboplastin R* and 1 volume of a 3.5 g/l solution of *calcium chloride R*; measure the coagulation times, i.e. the interval between the moment at which the calcium chloride solution is added and the 1st indication of the formation of fibrin, which may be observed visually or by means of a suitable apparatus.

In the same manner, determine the coagulation time of 4 twofold dilutions (1 in 10 to 1 in 80) of human normal plasma in *imidazole buffer solution pH 7.3 R*. 1 unit of factor V is equal to the activity of 1 ml of human normal plasma. Human normal plasma is prepared by pooling plasma units from not fewer than 30 donors and stored at −30 °C or lower.

Check the validity of the assay and calculate the potency of the test preparation by the usual statistical methods for a parallel-line assay (for example, *5.3*).

The estimated potency is not less than 0.5 IU/ml. The confidence limits ($P = 0.95$) are not less than 80 per cent and not more than 120 per cent of the estimated potency.

Factor XI. Carry out the assay of human coagulation factor XI (*2.7.22*) using a reference plasma calibrated against the International Standard for blood coagulation factor XI in plasma.

The estimated potency is not less than 0.5 IU/ml. The confidence limits ($P = 0.95$) are not less than 80 per cent and not more than 125 per cent of the estimated potency.

Protein C. Carry out the assay of human protein C (*2.7.30*) using a reference plasma calibrated against the International Standard for human protein C in plasma.

The estimated potency is not less than 0.7 IU/ml. The confidence limits ($P = 0.95$) are not less than 80 per cent and not more than 120 per cent of the estimated potency.

Protein S. Carry out the assay of human protein S (*2.7.31*) using a reference plasma calibrated against the International Standard for human protein S in plasma.

The estimated potency is within the limits approved for the particular product. The confidence limits ($P = 0.95$) are not less than 80 per cent and not more than 120 per cent of the estimated potency.

Plasmin inhibitor (α_2-antiplasmin). Carry out the assay of human plasmin inhibitor (*2.7.25*) using a reference plasma calibrated against a suitable reference standard for human plasmin inhibitor (α_2-antiplasmin) in plasma.

The estimated potency is not less than 0.2 units/ml. The confidence limits ($P = 0.95$) are not less than 80 per cent and not more than 120 per cent of the estimated potency.

LABELLING

The label states:

– the ABO blood group;

– the method used for virus inactivation.

07/2008:2387

HUMAN α-1-PROTEINASE INHIBITOR

α-1-Proteinasi inhibitor humanum

DEFINITION

Human α-1-proteinase inhibitor is a plasma protein fraction containing mainly human α-1-proteinase inhibitor (also known as human α-1-antitrypsin or α-1-antiproteinase). Human α-1-proteinase inhibitor is a glycoprotein existing in isoforms with different isoelectric points and is the most abundant multifunctional serine proteinase inhibitor in human plasma. It is obtained from human plasma that complies with the monograph *Human plasma for fractionation (0853)*, using a suitable fractionation process and further purification steps. Other plasma proteins may be present.

PRODUCTION

GENERAL PROVISIONS

The method of preparation includes steps that have been shown to remove or to inactivate known agents of infection. The subsequent purification procedure must be validated to demonstrate that the concentration of any substances used for inactivation of viruses during production is reduced to a suitable level and that any residues are such as not to compromise the safety of the preparation for patients.

The specific activity is not less than 0.35 mg of active human α-1-proteinase inhibitor per milligram of total protein. Ratio of human α-1 proteinase inhibitor activity to human α-1-proteinase inhibitor antigen is not less than 0.7.

Buffering and other auxiliary substances such as a stabiliser may be included. No antimicrobial preservative is added. The solution is passed through a bacteria-retentive filter and distributed aseptically into the final containers. The product may be freeze-dried.

CONSISTENCY OF THE METHOD OF PRODUCTION
The consistency of the method of production, including demonstration that the manufacturing process yields a product with a consistent composition and maintains the functional integrity of human α-1-proteinase inhibitor, is evaluated by suitable analytical procedures that are determined during process development, and which include:

- assay of human α-1-proteinase inhibitor activity;
- determination of specific human α-1-proteinase inhibitor activity, expressed as the ratio of active human α-1-proteinase inhibitor to total protein;
- characterisation of isoform composition and protein structure by suitable methods such as isoelectric focusing (*2.2.54*), spectrometric methods (for example, mass spectrometry) or capillary electrophoresis (*2.2.47*);
- determination of the ratio of human α-1-proteinase inhibitor activity to human α-1-proteinase inhibitor antigen;
- characterisation of accompanying plasma proteins that might be present, by a set of suitable methods such as SDS-PAGE, cellulose acetate electrophoresis or capillary zone electrophoresis (*2.2.31*) and quantitative determination of relevant accompanying plasma proteins;
- determination of molecular-size distribution, used to quantify the polymeric forms of human α-1-proteinase inhibitor; consideration is given to the potential presence of accompanying proteins that might affect the results.

CHARACTERS

Appearance: freeze-dried products are hygroscopic, white or pale yellow or pale brown powders or friable solids; liquid products are clear or slightly opalescent, colourless or pale yellow or pale green or pale brown.

If the preparation to be examined is freeze-dried, reconstitute it as stated on the label immediately before carrying out the identification, tests (except those for solubility and water) and assay.

IDENTIFICATION

The assay of human α-1-proteinase inhibitor activity serves to identify the preparation.

TESTS

pH (*2.2.3*): 6.5 to 7.8.

Solubility. To a container of the preparation to be examined add the volume of the liquid stated on the label at room temperature. The preparation dissolves completely when reconstituted according to the instructions for use, giving a clear, colourless or pale green or pale yellow or pale brown solution.

Osmolality (*2.2.35*): minimum 210 mosmol/kg.

Total protein. Dilute the preparation to be examined with a 9 g/l solution of *sodium chloride R* to obtain a solution containing about 15 mg of protein in 2 ml. To 2.0 ml of this solution in a round-bottomed centrifuge tube add 2 ml of a 75 g/l solution of *sodium molybdate R* and 2 ml of a mixture of 1 volume of *nitrogen-free sulphuric acid R* and 30 volumes of *water R*. Shake, centrifuge for 5 min, decant the supernatant and allow the inverted tube to drain on filter paper. Determine the nitrogen in the residue by the method of sulphuric acid digestion (*2.5.9*) and calculate the protein content by multiplying by 6.25.

Water. Determined by a suitable method, such as the semi-micro determination of water (*2.5.12*), loss on drying (*2.2.32*) or near-infrared spectrophotometry (*2.2.40*), the water content is within the limits approved by the competent authority.

Sterility (*2.6.1*). It complies with the test.

Pyrogens (*2.6.8*). It complies with the test. Inject per kilogram of the rabbit's mass a volume equivalent to not less than 60 mg of human α-1-proteinase inhibitor.

ASSAY

Carry out the assay of human α-1-proteinase inhibitor (*2.7.32*). The estimated potency is not less than 80 per cent and not more than 120 per cent of the stated potency. The confidence limits ($P = 0.95$) are not less than 80 per cent and not more than 120 per cent of the estimated potency.

STORAGE

Unless otherwise justified and authorised, in an airtight and sterile container, at a temperature not exceeding 25 °C.

LABELLING

The label states:

- the potency of active (functional) human α-1-proteinase inhibitor per container;
- the name and quantity of any added substances;
- the quantity of protein per container;
- where applicable, the name and volume of the liquid to be used for reconstitution;
- that the transmission of infectious agents cannot be totally excluded when medicinal products prepared from human blood or plasma are administered.

07/2008:1804

HYDROXYPROPYLBETADEX

Hydroxypropylbetadexum

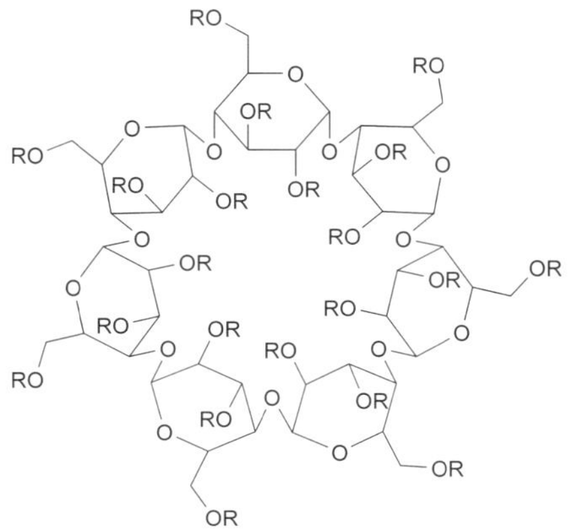

R = -[CH2-CH(CH3)-O]n-H   n = 0, 1, 2...

$C_{42}H_{70}O_{35}(C_3H_6O)_x$ with x = 7 *MS*

DEFINITION

Hydroxypropylbetadex (β-cyclodextrin, 2-hydroxypropyl ether) is a partially substituted poly(hydroxypropyl) ether of betadex. The number of hydroxypropyl groups per anhydroglucose unit, expressed as molar substitution (*MS*), is not less than 0.40 and not more than 1.50 and is within 10 per cent of the value stated on the label.

CHARACTERS

Appearance: white or almost white, amorphous or crystalline powder.

Solubility: freely soluble in water and in propylene glycol.

IDENTIFICATION

A. Infrared absorption spectrophotometry (*2.2.24*).

Comparison: *hydroxypropylbetadex CRS*.

Results: the spectrum obtained with the substance to be examined shows the same absorption bands as the spectrum obtained with *hydroxypropylbetadex CRS*. Due to the difference in the substitution of the substance, the intensity of some absorption bands can vary.

B. Appearance of solution (see Tests).

TESTS

Solution S. Dissolve 5.0 g in *carbon dioxide-free water R* prepared from *distilled water R* and dilute to 50.0 ml with the same solvent.

Appearance of solution. The solution is clear (*2.2.1*) and colourless (*2.2.2, Method II*), and remains so after cooling to room temperature.

Dissolve 1.0 g in 2.0 ml of *water R*, with heating.

Conductivity (*2.2.38*): maximum 200 μS·cm^{-1}.

Measure the conductivity of solution S, while gently stirring with a magnetic stirrer.

Related substances. Liquid chromatography (*2.2.29*).

Test solution. Dissolve 2.50 g of the substance to be examined in *water R* with heating, cool, and dilute to 25.0 ml with the same solvent.

Reference solution (a). Dissolve 0.15 g of *betadex CRS* and 0.25 g of *propylene glycol R* in *water R* and dilute to 10.0 ml with the same solvent.

Reference solution (b). Dilute 5.0 ml of reference solution (a) to 50.0 ml with *water R*.

Precolumn:

- *stationary phase*: *phenylsilyl silica gel for chromatography R*.

Column:

- *size*: *l* = 0.30 m, Ø = 3.9 mm;
- *stationary phase*: *phenylsilyl silica gel for chromatography R*;
- *temperature*: 40 °C.

Mobile phase: *water for chromatography R*.

Flow rate: 1.5 ml/min.

Detection: differential refractometer, at 40 °C.

Injection: 20 μl.

Run time: 6 times the retention time of impurity A.

Relative retention with reference to impurity B (retention time = about 2.5 min): impurity A = about 4.2; hydroxypropylbetadex = about 6 for the beginning of the elution.

Hydroxypropylbetadex elutes as a very wide peak or several peaks.

System suitability: reference solution (a):

- *resolution*: minimum 4 between the peaks due to impurities A and B.

Limits:

- *impurity A*: not more than the area of the corresponding peak in the chromatogram obtained with reference solution (b) (1.5 per cent);
- *impurity B*: not more than the area of the corresponding peak in the chromatogram obtained with reference solution (b) (2.5 per cent);
- *any other impurity*: for each impurity, not more than 0.04 times the area of the peak due to impurity B in the chromatogram obtained with reference solution (b) (0.1 per cent);
- *sum of impurities other than A and B*: not more than 0.4 times the area of the peak due to impurity B in the chromatogram obtained with reference solution (b) (1.0 per cent);
- *disregard limit*: 0.02 times the area of the peak due to impurity B in the chromatogram obtained with reference solution (b) (0.05 per cent); disregard any peak eluting before impurity B or after impurity A.

Heavy metals (*2.4.8*): maximum 20 ppm.

12 ml of solution S complies with test A. Prepare the reference solution using *lead standard solution (2 ppm Pb) R*.

Loss on drying (*2.2.32*): maximum 10.0 per cent, determined on 1.000 g by drying in an oven at 120 °C for 2 h.

Molar substitution. Nuclear magnetic resonance spectrometry (*2.2.33*).

The molar substitution (*MS*) is calculated from the ratio between the signal from the 3 protons of the methyl group that is part of the hydroxypropyl group and the signal from the proton attached to the C1 carbon (glycosidic proton) of the anhydroglucose units.

Use a Fourier transform nuclear magnetic resonance spectrometer of minimum frequency 250 MHz, suited to record a proton spectrum and to carry out quantitative analysis, at a temperature of at least 25 °C.

Introduce not less than the equivalent of 10.0 mg of the substance to be examined (dried substance) into a 5 mm NMR tube, equipped with a spinner in order to record the spectrum in rotation. Add approximately 0.75 ml of *deuterium oxide R1*. Cap the tube, mix thoroughly and adapt the spinner.

Make the appropriate instrument settings (frequency, gain, digital resolution, sample rotation, shims, probe tuning, resolution/data point, receiver gain etc.) so as to obtain a suitable spectrum for quantitative analysis (good FID (Free Induction Decay), no distortion of the spectrum after Fourier transform and phase corrections). The relaxation delay must be adapted to the pulse angle in order to have sufficient relaxation of the protons concerned between 2 pulses (for example: 10 s for a 90° pulse).

Record the FID, with at least 8 scans, so as to obtain a spectral window comprised, at least, between 0 ppm and 6.2 ppm, referring to the signal of exchangeable protons (solvent) at 4.8 ppm (25 °C).

Make a zero filling of at least 3-fold in size relative to the acquisition data file and transform the FID to the spectrum without any correction of Gaussian broadening factor (GB = 0) and with a line broadening factor not greater than 0.2 (LB ≤ 0.2). Call the integration sub-routine after phase corrections and baseline correction between 0.5 ppm and 6.2 ppm.

Measure the peak areas of the doublet from the methyl groups at 1.2 ppm (A_1), and of the signals of the glycosidic protons between 5 ppm and 5.4 ppm (A_2).

The molar substitution is obtained using the following equation:

$$MS = \frac{A_1}{(3 \times A_2)}$$

A_1 = area of the signal due to the 3 protons of the methyl groups that are part of the hydroxypropyl groups;

A_2 = area of the signals due to the glycosidic protons.

The degree of substitution is the number of hydroxypropyl groups per molecule of β-cyclodextrin and is obtained by multiplying the *MS* by 7.

Microbial contamination. Total viable aerobic count (*2.6.12*) not more than 10^3 bacteria and 10^2 fungi per gram, determined by plate count. If intended for use in the manufacture of parenteral preparations, the total viable aerobic count is not more than 10^2 bacteria and 10^2 fungi per gram. It complies with the tests for *Escherichia coli* and *Salmonella* (*2.6.13*).

Bacterial endotoxins (*2.6.14*): less than 10 IU/g, if intended for use in the manufacture of parenteral preparations without a further appropriate procedure for the removal of bacterial endotoxins.

LABELLING

The label states:

– the molar substitution (*MS*);

– where applicable, that the substance is suitable for use in the manufacture of parenteral preparations.

IMPURITIES

A. betadex,

B. propylene glycol.

Monographs D-K

I

07/2008:0029

IMIPRAMINE HYDROCHLORIDE

Imipramini hydrochloridum

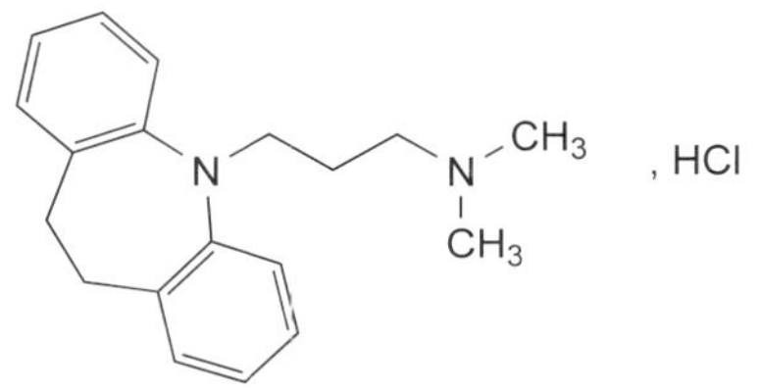

$C_{19}H_{25}ClN_2$ M_r 316.9
[113-52-0]

DEFINITION

3-(10,11-Dihydro-5*H*-dibenzo[*b,f*]azepin-5-yl)-*N,N*-dimethylpropan-1-amine hydrochloride.

Content: 98.5 per cent to 101.0 per cent (dried substance).

CHARACTERS

Appearance: white or slightly yellow, crystalline powder.

Solubility: freely soluble in water and in ethanol (96 per cent).

IDENTIFICATION

First identification: B, D.

Second identification: A, C, D.

A. Melting point (*2.2.14*): 170 °C to 174 °C.

B. Infrared absorption spectrophotometry (*2.2.24*).
Comparison: *imipramine hydrochloride CRS.*

C. Dissolve about 5 mg in 2 ml of *nitric acid R*. An intense blue colour develops.

D. About 20 mg gives reaction (a) of chlorides (*2.3.1*).

TESTS

Solution S. To 3.0 g add 20 ml of *carbon dioxide-free water R*, dissolve rapidly by shaking and triturating with a glass rod and dilute to 30 ml with the same solvent.

Appearance of solution. Solution S is clear (*2.2.1*). Immediately after preparation, dilute solution S with an equal volume of *water R*. This solution is not more intensely coloured than reference solution BY_6 (*2.2.2, Method II*).

pH (*2.2.3*): 3.6 to 5.0 for solution S, measured immediately after preparation.

Related substances. Liquid chromatography (*2.2.29*).

Test solution. Dissolve 50.0 mg of the substance to be examined in the mobile phase and dilute to 50.0 ml with the mobile phase.

Reference solution. Dissolve 5 mg of *imipramine for system suitability CRS* (containing impurity B) in the mobile phase and dilute to 5.0 ml with the mobile phase.

Column:
- *size*: *l* = 0.15 m, Ø = 4.6 mm;
- *stationary phase*: *end-capped polar-embedded octadecylsilyl amorphous organosilica polymer R* (5 µm);
- *temperature*: 40 °C.

Mobile phase: mix 40 volumes of *acetonitrile R1* with 60 volumes of a 5.2 g/l solution of *dipotassium hydrogen phosphate R* previously adjusted to pH 7.0 with *phosphoric acid R*.

Flow rate: 1.0 ml/min.

Detection: spectrophotometer at 220 nm.

Injection: 10 µl.

Run time: 2.5 times the retention time of imipramine.

Relative retention with reference to imipramine (retention time = about 7 min): impurity B = about 0.7.

System suitability: reference solution:
- *resolution*: minimum 5.0 between the peaks due to impurity B and imipramine.

Limits:
- *impurity B*: not more than the area of the corresponding peak in the chromatogram obtained with the reference solution (0.1 per cent);
- *unspecified impurities*: for each impurity, not more than the area of the peak due to imipramine in the chromatogram obtained with the reference solution (0.10 per cent);
- *total*: not more than 3 times the area of the peak due to imipramine in the chromatogram obtained with the reference solution (0.3 per cent);
- *disregard limit*: 0.5 times the area of the peak due to imipramine in the chromatogram obtained with the reference solution (0.05 per cent).

Heavy metals (*2.4.8*): maximum 20 ppm.

Test solution. Dissolve 0.500 g of the substance to be examined in 20 ml of *water R*.

Reference solution. Dilute 10 ml of *lead standard solution (1 ppm Pb) R* to 20 ml with *water R*.

Blank solution. 20 ml of *water R*.

Monitor solution. Dissolve 0.500 g of the substance to be examined in 10 ml of *lead standard solution (1 ppm Pb) R* and dilute to 20 ml of *water R*.

To each solution add 2 ml of *buffer solution pH 3.5 R*. Mix and add to 1.2 ml of *thioacetamide reagent R*. Mix immediately. Filter the solutions through a suitable membrane filter (pore size 0.45 µm). Compare the spots on the filters obtained with the different solutions. The test is invalid if the reference solution and the monitor solution do not show a slight brown colour compared to the blank solution. The substance to be examined complies with the test if the brown colour of the spot resulting from the test solution is not more intense than that of the spot resulting from the reference solution.

Loss on drying (*2.2.32*): maximum 0.5 per cent, determined on 1.000 g by drying in an oven at 105 °C.

Sulphated ash (*2.4.14*): maximum 0.1 per cent, determined on 1.0 g.

ASSAY

Dissolve 0.250 g in 50 ml of *ethanol (96 per cent) R* and add 5.0 ml of *0.01 M hydrochloric acid*. Carry out a potentiometric titration (*2.2.20*), using *0.1 M sodium hydroxide*. Read the volume added between the 2 points of inflexion.

1 ml of *0.1 M sodium hydroxide* is equivalent to 31.69 mg of $C_{19}H_{25}ClN_2$.

STORAGE

Protected from light.

IMPURITIES

Specified impurities: B.

Other detectable impurities (the following substances would, if present at a sufficient level, be detected by one or other of the tests in the monograph. They are limited by the general acceptance criterion for other/unspecified impurities and/or by the general monograph *Substances for pharmaceutical use (2034)*. It is therefore not necessary to identify these impurities for demonstration of compliance. See also *5.10. Control of impurities in substances for pharmaceutical use*): *A, C*.

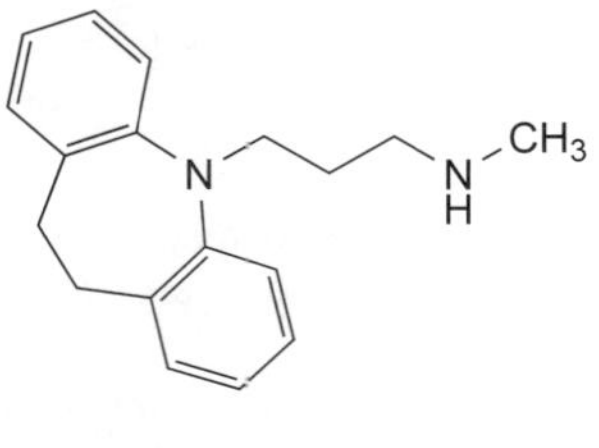

A. 3-(10,11-dihydro-5*H*-dibenzo[*b,f*]azepin-5-yl)-*N*-methylpropan-1-amine (desipramine),

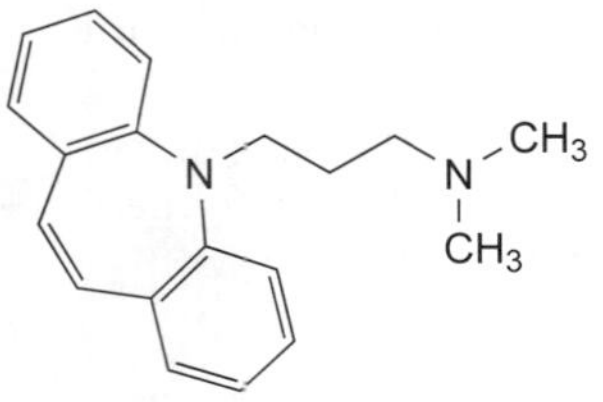

B. 3-(5*H*-dibenzo[*b,f*]azepin-5-yl)-*N,N*-dimethylpropan-1-amine (depramine),

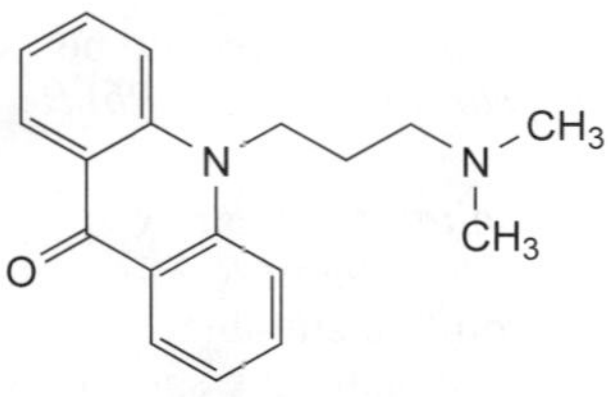

C. 10-[3-(dimethylamino)propyl]acridin-9(10*H*)-one.

01/2008:0093

IPECACUANHA, PREPARED

Ipecacuanhae pulvis normatus

DEFINITION

Ipecacuanha root powder (180) (*2.9.12*) adjusted, if necessary, by the addition of powdered lactose or ipecacuanha root powder with a lower alkaloidal content.

Content: 1.9 per cent to 2.1 per cent of total alkaloids, expressed as emetine ($C_{29}H_{40}N_2O_4$; M_r 480.7) (dried drug).

CHARACTERS

Appearance: light grey or yellowish-brown powder.

Slight odour.

IDENTIFICATION

A. Examine under a microscope, using *chloral hydrate solution R*. The powder shows the following diagnostic characters: parenchymatous cells, raphides of calcium oxalate up to 80 µm in length either in bundles or scattered throughout the powder; fragments of tracheids and vessels usually 10-20 µm in diameter, with bordered pits; larger vessels and sclereids from the rhizome. Examine under a microscope using a 50 per cent *V/V* solution of *glycerol R*. The powder shows simple or 2-8-compound starch granules contained in parenchymatous cells, the simple granules being up to 15 µm in diameter in *Cephaelis ipecacuanha* and up to 22 µm in diameter in *C. acuminata*. Examined in *glycerol (85 per cent) R*, it may be seen to contain lactose crystals.

B. Thin-layer chromatography (*2.2.27*).

Test solution. To 0.1 g of the drug to be examined in a test-tube add 0.05 ml of *concentrated ammonia R* and 5 ml of *ether R* and stir the mixture vigorously with a glass rod. Allow to stand for 30 min and filter.

Reference solution. Dissolve 2.5 mg of *emetine hydrochloride CRS* and 3 mg of *cephaeline hydrochloride CRS* in *methanol R* and dilute to 20 ml with the same solvent.

Plate: *TLC silica gel plate R*.

Mobile phase: *concentrated ammonia R, methanol R, ethyl acetate R, toluene R* (2:15:18:65 *V/V/V/V*).

Application: 10 µl, as bands.

Development: over a path of 10 cm.

Drying: in air.

Detection A: spray with a 5 g/l solution of *iodine R* in *ethanol (96 per cent) R*; heat at 60 °C for 10 min and examine in daylight.

Results A: the chromatograms obtained with the test solution and the reference solution show in the lower part a yellow zone due to emetine and below it a light brown zone due to cephaeline.

Detection B: examine in ultraviolet light at 365 nm.

Results B: the zone due to emetine shows an intense yellow fluorescence and that due to cephaeline a light blue fluorescence. The chromatogram obtained with the test solution also shows faint fluorescent zones.

With prepared *C. acuminata*, the principal zones in the chromatogram obtained with the test solution are similar in position, fluorescence and size to the zones in the chromatogram obtained with the reference solution.

With prepared *C. ipecacuanha*, the only difference is that the zone due to cephaeline in the chromatogram obtained with the test solution is much smaller than the corresponding zone in the chromatogram obtained with the reference solution.

TESTS

Loss on drying (*2.2.32*): maximum 5.0 per cent, determined on 1.000 g by drying in an oven at 105 °C.

Total ash (*2.4.16*): maximum 5.0 per cent.

Ash insoluble in hydrochloric acid (*2.8.1*): maximum 3.0 per cent.

ASSAY

To 7.5 g in a dry flask, add 100 ml of *ether R* and shake for 5 min. Add 5 ml of *dilute ammonia R1*, shake for 1 h, add 5 ml of *water R* and shake vigorously. Decant the ether layer into a flask through a plug of cotton. Wash the residue in the flask with 2 quantities, each of 25 ml, of *ether R*, decanting each portion through the same plug of cotton. Combine the ether solutions and eliminate the ether by distillation. Dissolve the residue in 2 ml of *ethanol (90 per cent V/V) R*, evaporate the ethanol to dryness and heat at 100 °C for 5 min. Dissolve the residue in 5 ml of previously neutralised *ethanol (90 per cent V/V) R*, warming on a water-bath, add 15.0 ml of *0.1 M hydrochloric acid* and titrate the excess acid with *0.1 M sodium hydroxide* using 0.5 ml of *methyl red mixed solution R* as indicator.

1 ml of *0.1 M hydrochloric acid* is equivalent to 24.03 mg of total alkaloids, expressed as emetine.

STORAGE

In an airtight container.

01/2008:0919
corrected 6.2

IPRATROPIUM BROMIDE

Ipratropii bromidum

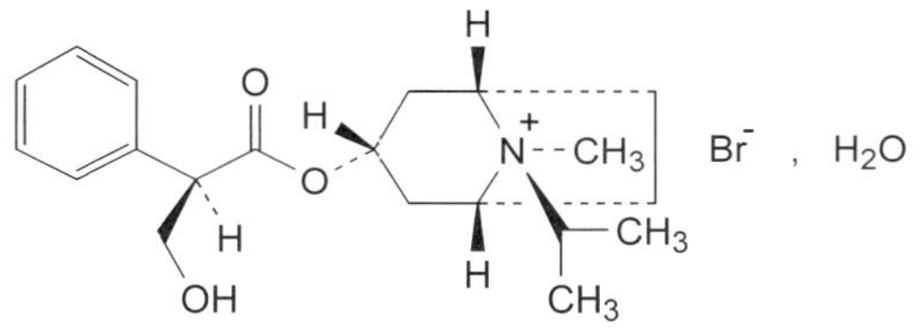

$C_{20}H_{30}BrNO_3,H_2O$ M_r 430.4
[66985-17-9]

DEFINITION

(1*R*,3*r*,5*S*,8*r*)-3-[[(2*RS*)-3-Hydroxy-2-phenylpropanoyl]oxy]-8-methyl-8-(1-methylethyl)-8-azoniabicyclo[3.2.1]octane bromide monohydrate.

Content: 99.0 per cent to 100.5 per cent (anhydrous substance).

CHARACTERS

Appearance: white or almost white, crystalline powder.

Solubility: soluble in water, freely soluble in methanol, slightly soluble in ethanol (96 per cent).

mp: about 230 °C, with decomposition.

IDENTIFICATION

First identification: A, E.

Second identification: B, C, D, E.

A. Infrared absorption spectrophotometry (*2.2.24*).

Comparison: *ipratropium bromide CRS*.

B. Examine the chromatograms obtained in the test for impurity A.

Results: the principal spot in the chromatogram obtained with the test solution is similar in position, colour and size to the principal spot in the chromatogram obtained with reference solution (a).

C. To 5 ml of solution S (see Tests), add 2 ml of *dilute sodium hydroxide solution R*. No precipitate is formed.

D. To about 1 mg add 0.2 ml of *nitric acid R* and evaporate to dryness on a water-bath. Dissolve the residue in 2 ml of *acetone R* and add 0.1 ml of a 30 g/l solution of *potassium hydroxide R* in *methanol R*. A violet colour develops.

E. It gives reaction (a) of bromides (*2.3.1*).

TESTS

Solution S. Dissolve 0.50 g in *carbon dioxide-free water R* and dilute to 50.0 ml with the same solvent.

Appearance of solution. Solution S is clear (*2.2.1*) and not more intensely coloured than reference solution GY_7 (*2.2.2, Method II*).

pH (*2.2.3*): 5.0 to 7.5 for solution S.

Impurity A. Thin-layer chromatography (*2.2.27*).

Test solution. Dissolve 20 mg of the substance to be examined in *methanol R* and dilute to 1.0 ml with the same solvent.

Reference solution (a). Dissolve 20 mg of *ipratropium bromide CRS* in *methanol R* and dilute to 1.0 ml with the same solvent.

Reference solution (b). Dissolve 20 mg of *methylatropine bromide CRS* in 1.0 ml of reference solution (a).

Reference solution (c). Dissolve 5 mg of *ipratropium impurity A CRS* in 100.0 ml of *methanol R*. Dilute 2.0 ml of the solution to 5.0 ml with *methanol R*.

Plate: *TLC silica gel plate R* (2-10 μm).

Mobile phase: *anhydrous formic acid R, water R, ethanol (96 per cent) R, methylene chloride R* (1:3:18:18 *V/V/V/V*).

Application: 1 μl.

Development: over a path of 6 cm.

Drying: at 60 °C for 15 min.

Detection: spray with *potassium iodobismuthate solution R*, allow the plate to dry in air, spray with a 50 g/l solution of *sodium nitrite R* and protect immediately with a sheet of glass.

System suitability: the chromatogram obtained with reference solution (b) shows 2 clearly separated principal spots.

Limit:

– *impurity A*: any spot due to impurity A is not more intense than the principal spot in the chromatogram obtained with reference solution (c) (0.1 per cent).

Related substances. Liquid chromatography (*2.2.29*).

Test solution. Dissolve 0.200 g of the substance to be examined in the mobile phase and dilute to 20.0 ml with the mobile phase.

Reference solution (a). Dissolve 10.0 mg of *ipratropium bromide CRS* in the mobile phase and dilute to 20.0 ml with the mobile phase. Dilute 1.0 ml of the solution to 50.0 ml with the mobile phase.

Reference solution (b). Dissolve 5 mg of *ipratropium bromide CRS* and 5 mg of *ipratropium impurity B CRS* in 1 ml of *methanol R* and dilute to 25.0 ml with the mobile phase. Dilute 1.0 ml of the solution to 20.0 ml with the mobile phase.

Column:

– *size*: *l* = 0.15 m, Ø = 3.9 mm;
– *stationary phase*: *octadecylsilyl silica gel for chromatography R* (5 μm);
– *temperature*: 30 °C.

Mobile phase: dissolve 12.4 g of *sodium dihydrogen phosphate R* and 1.7 g of *tetrapropylammonium chloride R* in 870 ml of *water R*; adjust to pH 5.5 with a 180 g/l solution of *disodium hydrogen phosphate R* and add 130 ml of *methanol R*.

Flow rate: 1.5 ml/min.

Detection: spectrophotometer at 220 nm.

Injection: 5 μl.

Run time: 6 times the retention time of ipratropium.

Relative retention with reference to ipratropium (retention time = about 4.9 min): impurity C = about 0.7; impurity B = about 1.2; impurity D = about 1.8; impurity E = about 2.3; impurity F = about 5.1.

System suitability: reference solution (b):
- *resolution*: minimum 3.0 between the peaks due to impurity B and ipratropium;
- *symmetry factor*: maximum 2.5 for the principal peak.

Limits:
- *correction factors*: for the calculation of content, multiply the peak areas of the following impurities by the corresponding correction factor: impurity C = 0.3; impurity D = 0.2; impurity F = 0.5;
- *impurity D*: not more than 0.5 times the area of the principal peak in the chromatogram obtained with reference solution (a) (0.05 per cent);
- *impurities B, C*: for each impurity, not more than the area of the principal peak in the chromatogram obtained with reference solution (a) (0.1 per cent);
- *unspecified impurities*: for each impurity, not more than the area of the principal peak in the chromatogram obtained with reference solution (a) (0.10 per cent);
- *total*: not more than 2.5 times the area of the principal peak in the chromatogram obtained with reference solution (a) (0.25 per cent);
- *disregard limit*: one-third of the area of the principal peak in the chromatogram obtained with reference solution (a) (0.03 per cent); disregard the peak due to the bromide ion.

Water (*2.5.12*): 3.9 per cent to 4.4 per cent, determined on 0.50 g.

Sulphated ash (*2.4.14*): maximum 0.1 per cent, determined on 1.0 g.

ASSAY

Dissolve 0.350 g in 50 ml of *water R* and add 3 ml of *dilute nitric acid R*. Titrate with *0.1 M silver nitrate*, determining the end-point potentiometrically (*2.2.20*).

1 ml of *0.1 M silver nitrate* is equivalent to 41.24 mg of $C_{20}H_{30}BrNO_3$.

IMPURITIES

Specified impurities: *A, B, C, D*.

Other detectable impurities (the following substances would, if present at a sufficient level, be detected by one or other of the tests in the monograph. They are limited by the general acceptance criterion for other/unspecified impurities and/or by the general monograph *Substances for pharmaceutical use (2034)*. It is therefore not necessary to identify these impurities for demonstration of compliance. See also *5.10. Control of impurities in substances for pharmaceutical use*): *E, F*.

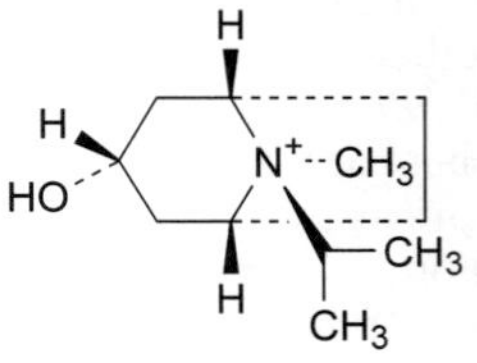

A. (1*R*,3*r*,5*S*,8*r*)-3-hydroxy-8-methyl-8-(1-methylethyl)-8-azoniabicyclo[3.2.1]octane,

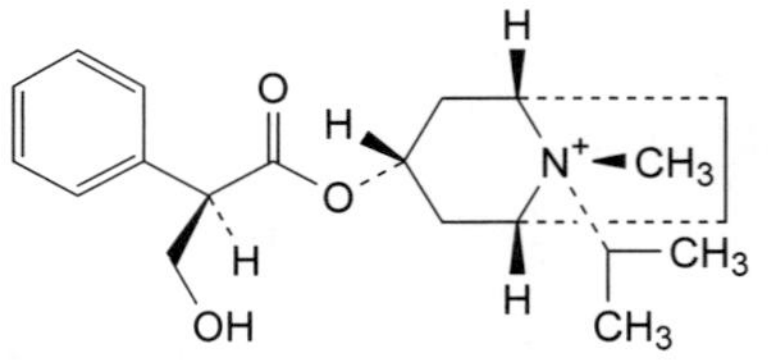
and enantiomer

B. (1*R*,3*r*,5*S*,8*s*)-3-[[(2*RS*)-3-hydroxy-2-phenylpropanoyl]oxy]-8-methyl-8-(1-methylethyl)-8-azoniabicyclo[3.2.1]octane,

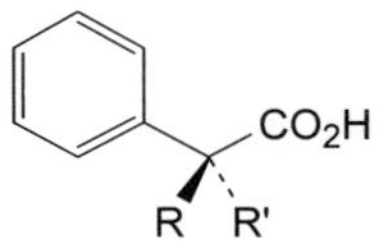
and enantiomer

C. R = CH_2-OH, R′ = H: (2*RS*)-3-hydroxy-2-phenylpropanoic acid (DL-tropic acid),

D. R + R′ = CH_2: 2-phenylpropenoic acid (atropic acid),

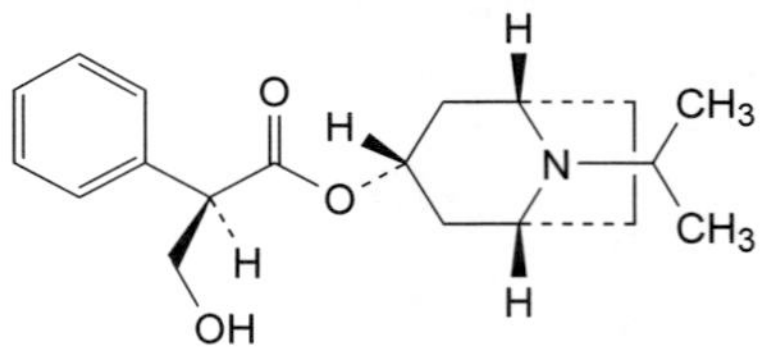
and enantiomer

E. (1*R*,3*r*,5*S*)-8-(1-methylethyl)-8-azabicyclo[3.2.1]oct-3-yl (2*RS*)-3-hydroxy-2-phenylpropanoate,

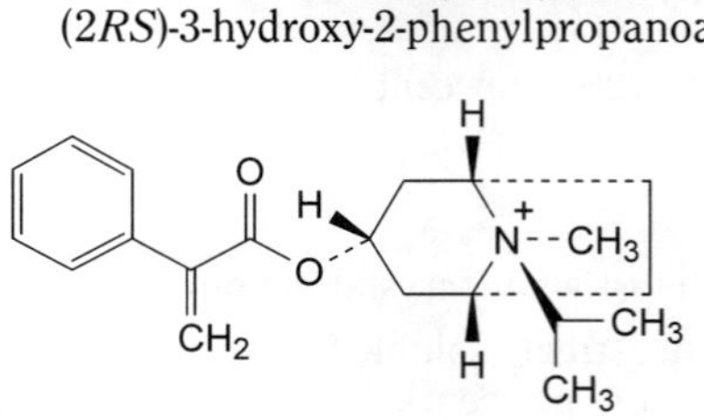

F. (1*R*,3*r*,5*S*,8*r*)-8-methyl-8-(1-methylethyl)-3-[(2-phenylpropenoyl)oxy]-8-azoniabicyclo[3.2.1]octane.

L

Monographs
L-P

01/2008:1536

LIQUORICE ETHANOLIC LIQUID EXTRACT, STANDARDISED

Liquiritiae extractum fluidum ethanolicum normatum

DEFINITION

Standardised ethanolic liquid extract produced from *Liquorice root (0277)*.

Content: 3.0 per cent to 5.0 per cent of glycyrrhizic acid ($C_{42}H_{62}O_{16}$; M_r 823).

PRODUCTION

The extract is produced from the herbal drug by a suitable procedure for liquid extracts using ethanol (70 per cent *V/V*).

CHARACTERS

Appearance: dark brown, clear liquid.

It has a faint characteristic odour and a sweet taste.

IDENTIFICATION

Thin-layer chromatography (*2.2.27*).

Test solution. Place 1.0 g of the extract to be examined in a 50 ml round-bottomed flask, add 16.0 ml of *water R* and 4.0 ml of *hydrochloric acid R1* and heat on a water-bath under a reflux condenser for 30 min. Allow to cool and filter. Dry the filter and the round-bottomed flask at 105 °C for 60 min. Transfer the filter to the round-bottomed flask, add 20 ml of *ether R* and heat in a water-bath at 40 °C under a reflux condenser for 5 min. Allow to cool and filter. Evaporate the filtrate to dryness and dissolve the residue in 5.0 ml of *ether R*.

Reference solution. Dissolve 5.0 mg of *glycyrrhetic acid R* and 5.0 mg of *thymol R* in 5 ml of *ether R*.

Plate: *TLC silica gel F_{254} plate R.*

Mobile phase: *concentrated ammonia R, water R, ethanol (96 per cent) R, ethyl acetate R* (1:9:25:65 *V/V/V/V*).

Application: 10 µl as bands.

Development: over a path of 15 cm.

Drying: in air for 5 min.

Detection A: examine in ultraviolet light at 254 nm.

Results A: the chromatograms obtained with the test solution and the reference solution show in the lower half a quenching zone due to glycyrrhetic acid.

Detection B: spray with *anisaldehyde solution R*; heat at 100-105 °C for 5-10 min and examine in daylight.

Results B: the chromatogram obtained with the reference solution shows in the lower half a violet zone (glycyrrhetic acid), and in the upper third a red zone (thymol); the chromatogram obtained with the test solution shows in the lower half a violet zone corresponding to glycyrrhetic acid in the chromatogram obtained with the reference solution, and in the upper third, below the zone of thymol in the chromatogram obtained with the reference solution, a yellow zone due to isoliquiritigenin; further zones are present.

TESTS

Ethanol (*2.9.10*): 52 per cent *V/V* to 65 per cent *V/V*.

Methanol and 2-propanol (*2.9.11*): maximum 0.05 per cent *V/V* of methanol and maximum 0.05 per cent *V/V* of 2-propanol.

ASSAY

Liquid chromatography (*2.2.29*).

Solvent mixture: *dilute ammonia R1, water R* (8:92 *V/V*).

Test solution. Dilute 1.000 g of the extract to be examined to 100 ml with the solvent mixture and centrifuge. Dilute 2.0 ml of the supernatant to 10.0 ml with the solvent mixture.

Stock solution. Dissolve 0.130 g of *monoammonium glycyrrhizate CRS* in the solvent mixture and dilute to 100.0 ml with the solvent mixture.

Reference solution (a). Dilute 5.0 ml of the stock solution to 100.0 ml with the solvent mixture.

Reference solution (b). Dilute 10.0 ml of the stock solution to 100.0 ml with the solvent mixture.

Reference solution (c). Dilute 15.0 ml of the stock solution to 100.0 ml with the solvent mixture.

Column:

- *size*: l = 0.10 m, Ø = 4 mm;
- *stationary phase*: *octadecylsilyl silica gel for chromatography R* (5 µm).

Mobile phase: *glacial acetic acid R, acetonitrile R, water R* (6:30:64 *V/V/V*).

Flow rate: 1.5 ml/min.

Detection: spectrophotometer at 254 nm.

Injection: 10 µl.

Establish a calibration curve with the concentrations of the reference solutions (g/100 ml) as the abscissa and the corresponding peak areas as the ordinate.

Using the retention times and the peak areas determined from the chromatograms obtained with the reference solutions, locate and integrate the peak due to glycyrrhizic acid in the chromatogram obtained with the test solution.

Calculate the percentage content of glycyrrhizic acid using the following expression:

$$A \times \frac{5}{m} \times B \times \frac{822}{840}$$

A = concentration of monoammonium glycyrrhizate in the test solution, determined from the calibration curve, in g/100 ml;

B = declared percentage content of *monoammonium glycyrrhizate CRS*;

m = mass of the extract to be examined, in grams;

822 = molecular mass of glycyrrhizic acid;

840 = molecular mass of monoammonium glycyrrhizate (without any water of crystallisation).

M

07/2008:0043

MAGNESIUM CARBONATE, HEAVY

Magnesii subcarbonas ponderosus

[546-93-0]

DEFINITION

Hydrated basic magnesium carbonate.

Content: 40.0 per cent to 45.0 per cent, calculated as MgO (M_r 40.30).

CHARACTERS

Appearance: white or almost white powder.

Solubility: practically insoluble in water. It dissolves in dilute acids with effervescence.

IDENTIFICATION

A. Bulk density (*2.9.34*): minimum 0.25 g/ml.

B. It gives the reaction of carbonates (*2.3.1*).

C. Dissolve about 15 mg in 2 ml of *dilute nitric acid R* and neutralise with *dilute sodium hydroxide solution R*. The solution gives the reaction of magnesium (*2.3.1*).

TESTS

Solution S. Dissolve 5.0 g in 100 ml of *dilute acetic acid R*. When the effervescence has ceased, boil for 2 min, allow to cool and dilute to 100 ml with *dilute acetic acid R*. Filter, if necessary, through a previously ignited and tared porcelain or silica filter crucible of suitable porosity to give a clear filtrate.

Appearance of solution. Solution S is not more intensely coloured than reference solution B_4 (*2.2.2, Method II*).

Soluble substances: maximum 1.0 per cent.

Mix 2.00 g with 100 ml of *water R* and boil for 5 min. Filter whilst hot through a sintered-glass filter (40) (*2.1.2*), allow to cool and dilute to 100 ml with *water R*. Evaporate 50 ml of the filtrate to dryness and dry at 100-105 °C. The residue weighs not more than 10 mg.

Substances insoluble in acetic acid: maximum 0.05 per cent.

Any residue obtained during the preparation of solution S, washed, dried, and ignited at 600 ± 50 °C, weighs not more than 2.5 mg.

Chlorides (*2.4.4*): maximum 700 ppm.

Dilute 1.5 ml of solution S to 15 ml with *water R*.

Sulphates (*2.4.13*): maximum 0.6 per cent.

Dilute 0.5 ml of solution S to 15 ml with *distilled water R*.

Arsenic (*2.4.2, Method A*): maximum 2 ppm, determined on 10 ml of solution S.

Calcium (*2.4.3*): maximum 0.75 per cent.

Dilute 2.6 ml of solution S to 150 ml with *distilled water R*. 15 ml of the solution complies with the test.

Iron (*2.4.9*): maximum 400 ppm.

Dissolve 0.1 g in 3 ml of *dilute hydrochloric acid R* and dilute to 10 ml with *water R*. Dilute 2.5 ml of the solution to 10 ml with *water R*.

Heavy metals (*2.4.8*): maximum 20 ppm.

To 20 ml of solution S add 15 ml of *hydrochloric acid R1* and shake with 25 ml of *methyl isobutyl ketone R* for 2 min. Allow to stand, separate the aqueous lower layer and evaporate to dryness. Dissolve the residue in 1 ml of *acetic acid R* and dilute to 20 ml with *water R*. 12 ml of the solution complies with test A. Prepare the reference solution using *lead standard solution (1 ppm Pb) R*.

ASSAY

Dissolve 0.150 g in a mixture of 2 ml of *dilute hydrochloric acid R* and 20 ml of *water R*. Carry out the complexometric titration of magnesium (*2.5.11*).

1 ml of *0.1 M sodium edetate* is equivalent to 4.030 mg of MgO.

FUNCTIONALITY-RELATED CHARACTERISTICS

This section provides information on characteristics that are recognised as being relevant control parameters for one or more functions of the substance when used as an excipient (see chapter 5.15). This section is a non-mandatory part of the monograph and it is not necessary to verify the characteristics to demonstrate compliance. Control of these characteristics can however contribute to the quality of a medicinal product by improving the consistency of the manufacturing process and the performance of the medicinal product during use. Where control methods are cited, they are recognised as being suitable for the purpose, but other methods can also be used. Wherever results for a particular characteristic are reported, the control method must be indicated.

The following characteristics may be relevant for heavy magnesium carbonate used as a filler in tablets.

Particle-size distribution (*2.9.31* or *2.9.38*).

Bulk and tapped density (*2.9.34*).

01/2008:1342
corrected 6.2

MAIZE OIL, REFINED

Maydis oleum raffinatum

DEFINITION

Fatty oil obtained from the seeds of *Zea mays* L. by expression or by extraction, then refined.

CHARACTERS

Appearance: clear, light yellow or yellow oil.

Solubility: practically insoluble in water and in ethanol (96 per cent), miscible with light petroleum (bp: 40-60 °C) and with methylene chloride.

Relative density: about 0.920.

Refractive index: about 1.474.

IDENTIFICATION

A. Identification of fatty oils by thin-layer chromatography (*2.3.2*).

Results: the chromatogram obtained with the test solution is similar to that obtained with the reference solution.

B. Composition of fatty acids (see Tests).

TESTS

Acid value (*2.5.1*): maximum 0.5, or maximum 0.3 if intended for use in the manufacture of parenteral preparations, determined on 10.0 g.

Peroxide value (*2.5.5, Method A*): maximum 10.0, or maximum 5.0 if intended for use in the manufacture of parenteral preparations.

Unsaponifiable matter (*2.5.7*): maximum 2.8 per cent, determined on 5.0 g.

Alkaline impurities (*2.4.19*). It complies with the test.

Composition of fatty acids (*2.4.22, Method A*). Use the mixture of calibrating substances in Table 2.4.22.-3.

Composition of the fatty-acid fraction of the oil:

- *fatty acids of chain length less than* C_{16}: maximum 0.6 per cent;
- *palmitic acid*: 8.6 per cent to 16.5 per cent;
- *stearic acid*: maximum 3.3 per cent;
- *oleic acid*: 20.0 per cent to 42.2 per cent;
- *linoleic acid*: 39.4 per cent to 65.6 per cent;
- *linolenic acid*: 0.5 per cent to 1.5 per cent;
- *arachidic acid*: maximum 0.8 per cent;
- *eicosenoic acid*: maximum 0.5 per cent;
- *behenic acid*: maximum 0.5 per cent;
- *other fatty acids*: maximum 0.5 per cent.

Sterols (*2.4.23*): maximum 0.3 per cent of brassicasterol in the sterol fraction of the oil.

Water (*2.5.32*): maximum 0.1 per cent if intended for use in the manufacture of parenteral preparations, determined on 5.00 g. Use a mixture of equal volumes of *anhydrous methanol R* and *decanol R* as the solvent.

STORAGE

Protected from light, at a temperature not exceeding 25 °C.

LABELLING

The label states:

- where applicable, that the substance is suitable for use in the manufacture of parenteral preparations;
- whether the oil is obtained by mechanical expression or by extraction.

01/2008:1544

MATRICARIA LIQUID EXTRACT

Matricariae extractum fluidum

DEFINITION

Liquid extract produced from *Matricaria flower (0404)*.

Content: minimum 0.30 per cent of blue residual oil.

PRODUCTION

The extract is produced from the herbal drug by a suitable procedure for liquid extracts using a mixture of 2.5 volumes of a 10 per cent *m/m* solution of ammonia (NH_3), 47.5 volumes of water and 50 volumes of ethanol (96 per cent).

CHARACTERS

Appearance: brownish, clear liquid.

Intense characteristic odour and characteristic bitter taste.

Solubility: miscible with water and with ethanol (96 per cent) with development of turbidity, soluble in ethanol (50 per cent *V/V*).

IDENTIFICATION

A. Thin-layer chromatography (*2.2.27*).

Test solution. Place 10 ml of the extract to be examined in a separating funnel and shake with 2 quantities, each of 10 ml, of *pentane R*. Combine the pentane layers, dry over 2 g of *anhydrous sodium sulphate R* and filter. Evaporate the filtrate to dryness on a water-bath and dissolve the residue in 0.5 ml of *toluene R*.

Reference solution. Dissolve 4 mg of *guaiazulene R*, 20 mg of *(-)-α-bisabolol R* and 20 mg of *bornyl acetate R* in 10 ml of *toluene R*.

Plate: *TLC silica gel* F_{254} *plate R*.

Mobile phase: *ethyl acetate R, toluene R* (5:95 *V/V*).

Application: 10 µl as bands.

Development: over a path of 10 cm.

Drying: in air.

Detection A: examine in ultraviolet light at 254 nm.

Results A: the chromatogram obtained with the test solution shows several quenching zones, of which 2 main zones are in the middle third (en-yne-dicycloether).

Detection B: examine in ultraviolet light at 365 nm.

Results B: the chromatogram obtained with the test solution shows in the middle part an intense blue fluorescent zone (herniarin).

Detection C: spray with *anisaldehyde solution R* and examine in daylight while heating at 100-105 °C for 5-10 min.

Results C: the chromatogram obtained with the reference solution shows in the lower third a reddish-violet or bluish-violet zone ((-)-α-bisabolol), in the middle third a yellowish-brown or greyish-green zone (bornyl acetate) and in the upper third a red or reddish-violet zone (guaiazulene). The chromatogram obtained with the test solution shows in the lower third yellowish-brown or greenish-yellow and violet zones and a reddish-violet or bluish-violet zone due to (-)-α-bisabolol in the chromatogram obtained with the reference solution; a brownish zone (en-yne-dicycloether) similar in position to the zone due to bornyl acetate in the chromatogram obtained with the reference solution; a red or reddish-violet zone (chamazulene) corresponding to guaiazulene in the chromatogram obtained with the reference solution and immediately above it 1 or 2 blue or bluish-violet zones; further weak zones may be present in the chromatogram obtained with the test solution.

B. Thin-layer chromatography (*2.2.27*).

Test solution. The extract to be examined.

Reference solution. Dissolve 1.0 mg of *chlorogenic acid R*, 2.5 mg of *hyperoside R* and 2.5 mg of *rutin R* in 10 ml of *methanol R*.

Plate: *TLC silica gel plate R*.

Mobile phase: *anhydrous formic acid R, glacial acetic acid R, water R, ethyl acetate R* (7.5:7.5:18:67 *V/V/V/V*).

Application: 10 µl as bands.

Development: over a path of 15 cm.

Drying: at 100-105 °C.

Detection: spray the warm plate with a 10 g/l solution of *diphenylboric acid aminoethyl ester R* in *methanol R*; subsequently spray with a 50 g/l solution of *macrogol 400 R* in *methanol R*; allow to dry in air for about 30 min and examine in ultraviolet light at 365 nm.

Results: the chromatogram obtained with the reference solution shows in the middle part a light blue fluorescent zone (chlorogenic acid), below it a yellowish-brown fluorescent zone (rutin) and above it a yellowish-brown fluorescent zone (hyperoside). The chromatogram obtained with the test solution shows a yellowish-brown fluorescent zone corresponding to the zone of rutin in the chromatogram obtained with the reference solution, a light blue fluorescent zone corresponding to the zone of chlorogenic acid in the chromatogram obtained with the reference solution, a yellowish-brown fluorescent zone similar in position to the zone of hyperoside in the chromatogram obtained with the reference solution; it also shows above the yellowish-brown fluorescent zone a green fluorescent zone, then several bluish or greenish fluorescent zones and near the solvent front a yellowish fluorescent zone.

TESTS

Ethanol (*2.9.10*): 38 per cent *V/V* to 53 per cent *V/V*.

Dry residue (*2.8.16*): minimum 12.0 per cent.

ASSAY

Place 20.0 g in a 1000 ml round-bottomed flask, add 300 ml of *water R* and distil until 200 ml has been collected in a flask. Transfer the distillate into a separating funnel. Dissolve 65 g of *sodium chloride R* in the distillate and shake with 3 quantities, each of 30 ml, of *pentane R* previously used to rinse the reflux condenser and the flask. Combine the pentane layers, dry over 2 g of *anhydrous sodium sulphate R* and filter into a tared 100 ml round-bottomed flask which has been dried in a desiccator for 3 h. Rinse the anhydrous sodium sulphate and the filter with 2 quantities, each of 20 ml, of *pentane R*. Evaporate the pentane in a water-bath at 45 °C. The residue of pentane is eliminated in a current of air for 3 min. Dry the flask in a desiccator for 3 h and weigh. The residual oil is blue (chamazulene).

01/2008:1128
corrected 6.2

METHACRYLIC ACID - ETHYL ACRYLATE COPOLYMER (1:1)

Acidi methacrylici et ethylis acrylatis polymerisatum 1:1

DEFINITION

Copolymer of methacrylic acid and ethyl acrylate having a mean relative molecular mass of about 250 000. The ratio of carboxylic groups to ester groups is about 1:1. The substance is in the acid form (type A) or partially neutralised using sodium hydroxide (type B). It may contain suitable surface-active agents such as sodium dodecyl sulphate and polysorbate 80.

Content:

- type A: 46.0 per cent to 50.6 per cent of methacrylic acid units (dried substance);
- type B: 43.0 per cent to 48.0 per cent of methacrylic acid units (dried substance).

CHARACTERS

Appearance: white or almost white, free-flowing powder.

Solubility: practically insoluble in water (type A) or dispersible in water (type B), freely soluble in anhydrous ethanol, practically insoluble in ethyl acetate. It is freely soluble in a 40 g/l solution of sodium hydroxide.

IDENTIFICATION

A. Infrared absorption spectrophotometry (*2.2.24*).

Preparation: dissolve 0.1 g of the substance to be examined in 1 ml of *ethanol (90 per cent V/V) R*, and place 2 drops of the solution on a sodium chloride plate; dry to allow the formation of a film and cover with another sodium chloride plate.

Comparison: *Methacrylic acid - ethyl acrylate copolymer (1:1) (type A or type B) CRS*.

B. It complies with the limits of the assay.

C. Sulphated ash (see Tests).

TESTS

Ethyl acrylate and methacrylic acid. Liquid chromatography (*2.2.29*).

Blank solution. To 50.0 ml of *methanol R* add 25.0 ml of the mobile phase.

Test solution. Dissolve 40 mg of the substance to be examined in 50.0 ml of *methanol R* and add 25.0 ml of the mobile phase.

Reference solution. Dissolve 10 mg of *ethyl acrylate R* and 10 mg of *methacrylic acid R* in *methanol R* and dilute to 50.0 ml with the same solvent. Dilute 0.1 ml of this solution to 50.0 ml with *methanol R* and add 25.0 ml of the mobile phase.

Column:

- *size*: l = 0.10 m, Ø = 4 mm;
- *stationary phase*: *octadecylsilyl silica gel for chromatography R* (5 μm).

Mobile phase: *methanol R, phosphate buffer solution pH 2.0 R* (30:70 *V/V*).

Flow rate: 2.5 ml/min.

Detection: spectrophotometer at 202 nm.

Injection: 50 μl.

System suitability:

- *resolution*: minimum 2.0 between the peaks due to ethyl acrylate and methacrylic acid in the chromatogram obtained with the reference solution;
- the chromatogram obtained with the blank solution does not show peaks with the same retention time as the peaks due to ethyl acrylate or methacrylic acid.

Limit:

- *sum of the contents of ethyl acrylate and methacrylic acid*: maximum 0.1 per cent.

Loss on drying (*2.2.32*): maximum 5.0 per cent, determined on 1.000 g by drying in an oven at 105 °C for 6 h.

Sulphated ash (*2.4.14*): maximum 0.4 per cent (type A) or 0.5 per cent to 3.0 per cent (type B), determined on 1.0 g.

ASSAY

Dissolve 1.000 g in a mixture of 40 ml of *water R* and 60 ml of *2-propanol R*. Titrate slowly while stirring with *0.5 M sodium hydroxide*, using *phenolphthalein solution R* as indicator.

1 ml of *0.5 M sodium hydroxide* is equivalent to 43.05 mg of $C_4H_6O_2$ (methacrylic acid units).

LABELLING

The label states the type (type A or type B).

FUNCTIONALITY-RELATED CHARACTERISTICS

This section provides information on characteristics that are recognised as being relevant control parameters for one or more functions of the substance when used as an excipient. This section is a non-mandatory part of the monograph and it is not necessary to verify the characteristics to demonstrate compliance. Control of these characteristics can however contribute to the quality of a medicinal product by improving the consistency of the manufacturing process and the performance of the medicinal product during use. Where control methods are cited, they are recognised as being suitable for the purpose, but other methods can also be used. Wherever results for a particular characteristic are reported, the control method must be indicated.

The following characteristics may be relevant for methacrylic acid - ethyl acrylate copolymer (1:1) used as gastro-resistant coating agent.

Apparent viscosity:

– *Type A*: 100 mPa·s to 200 mPa·s.

Dissolve a quantity of the substance to be examined corresponding to 37.5 g of the dried substance in a mixture of 7.9 g of *water R* and 254.6 g of *2-propanol R*. Determine the viscosity (*2.2.10*) at 20 °C using a rotating viscometer at a shear rate of 10 s^{-1}.

– *Type B*: not more than 100 mPa·s.

Disperse a quantity of the substance to be examined corresponding to 80.0 g of the dried substance in *water R* and make up to 320 g with the same solvent. Stir for 3 h and determine the viscosity (*2.2.10*) at 23 °C using a rotating viscometer and a spindle rotating at 100 r/min (rotor 2).

Solubility of a film. Place 1 ml of the solution (type A) or dispersion (type B) prepared for the test on apparent viscosity on a glass plate and allow to dry. A clear brittle film is formed. Take a piece of the film and place it in a flask containing phosphate buffer solution pH 6.8. It dissolves.

07/2008:0410

METHYLTESTOSTERONE

Methyltestosteronum

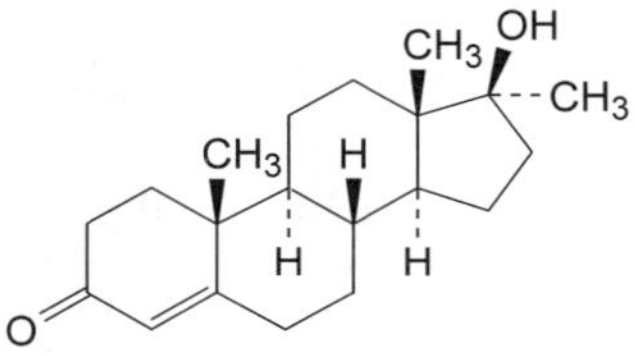

$C_{20}H_{30}O_2$ M_r 302.5
[58-18-4]

DEFINITION

17β-Hydroxy-17-methylandrost-4-en-3-one.

Content: 97.0 per cent to 103.0 per cent (dried substance).

CHARACTERS

Appearance: white or slightly yellowish-white, crystalline powder.

Solubility: practically insoluble in water, freely soluble in ethanol (96 per cent).

IDENTIFICATION

First identification: B.

Second identification: A, C.

A. Melting point (*2.2.14*): 162 °C to 168 °C.

B. Infrared absorption spectrophotometry (*2.2.24*).

Comparison: *methyltestosterone CRS.*

C. Thin-layer chromatography (*2.2.27*).

Test solution. Dissolve 0.2 g of the substance to be examined in a mixture of 1 volume of *methanol R* and 9 volumes of *chloroform R* and dilute to 10 ml with the same mixture of solvents.

Reference solution. Dissolve 20 mg of *methyltestosterone CRS* in 1 ml of a mixture of 1 volume of *methanol R* and 9 volumes of *chloroform R*.

Plate: *TLC silica gel F_{254} plate R.*

Mobile phase: *anhydrous acetic acid R, light petroleum R, butyl acetate R* (1:30:70 *V/V/V*).

Application: 5 µl.

Development: over 2/3 of the plate.

Drying: in air.

Detection: examine in ultraviolet light at 254 nm and spray with a saturated solution of *potassium dichromate R* in a mixture of 30 volumes of *water R* and 70 volumes of *sulphuric acid R*. Examine immediately in daylight.

Results: the principal spot in the chromatogram obtained with the test solution is similar in position, colour and size to the principal spot in the chromatogram obtained with the reference solution.

TESTS

Specific optical rotation (*2.2.7*): + 79 to + 85 (dried substance).

Dissolve 0.250 g in *ethanol (96 per cent) R* and dilute to 25.0 ml with the same solvent.

Related substances. Liquid chromatography (*2.2.29*).

Test solution. Dissolve 50 mg of the substance to be examined in *methanol R* and dilute to 100.0 ml with the same solvent.

Reference solution (a). Dilute 0.5 ml of the test solution to 100.0 ml with *methanol R*.

Reference solution (b). Dissolve 5 mg of *methyltestosterone for system suitability CRS* (containing impurity A) in *methanol R* and dilute to 10 ml with the same solvent.

Column:

– *size*: *l* = 0.15 m, Ø = 3.9 mm;

– *stationary phase*: *end-capped octadecylsilyl silica gel for chromatography R* (5 µm).

Mobile phase:

– *mobile phase A*: *water R;*

– *mobile phase B*: *methanol R;*

Time (min)	Mobile phase A (per cent *V/V*)	Mobile phase B (per cent *V/V*)
0 - 15	30	70
15 - 45	30 → 0	70 → 100
45 - 50	0	100

Flow rate: 1.5 ml/min.

Detection: spectrophotometer at 254 nm.

Injection: 20 µl.

Identification of impurities: use the chromatogram supplied with *methyltestosterone for system suitability CRS* and the chromatogram obtained with reference solution (b) to identify the peak due to impurity A.

Relative retention with reference to methyltestosterone (retention time = about 8 min): impurity A = about 1.5.

System suitability: reference solution (b):

– *resolution*: minimum 5 between the peaks due to methyltestosterone and impurity A.

Monographs L-P

Limits:
- *impurity A*: not more than the area of the principal peak in the chromatogram obtained with reference solution (a) (0.5 per cent);
- *unspecified impurities*: for each impurity, not more than 0.2 times the area of the principal peak in the chromatogram obtained with reference solution (a) (0.10 per cent);
- *total*: not more than twice the area of the principal peak in the chromatogram obtained with reference solution (a) (1.0 per cent);
- *disregard limit*: 0.1 times the area of the principal peak in the chromatogram obtained with reference solution (a) (0.05 per cent).

Loss on drying (*2.2.32*): maximum 2.0 per cent, determined on 0.500 g by drying in an oven at 105 °C for 2 h.

ASSAY

Dissolve 50.0 mg in *ethanol (96 per cent) R* and dilute to 50.0 ml with the same solvent. Dilute 10.0 ml of the solution to 100.0 ml with *ethanol (96 per cent) R*. Dilute 10.0 ml of this solution to 100.0 ml with *ethanol (96 per cent) R*. Measure the absorbance (*2.2.25*) at the absorption maximum at 241 nm.

Calculate the content of $C_{20}H_{30}O_2$, taking the specific absorbance to be 540.

STORAGE

Protected from light.

IMPURITIES

Specified impurities: A.

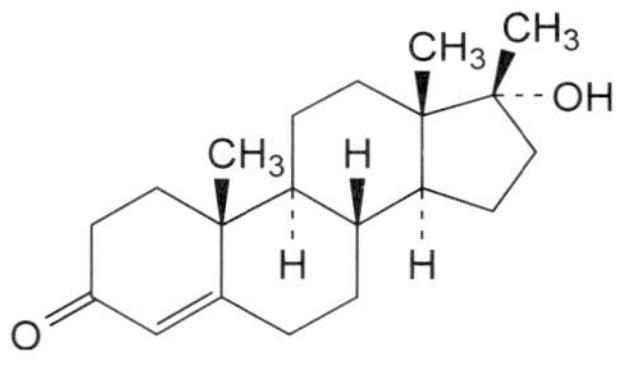

A. 17α-hydroxy-17-methylandrost-4-en-3-one.

07/2008:1348

METOCLOPRAMIDE

Metoclopramidum

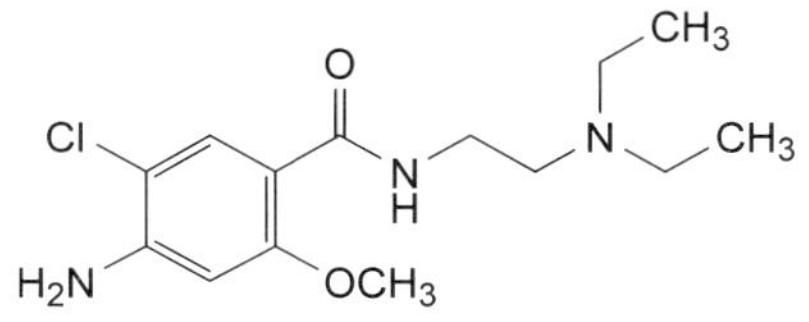

$C_{14}H_{22}ClN_3O_2$ M_r 299.8
[364-62-5]

DEFINITION

4-Amino-5-chloro-*N*-[2-(diethylamino)ethyl]-2-methoxybenzamide.

Content: 99.0 per cent to 101.0 per cent (dried substance).

CHARACTERS

Appearance: white or almost white, fine powder.

Solubility: practically insoluble in water, sparingly soluble or slightly soluble in ethanol (96 per cent), slightly soluble in methylene chloride.

It shows polymorphism (*5.9*).

IDENTIFICATION

First identification: A, B.

Second identification: A, C.

A. Melting point (*2.2.14*): 145 °C to 149 °C.

B. Infrared absorption spectrophotometry (*2.2.24*).

Comparison: *metoclopramide CRS.*

C. Examine the chromatograms obtained in test A for related substances.

Detection: examine in ultraviolet light at 254 nm before spraying with *dimethylaminobenzaldehyde solution R1.*

Results: the principal spot in the chromatogram obtained with test solution (a) is similar in position and size to the principal spot in the chromatogram obtained with reference solution (a).

TESTS

Appearance of solution. The freshly prepared solution is clear (*2.2.1*) and not more intensely coloured than reference solution Y_6 (*2.2.2, Method II*).

Dissolve 2.5 g in 25 ml of *1 M hydrochloric acid.*

Related substances

A. Thin-layer chromatography (*2.2.27*).

Test solution (a). Dissolve 40 mg of the substance to be examined in *methanol R* and dilute to 10 ml with the same solvent.

Test solution (b). Dissolve 0.160 g of the substance to be examined in *methanol R* and dilute to 10 ml with the same solvent.

Reference solution (a). Dissolve 20 mg of *metoclopramide CRS* and 10 mg of *sulpiride CRS* in *methanol R* and dilute to 5 ml with the same solvent.

Reference solution (b). Dissolve 20 mg of *N,N-diethylethane-1,2-diamine R* (impurity E) in *methanol R* and dilute to 50 ml with the same solvent. Dilute 2 ml of this solution to 25 ml with *methanol R.*

Plate: *TLC silica gel F_{254} plate R.*

Mobile phase: *concentrated ammonia R, dioxan R, methanol R, methylene chloride R* (2:10:14:90 *V/V/V/V*).

Application: 10 µl.

Development: over 2/3 of the plate.

Drying: in air.

Detection: examine in ultraviolet light at 254 nm (identification C), then spray with *dimethylaminobenzaldehyde solution R1* and allow to dry in air.

System suitability: reference solution (a):
- the chromatogram shows 2 clearly separated spots.

Limit: test solution (b):
- *impurity E*: any spot due to impurity E (not visualised in ultraviolet light at 254 nm) is not more intense than the corresponding spot in the chromatogram obtained with reference solution (b) (0.2 per cent).

B. Liquid chromatography (*2.2.29*).

Test solution. Dissolve 10.0 mg of the substance to be examined in the mobile phase and dilute to 10.0 ml with the mobile phase.

Reference solution (a). Dilute 0.2 ml of the test solution to 100.0 ml with the mobile phase.

Reference solution (b). Dissolve 10 mg of *metoclopramide impurity A CRS* in the mobile phase and dilute to 100 ml with the mobile phase. Mix 1 ml of this solution with 0.1 ml of the test solution and dilute to 10 ml with the mobile phase.

Column:

- *size*: *l* = 0.25 m, Ø = 4.6 mm;
- *stationary phase*: *octylsilyl silica gel for chromatography R* (5 μm).

Mobile phase: dissolve 6.8 g of *potassium dihydrogen phosphate R* in 700 ml of *water R*; add 0.2 ml of *N,N-dimethyloctylamine R* and adjust to pH 4.0 with *dilute phosphoric acid R*; dilute to 1000 ml with *water R*, add 250 ml of *acetonitrile R* and mix.

Flow rate: 1.5 ml/min.

Detection: spectrophotometer at 240 nm.

Injection: 10 μl.

Run time: 8 times the retention time of metoclopramide.

Relative retention with reference to metoclopramide (retention time = about 3.6 min): impurity A = about 0.82; impurity F = about 0.89; impurity H = about 0.91; impurity G = about 1.7; impurity C = about 2.7; impurity D = about 2.8; impurity B = about 6.4.

System suitability: reference solution (b):

- *resolution*: minimum 2.0 between the peaks due to impurity A and metoclopramide .

Limits:

- *impurities A, B, C, D, F, G, H*: for each impurity, not more than the area of the principal peak in the chromatogram obtained with reference solution (a) (0.2 per cent);
- *total*: not more than 3 times the area of the principal peak in the chromatogram obtained with reference solution (a) (0.6 per cent);
- *disregard limit*: 0.1 times the area of the principal peak in the chromatogram obtained with reference solution (a) (0.02 per cent).

Heavy metals (*2.4.8*): maximum 20 ppm.

1.0 g complies with test C. Prepare the reference solution using 2 ml of *lead standard solution (10 ppm Pb) R*.

Loss on drying (*2.2.32*): maximum 1.0 per cent, determined on 1.000 g by drying in an oven at 105 °C.

Sulphated ash (*2.4.14*): maximum 0.1 per cent, determined on 1.0 g.

ASSAY

Dissolve 0.250 g in 50 ml of *anhydrous acetic acid R* and add 5 ml of *acetic anhydride R*. Titrate with *0.1 M perchloric acid*, determining the end-point potentiometrically (*2.2.20*).

1 ml of *0.1 M perchloric acid* is equivalent to 29.98 mg of $C_{14}H_{22}ClN_3O_2$.

IMPURITIES

Specified impurities: A, B, C, D, E, F, G, H.

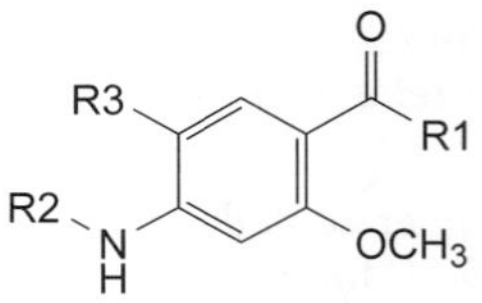

A. R1 = NH-CH_2-CH_2-N(C_2H_5)$_2$, R2 = CO-CH_3, R3 = Cl: 4-(acetylamino)-5-chloro-*N*-[2-(diethylamino)ethyl]-2-methoxybenzamide,

B. R1 = OCH_3, R2 = CO-CH_3, R3 = Cl: methyl 4-(acetylamino)-5-chloro-2-methoxybenzoate,

C. R1 = OH, R2 = H, R3 = Cl: 4-amino-5-chloro-2-methoxybenzoic acid,

D. R1 = OCH_3, R2 = CO-CH_3, R3 = H: methyl 4-(acetylamino)-2-methoxybenzoate,

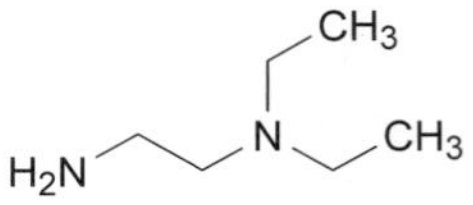

E. *N,N*-diethylethane-1,2-diamine,

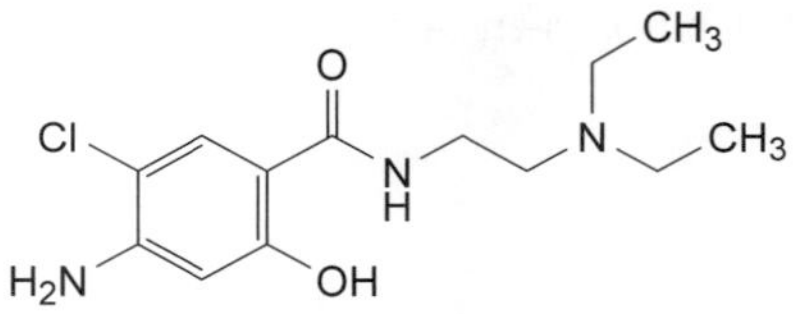

F. 4-amino-5-chloro-*N*-[2-(diethylamino)ethyl]-2-hydroxybenzamide,

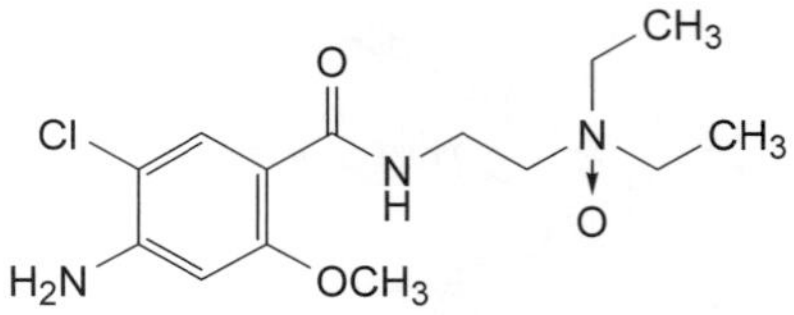

G. *N'*-(4-amino-5-chloro-2-methoxybenzoyl)-*N,N*-diethylethane-1,2-diamine *N*-oxide,

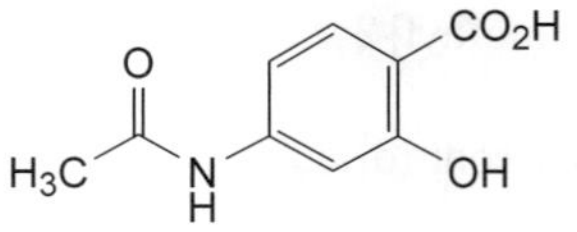

H. 4-(acetylamino)-2-hydroxybenzoic acid.

04/2008:1244
corrected 6.2

MORPHINE SULPHATE

Morphini sulfas

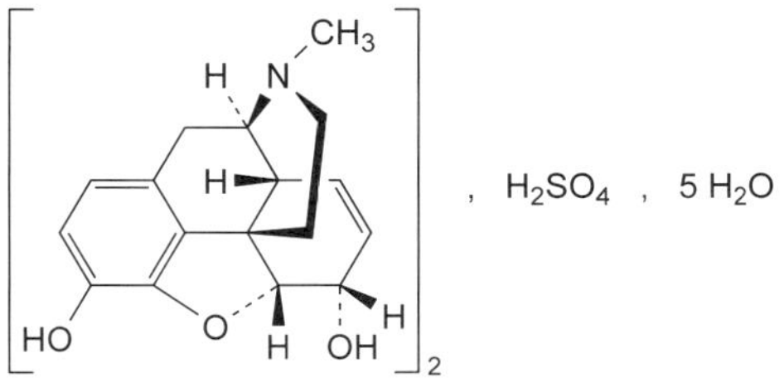

$C_{34}H_{40}N_2O_{10}S,5H_2O$ M_r 759
[6211-15-0]

DEFINITION

Di(7,8-didehydro-4,5α-epoxy-17-methylmorphinan-3,6α-diol) sulphate pentahydrate.

Content: 98.0 per cent to 102.0 per cent (anhydrous substance).

CHARACTERS

Appearance: white or almost white, crystalline powder.

Solubility: soluble in water, very slightly soluble in ethanol (96 per cent), practically insoluble in toluene.

IDENTIFICATION

First identification: A, E.

Second identification: B, C, D, E.

A. Infrared absorption spectrophotometry (*2.2.24*).

Preparation: dissolve 20 mg in 1 ml of *water R*, add 0.05 ml of *1 M sodium hydroxide* and shake. A precipitate is formed. Filter, wash with 2 quantities, each of 0.5 ml, of *water R* and dry the precipitate at 145 °C for 1 h. Prepare discs using the dried precipitate.

Comparison: repeat the operations using 20 mg of *morphine sulphate CRS*.

B. Ultraviolet and visible absorption spectrophotometry (*2.2.25*).

Solution A. Dissolve 25.0 mg in *water R* and dilute to 25.0 ml with the same solvent.

Test solution (a). Dilute 10.0 ml of solution A to 100.0 ml with *water R*.

Test solution (b). Dilute 10.0 ml of solution A to 100.0 ml with *0.1 M sodium hydroxide*.

Spectral range: 250-350 nm for test solutions (a) and (b).

Absorption maximum: at 285 nm for test solution (a); at 298 nm for test solution (b).

Specific absorbance at the absorption maximum: 37 to 43 for test solution (a); 64 to 72 for test solution (b).

C. To about 1 mg of powdered substance in a porcelain dish add 0.5 ml of *sulphuric acid-formaldehyde reagent R*. A purple colour develops and becomes violet.

D. It gives the reaction of alkaloids (*2.3.1*).

E. It gives the reactions of sulphates (*2.3.1*).

TESTS

Solution S. Dissolve 0.500 g in *carbon dioxide-free water R* and dilute to 25.0 ml with the same solvent.

Appearance of solution. Solution S is clear (*2.2.1*) and not more intensely coloured than reference solution Y_6 or BY_6 (*2.2.2, Method II*).

Acidity or alkalinity. To 10 ml of solution S add 0.05 ml of *methyl red solution R*. Not more than 0.2 ml of *0.02 M sodium hydroxide* or *0.02 M hydrochloric acid* is required to change the colour of the indicator.

Specific optical rotation (*2.2.7*): – 107 to – 110 (anhydrous substance), determined on solution S.

Related substances. Liquid chromatography (*2.2.29*).

Test solution. Dissolve 0.125 g of the substance to be examined in a 1 per cent *V/V* solution of *acetic acid R* and dilute to 50 ml with the same solution.

Reference solution (a). Dilute 1.0 ml of the test solution to 100.0 ml with a 1 per cent *V/V* solution of *acetic acid R*. Dilute 2.0 ml of this solution to 10.0 ml with a 1 per cent *V/V* solution of *acetic acid R*.

Reference solution (b). Dissolve 5 mg of *morphine for system suitability CRS* (containing impurities B, C, E and F) in a 1 per cent *V/V* solution of *acetic acid R* and dilute to 2 ml with the same solution.

Column:
- *size*: *l* = 0.15 m, Ø = 4.6 mm;
- *stationary phase*: *end-capped octadecylsilyl silica gel for chromatography R* (5 µm);
- *temperature*: 35 °C.

Mobile phase:
- *mobile phase A*: 1.01 g/l solution of *sodium heptanesulphonate R* adjusted to pH 2.6 with a 50 per cent *V/V* solution of *phosphoric acid R*;
- *mobile phase B*: *methanol R*;

Time (min)	Mobile phase A (per cent *V/V*)	Mobile phase B (per cent *V/V*)
0 - 2	85	15
2 - 35	85 → 50	15 → 50
35 - 40	50	50

Flow rate: 1.5 ml/min.

Detection: spectrophotometer at 230 nm.

Injection: 10 µl.

Identification of impurities: use the chromatogram supplied with *morphine for system suitability CRS* and the chromatogram obtained with reference solution (b) to identify the peaks due to impurities B, C, E and F.

Relative retention with reference to morphine (retention time = about 12.5 min): impurity F = about 0.95; impurity E = about 1.1; impurity C = about 1.6; impurity B = about 1.9.

System suitability: reference solution (b):
- *peak-to-valley ratio*: minimum 2, where H_p = height above the baseline of the peak due to impurity F and H_v = height above the baseline of the lowest point of the curve separating this peak from the peak due to morphine.

Limits:
- *correction factors*: for the calculation of content, multiply the peak areas of the following impurities by the corresponding correction factor: impurity B = 0.25; impurity C = 0.4; impurity E = 0.5;
- *impurity B*: not more than twice the area of the principal peak in the chromatogram obtained with reference solution (a) (0.4 per cent);

Monographs L-P

- *impurities C, E*: for each impurity, not more than the area of the principal peak in the chromatogram obtained with reference solution (a) (0.2 per cent);
- *any other impurity*: for each impurity, not more than the area of the principal peak in the chromatogram obtained with reference solution (a) (0.2 per cent);
- *total*: not more than 5 times the area of the principal peak in the chromatogram obtained with reference solution (a) (1.0 per cent);
- *disregard limit*: 0.25 times the area of the principal peak in the chromatogram obtained with reference solution (a) (0.05 per cent).

The thresholds indicated under Related substances (Table 2034.-1) in the general monograph *Substances for pharmaceutical use (2034)* do not apply.

Iron (*2.4.9*): maximum 5 ppm.

Dissolve the residue from the test for sulphated ash in *water R* and dilute to 10.0 ml with the same solvent.

Water (*2.5.12*): 10.4 per cent to 13.4 per cent, determined on 0.10 g.

Sulphated ash (*2.4.14*): maximum 0.1 per cent, determined on 2.0 g.

ASSAY

Dissolve 0.500 g in 120 ml of *anhydrous acetic acid R.* Titrate with *0.1 M perchloric acid,* determining the end-point potentiometrically (*2.2.20*).

1 ml of *0.1 M perchloric acid* is equivalent to 66.88 mg of $C_{34}H_{40}N_2O_{10}S$.

STORAGE

Protected from light.

IMPURITIES

Specified impurities: *B, C, E.*

Other detectable impurities (the following substances would, if present at a sufficient level, be detected by one or other of the tests in the monograph. They are limited by the general acceptance criterion for other/unspecified impurities and/or by the general monograph *Substances for pharmaceutical use (2034).* It is therefore not necessary to identify these impurities for demonstration of compliance. See also *5.10. Control of impurities in substances for pharmaceutical use*): *A, D, F.*

A. codeine,

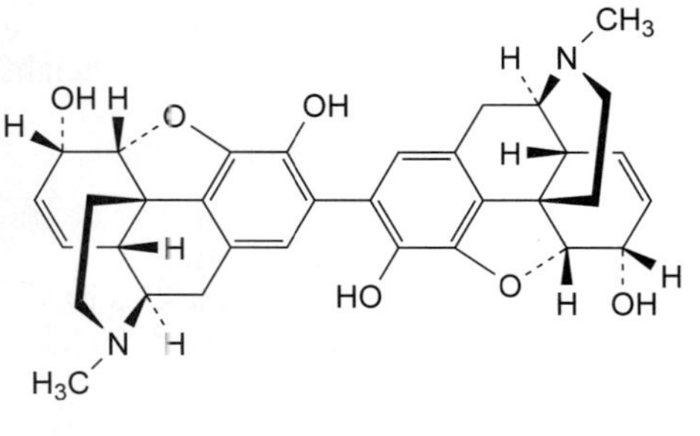

B. 7,7′,8,8′-tetradehydro-4,5α:4′,5′α-diepoxy-17,17′-dimethyl-2,2′-bimorphinanyl-3,3′,6α,6′α-tetrol (2,2′-bimorphine),

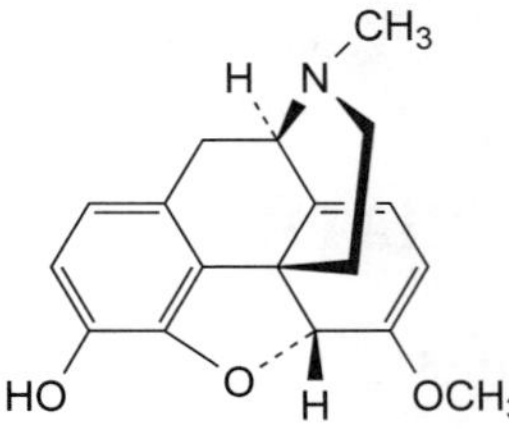

C. 6,7,8,14-tetradehydro-4,5α-epoxy-6-methoxy-17-methylmorphinan-3-ol (oripavine),

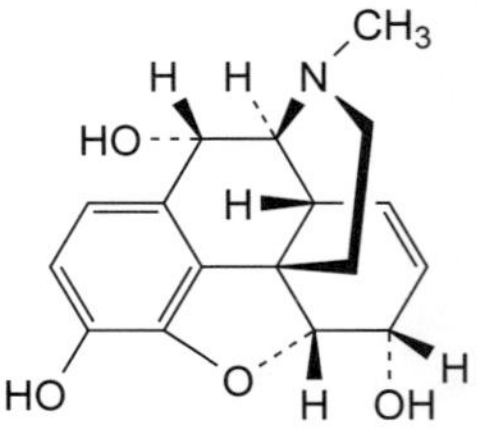

D. 7,8-didehydro-4,5α-epoxy-17-methylmorphinan-3,6α,10α-triol (10*S*-hydroxymorphine),

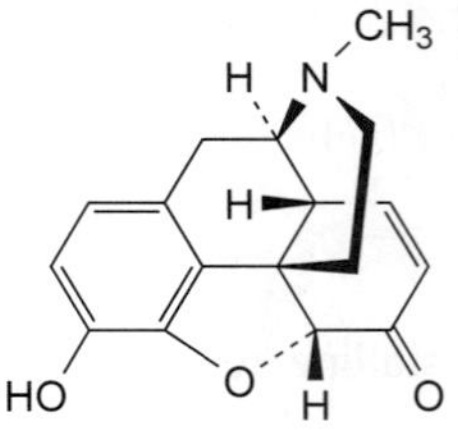

E. 7,8-didehydro-4,5α-epoxy-3-hydroxy-17-methylmorphinan-6-one (morphinone),

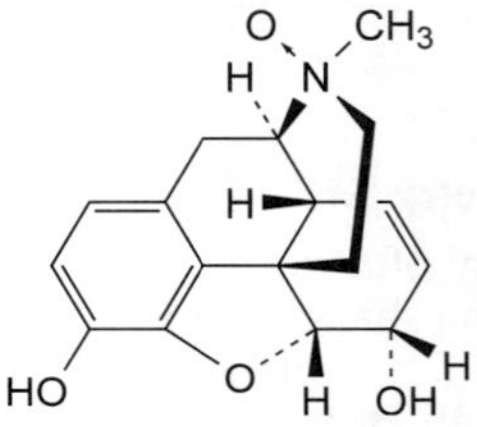

F. (17*S*)-7,8-didehydro-4,5α-epoxy-17-methylmorphinan-3, 6α-diol 17-oxide (morphine *N*-oxide).

01/2008:2254
corrected 6.2

MOXIFLOXACIN HYDROCHLORIDE

Moxifloxacini hydrochloridum

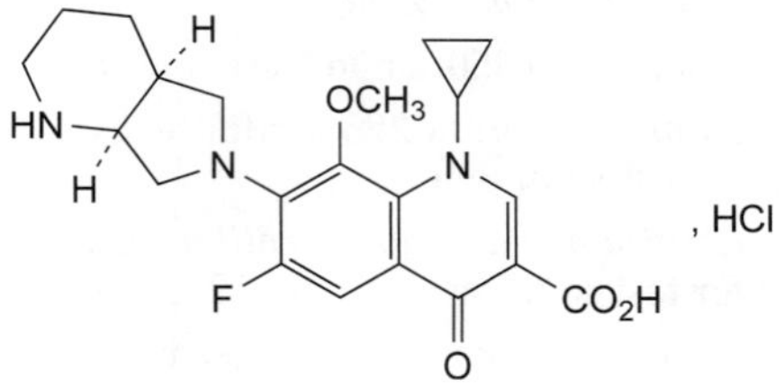

$C_{21}H_{25}ClFN_3O_4$ M_r 437.9

DEFINITION

1-Cyclopropyl-6-fluoro-8-methoxy-7-[(4a*S*,7a*S*)-octahydro-6*H*-pyrrolo[3,4-*b*]pyridin-6-yl]-4-oxo-1,4-dihydroquinoline-3-carboxylic acid hydrochloride.

Content: 98.0 per cent to 102.0 per cent (anhydrous substance).

PRODUCTION

The production method is validated to demonstrate the satisfactory enantiomeric purity of the final product.

CHARACTERS

Appearance: light yellow or yellow powder or crystals, slightly hygroscopic.

Solubility: sparingly soluble in water, slightly soluble in ethanol (96 per cent), practically insoluble in acetone.

IDENTIFICATION

A. Specific optical rotation (see Tests).

B. Infrared absorption spectrophotometry (*2.2.24*).

Comparison: *moxifloxacin hydrochloride CRS*.

C. Dissolve 50 mg in 5 ml of *water R*, add 1 ml of *dilute nitric acid R*, mix, allow to stand for 5 min and filter. The filtrate gives reaction (a) of chlorides (*2.3.1*).

TESTS

Appearance of solution. The solution is not more opalescent than reference suspension II (*2.2.1*) and not more intensely coloured than reference solution GY_2 (*2.2.2, Method II*). If intended for use in the manufacture of parenteral dosage forms, the solution is clear (*2.2.1*) and not more intensely coloured than reference solution GY_2 (*2.2.2, Method II*).

Dissolve 1.0 g in 20 ml of *dilute sodium hydroxide solution R*.

pH (*2.2.3*): 3.9 to 4.6.

Dissolve 0.10 g in 50 ml of *carbon dioxide-free water R*.

Specific optical rotation (*2.2.7*): – 125 to – 138 (anhydrous substance).

Dissolve 0.200 g in 20.0 ml of a mixture of equal volumes of *acetonitrile R* and *water R*.

Related substances. Liquid chromatography (*2.2.29*). *Carry out the test protected from light.*

Solution A. Dissolve 0.50 g of *tetrabutylammonium hydrogen sulphate R* and 1.0 g of *potassium dihydrogen phosphate R* in about 500 ml of *water R*. Add 2 ml of *phosphoric acid R* and 0.050 g of *anhydrous sodium sulphite R*, then dilute to 1000.0 ml with *water R*.

Test solution (a). Dissolve 50.0 mg of the substance to be examined in solution A and dilute to 50.0 ml with the same solution.

Test solution (b). Dilute 2.0 ml of test solution (a) to 20.0 ml with solution A.

Reference solution (a). Dissolve 50.0 mg of *moxifloxacin hydrochloride CRS* in solution A and dilute to 50.0 ml with the same solution. Dilute 2.0 ml of this solution to 20.0 ml with solution A.

Reference solution (b). Dissolve 5 mg of *moxifloxacin for peak identification CRS* (containing impurities A, B, C, D and E) in solution A and dilute to 5.0 ml with the same solution.

Reference solution (c). Dilute 1.0 ml of test solution (a) to 100.0 ml with solution A. Dilute 1.0 ml of this solution to 10.0 ml with solution A.

Column:

- *size*: *l* = 0.25 m, Ø = 4.6 mm;
- *stationary phase*: *end-capped phenylsilyl silica gel for chromatography R* (5 µm);
- *temperature*: 45 °C.

Mobile phase: mix 28 volumes of *methanol R* and 72 volumes of a solution containing 0.5 g/l of *tetrabutylammonium hydrogen sulphate R*, 1.0 g/l of *potassium dihydrogen phosphate R* and 3.4 g/l of *phosphoric acid R*.

Flow rate: 1.3 ml/min.

Detection: spectrophotometer at 293 nm.

Injection: 10 µl of test solution (a) and reference solutions (b) and (c).

Run time: 2.5 times the retention time of moxifloxacin.

Identification of impurities: use the chromatogram supplied with *moxifloxacin for peak identification CRS* and the chromatogram obtained with reference solution (b) to identify the peaks due to impurities A, B, C, D and E.

Relative retention with reference to moxifloxacin (retention time = about 14 min): impurity A = about 1.1; impurity B = about 1.3; impurity C = about 1.4; impurity D = about 1.6; impurity E = about 1.7.

System suitability: reference solution (b):

- *resolution*: minimum 1.5 between the peaks due to moxifloxacin and impurity A;
- the chromatogram obtained is similar to the chromatogram supplied with *moxifloxacin for peak identification CRS*.

Limits:

- *correction factors*: for the calculation of content, multiply the peak areas of the following impurities by the corresponding correction factor: impurity B = 1.4; impurity E = 3.5;
- *impurities A, B, C, D, E*: for each impurity, not more than the area of the principal peak in the chromatogram obtained with reference solution (c) (0.1 per cent);
- *unspecified impurities*: for each impurity, not more than the area of the principal peak in the chromatogram obtained with reference solution (c) (0.10 per cent);
- *total*: not more than 3 times the area of the principal peak in the chromatogram obtained with reference solution (c) (0.3 per cent);
- *disregard limit*: 0.5 times the area of the principal peak in the chromatogram obtained with reference solution (c) (0.05 per cent).

Water (*2.5.12*): maximum 4.5 per cent, determined on 0.200 g.

Sulphated ash (*2.4.14*): maximum 0.1 per cent, determined on 1.0 g in a platinum crucible.

ASSAY

Liquid chromatography (*2.2.29*) as described in the test for related substances with the following modification.

Injection: test solution (b) and reference solution (a).

Calculate the percentage content of $C_{21}H_{25}ClFN_3O_4$ from the declared content of *moxifloxacin hydrochloride CRS*.

STORAGE

In an airtight container, protected from light.

LABELLING

The label states, where applicable, that the substance is suitable for use in the manufacture of parenteral dosage forms.

IMPURITIES

Specified impurities: A, B, C, D, E.

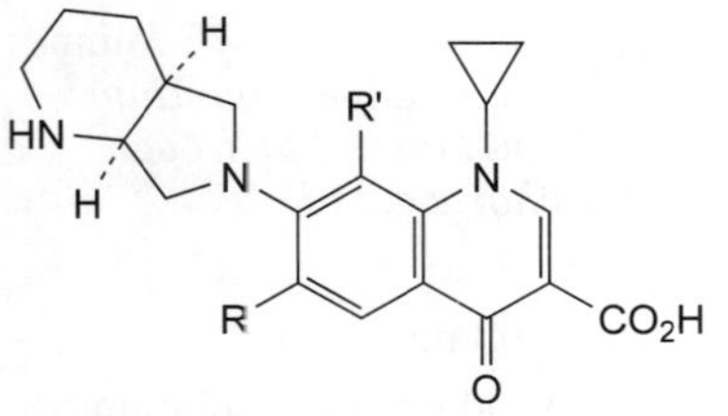

A. R = R′ = F: 1-cyclopropyl-6,8-difluoro-7-[(4a*S*,7a*S*)-octahydro-6*H*-pyrrolo[3,4-*b*]pyridin-6-yl]-4-oxo-1,4-dihydroquinoline-3-carboxylic acid,

B. R = R′ = OCH_3: 1-cyclopropyl-6,8-dimethoxy-7-[(4a*S*,7a*S*)-octahydro-6*H*-pyrrolo[3,4-*b*]pyridin-6-yl]-4-oxo-1,4-dihydroquinoline-3-carboxylic acid,

C. R = F, R′ = OC_2H_5: 1-cyclopropyl-8-ethoxy-6-fluoro-7-[(4a*S*,7a*S*)-octahydro-6*H*-pyrrolo[3,4-*b*]pyridin-6-yl]-4-oxo-1,4-dihydroquinoline-3-carboxylic acid,

D. R = OCH_3, R′ = F: 1-cyclopropyl-8-fluoro-6-methoxy-7-[(4a*S*,7a*S*)-octahydro-6*H*-pyrrolo[3,4-*b*]pyridin-6-yl]-4-oxo-1,4-dihydroquinoline-3-carboxylic acid,

E. R = F, R′ = OH: 1-cyclopropyl-6-fluoro-8-hydroxy-7-[(4a*S*,7a*S*)-octahydro-6*H*-pyrrolo[3,4-*b*]pyridin-6-yl]-4-oxo-1,4-dihydroquinoline-3-carboxylic acid.

Monographs L-P

N

07/2008:0731

NAPROXEN

Naproxenum

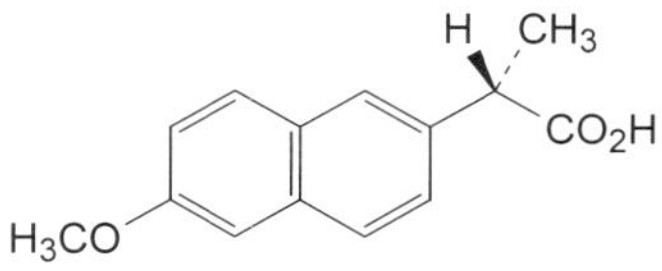

$C_{14}H_{14}O_3$ M_r 230.3
[22204-53-1]

DEFINITION

(2*S*)-2-(6-Methoxynaphthalen-2-yl)propanoic acid.

Content: 99.0 per cent to 101.0 per cent (dried substance).

CHARACTERS

Appearance: white or almost white, crystalline powder.

Solubility: practically insoluble in water, soluble in ethanol (96 per cent) and in methanol.

IDENTIFICATION

First identification: A, D.

Second identification: A, B, C.

A. Specific optical rotation (*2.2.7*): + 59 to + 62 (dried substance).

   Dissolve 0.50 g in *ethanol (96 per cent) R* and dilute to 25.0 ml with the same solvent.

B. Melting point (*2.2.14*): 154 °C to 158 °C.

C. Dissolve 40.0 mg in *methanol R* and dilute to 100.0 ml with the same solvent. Dilute 10.0 ml of this solution to 100.0 ml with *methanol R*. Examined between 230 nm and 350 nm (*2.2.25*), the solution shows 4 absorption maxima, at 262 nm, 271 nm, 316 nm and 331 nm. The specific absorbances at the absorption maxima are 216 to 238, 219 to 241, 61 to 69 and 79 to 87, respectively.

D. Infrared absorption spectrophotometry (*2.2.24*).

   Comparison: *naproxen CRS*.

TESTS

Appearance of solution. The solution is clear (*2.2.1*) and not more intensely coloured than reference solution BY_7 (*2.2.2, Method II*).

Dissolve 1.25 g in *methanol R* and dilute to 25 ml with the same solvent.

Enantiomeric purity. Liquid chromatography (*2.2.29*). *Protect the solutions from light.*

Test solution. Dissolve 25.0 mg of the substance to be examined in *tetrahydrofuran R* and dilute to 50.0 ml with the same solvent. Dilute 2.0 ml of this solution to 20.0 ml with the mobile phase.

Reference solution (a). Dilute 2.5 ml of the test solution to 100.0 ml with the mobile phase.

Reference solution (b). Dissolve 5 mg of *racemic naproxen CRS* in 10 ml of *tetrahydrofuran R* and dilute to 100 ml with the mobile phase.

Column:

- *size*: *l* = 0.25 m, Ø = 4.6 mm;
- *stationary phase*: *silica gel π-acceptor/π-donor for chiral separations R* (5 μm) (S,S);
- *temperature*: 25 °C.

Mobile phase: *glacial acetic acid R, acetonitrile R, 2-propanol R, hexane R* (5:50:100:845 *V/V/V/V*).

Flow rate: 2 ml/min.

Detection: spectrophotometer at 263 nm.

Injection: 20 μl.

Run time: 1.5 times the retention time of naproxen (retention time = about 5 min).

System suitability: reference solution (b):

- *resolution*: minimum 3 between the peaks due to impurity G and naproxen.

Limit:

- *impurity G*: not more than the area of the principal peak in the chromatogram obtained with reference solution (a) (2.5 per cent).

Related substances. Liquid chromatography (*2.2.29*). *Protect the solutions from light.*

Test solution. Dissolve 12 mg of the substance to be examined in the mobile phase and dilute to 20 ml with the mobile phase.

Reference solution (a). Dilute 1.0 ml of the test solution to 50.0 ml with the mobile phase. Dilute 1.0 ml of this solution to 20.0 ml with the mobile phase.

Reference solution (b). Dissolve 6 mg of *bromomethoxynaphthalene R* (impurity N), 6 mg of *1-(6-methoxynaphthalen-2-yl)ethanone R* (impurity L) and 6 mg of *(1RS)-1-(6-methoxynaphthalen-2-yl)ethanol R* (impurity K) in *acetonitrile R* and dilute to 10 ml with the same solvent. To 1 ml of this solution add 1 ml of the test solution and dilute to 50 ml with the mobile phase. Dilute 1 ml of this solution to 20 ml with the mobile phase.

Column:

- *size*: *l* = 0.10 m, Ø = 4.0 mm;
- *stationary phase*: *octadecylsilyl silica gel for chromatography R* (3 μm);
- *temperature*: 50 °C.

Mobile phase: mix 42 volumes of *acetonitrile R* and 58 volumes of a 1.36 g/l solution of *potassium dihydrogen phosphate R* previously adjusted to pH 2.0 with *phosphoric acid R*.

Flow rate: 1.5 ml/min.

Detection: spectrophotometer at 230 nm.

Injection: 20 μl.

Run time: 1.5 times the retention time of impurity N.

Relative retention with reference to naproxen (retention time = about 2.5 min): impurity K = about 0.9; impurity L = about 1.4; impurity N = about 5.3.

System suitability: reference solution (b):

- *resolution*: minimum 2.2 between the peaks due to impurity K and naproxen.

Limits:

- *impurity L*: not more than the area of the corresponding peak in the chromatogram obtained with reference solution (b) (0.1 per cent);
- *unspecified impurities*: for each impurity, not more than the area of the principal peak in the chromatogram obtained with reference solution (a) (0.10 per cent);
- *total*: not more than 3 times the area of the principal peak in the chromatogram obtained with reference solution (a) (0.3 per cent);
- *disregard limit*: 0.5 times the area of the principal peak in the chromatogram obtained with reference solution (a) (0.05 per cent).

Heavy metals (*2.4.8*): maximum 20 ppm.

1.0 g complies with limit test C. Prepare the reference solution using 2 ml of *lead standard solution (10 ppm Pb) R*.

Loss on drying (*2.2.32*): maximum 0.5 per cent, determined on 1.000 g by drying in an oven at 105 °C for 3 h.

Sulphated ash (*2.4.14*): maximum 0.1 per cent, determined on 1.0 g.

ASSAY

Dissolve 0.200 g in a mixture of 25 ml of *water R* and 75 ml of *methanol R*. Titrate with *0.1 M sodium hydroxide*, using 1 ml of *phenolphthalein solution R* as indicator.

1 ml of *0.1 M sodium hydroxide* is equivalent to 23.03 mg of $C_{14}H_{14}O_3$.

STORAGE

Protected from light.

IMPURITIES

Specified impurities: *G, L*.

Other detectable impurities (the following substances would, if present at a sufficient level, be detected by one or other of the tests in the monograph. They are limited by the general acceptance criterion for other/unspecified impurities and/or by the general monograph *Substances for pharmaceutical use (2034)*. It is therefore not necessary to identify these impurities for demonstration of compliance. See also *5.10. Control of impurities in substances for pharmaceutical use*): *A, B, C, D, E, F, H, I, J, K, M, N*.

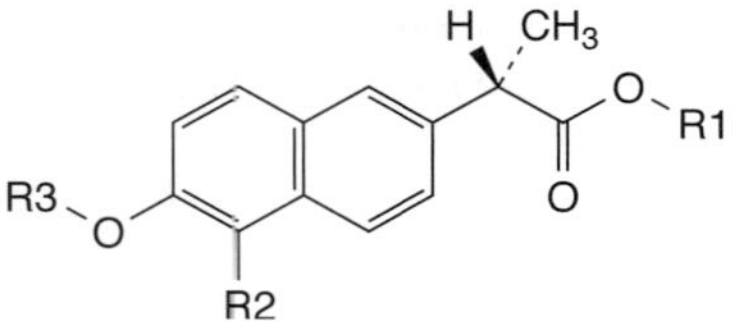

A. R1 = R2 = R3 = H: (2*S*)-2-(6-hydroxynaphthalen-2-yl)propanoic acid,

B. R1 = H, R2 = Cl, R3 = CH_3: (2*S*)-2-(5-chloro-6-methoxynaphthalen-2-yl)propanoic acid,

C. R1 = H, R2 = Br, R3 = CH_3: (2*S*)-2-(5-bromo-6-methoxynaphthalen-2-yl)propanoic acid,

D. R1 = H, R2 = I, R3 = CH_3: (2*S*)-2-(5-iodo-6-methoxynaphthalen-2-yl)propanoic acid,

E. R1 = R3 = CH_3, R2 = H: methyl (2*S*)-2-(6-methoxynaphthalen-2-yl)propanoate,

F. R1 = C_2H_5, R2 = H, R3 = CH_3: ethyl (2*S*)-2-(6-methoxynaphthalen-2-yl)propanoate,

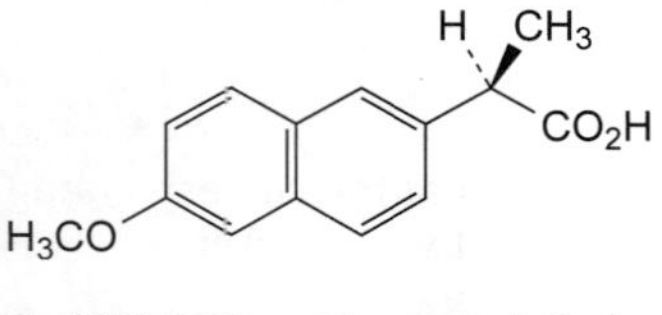

G. (2*R*)-2-(6-methoxynaphthalen-2-yl)propanoic acid ((*R*)-enantiomer),

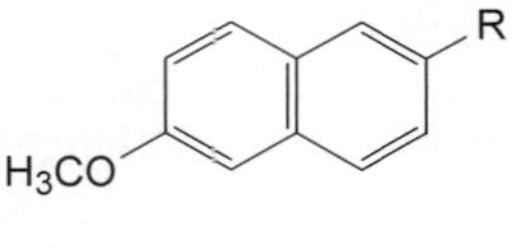

H. R = OH: 6-methoxynaphthalen-2-ol,

I. R = CH_2-CO_2H: (6-methoxynaphthalen-2-yl)acetic acid,

J. R = C_2H_5: 2-ethyl-6-methoxynaphthalene,

K. R = CHOH-CH_3: (1*RS*)-1-(6-methoxynaphthalen-2-yl)ethanol,

M. R = H: 2-methoxynaphthalene (nerolin),

N. R = Br: 2-bromo-6-methoxynaphthalene,

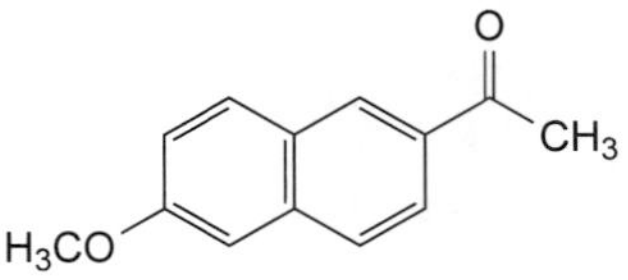

L. 1-(6-methoxynaphthalen-2-yl)ethanone.

07/2008:2256

NILUTAMIDE

Nilutamidum

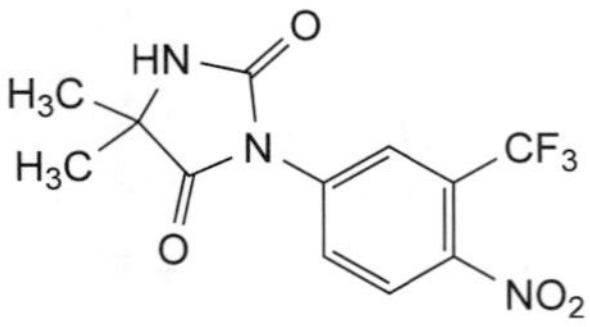

$C_{12}H_{10}F_3N_3O_4$ M_r 317.2
[63612-50-0]

DEFINITION

5,5-Dimethyl-3-[4-nitro-3-(trifluoromethyl)phenyl]-imidazolidine-2,4-dione.

Content: 98.0 per cent to 102.0 per cent (anhydrous substance).

CHARACTERS

Appearance: white or almost white powder.

Solubility: very slightly soluble in water, freely soluble in acetone, soluble in anhydrous ethanol.

IDENTIFICATION

Infrared absorption spectrophotometry (*2.2.24*).

Comparison: *nilutamide CRS*.

TESTS

Related substances. Liquid chromatography (*2.2.29*). *Prepare the solutions immediately before use.*

Solvent mixture: *acetonitrile for chromatography R, water R* (35:65 *V/V*).

Test solution. Dissolve 0.10 g of the substance to be examined in the solvent mixture and dilute to 100 ml with the solvent mixture.

Reference solution (a). Dilute 20.0 ml of the test solution to 100.0 ml with the solvent mixture. Dilute 1.0 ml of this solution to 100.0 ml with the solvent mixture.

Reference solution (b). Dissolve 2 mg of the substance to be examined and 2 mg of *nilutamide impurity B CRS* in the solvent mixture and dilute to 50 ml with the solvent mixture.

Column:

– *size*: *l* = 0.15 m, Ø = 4.6 mm;
– *stationary phase*: spherical *octadecylsilyl silica gel for chromatography R* (5 μm).

Mobile phase:

- *mobile phase A*: 2.0 g/l solution of *potassium dihydrogen phosphate R* adjusted to pH 7.5 with *1 M sodium hydroxide*;
- *mobile phase B*: *acetonitrile for chromatography R*;

Time (min)	Mobile phase A (per cent *V/V*)	Mobile phase B (per cent *V/V*)
0 - 8	55	45
8 - 30	55 → 30	45 → 70
30 - 31	30 → 55	70 → 45
31 - 45	55	45

Flow rate: 1.5 ml/min.

Detection: spectrophotometer at 230 nm.

Injection: 20 μl.

Relative retention with reference to nilutamide (retention time = about 5.3 min): impurity B = about 0.9.

System suitability: reference solution (b):

- *resolution*: minimum 3.0 between the peaks due to impurity B and nilutamide.

Limits:

- *unspecified impurities*: for each impurity, not more than 0.5 times the area of the principal peak in the chromatogram obtained with reference solution (a) (0.10 per cent);
- *total*: not more than 1.5 times the area of the principal peak in the chromatogram obtained with reference solution (a) (0.3 per cent);
- *disregard limit*: 0.25 times the area of the principal peak in the chromatogram obtained with reference solution (a) (0.05 per cent).

Heavy metals (*2.4.8*): maximum 20 ppm.

It complies with test B with the following modifications.

Prescribed solution. Dissolve 0.5 g in a mixture of 10 volumes of *water R* and 90 volumes of *acetone R* and dilute to 20 ml with the same mixture of solvents.

Test solution. 12 ml of the prescribed solution.

Reference solution. Dilute 0.5 ml of *lead standard solution (10 ppm Pb) R* to 10 ml with a mixture of 10 volumes of *water R* and 90 volumes of *acetone R* and add 2 ml of the prescribed solution.

Filter the solutions through a membrane filter (0.45 μm). Compare the spots on the filters obtained with the different solutions. The substance to be examined complies with the test if the brown colour of the spot obtained with the test solution is not more intense than that of the spot obtained with the reference solution.

Water (*2.5.12*): maximum 0.5 per cent, determined on 0.500 g.

Sulphated ash (*2.4.14*): maximum 0.1 per cent, determined on 1.0 g in a platinum crucible.

ASSAY

Liquid chromatography (*2.2.29*). *The solutions are stable for 24 h at room temperature and in daylight.*

Solvent mixture: *acetonitrile for chromatography R*, *water R* (35:65 *V/V*).

Test solution. Dissolve 50.0 mg of the substance to be examined in the solvent mixture and dilute to 100.0 ml with the solvent mixture.

Reference solution. Dissolve 50.0 mg of *nilutamide CRS* in the solvent mixture and dilute to 100.0 ml with the solvent mixture.

Column:

- *size*: *l* = 0.15 m, Ø = 4.6 mm;
- *stationary phase*: spherical *octadecylsilyl silica gel for chromatography R* (5 μm).

Mobile phase: mix 40 volumes of *acetonitrile R* and 60 volumes of a 2.0 g/l solution of *potassium dihydrogen phosphate R* adjusted to pH 7.5 with *1 M sodium hydroxide*.

Flow rate: 1.5 ml/min.

Detection: spectrophotometer at 267 nm.

Injection: 20 μl.

Retention time: about 9 min.

Calculate the percentage content of $C_{12}H_{10}F_3N_3O_4$ from the declared content of *nilutamide CRS*.

STORAGE

Protected from light.

IMPURITIES

Other detectable impurities (the following substances would, if present at a sufficient level, be detected by one or other of the tests in the monograph. They are limited by the general acceptance criterion for other/unspecified impurities and/or by the general monograph *Substances for pharmaceutical use (2034)*. It is therefore not necessary to identify these impurities for demonstration of compliance. See also *5.10. Control of impurities in substances for pharmaceutical use*): *A, B, C, D*.

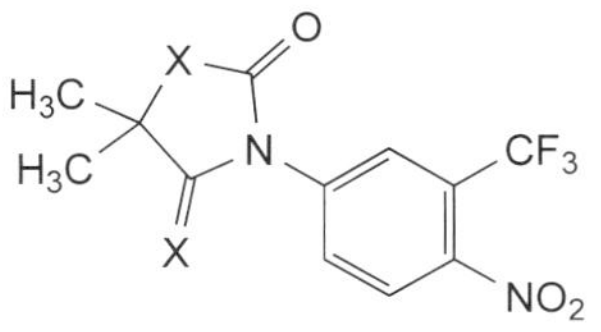

A. X = NH: 5-imino-4,4-dimethyl-1-[4-nitro-3-(trifluoromethyl)phenyl]imidazolidin-2-one,

C. X = O: 5,5-dimethyl-3-[4-nitro-3-(trifluoromethyl)phenyl]-oxazolidine-2,4-dione,

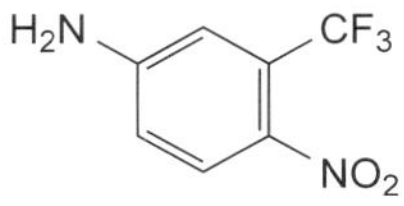

B. 4-nitro-3-(trifluoromethyl)aniline (nifeline),

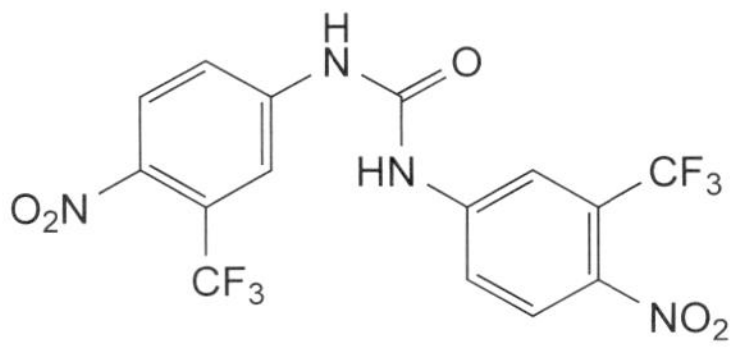

D. 1,3-bis[4-nitro-3-(trifluoromethyl)phenyl]urea.

01/2008:1550

NITRIC OXIDE

Nitrogenii oxidum

NO M_r 30.01

[10102-43-9]

DEFINITION

Content: minimum 99.0 per cent *V/V* of NO.

This monograph applies to nitric oxide for medicinal use.

CHARACTERS

Appearance: colourless gas which turns brown when exposed to air.

Solubility: at 20 °C and at a pressure of 101 kPa, 1 volume dissolves in about 21 volumes of water.

PRODUCTION

Carbon dioxide. Gas chromatography (*2.2.28*).

Gas to be examined. The substance to be examined.

Reference gas: mixture containing 3000 ppm *V/V* of *carbon dioxide R1* in *nitrogen R*.

Column:

- *material*: stainless steel;
- *size*: *l* = 3.5 m, Ø = 2 mm;
- *stationary phase*: *ethylvinylbenzene-divinylbenzene copolymer R*;
- *temperature*: 50 °C.

Carrier gas: *helium for chromatography R*.

Flow rate: 15 ml/min.

Detection: thermal conductivity.

Injection: loop injector.

System suitability:

- the chromatograms obtained show a clear separation of carbon dioxide from nitric oxide.

Limit:

- *carbon dioxide*: not more than the area of the corresponding peak in the chromatogram obtained with the reference gas (3000 ppm *V/V*).

Nitrogen. Gas chromatography (*2.2.28*).

Gas to be examined. The substance to be examined.

Reference gas: mixture containing 3000 ppm *V/V* of *nitrogen R* in *helium for chromatography R*.

Column:

- *material*: stainless steel;
- *size*: *l* = 3.5 m, Ø = 2 mm;
- *stationary phase*: *molecular sieve for chromatography R* (0.5 nm);
- *temperature*: 50 °C.

Carrier gas: *helium for chromatography R*.

Flow rate: 15 ml/min.

Detection: thermal conductivity.

Injection: loop injector.

System suitability:

- the chromatograms obtained show a clear separation of nitrogen from nitric oxide.

Limit:

- *nitrogen*: not more than the area of the corresponding peak in the chromatogram obtained with the reference gas (3000 ppm *V/V*).

Nitrogen dioxide: maximum 400 ppm *V/V*.

Ultraviolet absorption spectrophotometry analyser.

Gas to be examined. The substance to be examined.

Reference gas (a): *nitrogen R1*.

Reference gas (b): mixture containing 400 ppm *V/V* of *nitrogen dioxide R* in *nitrogen R*.

Apparatus:

- an ultraviolet-visible light source (analytical wavelength about 400 nm);
- a sample gas cell through which the feed gas flows;
- a closed reference gas cell containing *nitrogen R1* in parallel with the sample gas cell;
- a rotating chopper which feeds light alternately through the reference gas cell and the sample gas cell;
- a semiconductor detector which generates a frequency modulated output whose amplitude is a measure of the difference of absorption of the sample gas and the reference gas.

Analysis:

- set the zero of the instrument using reference gas (a) through the sample gas cell at a flow rate of 1 litre/min;
- adjust the span while feeding reference gas (b) through the sample gas cell at a flow rate of 1 litre/min;
- feed the gas to be examined through the sample gas cell at a flow rate of 1 litre/min, read the value from the instrument output and calculate, if necessary, the concentration of nitrogen dioxide.

Nitrous oxide. Gas chromatography (*2.2.28*).

Gas to be examined. The substance to be examined.

Reference gas: mixture containing 3000 ppm *V/V* of *nitrous oxide R* in *nitrogen R*.

Column:

- *material*: stainless steel;
- *size*: *l* = 3.5 m, Ø = 2 mm;
- *stationary phase*: *ethylvinylbenzene-divinylbenzene copolymer R*;
- *temperature*: 50 °C.

Carrier gas: *helium for chromatography R*.

Flow rate: 15 ml/min.

Detection: thermal conductivity.

Injection: loop injector.

System suitability:

- the chromatograms obtained show a clear separation of nitrous oxide from nitric oxide.

Limit:

- *nitrous oxide*: not more than the area of the corresponding peak in the chromatogram obtained with the reference gas (3000 ppm *V/V*).

Water (*2.5.28*): maximum 100 ppm *V/V*.

Assay. Determine the content of nitric oxide by difference using the mass balance equation after determining the sum of the impurities described under Production.

IDENTIFICATION

Infrared absorption spectrophotometry (*2.2.24*).

Comparison: *Ph. Eur. reference spectrum of nitric oxide.*

STORAGE

Compressed at a pressure not exceeding 2.5 MPa (25 bars) measured at 15 °C, in suitable containers complying with the legal regulations.

IMPURITIES

Specified impurities: A, B, C, D, E.

A. carbon dioxide,

B. nitrogen,

C. nitrogen dioxide,

D. nitrous oxide,

E. water.

01/2008:1247

NITROGEN

Nitrogenium

N_2 M_r 28.01
[7727-37-9]

DEFINITION

Content: minimum 99.5 per cent *V/V* of N_2.

This monograph applies to nitrogen for medicinal use.

CHARACTERS

Appearance: colourless, odourless gas.

Solubility: at 20 °C and at a pressure of 101 kPa, 1 volume dissolves in about 62 volumes of water and about 10 volumes of ethanol (96 per cent).

PRODUCTION

Carbon dioxide: maximum 300 ppm *V/V*, determined using an infrared analyser (*2.5.24*).

Gas to be examined. The substance to be examined. It must be filtered to avoid stray light phenomena.

Reference gas (a). Nitrogen R1.

Reference gas (b). Mixture containing 300 ppm *V/V* of *carbon dioxide R1* in *nitrogen R1.*

Calibrate the apparatus and set the sensitivity using reference gases (a) and (b). Measure the content of carbon dioxide in the gas to be examined.

Carbon monoxide: maximum 5 ppm *V/V*, determined using an infrared analyser (*2.5.25*).

Gas to be examined. The substance to be examined. It must be filtered to avoid stray light phenomena.

Reference gas (a). Nitrogen R1.

Reference gas (b). Mixture containing 5 ppm *V/V* of *carbon monoxide R* in *nitrogen R1.*

Calibrate the apparatus and set the sensitivity using reference gases (a) and (b). Measure the content of carbon monoxide in the gas to be examined.

Oxygen: maximum 50 ppm *V/V*, determined using an oxygen analyser with a detector scale ranging from 0-100 ppm *V/V* and equipped with an electrochemical cell.

The gas to be examined passes through a detection cell containing an aqueous solution of an electrolyte, generally potassium hydroxide. The presence of oxygen in the gas to be examined produces variation in the electric signal recorded at the outlet of the cell that is proportional to the oxygen content.

Calibrate the analyser according to the instructions of the manufacturer. Pass the gas to be examined through the analyser using a suitable pressure regulator and airtight metal tubes and operating at the prescribed flow-rates until constant readings are obtained.

Water (*2.5.28*): maximum 67 ppm *V/V.*

Assay. Gas chromatography (*2.2.28*).

Gas to be examined. The substance to be examined.

Reference gas (a). Ambient air.

Reference gas (b). Nitrogen R1.

Column:

- *material*: stainless steel;
- *size*: *l* = 2 m, Ø = 2 mm;
- *stationary phase*: *molecular sieve for chromatography R* (0.5 nm).

Carrier gas: *helium for chromatography R.*

Flow rate: 40 ml/min.

Temperature:

- *column*: 50 °C;
- *detection*: 130 °C.

Detection: thermal conductivity.

Injection: loop injector.

Inject reference gas (a). Adjust the injected volumes and operating conditions so that the height of the peak due to nitrogen in the chromatogram obtained with the reference gas is at least 35 per cent of the full scale of the recorder.

System suitability:

- the chromatograms obtained show a clear separation of oxygen and nitrogen.

Calculate the content of N_2 in the gas to be examined.

IDENTIFICATION

First identification: A.

Second identification: B, C.

A. Examine the chromatograms obtained in the assay (see Production).

   Results: the principal peak in the chromatogram obtained with the substance to be examined is similar in retention time to the principal peak in the chromatogram obtained with reference gas (b).

B. In a 250 ml conical flask replace the air by the substance to be examined. Place a burning or glowing splinter of wood in the flask. The splinter is extinguished.

C. In a suitable test tube, place 0.1 g of *magnesium R* in turnings. Close the tube with a two-hole stopper fitted with a glass tube reaching about 1 cm above the turnings. Pass the substance to be examined through the glass tube for 1 min without heating, then for 15 min while heating the test tube to a red glow. After cooling, add 5 ml of *dilute sodium hydroxide solution R*. The evolving vapours change the colour of moistened *red litmus paper R* blue.

TESTS

Carbon dioxide (*2.1.6*): maximum 300 ppm *V/V*, determined using a carbon dioxide detector tube.

Carbon monoxide (*2.1.6*): maximum 5 ppm *V/V*, determined using a carbon monoxide detector tube.

Water vapour (*2.1.6*): maximum 67 ppm *V/V*, determined using a water vapour detector tube.

STORAGE

As a compressed gas or a liquid in appropriate containers complying with the legal regulations.

IMPURITIES

Specified impurities: A, B, C, D.

A. carbon dioxide,

B. carbon monoxide,

C. oxygen,

D. water.

07/2008:1248

NORFLOXACIN

Norfloxacinum

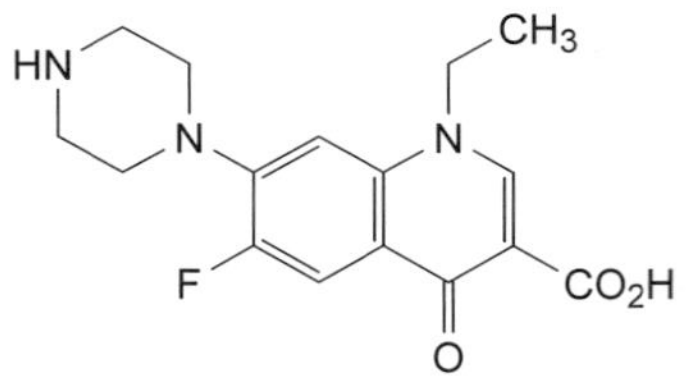

$C_{16}H_{18}FN_3O_3$ M_r 319.3
[70458-96-7]

DEFINITION

1-Ethyl-6-fluoro-4-oxo-7-(piperazin-1-yl)-1,4-dihydroquinoline-3-carboxylic acid.

Content: 99.0 per cent to 101.0 per cent (dried substance).

CHARACTERS

Appearance: white or pale yellow, hygroscopic, photosensitive, crystalline powder.

Solubility: very slightly soluble in water, slightly soluble in acetone and in ethanol (96 per cent).

IDENTIFICATION

Infrared absorption spectrophotometry (*2.2.24*).

Comparison: *norfloxacin CRS.*

TESTS

Appearance of solution. Dissolve 0.5 g in a previously filtered 4 g/l solution of *sodium hydroxide R* in *methanol R* and dilute to 50 ml with the same solution. The solution is not more opalescent than reference suspension II (*2.2.1*) and not more intensely coloured than reference solution B_7 (*2.2.2, Method II*).

Related substances. Liquid chromatography (*2.2.29*).

Solution A. Mix 5 volumes of *acetonitrile R* and 95 volumes of *water R* previously adjusted to pH 2.0 with *phosphoric acid R*.

Test solution. Dissolve 20 mg of the substance to be examined in 25 ml of solution A. Sonicate for 5 min and dilute to 50.0 ml with solution A.

Reference solution (a). Dilute 1.0 ml of the test solution to 100.0 ml with solution A. Dilute 1.0 ml of this solution to 10.0 ml with solution A.

Reference solution (b). Dissolve 4 mg of *norfloxacin for system suitability CRS* (containing impurities A, E and H) in 5 ml of solution A. Sonicate for 5 min and dilute to 10 ml with solution A.

Column:

- *size*: *l* = 0.25 m, Ø = 4.6 mm;
- *stationary phase*: *end-capped hexadecylamidylsilyl silica gel for chromatography R* (5 µm);
- *temperature*: 60 °C.

Mobile phase:

- *mobile phase A*: *water R* adjusted to pH 2.0 with *phosphoric acid R*;
- *mobile phase B*: *acetonitrile R*;

Time (min)	Mobile phase A (per cent *V/V*)	Mobile phase B (per cent *V/V*)
0 - 5	95	5
5 - 7	95 → 93	5 → 7
7 - 10	93 → 87	7 → 13
10 - 15	87 → 47	13 → 53
15 - 20	47 → 10	53 → 90

Flow rate: 1.4 ml/min.

Detection: spectrophotometer at 265 nm.

Injection: 20 µl.

Identification of impurities: use the chromatogram supplied with *norfloxacin for system suitability CRS* and the chromatogram obtained with reference solution (b) to identify the peaks due to impurities A, E and H.

Relative retention with reference to norfloxacin (retention time = about 11 min): impurity E = about 0.97; impurity A = about 1.5; impurity H = about 1.6.

System suitability: reference solution (b):

- *resolution*: minimum 3.0 between the peaks due to impurities A and H;
- *peak-to-valley ratio*: minimum 5, where H_p = height above the baseline of the peak due to impurity E and H_v = height above the baseline of the lowest point of the curve separating this peak from the peak due to norfloxacin.

Limits:

- *impurity E*: not more than the area of the principal peak in the chromatogram obtained with reference solution (a) (0.1 per cent);
- *unspecified impurities*: for each impurity, not more than the area of the principal peak in the chromatogram obtained with reference solution (a) (0.10 per cent);
- *total*: not more than 5 times the area of the principal peak in the chromatogram obtained with reference solution (a) (0.5 per cent);
- *disregard limit*: 0.5 times the area of the principal peak in the chromatogram obtained with reference solution (a) (0.05 per cent).

Heavy metals (*2.4.8*): maximum 15 ppm.

2.0 g complies with test D. Prepare the reference solution using 3 ml of *lead standard solution (10 ppm Pb) R.*

Loss on drying (*2.2.32*): maximum 1.0 per cent, determined on 1.000 g by drying under high vacuum at 105 °C for 2 h.

Sulphated ash (*2.4.14*): maximum 0.1 per cent, determined on 1.0 g in a platinum crucible.

ASSAY

Dissolve 0.240 g in 80 ml of *anhydrous acetic acid R*. Titrate with *0.1 M perchloric acid,* determining the end-point potentiometrically (*2.2.20*).

1 ml of *0.1 M perchloric acid* is equivalent to 31.93 mg of $C_{16}H_{18}FN_3O_3$.

STORAGE

In an airtight container, protected from light.

IMPURITIES

Specified impurities: E.

Other detectable impurities (the following substances would, if present at a sufficient level, be detected by one or other of the tests in the monograph. They are limited by the general acceptance criterion for other/unspecified impurities and/or by the general monograph *Substances for pharmaceutical use (2034)*. It is therefore not necessary to identify these impurities for demonstration of compliance. See also *5.10. Control of impurities in substances for pharmaceutical use*): *A, B, C, D, F, G, H, I, J.*

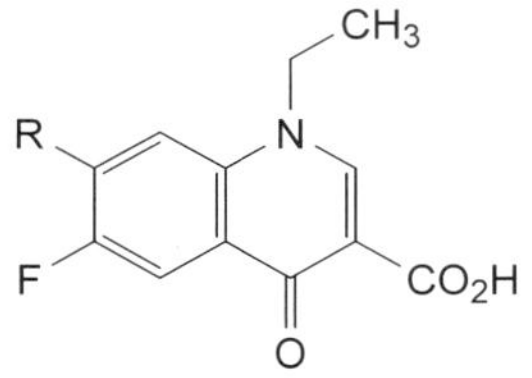

A. R = Cl: 7-chloro-1-ethyl-6-fluoro-4-oxo-1,4-dihydroquinoline-3-carboxylic acid,

B. R = $NH-CH_2-CH_2-NH_2$: 7-[(2-aminoethyl)amino]-1-ethyl-6-fluoro-4-oxo-1,4-dihydroquinoline-3-carboxylic acid,

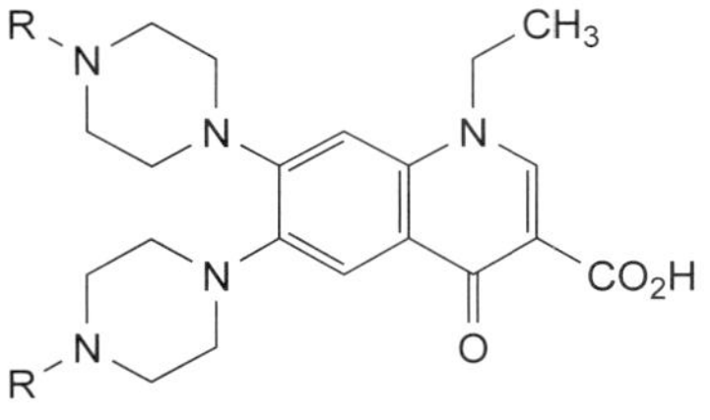

C. R = H: 1-ethyl-4-oxo-6,7-bis(piperazin-1-yl)-1,4-dihydroquinoline-3-carboxylic acid,

J. R = $CO-O-C_2H_5$: 6,7-bis[4-(ethoxycarbonyl)piperazin-1-yl]-1-ethyl-4-oxo-1,4-dihydroquinoline-3-carboxylic acid,

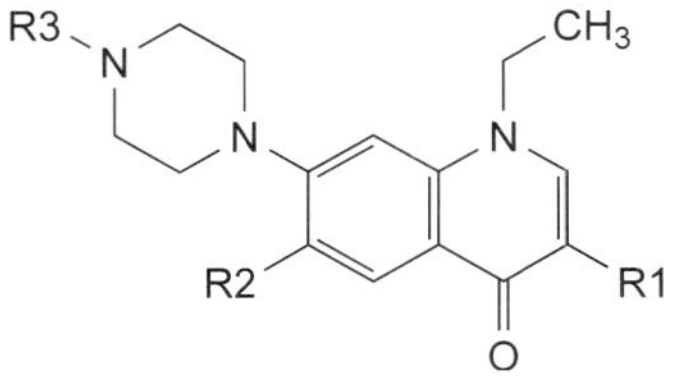

D. R1 = R3 = H, R2 = F: 1-ethyl-6-fluoro-7-(piperazin-1-yl)quinolin-4(1*H*)-one,

F. R1 = CO_2H, R2 = Cl, R3 = H: 6-chloro-1-ethyl-4-oxo-7-(piperazin-1-yl)-1,4-dihydroquinoline-3-carboxylic acid,

G. R1 = CO_2H, R2 = F, R3 = CHO: 1-ethyl-6-fluoro-7-(4-formylpiperazin-1-yl)-4-oxo-1,4-dihydroquinoline-3-carboxylic acid,

H. R1 = CO_2H, R2 = F, R3 = $CO-O-C_2H_5$: 7-[4-(ethoxycarbonyl)piperazin-1-yl]-1-ethyl-6-fluoro-4-oxo-1,4-dihydroquinoline-3-carboxylic acid,

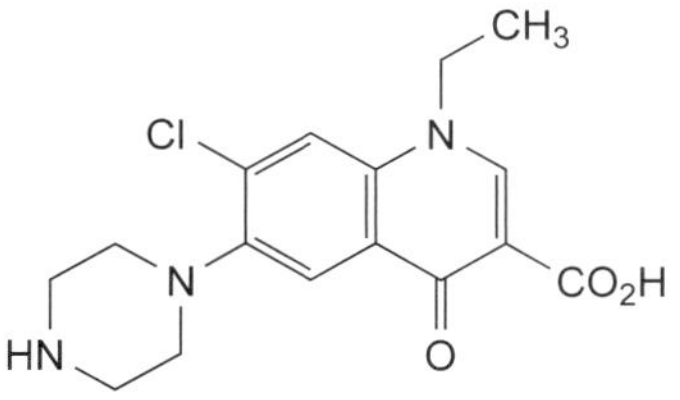

E. 7-chloro-1-ethyl-4-oxo-6-(piperazin-1-yl)-1,4-dihydroquinoline-3-carboxylic acid,

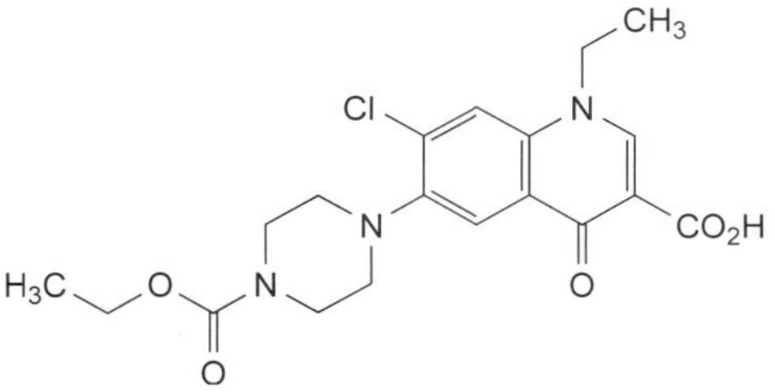

I. 7-chloro-6-[4-(ethoxycarbonyl)piperazin-1-yl]-1-ethyl-4-oxo-1,4-dihydroquinoline-3-carboxylic acid.

01/2008:1552

NUTMEG OIL

Myristicae fragrantis aetheroleum

DEFINITION

Essential oil obtained by steam distillation of the dried and crushed kernels of *Myristica fragrans* Houtt.

CHARACTERS

Appearance: colourless or pale yellow liquid.

Spicy odour.

IDENTIFICATION

First identification: B.

Second identification: A.

A. Thin-layer chromatography (*2.2.27*).

Test solution. Dissolve 1 ml of the substance to be examined in *toluene R* and dilute to 10 ml with the same solvent.

Reference solution. Dissolve 20 µl of *myristicine R* in 10 ml of *toluene R*.

Plate: *TLC silica gel plate R.*

Mobile phase: *ethyl acetate R, toluene R* (5:95 *V/V*).

Application: 10 µl as bands.

Development: over a path of 15 cm.

Drying: in air.

Detection: spray with *vanillin reagent R,* heat at 100-105 °C for 10 min and examine in daylight.

Results: the chromatogram obtained with the reference solution shows in the upper third a pink or reddish-brown zone (myristicine); the chromatogram obtained with the test solution shows a series of zones of which 1 is similar in position and colour to the zone in the chromatogram obtained with the reference solution; above this zone a brownish zone (safrole) and a violet zone (hydrocarbons) are present; below the myristicine zone, 5 blue zones of variable intensity are present.

B. Examine the chromatograms obtained in the test for chromatographic profile.
Results: the principal peaks in the chromatogram obtained with the test solution are similar in retention time to those in the chromatogram obtained with the reference solution.

TESTS

Relative density (*2.2.5*): 0.885 to 0.905.

Refractive index (*2.2.6*): 1.475 to 1.485.

Optical rotation (*2.2.7*): + 8° to + 18°.

Chromatographic profile. Gas chromatography (*2.2.28*): use the normalisation procedure.

Test solution. The substance to be examined.

Reference solution. Dissolve 15 µl of *α-pinene R,* 15 µl of *β-pinene R,* 15 µl of *sabinene R,* 5 µl of *car-3-ene R,* 5 µl of *limonene R,* 5 µl of *γ-terpinene R,* 5 µl of *terpinen-4-ol R,* 5 µl of *safrole R* and 10 µl of *myristicine R* in 1 ml of *hexane R.*

Column:
- *material*: fused silica;
- *size*: *l* = 25-60 m, Ø = about 0.3 mm;
- *stationary phase*: bonded *macrogol 20 000 R.*

Carrier gas: *helium for chromatography R.*

Flow rate: 1.5 ml/min.

Split ratio: 1:100.

Temperature:

	Time (min)	Temperature (°C)
Column	0 - 10	50
	10 - 75	50 → 180
	75 - 130	180
Injection port		200 - 220
Detector		240 - 250

Detection: flame ionisation.

Injection: 0.2 µl.

Elution order: order indicated in the composition of the reference solution; record the retention times of these substances.

System suitability: reference solution:
- *resolution*: minimum 1.5 between the peaks due to β-pinene and sabinene.

Identification of components: using the retention times determined from the chromatogram obtained with the reference solution, locate the components of the reference solution in the chromatogram obtained with the test solution.

Determine the percentage content of each of these components. The percentages are within the following ranges:
- *α-pinene*: 15 per cent to 28 per cent;
- *β-pinene*: 13 per cent to 18 per cent;
- *sabinene*: 14 per cent to 29 per cent;
- *car-3-ene*: 0.5 per cent to 2.0 per cent;
- *limonene*: 2.0 per cent to 7.0 per cent;
- *γ-terpinene*: 2.0 per cent to 6.0 per cent;
- *terpinen-4-ol*: 2.0 per cent to 6.0 per cent;
- *safrole*: less than 2.5 per cent;
- *myristicine*: 5.0 per cent to 12.0 per cent.

STORAGE

Protected from heat.

Monographs L-P

O

07/2008:1455

OFLOXACIN

Ofloxacinum

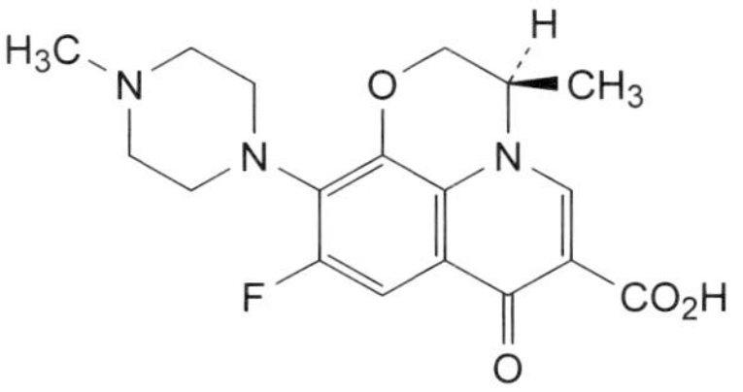

and enantiomer

$C_{18}H_{20}FN_3O_4$ M_r 361.4

[82419-36-1]

DEFINITION

(*RS*)-9-Fluoro-3-methyl-10-(4-methylpiperazin-1-yl)-7-oxo-2,3-dihydro-7*H*-pyrido[1,2,3-*de*]-1,4-benzoxazine-6-carboxylic acid.

Content: 99.0 per cent to 101.0 per cent (dried substance).

CHARACTERS

Appearance: pale yellow or bright yellow, crystalline powder.

Solubility: slightly soluble in water, soluble in glacial acetic acid, slightly soluble or soluble in methylene chloride, slightly soluble in methanol.

IDENTIFICATION

Infrared absorption spectrophotometry (*2.2.24*).

Comparison: *ofloxacin CRS.*

TESTS

Optical rotation (*2.2.7*): – 0.10° to + 0.10°.

Dissolve 0.300 g in a mixture of 10 volumes of *methanol R* and 40 volumes of *methylene chloride R* and dilute to 10 ml with the same mixture of solvents.

Absorbance (*2.2.25*): maximum 0.25 at 440 nm.

Dissolve 0.5 g in *0.1 M hydrochloric acid* and dilute to 100 ml with the same solvent.

Impurity A. Thin-layer chromatography (*2.2.27*).

Solvent mixture: *methanol R, methylene chloride R* (10:40 *V/V*).

Test solution. Dissolve 0.250 g of the substance to be examined in the solvent mixture and dilute to 5.0 ml with the solvent mixture.

Reference solution. Dissolve 10.0 mg of *ofloxacin impurity A CRS* in the solvent mixture and dilute to 100.0 ml with the solvent mixture.

Plate: *TLC silica gel GF_{254} plate R* (2-10 µm).

Mobile phase: *glacial acetic acid R, water R, ethyl acetate R* (10:10:20 *V/V/V*).

Application: 10 µl.

Development: over 2/3 of the plate.

Drying: in air.

Detection: examine in ultraviolet light at 254 nm.

Limit:

– *impurity A*: any spot due to impurity A is not more intense than the corresponding spot in the chromatogram obtained with the reference solution (0.2 per cent).

Related substances. Liquid chromatography (*2.2.29*). *Prepare the solutions immediately before use.*

Solvent mixture: *acetonitrile R, water R* (10:60 *V/V*).

Test solution. Dissolve 10.0 mg of the substance to be examined in the solvent mixture and dilute to 50.0 ml with the solvent mixture.

Reference solution (a). Dilute 1.0 ml of the test solution to 50.0 ml with the solvent mixture. Dilute 1.0 ml of this solution to 10.0 ml with the solvent mixture.

Reference solution (b). Dissolve 10 mg of *ofloxacin impurity E CRS* in the solvent mixture and dilute to 100 ml with the solvent mixture. Mix 10 ml of the solution with 5 ml of the test solution and dilute to 50 ml with the solvent mixture. Dilute 1 ml of this solution to 50 ml with the solvent mixture.

Column:

– *size*: *l* = 0.15 m, Ø = 4.6 mm;

– *stationary phase*: *octadecylsilyl silica gel for chromatography R* (5 µm);

– *temperature*: 45 °C.

Mobile phase: dissolve 4.0 g of *ammonium acetate R* and 7.0 g of *sodium perchlorate R* in 1300 ml of *water R*; adjust to pH 2.2 with *phosphoric acid R* and add 240 ml of *acetonitrile R.*

Flow rate: adjust so that a retention time of about 20 min is obtained for ofloxacin.

Detection: spectrophotometer at 294 nm.

Injection: 10 µl.

Run time: 2.5 times the retention time of ofloxacin.

Relative retention with reference to ofloxacin (retention time = about 20 min): impurity B = about 0.3; impurity C = about 0.5; impurity D = about 0.7; impurity E = about 0.9; impurity F = about 1.6.

System suitability: reference solution (b):

– *resolution*: minimum 2.0 between the peaks due to impurity E and ofloxacin.

Limits:

– *impurities B, C, D, E, F*: for each impurity, not more than the area of the principal peak in the chromatogram obtained with reference solution (a) (0.2 per cent);

– *total*: not more than 2.5 times the area of the principal peak in the chromatogram obtained with reference solution (a) (0.5 per cent);

– *disregard limit*: 0.1 times the area of the principal peak in the chromatogram obtained with reference solution (a) (0.02 per cent).

Heavy metals (*2.4.8*): maximum 10 ppm.

2.0 g complies with test C. Prepare the reference solution using 2 ml of *lead standard solution (10 ppm Pb) R.*

Loss on drying (*2.2.32*): maximum 0.2 per cent, determined on 1.000 g by drying at 105 °C for 4 h.

Sulphated ash (*2.4.14*): maximum 0.1 per cent, determined on 1.0 g.

ASSAY

Dissolve 0.300 g in 100 ml of *anhydrous acetic acid R.* Titrate with *0.1 M perchloric acid* determining the end-point potentiometrically (*2.2.20*).

1 ml of *0.1 M perchloric acid* is equivalent to 36.14 mg of $C_{18}H_{20}FN_3O_4$.

STORAGE

In an airtight container, protected from light.

IMPURITIES

Specified impurities: A, B, C, D, E, F.

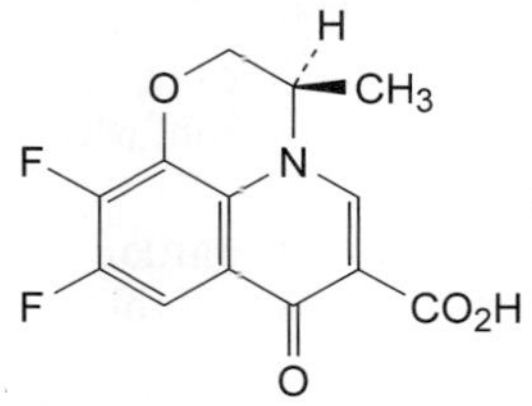

and enantiomer

A. (*RS*)-9,10-difluoro-3-methyl-7-oxo-2,3-dihydro-7*H*-pyrido-[1,2,3-*de*]-1,4-benzoxazine-6-carboxylic acid (FPA),

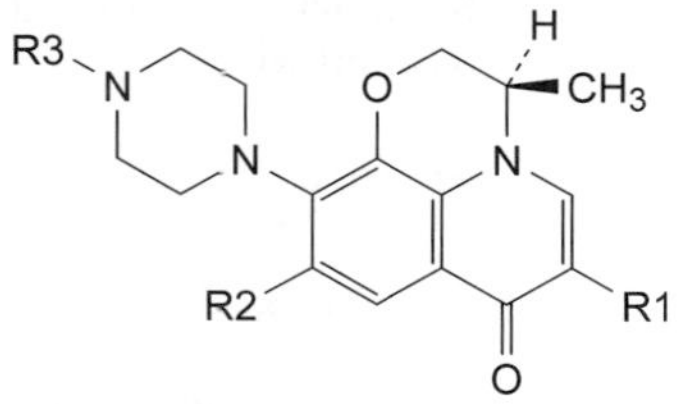

and enantiomer

B. R1 = H, R2 = F, R3 = CH_3: (*RS*)-9-fluoro-3-methyl-10-(4-methylpiperazin-1-yl)-2,3-dihydro-7*H*-pyrido[1,2,3-*de*]-1,4-benzoxazin-7-one,

C. R1 = CO_2H, R2 = H, R3 = CH_3: (*RS*)-3-methyl-10-(4-methylpiperazin-1-yl)-7-oxo-2,3-dihydro-7*H*-pyrido-[1,2,3-*de*]-1,4-benzoxazine-6-carboxylic acid,

E. R1 = CO_2H, R2 = F, R3 = H: (*RS*)-9-fluoro-3-methyl-7-oxo-10-(piperazin-1-yl)-2,3-dihydro-7*H*-pyrido[1,2,3-*de*]-1,4-benzoxazine-6-carboxylic acid,

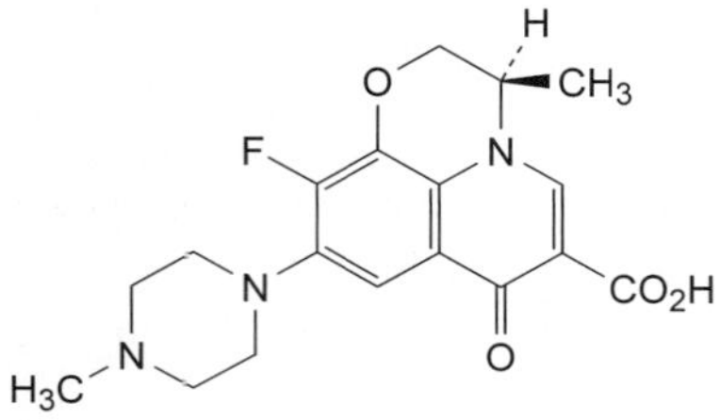

and enantiomer

D. (*RS*)-10-fluoro-3-methyl-9-(4-methylpiperazin-1-yl)-7-oxo-2,3-dihydro-7*H*-pyrido[1,2,3-*de*]-1,4-benzoxazine-6-carboxylic acid,

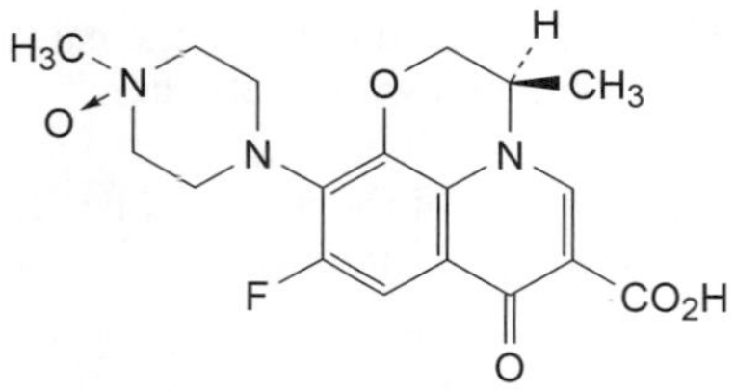

and enantiomer

F. 4-[(*RS*)-6-carboxy-9-fluoro-3-methyl-7-oxo-2,3-dihydro-7*H*-pyrido[1,2,3-*de*]-1,4-benzoxazine-10-yl]-1-methylpiperazine 1-oxide.

01/2008:1456
corrected 6.2

OLIVE OIL, REFINED

Olivae oleum raffinatum

DEFINITION

Fatty oil obtained by refining of crude olive oil, obtained by cold expression or other suitable mechanical means from the ripe drupes of *Olea europaea* L. A suitable antioxidant may be added.

CHARACTERS

Appearance: clear, colourless or greenish-yellow transparent liquid.

Solubility: practically insoluble in ethanol (96 per cent), miscible with light petroleum (50-70 °C).

When cooled, it begins to become cloudy at 10 °C and becomes a butter-like mass at about 0 °C.

Relative density: about 0.913.

IDENTIFICATION

A. Acid value (see Tests).

B. Identification of fatty oils by thin-layer chromatography (*2.3.2*).

Results: the chromatogram obtained shows spots corresponding to those in the typical chromatogram for olive oil (see Figure 2.3.2.-1). For certain types of olive oil, the difference in the size of spots E and F is less pronounced than in the typical chromatogram.

TESTS

Acid value (*2.5.1*): maximum 0.3, determined on 10.0 g.

Peroxide value (*2.5.5, Method A*): maximum 10.0. If intended for use in the manufacture of parenteral preparations: maximum 5.0.

Unsaponifiable matter: maximum 1.5 per cent.

Place 5.0 g (*m* g) in a 150 ml flask fitted with a reflux condenser. Add 50 ml of *2 M alcoholic potassium hydroxide R* and heat on a water-bath for 1 h, shaking frequently. Add 50 ml of *water R* through the top of the condenser, shake, allow to cool and transfer the contents of the flask to a separating funnel. Rinse the flask with several portions totalling 50 ml of *light petroleum R1* and add the rinsings to the separating funnel. Shake vigorously for 1 min. Allow to separate and transfer the aqueous layer to a 2nd separating funnel. If an emulsion forms, add small quantities of *ethanol (96 per cent) R* or a concentrated solution of *potassium hydroxide R*. Shake the aqueous layer with 2 quantities, each of 50 ml, of *light petroleum R1*. Combine the light petroleum layers in a 3rd separating funnel and wash with 3 quantities, each of 50 ml, of *ethanol (50 per cent V/V) R*. Transfer the light petroleum layer to a tared 250 ml flask. Rinse the separating funnel with small quantities of *light petroleum R1* and add to the flask. Evaporate the light petroleum on a water-bath and dry the residue at 100-105 °C for 15 min, keeping the flask horizontal. Allow to cool in a desiccator and weigh (*a* g). Repeat the drying for successive periods of 15 min until the loss of mass between 2 successive weighings does not exceed 0.1 per cent. Dissolve the residue in 20 ml of *ethanol (96 per cent) R*, previously neutralised to 0.1 ml of *bromophenol blue solution R*. If necessary, titrate with *0.1 M hydrochloric acid* (*b* ml).

Calculate the percentage content of unsaponifiable matter using the following expression:

$$\frac{100\,(a - 0.032b)}{m}$$

If 0.032*b* is greater than 5 per cent of *a*, the test is not valid and must be repeated.

Alkaline impurities (*2.4.19*). It complies with the test.

Specific absorbance (*2.2.25*): maximum 1.20, determined at 270 nm.

Dissolve 1.00 g in *cyclohexane R* and dilute to 100.0 ml with the same solvent.

Composition of fatty acids (*2.4.22, Method A*). Use the mixture of calibrating substances in Table 2.4.22.-3.

Composition of the fatty-acid fraction of the oil:

- *saturated fatty acids of chain length less than* C_{16}: maximum 0.1 per cent;
- *palmitic acid*: 7.5 per cent to 20.0 per cent;
- *palmitoleic acid* : maximum 3.5 per cent;
- *stearic acid*: 0.5 per cent to 5.0 per cent;
- *oleic acid* : 56.0 per cent to 85.0 per cent;
- *linoleic acid* : 3.5 per cent to 20.0 per cent;
- *linolenic acid* : maximum 1.2 per cent;
- *arachidic acid*: maximum 0.7 per cent;
- *eicosenoic acid* : maximum 0.4 per cent;
- *behenic acid*: maximum 0.2 per cent;
- *lignoceric acid*: maximum 0.2 per cent.

Sterols (*2.4.23*).

Composition of the sterol fraction of the oil:

- *cholesterol*: maximum 0.5 per cent;
- *campesterol*: maximum 4.0 per cent;
- *Δ7-stigmasterol*: maximum 0.5 per cent;
- *sum of contents of Δ5,23-stigmastadienol, clerosterol, β-sitosterol, sitostanol, Δ5-avenasterol and Δ5,24-stigmastadienol*: minimum 93.0 per cent.

The content of stigmasterol is not greater than that of campesterol.

Sesame oil. In a ground-glass-stoppered cylinder shake 10 ml for about 1 min with a mixture of 0.5 ml of a 0.35 per cent *V/V* solution of *furfural R* in *acetic anhydride R* and 4.5 ml of *acetic anhydride R*. Filter through a filter paper impregnated with *acetic anhydride R*. To the filtrate add 0.2 ml of *sulphuric acid R*. No bluish-green colour develops.

Water (*2.5.32*): maximum 0.1 per cent, determined on 5.0 g, if intended for use in the manufacture of parenteral preparations. Use a mixture of equal volumes of *anhydrous methanol R* and *decanol R* as solvent.

STORAGE

In a well-filled container, protected from light, at a temperature not exceeding 25 °C. If intended for use in the manufacture of parenteral preparations, store under an inert gas.

LABELLING

The label states:

- where applicable, that the substance is suitable for use in the manufacture of parenteral preparations;
- the name of the inert gas.

01/2008:0518
corrected 6.2

OLIVE OIL, VIRGIN

Olivae oleum virginale

DEFINITION

Fatty oil obtained by cold expression or other suitable mechanical means from the ripe drupes of *Olea europaea* L.

CHARACTERS

Appearance: clear, transparent, yellow or greenish-yellow liquid.

Solubility: practically insoluble in ethanol (96 per cent), miscible with light petroleum (50-70 °C).

It has a characteristic odour.

When cooled, it begins to become cloudy at 10 °C and becomes a butter-like mass at about 0 °C.

Relative density: about 0.913.

IDENTIFICATION

Identification of fatty oils by thin-layer chromatography (*2.3.2*).

Results: the chromatogram obtained shows spots corresponding to those in the typical chromatogram for olive oil (see Figure 2.3.2.-1). For certain types of olive oil, the difference in the size of spots E and F is less pronounced than in the typical chromatogram.

TESTS

Acid value (*2.5.1*): maximum 2.0, determined on 5.0 g.

Peroxide value (*2.5.5, Method A*): maximum 20.0.

Unsaponifiable matter: maximum 1.5 per cent.

Place 5.0 g (*m* g) in a 150 ml flask fitted with a reflux condenser. Add 50 ml of *2 M alcoholic potassium hydroxide R* and heat on a water-bath for 1 h, shaking frequently. Add 50 ml of *water R* through the top of the condenser, shake, allow to cool and transfer the contents of the flask to a separating funnel. Rinse the flask with several portions totalling 50 ml of *light petroleum R1* and add the rinsings to the separating funnel. Shake vigorously for 1 min. Allow to separate and transfer the aqueous layer to a 2nd separating funnel. If an emulsion forms, add small quantities of *ethanol (96 per cent) R* or a concentrated solution of *potassium hydroxide R*. Shake the aqueous layer with 2 quantities, each of 50 ml, of *light petroleum R1*. Combine the light petroleum layers in a 3rd separating funnel and wash with 3 quantities, each of 50 ml, of *ethanol (50 per cent V/V) R*. Transfer the light petroleum layer to a tared 250 ml flask. Rinse the separating funnel with small quantities of *light petroleum R1* and add to the flask. Evaporate the light petroleum on a water-bath and dry the residue at 100-105 °C for 15 min, keeping the flask horizontal. Allow to cool in a desiccator and weigh (*a* g). Repeat the drying for successive periods of 15 min until the loss of mass between 2 successive weighings does not exceed 0.1 per cent. Dissolve the residue in 20 ml of *ethanol (96 per cent) R*, previously neutralised to 0.1 ml of *bromophenol blue solution R*. If necessary, titrate with *0.1 M hydrochloric acid* (*b* ml).

Calculate the percentage content of unsaponifiable matter using the following expression:

$$\frac{100\,(a - 0.032b)}{m}$$

If 0.032*b* is greater than 5 per cent of *a*, the test is not valid and must be repeated.

Absorbance (*2.2.25*): maximum 0.20 at 270 nm. The ratio of the absorbance at 232 nm to that at 270 nm is greater than 8.

Dissolve 1.00 g in *cyclohexane R* and dilute to 100.0 ml with the same solvent.

Composition of fatty acids (*2.4.22, Method A*). Use the mixture of calibrating substances in Table 2.4.22.-3.

Composition of the fatty-acid fraction of the oil:

- *saturated fatty acids of chain length less than* C_{16}: maximum 0.1 per cent;
- *palmitic acid*: 7.5 per cent to 20.0 per cent;
- *palmitoleic acid* : maximum 3.5 per cent;
- *stearic acid*: 0.5 per cent to 5.0 per cent;
- *oleic acid* : 56.0 per cent to 85.0 per cent;

- *linoleic acid* : 3.5 per cent to 20.0 per cent;
- *linolenic acid* : maximum 1.2 per cent;
- *arachidic acid*: maximum 0.7 per cent;
- *eicosenoic acid* : maximum 0.4 per cent;
- *behenic acid*: maximum 0.2 per cent;
- *lignoceric acid*: maximum 0.2 per cent.

Sterols (*2.4.23*).

Composition of the sterol fraction of the oil:
- *cholesterol*: maximum 0.5 per cent;
- *campesterol*: maximum 4.0 per cent;
- *Δ7-stigmasterol*: maximum 0.5 per cent;
- *sum of contents of Δ5,23-stigmastadienol, clerosterol, β-sitosterol, sitostanol, Δ5-avenasterol and Δ5,24-stigmastadienol*: minimum 93.0 per cent.

The content of stigmasterol is not greater than that of campesterol.

Sesame oil. In a ground-glass-stoppered cylinder shake 10 ml for about 1 min with a mixture of 0.5 ml of a 0.35 per cent *V/V* solution of *furfural R* in *acetic anhydride R* and 4.5 ml of *acetic anhydride R*. Filter through a filter paper impregnated with *acetic anhydride R*. To the filtrate add 0.2 ml of *sulphuric acid R*. No bluish-green colour develops.

STORAGE

In a well-filled container, protected from light, at a temperature not exceeding 25 °C.

07/2008:1033

ORCIPRENALINE SULPHATE

Orciprenalini sulfas

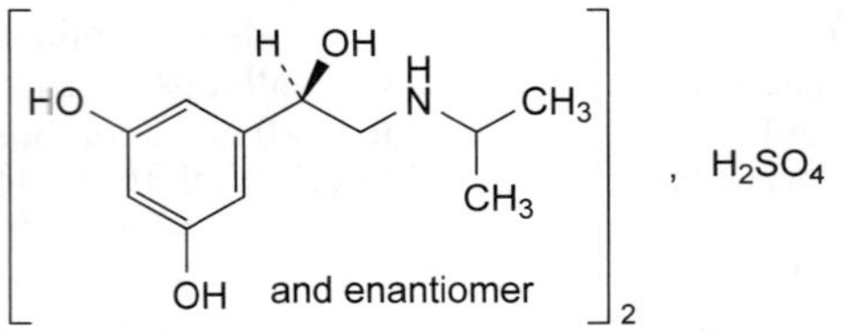

$C_{22}H_{36}N_2O_{10}S$ M_r 520.6

[5874-97-5]

DEFINITION

Bis[5-[(1*RS*)-1-hydroxy-2-[(1-methylethyl)amino]ethyl]-benzene-1,3-diol] sulphate.

Content: 98.0 per cent to 102.0 per cent (anhydrous substance).

CHARACTERS

Appearance: white or almost white, slightly hygroscopic, crystalline powder.

Solubility: freely soluble in water, slightly soluble in ethanol (96 per cent), practically insoluble in methylene chloride.

IDENTIFICATION

First identification: *B, E.*

Second identification: *A, C, D, E.*

A. Ultraviolet and visible absorption spectrophotometry (*2.2.25*).

Test solution. Dissolve 50.0 mg in a 0.04 per cent *V/V* solution of *hydrochloric acid R* and dilute to 50.0 ml with the same solution. Dilute 5.0 ml of this solution to 50.0 ml with a 0.04 per cent *V/V* solution of *hydrochloric acid R*.

Spectral range: 240-350 nm.

Absorption maximum: at 278 nm.

Specific absorbance at the absorption maximum: 68.5 to 76.0 (anhydrous substance).

B. Infrared absorption spectrophotometry (*2.2.24*).

Comparison: *orciprenaline sulphate CRS.*

If the spectra obtained show differences, dissolve separately, with heating, 50 mg of the substance to be examined and 50 mg of the reference substance, in the minimum volume of *water R*. Add 10 ml of *acetone R* and centrifuge. Dry the precipitates at 40 °C under reduced pressure for 3 h and record new spectra using the residues.

C. Thin-layer chromatography (*2.2.27*).

Test solution. Dissolve 10 mg of the substance to be examined in *ethanol (96 per cent) R* and dilute to 10 ml with the same solvent.

Reference solution (a). Dissolve 10 mg of *orciprenaline sulphate CRS* in *ethanol (96 per cent) R* and dilute to 10 ml with the same solvent.

Reference solution (b). Dissolve 10 mg of *orciprenaline sulphate CRS* and 10 mg of *salbutamol CRS* in *ethanol (96 per cent) R* and dilute to 10 ml with the same solvent.

Plate: *TLC silica gel G plate R.*

Mobile phase: *ammonia R, water R, aldehyde-free methanol R* (1.5:10:90 *V/V/V*).

Application: 2 μl.

Development: over 2/3 of the plate.

Drying: in air.

Detection: spray with a 10 g/l solution of *potassium permanganate R.*

System suitability: reference solution (b):
- the chromatogram shows 2 clearly separated principal spots.

Results: the principal spot in the chromatogram obtained with the test solution is similar in position, colour and size to the principal spot in the chromatogram obtained with reference solution (a).

D. Dissolve about 20 mg in 2 ml of *ethanol (96 per cent) R*. Add 2 ml of a 1 g/l solution of *dichloroquinonechlorimide R* in *ethanol (96 per cent) R* and 1 ml of *sodium carbonate solution R*. A violet colour is produced, turning to brown.

E. It gives reaction (a) of sulphates (*2.3.1*).

TESTS

Solution S. Dissolve 2.0 g in *carbon dioxide-free water R* and dilute to 20 ml with the same solvent.

Appearance of solution. Solution S is clear (*2.2.1*) and colourless (*2.2.2, Method II*).

pH (*2.2.3*): 4.0 to 5.5 for solution S.

Related substances. Liquid chromatography (*2.2.29*).

Test solution. Dissolve 20 mg of the substance to be examined in the mobile phase and dilute to 20 ml with the mobile phase.

Monographs L-P

Reference solution (a). Dilute 1.0 ml of the test solution to 100.0 ml with the mobile phase. Dilute 1.0 ml of this solution to 10.0 ml with the mobile phase.

Reference solution (b). Dissolve 2 mg of *orciprenaline for system suitability CRS* (containing impurities A and B) in 2.0 ml of the mobile phase.

Column:

- *size*: *l* = 0.125 m, Ø = 4.0 mm;
- *stationary phase*: spherical *end-capped octadecylsilyl silica gel for chromatography R* (5 μm);
- *temperature*: 45 °C.

Mobile phase. Dissolve 9.1 g of *potassium dihydrogen phosphate R* and 4.6 g of *sodium octanesulphonate R* in *water R*, adjust to pH 4.0 with *dilute phosphoric acid R* and dilute to 1000 ml with *water R*. Add 140 ml of *acetonitrile R*.

Flow rate: 1.5 ml/min.

Detection: spectrophotometer at 280 nm.

Injection: 10 μl.

Run time: twice the retention time of orciprenaline.

Identification of impurities: use the chromatogram supplied with *orciprenaline for system suitability CRS* and the chromatogram obtained with reference solution (b) to identify the peaks due to impurities A and B.

Relative retention with reference to orciprenaline (retention time = about 7 min): impurity A = about 0.9; impurity B = about 1.3.

System suitability: reference solution (b):

- *resolution*: minimum 2.0 between the peaks due to impurity A and orciprenaline.

Limits:

- *correction factor*: for the calculation of content, multiply the peak area of impurity B by 0.3;
- *impurities A, B*: for each impurity, not more than the area of the principal peak in the chromatogram obtained with reference solution (a) (0.1 per cent);
- *unspecified impurities*: for each impurity, not more than the area of the principal peak in the chromatogram obtained with reference solution (a) (0.10 per cent);
- *total*: not more than twice the area of the principal peak in the chromatogram obtained with reference solution (a) (0.2 per cent);
- *disregard limit*: 0.5 times the area of the principal peak in the chromatogram obtained with reference solution (a) (0.05 per cent).

Phenone: maximum 0.1 per cent.

Dissolve 0.50 g in a 0.04 per cent *V/V* solution of *hydrochloric acid R* and dilute to 25.0 ml with the same solution. The absorbance (*2.2.25*) of the solution measured at 328 nm is not greater than 0.16.

Iron (*2.4.9*): maximum 20 ppm.

The residue obtained in the test for sulphated ash complies with the test. Prepare the reference solution using *iron standard solution (2 ppm Fe) R*.

Heavy metals: maximum 20 ppm.

1.0 g complies with test C. Prepare the reference solution using 2 ml of *lead standard solution (10 ppm Pb) R*.

Water (*2.5.12*): maximum 2.0 per cent, determined on 1.000 g.

Sulphated ash (*2.4.14*): maximum 0.1 per cent, determined on 1.0 g.

ASSAY

Dissolve 0.400 g in 5 ml of *anhydrous formic acid R* and add 30 ml of *anhydrous acetic acid R*. Titrate with *0.1 M perchloric acid* using 0.1 ml of *crystal violet solution R* as indicator.

1 ml of *0.1 M perchloric acid* is equivalent to 52.06 mg of $C_{22}H_{36}N_2O_{10}S$.

STORAGE

In an airtight container, protected from light.

IMPURITIES

Specified impurities: A, B.

Other detectable impurities (the following substances would, if present at a sufficient level, be detected by one or other of the tests in the monograph. They are limited by the general acceptance criterion for other/unspecified impurities and/or by the general monograph *Substances for pharmaceutical use (2034)*. It is therefore not necessary to identify these impurities for demonstration of compliance. See also *5.10. Control of impurities in substances for pharmaceutical use*): *C*.

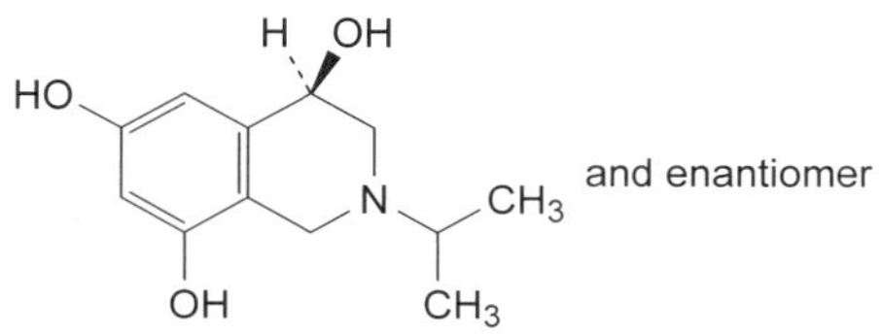

A. (4*RS*)-2-(1-methylethyl)-1,2,3,4-tetrahydroisoquinoline-4,6,8-triol,

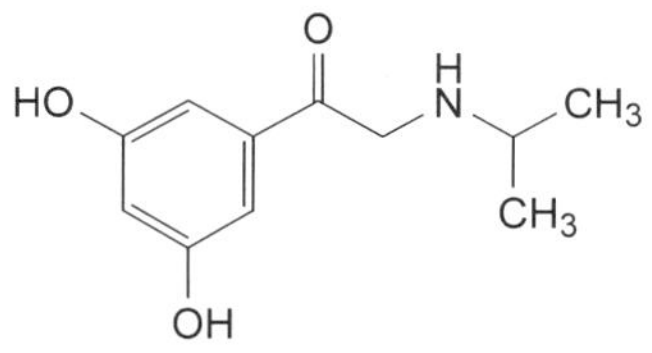

B. 1-(3,5-dihydroxyphenyl)-2-[(1-methylethyl)amino]ethanone,

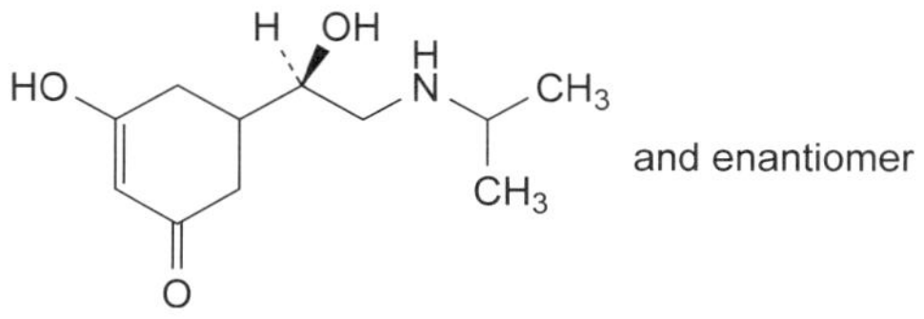

C. 3-hydroxy-5-[(1*RS*)-1-hydroxy-2-[(1-methylethyl)amino]-ethyl]cyclohex-2-enone.

Monographs L-P

07/2008:2260

OXACILLIN SODIUM MONOHYDRATE

Oxacillinum natricum monohydricum

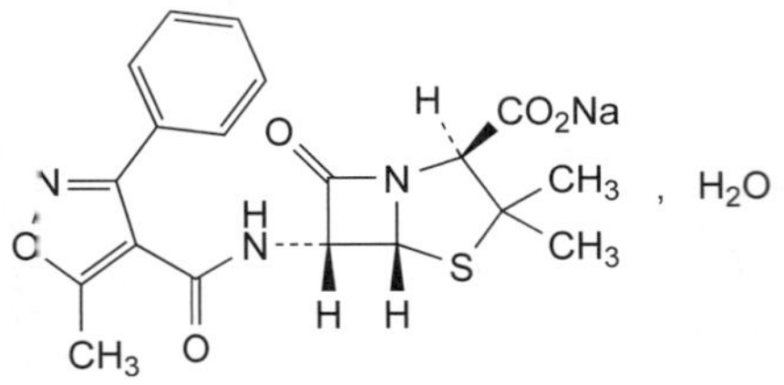

$C_{19}H_{18}N_3NaO_5S,H_2O$ M_r 441.4
[7240-38-2]

DEFINITION

Sodium (2*S*,5*R*,6*R*)-3,3-dimethyl-6-[[(5-methyl-3-phenylisoxazol-4-yl)carbonyl]amino]-7-oxo-4-thia-1-azabicyclo[3.2.0]heptane-2-carboxylate monohydrate.

Semi-synthetic product derived from a fermentation product.

Content: 95.0 per cent to 102.0 per cent (anhydrous substance).

CHARACTERS

Appearance: white or almost white powder.

Solubility: freely soluble in water, soluble in methanol, practically insoluble in methylene chloride.

IDENTIFICATION

A. Infrared absorption spectrophotometry (*2.2.24*).

Comparison: *oxacillin sodium monohydrate CRS*.

B. It gives reaction (a) of sodium (*2.3.1*).

TESTS

Appearance of solution. The solution is clear (*2.2.1*) and its absorbance (*2.2.25*) at 430 nm is not greater than 0.10.

Dissolve 2.50 g in *water R* and dilute to 25.0 ml with the same solvent.

pH (*2.2.3*): 4.5 to 7.5.

Dissolve 0.30 g in *carbon dioxide-free water R* and dilute to 10 ml with the same solvent.

Specific optical rotation (*2.2.7*): + 196 to + 212 (anhydrous substance).

Dissolve 0.250 g in *water R* and dilute to 25.0 ml with the same solvent.

Related substances. Liquid chromatography (*2.2.29*).

Test solution (a). Dissolve 50.0 mg of the substance to be examined in the mobile phase and dilute to 50.0 ml with the mobile phase.

Test solution (b). Dilute 5.0 ml of test solution (a) to 50.0 ml with the mobile phase.

Reference solution (a). Dissolve 50.0 mg of *oxacillin sodium monohydrate CRS* in the mobile phase and dilute to 50.0 ml with the mobile phase. Dilute 5.0 ml of this solution to 50.0 ml with the mobile phase.

Reference solution (b). Dilute 5.0 ml of test solution (b) to 50.0 ml with the mobile phase.

Reference solution (c). Dissolve 5 mg of *cloxacillin sodium CRS* (impurity E) and 5 mg of *oxacillin sodium monohydrate CRS* in the mobile phase and dilute to 50.0 ml with the mobile phase.

Reference solution (d). In order to prepare impurities B and D *in situ*, dissolve 25 mg of the substance to be examined in 1 ml of *0.05 M sodium hydroxide*, allow to stand for 3 min, then dilute to 100 ml with the mobile phase. Inject immediately.

Reference solution (e). Dissolve 5 mg of *oxacillin for peak identification CRS* (containing impurities E, F, G, I and J) in 5 ml of the mobile phase.

Column:

- *size*: l = 0.25 m, Ø = 4.0 mm;
- *stationary phase*: *octadecylsilyl silica gel for chromatography R* (5 µm).

Mobile phase: mix 25 volumes of *acetonitrile R* and 75 volumes of a 2.7 g/l solution of *potassium dihydrogen phosphate R* previously adjusted to pH 5.0 with *dilute sodium hydroxide solution R*.

Flow rate: 1.0 ml/min.

Detection: spectrophotometer at 225 nm.

Injection: 20 µl of test solution (a) and reference solutions (b), (c), (d) and (e).

Run time: 7 times the retention time of oxacillin.

Identification of impurities:

- in the chromatogram obtained with reference solution (d), the 2 principal peaks eluting before the main peak are due to impurities B and D respectively;
- use the chromatogram supplied with *oxacillin for peak identification CRS* and the chromatogram obtained with reference solution (e) to identify the peaks due to impurities E, F, G, I and J.

Relative retention with reference to oxacillin (retention time = about 5 min): impurity A = about 0.3; impurity B (isomer 1) = about 0.4; impurity B (isomer 2) = about 0.5; impurity C = about 0.65; impurity D (2 isomers) = about 0.9; impurity E = about 1.5; impurity F = about 1.9; impurity G = about 2.1; impurity H = about 3.5; impurity I = about 3.8; impurity J = about 5.8.

System suitability:

- *resolution*: minimum 2.5 between the peaks due to oxacillin and impurity E in the chromatogram obtained with reference solution (c);
- the chromatogram obtained with reference solution (e) is similar to the chromatogram supplied with *oxacillin for peak identification CRS*.

Limits:

- *impurity B*: for the sum of the areas of the 2 isomer peaks, not more than 1.5 times the area of the principal peak in the chromatogram obtained with reference solution (b) (1.5 per cent);
- *impurity E*: not more than the area of the principal peak in the chromatogram obtained with reference solution (b) (1.0 per cent);
- *impurities D (sum of the 2 isomers), F, G, I, J*: for each impurity, not more than 0.5 times the area of the principal peak in the chromatogram obtained with reference solution (b) (0.5 per cent);
- *any other impurity*: for each impurity, not more than 0.5 times the area of the principal peak in the chromatogram obtained with reference solution (b) (0.5 per cent);
- *total*: not more than 3 times the area of the principal peak in the chromatogram obtained with reference solution (b) (3.0 per cent);

Monographs L-P

– *disregard limit*: 0.05 times the area of the principal peak in the chromatogram obtained with reference solution (b) (0.05 per cent).

Ethyl acetate and butyl acetate. Head-space gas chromatography (*2.2.28*).

Test solution. Dissolve 0.200 g of the substance to be examined in 6.0 ml of *water R*.

Reference solution. Dissolve 83 mg of *ethyl acetate R* and 83 mg of *butyl acetate R* in *water R* and dilute to 250.0 ml with the same solvent. Use 6.0 ml of this solution.

Close the vials immediately with a rubber membrane stopper coated with polytetrafluoroethylene and secured with an aluminium crimped cap. Mix to obtain a homogeneous solution.

Column:

– *material*: fused silica;
– *size*: *l* = 50 m, Ø = 0.32 mm;
– *stationary phase*: *poly(dimethyl)siloxane R* (film thickness 5 μm).

Carrier gas: *helium for chromatography R*.

Flow rate: 2 ml/min.

Static head-space conditions that may be used:

– *equilibration temperature*: 80 °C;
– *equilibration time*: 60 min;
– *transfer-line temperature*: 140 °C;
– *pressurisation time*: 30 s.

Temperature:

	Time (min)	Temperature (°C)
Column	0 - 6	70
	6 - 16	70 → 220
	16 - 18	220
Injection port		140
Detector		250

Detection: flame ionisation.

Retention time: ethyl acetate = about 10 min; butyl acetate = about 15.5 min.

Limits:

– *ethyl acetate*: maximum 1.0 per cent,
– *butyl acetate*: maximum 1.0 per cent.

***N,N*-Dimethylaniline** (*2.4.26, Method B*): maximum 20 ppm.

2-Ethylhexanoic acid (*2.4.28*): maximum 0.8 per cent.

Water (*2.5.12*): 3.5 per cent to 5.0 per cent, determined on 0.300 g.

Bacterial endotoxins (*2.6.14*): less than 0.20 IU/mg, if intended for use in the manufacture of parenteral preparations without a further appropriate procedure for the removal of bacterial endotoxins.

ASSAY

Liquid chromatography (*2.2.29*) as described in the test for related substances with the following modification.

Injection: test solution (b) and reference solution (a).

Calculate the percentage content of $C_{19}H_{18}N_3NaO_5S$ from the declared content of *oxacillin sodium monohydrate CRS*.

IMPURITIES

Specified impurities: *B, D, E, F, G, I, J*.

Other detectable impurities (the following substances would, if present at a sufficient level, be detected by one or other of the tests in the monograph. They are limited by the general acceptance criterion for other/unspecified impurities and/or by the general monograph *Substances for pharmaceutical use (2034)*. It is therefore not necessary to identify these impurities for demonstration of compliance. See also *5.10. Control of impurities in substances for pharmaceutical use*): *A, C, H*.

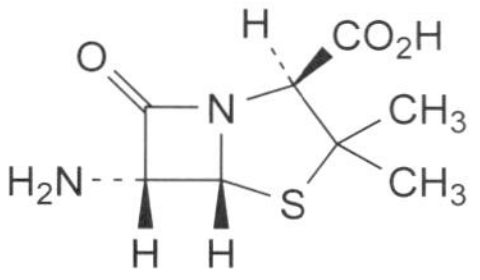

A. (2*S*,5*R*,6*R*)-6-amino-3,3-dimethyl-7-oxo-4-thia-1-azabicyclo[3.2.0]heptane-2-carboxylic acid (6-aminopenicillanic acid),

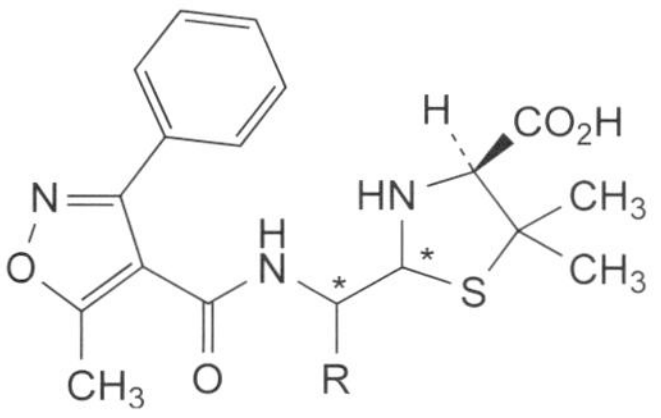

B. R = CO_2H: (4*S*)-2-[carboxy[[(5-methyl-3-phenylisoxazol-4-yl)carbonyl]amino]methyl]-5,5-dimethylthiazolidine-4-carboxylic acid (penicilloic acids of oxacillin),

D. R = H: (2*RS*,4*S*)-5,5-dimethyl-2-[[[(5-methyl-3-phenylisoxazol-4-yl)carbonyl]amino]methyl]thiazolidine-4-carboxylic acid (penilloic acids of oxacillin),

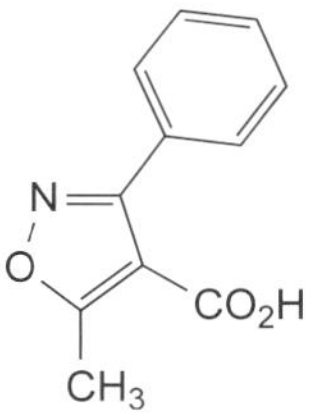

C. 5-methyl-3-phenylisoxazole-4-carboxylic acid,

E. cloxacillin,

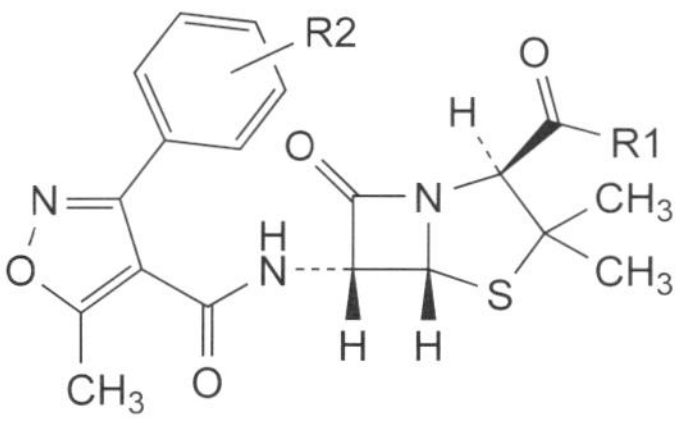

F. R1 = SH, R2 = H: (2*R*,5*R*,6*R*)-3,3-dimethyl-6-[[(5-methyl-3-phenylisoxazol-4-yl)carbonyl]amino]-7-oxo-4-thia-1-azabicyclo[3.2.0]heptane-2-carbothioic acid (thiooxacillin),

G. R1 = OH, R2 = Cl: (2*S*,5*R*,6*R*)-6-[[[3-(chlorophenyl)-5-methylisoxazol-4-yl]carbonyl]amino]-3,3-dimethyl-7-oxo-4-thia-1-azabicyclo[3.2.0]heptane-2-carboxylic acid (cloxacillin isomer),

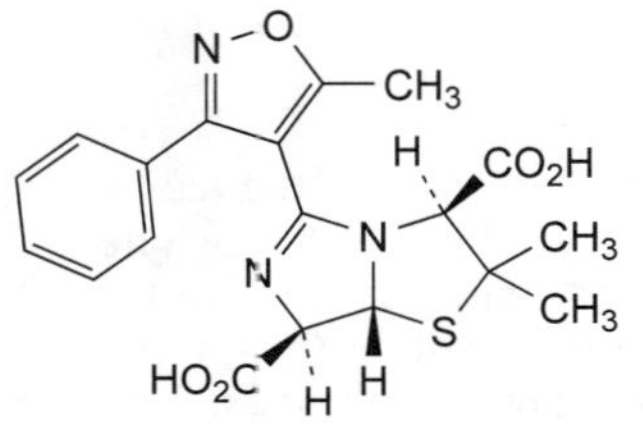

H. (3*S*,7*R*,7a*R*)-2,2-dimethyl-5-(5-methyl-3-phenylisoxazol-4-yl)-2,3,7,7a-tetrahydroimidazo[5,1-*b*]thiazole-3,7-dicarboxylic acid (penillic acid of oxacillin),

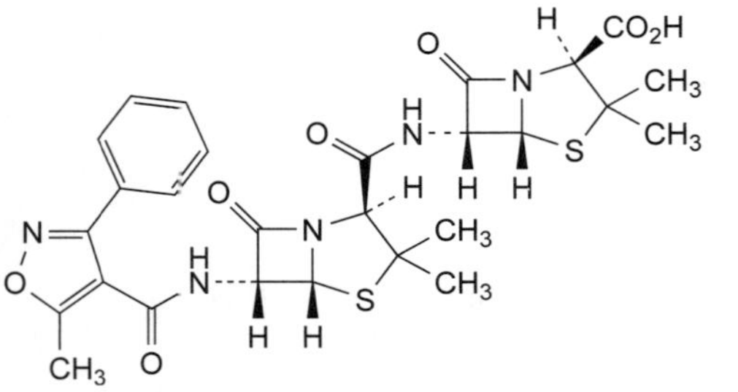

I. (2*S*,5*R*,6*R*)-6-[[(2*S*,5*R*,6*R*)-3,3-dimethyl-6-[[(5-methyl-3-phenylisoxazol-4-yl)carbonyl]amino]-7-oxo-4-thia-1-azabicyclo[3.2.0]heptane-2-carbonyl]amino]-3,3-dimethyl-7-oxo-4-thia-1-azabicyclo[3.2.0]heptane-2-carboxylic acid (6-APA oxacillin amide),

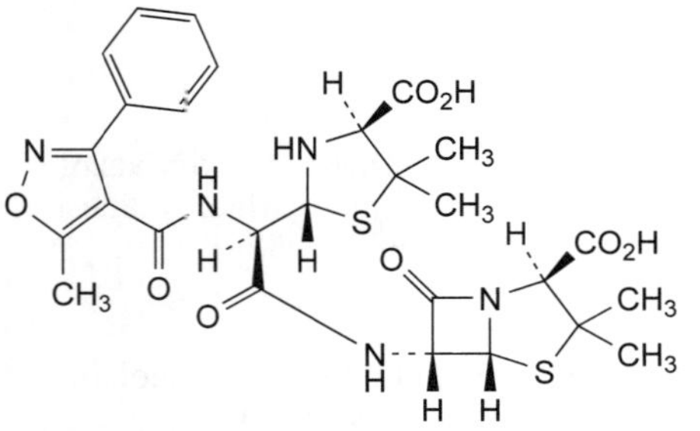

J. (2*S*,5*R*,6*R*)-6-[[(2*R*)-[(2*R*,4*S*)-4-carboxy-5,5-dimethylthiazolidin-2-yl][[(5-methyl-3-phenylisoxazol-4-yl)carbonyl]amino]acetyl]amino]-3,3-dimethyl-7-oxo-4-thia-1-azabicyclo[3.2.0]heptane-2-carboxylic acid (ozolamide of 6-APA dimer).

07/2008:1458

OXFENDAZOLE FOR VETERINARY USE

Oxfendazolum ad usum veterinarium

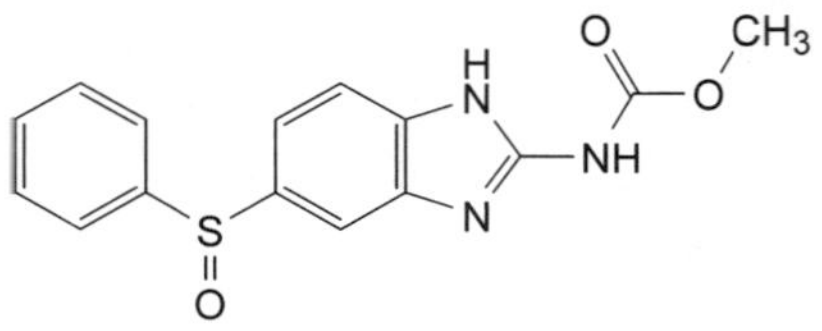

$C_{15}H_{13}N_3O_3S$ M_r 315.4

[53716-50-0]

DEFINITION

Methyl [5-(phenylsulphinyl)-1*H*-benzimidazol-2-yl]carbamate.

Content: 97.5 per cent to 100.5 per cent (dried substance).

CHARACTERS

Appearance: white or almost white powder.

Solubility: practically insoluble in water, slightly soluble in ethanol (96 per cent) and in methylene chloride.

It shows polymorphism (*5.9*).

IDENTIFICATION

Infrared absorption spectrophotometry (*2.2.24*).

Comparison: *oxfendazole CRS*.

If the spectra obtained in the solid state show differences, dissolve the substance to be examined and the reference substance separately in *ethanol (96 per cent) R*, evaporate to dryness and record new spectra using the residues.

TESTS

Related substances. Liquid chromatography (*2.2.29*).

Test solution. Dissolve 25.0 mg of the substance to be examined in the mobile phase and dilute to 100.0 ml with the mobile phase.

Reference solution (a). Dilute 1.0 ml of the test solution to 100.0 ml with the mobile phase.

Reference solution (b). To 10 ml of the test solution, add 0.25 ml of *strong hydrogen peroxide solution R* and dilute to 25 ml with the mobile phase.

Reference solution (c). Dissolve 5.0 mg of *fenbendazole CRS* (impurity A) and 10.0 mg of *oxfendazole impurity B CRS* in the mobile phase and dilute to 100.0 ml with the mobile phase. Dilute 1.0 ml of this solution to 20.0 ml with the mobile phase.

Reference solution (d). Dissolve 5 mg of *oxfendazole with impurity D CRS* in the mobile phase and dilute to 20 ml with the mobile phase (for identification of impurity D).

Column:

- *size*: l = 0.25 m, Ø = 4.6 mm;
- *stationary phase*: spherical *end-capped octadecylsilyl silica gel for chromatography R* (5 μm) with a specific surface area of 350 m^2/g, a pore size of 10 nm and a carbon loading of 14 per cent.

Mobile phase: mix 36 volumes of *acetonitrile R* and 64 volumes of a 2 g/l solution of *sodium pentanesulphonate R* previously adjusted to pH 2.7 with a 2.8 per cent *V/V* solution of *sulphuric acid R*.

Flow rate: 1 ml/min.

Detection: spectrophotometer at 254 nm.

Injection: 20 μl.

Run time: 4 times the retention time of oxfendazole.

Relative retention with reference to oxfendazole (retention time = about 6.5 min): impurity C = about 0.7; impurity B = about 1.5; impurity D = about 1.9; impurity A = about 3.4.

System suitability: reference solution (b):

- *resolution*: minimum 4.0 between the peaks due to impurity C and oxfendazole.

Limits:

- *impurity B*: not more than the area of the corresponding peak in the chromatogram obtained with reference solution (c) (2.0 per cent);
- *impurity A*: not more than the area of the corresponding peak in the chromatogram obtained with reference solution (c) (1.0 per cent);
- *impurities C, D*: for each impurity, not more than the area of the principal peak in the chromatogram obtained with reference solution (a) (1.0 per cent);

– *unspecified impurities*: not more than 0.1 times the area of the principal peak in the chromatogram obtained with reference solution (a) (0.10 per cent);
– *total*: not more than 3 times the area of the principal peak in the chromatogram obtained with reference solution (a) (3.0 per cent);
– *disregard limit*: 0.05 times the area of the principal peak in the chromatogram obtained with reference solution (a) (0.05 per cent).

Loss on drying (*2.2.32*): maximum 0.5 per cent, determined on 1.000 g by drying in an oven at 105 °C at a pressure not exceeding 0.7 kPa for 2 h.

Sulphated ash (*2.4.14*): maximum 0.2 per cent, determined on 1.0 g.

ASSAY

Dissolve 0.250 g in 3 ml of *anhydrous formic acid R*. Add 40 ml of *anhydrous acetic acid R*. Titrate with *0.1 M perchloric acid*, determining the end-point potentiometrically (*2.2.20*).

1 ml of *0.1 M perchloric acid* is equivalent to 31.54 mg of $C_{15}H_{13}N_3O_3S$.

STORAGE

Protected from light.

IMPURITIES

Specified impurities: A, B, C, D.

A. fenbendazole,

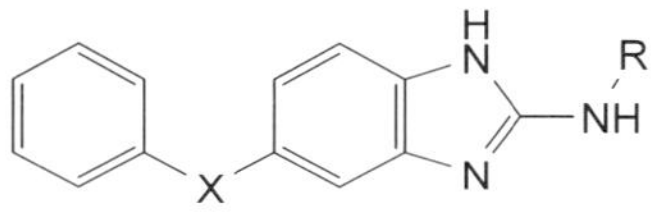

B. X = SO_2, R = CO_2-CH_3: methyl [5-(phenylsulphonyl)-1*H*-benzimidazol-2-yl]carbamate,

C. X = SO, R = H: 5-(phenylsulphinyl)-1*H*-benzimidazol-2-amine,

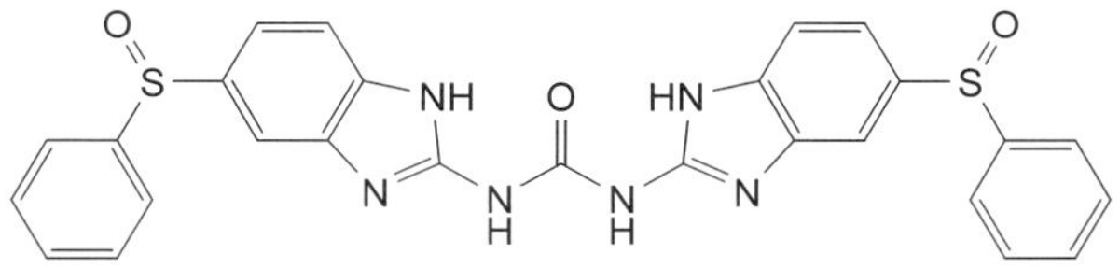

D. *N,N'*-bis[5-(phenylsulphinyl)-1*H*-benzimidazol-2-yl]urea.

01/2008:0417

OXYGEN

Oxygenium

O_2 M_r 32.00

[7782-44-7]

DEFINITION

Content: minimum 99.5 per cent *V/V* of O_2.

This monograph applies to oxygen for medicinal use.

CHARACTERS

Appearance: colourless, odourless gas.

Solubility: at 20 °C and at a pressure of 101 kPa, 1 volume dissolves in about 32 volumes of water.

PRODUCTION

Carbon dioxide: maximum 300 ppm *V/V*, determined using an infrared analyser (*2.5.24*).

Gas to be examined. The substance to be examined. It must be filtered to avoid stray light phenomena.

Reference gas (a). Oxygen R.

Reference gas (b). Mixture containing 300 ppm *V/V* of *carbon dioxide R1* in *nitrogen R1*.

Calibrate the apparatus and set the sensitivity using reference gases (a) and (b). Measure the content of carbon dioxide in the gas to be examined.

Carbon monoxide: maximum 5 ppm *V/V*, determined using an infrared analyser (*2.5.25*).

Gas to be examined. The substance to be examined. It must be filtered to avoid stray light phenomena.

Reference gas (a). Oxygen R.

Reference gas (b). Mixture containing 5 ppm *V/V* of *carbon monoxide R* in *nitrogen R1*.

Calibrate the apparatus and set the sensitivity using reference gases (a) and (b). Measure the content of carbon monoxide in the gas to be examined.

Water (*2.5.28*): maximum 67 ppm *V/V*.

Assay. Determine the concentration of oxygen using a paramagnetic analyser (*2.5.27*).

IDENTIFICATION

First identification: C.

Second identification: A, B.

A. Place a glowing splinter of wood in the substance to be examined. The splinter bursts into flame.

B. Shake with *alkaline pyrogallol solution R*. The substance to be examined is absorbed and the solution becomes dark brown.

C. It complies with the limits of the assay.

TESTS

Carbon dioxide (*2.1.6*): maximum 300 ppm *V/V*, determined using a carbon dioxide detector tube.

Carbon monoxide (*2.1.6*): maximum 5 ppm *V/V*, determined using a carbon monoxide detector tube.

Water vapour (*2.1.6*): maximum 67 ppm *V/V*, determined using a water vapour detector tube.

STORAGE

As a compressed gas or liquid in appropriate containers, complying with the legal regulations. Taps and valves are not to be greased or oiled.

IMPURITIES

Specified impurities: A, B, C.

A. carbon dioxide,

B. carbon monoxide,

C. water.

P

01/2008:0350
corrected 6.2

PANCREAS POWDER

Pancreatis pulvis

DEFINITION

Pancreas powder is prepared from the fresh or frozen pancreases of mammals. It contains various enzymes having proteolytic, lipolytic and amylolytic activities.

1 mg of pancreas powder contains not less than 1.0 Ph. Eur. U. of total proteolytic activity, 15 Ph. Eur. U. of lipolytic activity and 12 Ph. Eur. U. of amylolytic activity.

CHARACTERS

A slightly brown, amorphous powder, partly soluble in water, practically insoluble in ethanol (96 per cent).

IDENTIFICATION

A. Triturate 0.5 g with 10 ml of *water R* and adjust to pH 8 with *0.1 M sodium hydroxide*, using 0.1 ml of *cresol red solution R* as indicator. Divide the suspension into 2 equal parts (suspension (a) and suspension (b)). Boil suspension (a). To each suspension add 10 mg of *fibrin congo red R*, heat to 38-40 °C and maintain at this temperature for 1 h. Suspension (a) is colourless or slightly pink and suspension (b) is distinctly more red.

B. Triturate 0.25 g with 10 ml of *water R* and adjust to pH 8 with *0.1 M sodium hydroxide*, using 0.1 ml of *cresol red solution R* as indicator. Divide the suspension into 2 equal parts (suspension (a) and suspension (b)). Boil suspension (a). Dissolve 0.1 g of *soluble starch R* in 100 ml of boiling *water R*, boil for 2 min, cool and dilute to 150 ml with *water R*. To 75 ml of the starch solution add suspension (a) and to the remaining 75 ml add suspension (b). Heat each mixture to 38-40 °C and maintain at this temperature for 5 min.

   To 1 ml of each mixture add 10 ml of *iodine solution R2*. The mixture obtained with suspension (a) has an intense blue-violet colour; the mixture obtained with suspension (b) has the colour of the iodine solution.

TESTS

Fat content. In an extraction apparatus, treat 1.0 g with *light petroleum R1* for 3 h. Evaporate the solvent and dry the residue at 100-105 °C for 2 h. The residue weighs not more than 50 mg (5.0 per cent).

Loss on drying (*2.2.32*). Not more than 5.0 per cent, determined on 0.50 g by drying at 60 °C at a pressure not exceeding 670 Pa for 4 h.

Microbial contamination. Total viable aerobic count (*2.6.12*) not more than 10^4 micro-organisms per gram, determined by plate count. It complies with the tests for *Escherichia coli* and *Salmonella* (*2.6.13*).

ASSAY

Total proteolytic activity. The total proteolytic activity of pancreas powder is determined by comparing the quantity of peptides non-precipitable by a 50 g/l solution of *trichloroacetic acid R* released per minute from a substrate of casein solution with the quantity of such peptides released by *pancreas powder (protease) BRP* from the same substrate in the same conditions.

Casein solution. Suspend a quantity of *casein BRP* equivalent to 1.25 g of dried substance in 5 ml of *water R*, add 10 ml of *0.1 M sodium hydroxide* and stir for 1 min. (Determine the water content of *casein BRP* prior to the test by heating at 60 °C *in vacuo* for 4 h.) Add 60 ml of *water R* and stir with a magnetic stirrer until the solution is practically clear. Adjust to pH 8.0 with *0.1 M sodium hydroxide* or *0.1 M hydrochloric acid*. Dilute to 100.0 ml with *water R*. Use the solution on the day of preparation.

Enterokinase solution. Dissolve 50 mg of *enterokinase BRP* in *0.02 M calcium chloride solution R* and dilute to 50.0 ml with the same solvent. Use the solution on the day of preparation.

For the test suspension and the reference suspension, prepare the suspension and carry out the dilution at 0-4 °C.

Test suspension. Triturate 0.100 g of the substance to be examined for 5 min adding gradually 25 ml of *0.02 M calcium chloride solution R*. Transfer completely to a volumetric flask and dilute to 100.0 ml with *0.02 M calcium chloride solution R*. To 10.0 ml of this suspension add 10.0 ml of the enterokinase solution and heat on a water-bath at 35 ± 0.5 °C for 15 min. Cool and dilute with *borate buffer solution pH 7.5 R* at 5 ± 3 °C to a final concentration of about 0.065 Ph. Eur. U. of total proteolytic activity per millilitre calculated on the basis of the stated activity.

Reference suspension. Prepare a suspension of *pancreas powder (protease) BRP* as described for the test suspension but without the addition of enterokinase so as to obtain a known final concentration of about 0.065 Ph. Eur. U. per millilitre calculated on the basis of the stated activity.

Designate tubes in duplicate T, T_b, S_1, S_{1b}, S_2, S_{2b}, S_3, S_{3b}; designate a tube B.

Add *borate buffer solution pH 7.5 R* to the tubes as follows:

B: 3.0 ml,

S_1 and S_{1b}: 2.0 ml,

S_2, S_{2b}, T and T_b: 1.0 ml.

Add the reference suspension to the tubes as follows:

S_1 and S_{1b}: 1.0 ml,

S_2 and S_{2b}: 2.0 ml,

S_3 and S_{3b}: 3.0 ml.

Add 2.0 ml of the test suspension to tubes T and T_b.

Add 5.0 ml of a 50 g/l solution of *trichloroacetic acid R* to tubes B, S_{1b}, S_{2b}, S_{3b} and T_b. Mix by shaking.

Place the tubes and the casein solution in a water-bath at 35 ± 0.5 °C. Place a glass rod in each tube. When temperature equilibrium is reached, add 2.0 ml of the casein solution to tubes B, S_{1b}, S_{2b}, S_{3b} and T_b. Mix. At time zero, add 2.0 ml of casein solution successively and at intervals of 30 s to tubes S_1, S_2, S_3 and T. Mix immediately after each addition. Exactly 30 min after addition of the casein solution, taking into account the regular interval adopted, add 5.0 ml of a 50 g/l solution of *trichloroacetic acid R* to tubes S_1, S_2, S_3 and T. Mix. Withdraw the tubes from the water-bath and allow to stand at room temperature for 20 min.

Filter the contents of each tube twice through the same suitable filter paper previously washed with a 50 g/l solution of *trichloroacetic acid R*, then with *water R* and dried.

A suitable filter paper complies with the following test: filter 5 ml of a 50 g/l solution of *trichloroacetic acid R* on a 7 cm disc of white filter paper; the absorbance (*2.2.25*) of the filtrate, measured at 275 nm using unfiltered trichloroacetic acid solution as the compensation liquid, is less than 0.04.

A schematic presentation of the above operations is shown in Table 0350.-1.

Table 0350.-1

	Tubes								
	S_1	S_{1b}	S_2	S_{2b}	S_3	S_{3b}	T	T_b	B
Buffer solution	2	2	1	1			1	1	3
Reference suspension	1	1	2	2	3	3			
Test suspension							2	2	
Trichloroacetic acid solution		5		5		5		5	5
Mix		+		+		+		+	+
Water-bath 35 °C	+	+	+	+	+	+	+	+	+
Casein solution		2		2		2		2	2
Mix		+		+		+		+	+
Casein solution	2		2		2		2		
Mix	+		+		+		+		
Water-bath 35 °C 30 min	+	+	+	+	+	+	+	+	+
Trichloroacetic acid solution	5		5		5		5		
Mix	+		+		+		+		
Room temperature 20 min	+	+	+	+	+	+	+	+	+
Filter	+	+	+	+	+	+	+	+	+

Measure the absorbance (*2.2.25*) of the filtrates at 275 nm using the filtrate obtained from tube B as the compensation liquid.

Correct the average absorbance values for the filtrates obtained from tubes S_1, S_2 and S_3 by subtracting the average values obtained for the filtrates from tubes S_{1b}, S_{2b} and S_{3b} respectively. Draw a calibration curve of the corrected values against volume of reference suspension used.

Determine the activity of the substance to be examined using the corrected absorbance for the test suspension ($T - T_b$) and the calibration curve and taking into account the dilution factors.

The test is not valid unless the corrected absorbance values are between 0.15 and 0.60.

Lipolytic activity. The lipolytic activity is determined by comparing the rate at which a suspension of pancreas powder hydrolyses a substrate of olive oil emulsion with the rate at which a suspension of *pancreas powder (amylase and lipase) BRP* hydrolyses the same substrate under the same conditions. *The test is carried out under nitrogen.*

Olive oil stock emulsion. In an 800 ml beaker 9 cm in diameter, place 40 ml of *olive oil R*, 330 ml of *acacia solution R* and 30 ml of *water R*. Place an electric mixer at the bottom of the beaker. Place the beaker in a vessel containing *ethanol (96 per cent) R* and a sufficient quantity of ice as a cooling mixture. Emulsify using the mixer at an average speed of 1000-2000 r/min. Cool to 5-10 °C. Increase the mixing speed to 8000 r/min. Mix for 30 min keeping the temperature below 25 °C by the continuous addition of crushed ice into the cooling mixture. (A mixture of calcium chloride and crushed ice is also suitable). Store the stock emulsion in a refrigerator and use within 14 days. The emulsion must not separate into 2 distinct layers. Check the diameter of the globules of the emulsion under a microscope. At least 90 per cent have a diameter below 3 μm and none has a diameter greater than 10 μm. Shake the emulsion thoroughly before preparing the emulsion substrate.

Olive oil emulsion. For 10 determinations, mix the following solutions in the order indicated: 100 ml of the stock emulsion, 80 ml of *tris(hydroxymethyl)aminomethane solution R1*, 20 ml of a freshly prepared 80 g/l of *sodium taurocholate BRP* and 95 ml of *water R*. Use on the day of preparation.

Apparatus. Use a reaction vessel of about 50 ml capacity provided with:

- a device that will maintain a temperature of 37 ± 0.5 °C;
- a magnetic stirrer;
- a lid with holes for the insertion of electrodes, the tip of a burette, a tube for the admission of nitrogen and the introduction of reagents.

An automatic or manual titration apparatus may be used. In the latter case, the burette is graduated in 0.005 ml and the pH-meter is provided with a wide reading scale and glass-calomel or glass-silver-silver chloride electrodes. After each test the reaction vessel is evacuated by suction and washed several times with *water R*, the washings being removed each time by suction.

Test suspension. In a small mortar cooled to 0-4 °C, triturate carefully a quantity of the substance to be examined equivalent to about 2500 Ph. Eur. U. of lipolytic activity with 1 ml of cooled *maleate buffer solution pH 7.0 R* (lipase solvent) until a very fine suspension is obtained. Dilute the suspension with cold *maleate buffer solution pH 7.0 R*, transfer quantitatively to a volumetric flask and dilute to 100.0 ml with the cold buffer solution. Keep the flask containing the test suspension in iced water during the titration.

Reference suspension. To avoid absorption of water formed by condensation, allow the reference preparation to reach room temperature before opening the container. Prepare a suspension of *pancreas powder (amylase and lipase) BRP* as described for the test suspension using a quantity equivalent to about 2500 Ph. Eur. U.

Carry out the titrations immediately after preparation of the test suspension and the reference suspension. Place 29.5 ml of olive oil emulsion in the reaction vessel equilibrated at 37 ± 0.5 °C. Fit the vessel with the electrodes, a stirrer and the burette (the tip being immersed in the olive oil emulsion).

Put the lid in place and switch on the apparatus. Carefully add *0.1 M sodium hydroxide* with stirring to adjust to pH 9.2. Using a rapid-flow graduated pipette transfer about 0.5 ml of the previously homogenised reference suspension, start the chronometer and add continuously *0.1 M sodium hydroxide* to maintain the pH at 9.0. After exactly 1 min, note the volume of *0.1 M sodium hydroxide* used. Carry out the measurement a further 4 times. Discard the first reading and determine the average of the 4 others (S_1). Make 2 further determinations (S_2 and S_3). Calculate the average of the values S_1, S_2 and S_3. The average volume of *0.1 M sodium hydroxide* used should be about 0.12 ml per minute with limits of 0.08 ml to 0.16 ml.

Carry out 3 determinations in the same manner for the test suspension (T_1, T_2 and T_3). If the quantity of *0.1 M sodium hydroxide* used is outside the limits of 0.08 ml to 0.16 ml per minute, the assay is repeated with a quantity of test suspension that is more suitable but situated between 0.4 ml and 0.6 ml. Otherwise the quantity of the substance to be examined is adjusted to comply with the conditions of the test. Calculate the average of the values T_1, T_2 and T_3.

Calculate the activity in European Pharmacopoeia Units per milligram using the following expression:

$$\frac{n \times m_1}{n_1 \times m} \times A$$

n = average volume of *0.1 M sodium hydroxide* used per minute during the titration of the test suspension, in millilitres;

n_1 = average volume of *0.1 M sodium hydroxide* used per minute during the titration of the reference suspension, in millilitres;

m = mass of the substance to be examined, in milligrams;

m_1 = mass of the reference preparation, in milligrams;

A = activity of *pancreas powder (amylase and lipase) BRP*, in European Pharmacopoeia Units per milligram.

Amylolytic activity. The amylolytic activity is determined by comparing the rate at which a suspension of pancreas powder hydrolyses a substrate of starch solution with the rate at which a suspension of *pancreas powder (amylase and lipase) BRP* hydrolyses the same substrate under the same conditions.

Starch solution. To a quantity of *starch BRP* equivalent to 2.0 g of the dried substance add 10 ml of *water R* and mix. (Determine the water content of *starch BRP* prior to the test by heating at 120 °C for 4 h). Add this suspension, whilst stirring continuously, to 160 ml of boiling *water R*. Wash the container several times with successive quantities, each of 10 ml, of *water R* and add the washings to the hot starch solution. Heat to boiling, stirring continuously. Cool to room temperature and dilute to 200 ml with *water R*. Use the solution on the day of preparation.

For the test suspension and the reference suspension, prepare the suspension and carry out the dilution at 0-4 °C.

Test suspension. Triturate a quantity of the substance to be examined equivalent to about 1500 Ph. Eur. U. of amylolytic activity with 60 ml of *phosphate buffer solution pH 6.8 R1* for 15 min. Transfer quantitatively to a volumetric flask and dilute to 100.0 ml with *phosphate buffer solution pH 6.8 R1*.

Reference suspension. Prepare a suspension of *pancreas powder (amylase and lipase) BRP* as described for the test suspension, using a quantity equivalent to about 1500 Ph. Eur. U.

In a test tube 200 mm long and 22 mm in diameter, fitted with a ground-glass stopper, place 25.0 ml of starch solution, 10.0 ml of *phosphate buffer solution pH 6.8 R1* and 1.0 ml of an 11.7 g/l solution of *sodium chloride R*. Close the tube, shake and place in a water-bath at 25.0 ± 0.1 °C. When the temperature equilibrium has been reached, add 1.0 ml of the test suspension and start the chronometer. Mix and place the tube in the water-bath. After exactly 10 min, add 2 ml of *1 M hydrochloric acid*. Transfer the mixture quantitatively to a 300 ml conical flask fitted with a ground-glass stopper. Whilst shaking continuously, add 10.0 ml of *0.05 M iodine* immediately followed by 45 ml of *0.1 M sodium hydroxide*. Allow to stand in the dark at a temperature between 15 °C and 25 °C for 15 min. Add 4 ml of a mixture of 1 volume of *sulphuric acid R* and 4 volumes of *water R*. Titrate the excess of iodine with *0.1 M sodium thiosulphate* using a microburette. Carry out a blank titration adding the 2 ml of *1 M hydrochloric acid* before introducing the test suspension. Carry out the titration of the reference suspension in the same manner.

Calculate the amylolytic activity in European Pharmacopoeia Units per milligram using the following expression:

$$\frac{(n' - n)\, m_1}{(n'_1 - n_1)\, m} \times A$$

n = volume of *0.1 M sodium thiosulphate* used in the titration of the test suspension, in millilitres;

n_1 = volume of *0.1 M sodium thiosulphate* used in the titration of the reference suspension, in millilitres;

n' = volume of *0.1 M sodium thiosulphate* used in the blank titration of the test suspension, in millilitres;

n'_1 = volume of *0.1 M sodium thiosulphate* used in the blank titration of the reference suspension, in millilitres;

m = mass of the substance to be examined, in milligrams;

m_1 = mass of the reference preparation, in milligrams;

A = activity of *pancreas powder (amylase and lipase) BRP*, in European Pharmacopoeia Units per milligram.

STORAGE

Store in an airtight container.

07/2008:1799

PARAFFIN, WHITE SOFT

Vaselinum album

DEFINITION

Purified and wholly or nearly decolorised mixture of semi-solid hydrocarbons, obtained from petroleum. It may contain a suitable antioxidant. White soft paraffin described in this monograph is not suitable for oral use.

CHARACTERS

Appearance: white or almost white, translucent, soft unctuous mass, slightly fluorescent in daylight when melted.

Solubility: practically insoluble in water, slightly soluble in methylene chloride, practically insoluble in ethanol (96 per cent) and in glycerol.

IDENTIFICATION

First identification: A, B, D.

Second identification: A, C, D.

A. The drop point is between 35 °C and 70 °C and does not differ by more than 5 °C from the value stated on the label, according to method (*2.2.17*) with the following modification to fill the cup: heat the substance to be examined at a temperature not exceeding 80 °C, with stirring to ensure uniformity. Warm the metal cup at a temperature not exceeding 80 °C in an oven, remove it from the oven, place on a clean plate or ceramic tile and pour a sufficient quantity of the melted sample into the cup to fill it completely. Allow the filled cup to cool for 30 min on the plate or the ceramic tile and place it in a water bath at 24-26 °C for 30-40 min. Level the surface of the sample with a single stroke of a knife or razor blade, avoiding compression of the sample.

B. Infrared absorption spectrophotometry (*2.2.24*).

Preparation: place about 2 mg on a *sodium chloride R* plate, spread the substance with another *sodium chloride R* plate and remove 1 of the plates.

Comparison: repeat the operations using *white soft paraffin CRS*.

C. Melt 2 g and when a homogeneous phase is obtained, add 2 ml of *water R* and 0.2 ml of *0.05 M iodine*. Shake. Allow to cool. The solid upper layer is violet-pink or brown.

D. Appearance (see Tests).

TESTS

Appearance. The substance is white. Melt 12 g on a water-bath. The melted mass is not more intensely coloured than a mixture of 1 volume of yellow primary solution and 9 volumes of a 10 g/l solution of *hydrochloric acid R* (*2.2.2, Method II*).

Acidity or alkalinity. To 10 g add 20 ml of boiling *water R* and shake vigorously for 1 min. Allow to cool and decant. To 10 ml of the aqueous layer add 0.1 ml of *phenolphthalein solution R*. The solution is colourless. Not more than 0.5 ml of *0.01 M sodium hydroxide* is required to change the colour of the indicator to red.

Consistency (*2.9.9*): 60 to 300.

Polycyclic aromatic hydrocarbons: maximum 300 ppm.

Use reagents for ultraviolet spectrophotometry. Dissolve 1.0 g in 50 ml of *hexane R* which has been previously shaken twice with 10 ml of *dimethyl sulphoxide R*. Transfer the solution to a 125 ml separating funnel with unlubricated ground-glass parts (stopper, stopcock). Add 20 ml of *dimethyl sulphoxide R*. Shake vigorously for 1 min and allow to stand until 2 clear layers are formed. Transfer the lower layer to a second separating funnel. Repeat the extraction with a further 20 ml of *dimethyl sulphoxide R*. Shake vigorously the combined lower layers with 20 ml of *hexane R* for 1 min. Allow to stand until 2 clear layers are formed. Separate the lower layer and dilute to 50.0 ml with *dimethyl sulphoxide R*. Measure the absorbance (*2.2.25*) over the range 260 nm to 420 nm using a path length of 4 cm and as compensation liquid the clear lower layer obtained by vigorously shaking 10 ml of *dimethyl sulphoxide R* with 25 ml of *hexane R* for 1 min. Prepare a reference solution in *dimethyl sulphoxide R* containing 6.0 mg of *naphthalene R* per litre and measure the absorbance of the solution at the maximum at 278 nm using a path length of 4 cm and *dimethyl sulphoxide R* as compensation liquid. At no wavelength in the range 260 nm to 420 nm does the absorbance of the test solution exceed that of the reference solution at 278 nm.

Sulphated ash (*2.4.14*): maximum 0.05 per cent, determined on 2.0 g.

STORAGE

Protected from light.

LABELLING

The label states the nominal drop point.

07/2008:1554

PARAFFIN, YELLOW SOFT

Vaselinum flavum

DEFINITION

Yellow soft paraffin is a purified mixture of semi-solid hydrocarbons, obtained from petroleum. It may contain a suitable antioxidant.

CHARACTERS

A yellow, translucent, unctuous mass, slightly fluorescent in daylight when melted, practically insoluble in water, slightly soluble in methylene chloride, practically insoluble in ethanol (96 per cent) and in glycerol.

IDENTIFICATION

First identification: A, B, D.

Second identification: A, C, D.

A. The drop point (*2.2.17*) is 40 °C to 60 °C and does not differ by more than 5 °C from the value stated on the label, with the following modification to fill the cup: heat the substance to be examined at 118-22 °C, with stirring to ensure uniformity, then cool to 100-107 °C. Warm the metal cup at 103-107 °C in an oven, remove it from the oven, place on a clean plate or ceramic tile and pour a sufficient quantity of the melted sample into the cup to fill it completely. Allow the filled cup to cool for 30 min on the ceramic tile and place it in a water-bath at 24-26 °C for a further 30-40 min. Level the surface of the sample with a single stroke of a knife or razor blade, avoiding compression of the sample.

B. Examine by infrared absorption spectrophotometry (*2.2.24*).

Preparation: place about 2 mg on a *sodium chloride R* plate, spread the substance with another *sodium chloride R* plate and remove 1 of the plates.

Comparison: repeat the operations using *yellow soft paraffin CRS*.

C. Melt 2 g and when a homogeneous phase is obtained, add 2 ml of *water R* and 0.2 ml of *0.05 M iodine*. Shake. Allow to cool. The solid upper layer is violet-pink or brown.

D. Appearance (see Tests).

TESTS

Appearance. The substance is yellow. Melt 12 g on a water-bath. The melted mass is not more intensely coloured than a mixture of 7.6 volumes of yellow primary solution and 2.4 volumes of red primary solution (*2.2.2, Method II*).

Acidity or alkalinity. To 10 g add 20 ml of boiling *water R* and shake vigorously for 1 min. Allow to cool and decant. To 10 ml of the aqueous layer add 0.1 ml of *phenolphthalein solution R*. The solution is colourless. Not more than 0.5 ml of *0.01 M sodium hydroxide* is required to change the colour of the indicator to red.

Consistency (*2.9.9*). The consistency is 100 to 300.

Polycyclic aromatic hydrocarbons. *Use reagents for ultraviolet absorption spectrophotometry.* Dissolve 1.0 g in 50 ml of *hexane R* which has been previously shaken twice with one-fifth its volume of *dimethyl sulphoxide R*. Transfer the solution to a 125 ml separating funnel with unlubricated ground-glass parts (stopper, stopcock). Add 20 ml of *dimethyl sulphoxide R*. Shake vigorously for 1 min and allow to stand until two clear layers are formed. Transfer the lower layer to a second separating funnel. Repeat the extraction with a further 20 ml of *dimethyl sulphoxide R*.

Shake vigorously the combined lower layers with 20 ml of *hexane R* for 1 min. Allow to stand until two clear layers are formed. Separate the lower layer and dilute to 50.0 ml with *dimethyl sulphoxide R*. Measure the absorbance (*2.2.25*) between 260 nm and 420 nm using a path length of 4 cm and using as the compensation liquid the clear lower layer obtained by vigorously shaking 10 ml of *dimethyl sulphoxide R* with 25 ml of *hexane R* for 1 min. Prepare a 9.0 mg/l reference solution of *naphthalene R* in *dimethyl sulphoxide R* and measure the absorbance of this solution at the maximum at 278 nm using a path length of 4 cm and using *dimethyl sulphoxide R* as the compensation liquid. At no wavelength in the range of 260 nm to 420 nm does the absorbance of the test solution exceed that of the reference solution at 278 nm.

Sulphated ash (*2.4.14*). Not more than 0.05 per cent, determined on 2.0 g.

STORAGE

Store protected from light.

LABELLING

The label states the nominal drop point.

01/2008:0754

PERU BALSAM

Balsamum peruvianum

DEFINITION

Balsam obtained from the scorched and wounded trunk of *Myroxylon balsamum* (L.) Harms var. *pereirae* (Royle) Harms.

Content: 45.0 per cent *m/m* to 70.0 per cent *m/m* of esters, mainly benzyl benzoate and benzyl cinnamate.

CHARACTERS

Appearance: dark brown, viscous liquid which is transparent and yellowish-brown when viewed in a thin layer; it is not sticky, non-drying and does not form threads.

Solubility: practically insoluble in water, freely soluble in anhydrous ethanol, not miscible with fatty oils, except for castor oil.

IDENTIFICATION

A. Dissolve 0.20 g in 10 ml of *ethanol (96 per cent) R*. Add 0.2 ml of *ferric chloride solution R1*. A green or yellowish-green colour develops.

B. Thin-layer chromatography (*2.2.27*).

Test solution. Dissolve 0.5 g of the substance to be examined in 10 ml of *ethyl acetate R*.

Reference solution. Dissolve 4 mg of *thymol R*, 30 mg of *benzyl cinnamate R* and 80 µl of *benzyl benzoate R* in 5 ml of *ethyl acetate R*.

Plate: *TLC silica gel GF_{254} plate R*.

Mobile phase: *glacial acetic acid R, ethyl acetate R, hexane R* (0.5:10:90 *V/V/V*).

Application: 10 µl, as bands of 20 mm by 3 mm.

Development: twice over a path of 10 cm.

Drying: in air.

Detection A: examine in ultraviolet light at 254 nm and mark the quenching zones.

Results A: the chromatogram obtained with the reference solution shows in the upper third 2 quenching zones, the higher one due to benzyl benzoate and the lower one due to benzyl cinnamate. The chromatogram obtained with the test solution shows 2 quenching zones at the same levels and of approximately the same size.

Detection B: spray with a freshly prepared 200 g/l solution of *phosphomolybdic acid R* in *ethanol (96 per cent) R*, using 10 ml for a plate 200 mm square and examine in daylight while heating at 100-105 °C for 5-10 min.

Results B: the zones due to benzyl benzoate and benzyl cinnamate are blue against a yellow background. The chromatogram obtained with the reference solution shows at about the middle a violet-grey zone (thymol). In the chromatogram obtained with the test solution, a blue zone (nerolidol) is seen just below the level of the zone due to thymol in the chromatogram obtained with the reference solution. Just below the zone due to nerolidol, no blue zone is seen corresponding to a quenching zone seen when examined in ultraviolet light at 254 nm (colophony). In the upper and lower part of the chromatogram obtained with the test solution, other faint blue zones may be seen.

TESTS

Relative density (*2.2.5*): 1.14 to 1.17.

Saponification value (*2.5.6*): 230 to 255, determined on the residue obtained in the assay.

Artificial balsams. Shake 0.20 g with 6 ml of *light petroleum R1*. The light petroleum solution is clear and colourless and the whole of the insoluble parts of the balsam stick to the wall of the test-tube.

Fatty oils. Shake 1 g with 3 ml of a 1000 g/l solution of *chloral hydrate R*. The resulting solution is as clear as the 1000 g/l solution of *chloral hydrate R*.

Turpentine. Evaporate to dryness 4 ml of the solution obtained in the test for artificial balsams. The residue has no odour of turpentine.

ASSAY

To 2.50 g in a separating funnel add 7.5 ml of *dilute sodium hydroxide solution R* and 40 ml of *peroxide-free ether R* and shake vigorously for 10 min. Separate the lower layer and shake it with 3 quantities, each of 15 ml, of *peroxide-free ether R*. Combine the ether layers, dry over 10 g of *anhydrous sodium sulphate R* and filter. Wash the sodium sulphate with 2 quantities, each of 10 ml, of *peroxide-free ether R*. Combine the ether layers and evaporate to dryness. Dry the residue (esters) at 100-105 °C for 30 min and weigh.

STORAGE

Protected from light.

01/2008:2152
corrected 6.2

POLY(VINYL ACETATE) DISPERSION 30 PER CENT

Poly(vinylis acetas) dispersio 30 per centum

DEFINITION

Dispersion in water of poly(vinyl acetate) having a mean relative molecular mass of about 450 000. It may contain *Povidone (0685)* and a suitable surface-active agent, such as *Sodium laurilsulphate (0098)*, as stabilisers.

Content: 25.0 per cent to 30.0 per cent of poly(vinyl acetate).

CHARACTERS

Appearance: opaque, white or almost white, slightly viscous liquid.

Solubility: miscible with water and with ethanol (96 per cent).

It is sensitive to spoilage by microbial contaminants.

IDENTIFICATION

A. Infrared absorption spectrophotometry (*2.2.24*).

Preparation: dry 1 ml *in vacuo*, dissolve the residue in *acetone R*, and spread 1 drop of the solution between 2 *sodium chloride R* plates; remove 1 plate and allow the solvent to evaporate.

Comparison: repeat the operation using *poly(vinyl acetate) dispersion 30 per cent CRS*.

B. Place 3 ml on a glass plate and allow to dry. A clear film is formed.

C. 50 mg gives the reaction of acetyl (*2.3.1*).

TESTS

Agglomerates. Filter 100.0 g through a tared stainless steel sieve (90). Rinse with *water R* until a clear filtrate is obtained and dry to constant mass at 100-105 °C. The mass of the residue is not greater than 0.500 g.

Vinyl acetate. Liquid chromatography (*2.2.29*).

Test solution. Introduce 0.250 g into a 10 ml volumetric flask and add about 1 ml of *methanol R2*. Sonicate. Add about 8 ml of *water for chromatography R*. Sonicate and dilute to 10.0 ml with *water for chromatography R*. Centrifuge for about 10 min and filter.

Reference solution (a). Dissolve 5.0 mg of *vinyl acetate CRS* in *methanol R2* and dilute to 10.0 ml with the same solvent. Dilute 1.0 ml of the solution to 20.0 ml with mobile phase A. Dilute 1.0 ml of this solution to 10.0 ml with mobile phase A.

Reference solution (b). To 5 mg of *vinyl acetate R* and 5 mg of *1-vinylpyrrolidin-2-one R*, add 10 ml of *methanol R2* and sonicate. Dilute to 50 ml with mobile phase A. Dilute 1 ml of this solution to 20 ml with mobile phase A.

A precolumn containing *octadecylsilyl silica gel for chromatography R* (5 µm) may be used if a matrix effect is observed.

Column:

– *size*: *l* = 0.25 m, Ø = 4.0 mm;
– *stationary phase*: *octadecylsilyl silica gel for chromatography R* (5 µm);
– *temperature*: 30 °C.

Mobile phase:

– *mobile phase A*: *acetonitrile for chromatography R, methanol R2, water for chromatography R* (5:5:90 *V/V/V*);
– *mobile phase B*: *methanol R2, acetonitrile for chromatography R, water for chromatography R* (5:45:50 *V/V/V*);

Time (min)	Mobile phase A (per cent *V/V*)	Mobile phase B (per cent *V/V*)
0 - 2	100	0
2 - 26	100 → 80	0 → 20
26 - 27	80 → 0	20 → 100
27 - 30	0 → 100	100 → 0

Flow rate: 1.0 ml/min.

Detection: spectrophotometer at 205 nm.

Injection: 10 µl of the test solution and reference solutions (a) and (b).

System suitability: reference solution (b):

– *resolution*: minimum 5.0 between the peaks due to vinyl acetate and 1-vinylpyrrolidin-2-one.

Limit:

– *vinyl acetate*: not more than the area of the principal peak in the chromatogram obtained with reference solution (a) (100 ppm).

Povidone: maximum 4.0 per cent.

Carry out the determination of nitrogen by sulphuric acid digestion (*2.5.9*) on 0.25 g. Calculate the percentage content of povidone using the following expression:

$$\frac{N}{0.126}$$

N = percentage content of nitrogen.

Acetic acid. Liquid chromatography (*2.2.29*).

Test solution. Mix 0.200 g with *water for chromatography R*. Sonicate for about 10 min and dilute to 10.0 ml with *water for chromatography R*.

Reference solution. Dissolve 30.0 mg of *acetic acid R* and 30 mg of *citric acid R* in the mobile phase. Shake gently to dissolve and dilute to 100.0 ml with the mobile phase.

Column:

– *size*: *l* = 0.25 m, Ø = 4.6 mm;
– *stationary phase*: *octadecylsilyl silica gel for chromatography R* (5 µm).

Mobile phase: *0.005 M sulphuric acid.*

Flow rate: 1.0 ml/min.

Detection: spectrophotometer at 205 nm.

Injection: 20 µl. After each injection, rinse the column with a mixture of equal volumes of *acetonitrile for chromatography R* and *0.005 M sulphuric acid.*

Retention time: acetic acid = about 6 min; citric acid = about 8 min.

System suitability: reference solution:

– *resolution*: minimum 2.0 between the peaks due to citric acid and acetic acid.

Limit:

– *acetic acid*: not more than the area of the corresponding peak in the chromatogram obtained with the reference solution (1.5 per cent).

Residue on evaporation: 0.285 g to 0.315 g, determined on 1.000 g at 110 °C for 5 h.

Sulphated ash: maximum 0.5 per cent, determined on 1.0 g. Heat a silica crucible to redness for 30 min, allow to cool in a desiccator and weigh. Evenly distribute 1.00 g of the preparation to be examined in the crucible and weigh. Dry at 100-105 °C for 1 h and ignite in a muffle furnace at 600 °C ± 25 °C, until the substance is thoroughly charred. Carry out the test for sulphated ash (*2.4.14*) on the residue obtained, starting with "Moisten the substance to be examined...".

Microbial contamination. Total viable aerobic count (*2.6.12*) not more than 10^3 micro-organisms per gram, determined by plate count.

ASSAY

Determine the saponification value (*2.5.6*) on 1.5 g and calculate the percentage content of poly(vinyl acetate) using the following expression:

$$I_s \times 0.1534$$

I_s = saponification value.

STORAGE

At a temperature of 5 °C to 30 °C. Handle the substance so as to minimise microbial contamination.

FUNCTIONALITY-RELATED CHARACTERISTICS

This section provides information on characteristics that are recognised as being relevant control parameters for one or more functions of the substance when used as an excipient. This section is a non-mandatory part of the monograph and it is not necessary to verify the characteristics to demonstrate compliance. Control of these characteristics can however contribute to the quality of a medicinal product by improving the consistency of the manufacturing process and the performance of the medicinal product during use. Where control methods are cited, they are recognised as being suitable for the purpose, but other methods can also be used. Wherever results for a particular characteristic are reported, the control method must be indicated.

The following characteristics may be relevant for poly(vinyl acetate) dispersion 30 per cent used in the manufacture of modified-release dosage forms and to mask taste.

Solubility of a film. Place the film obtained in identification test B in 50 ml of *phosphate buffer solution pH 6.8 R* whilst stirring continuously. The film does not dissolve within 30 min.

Apparent viscosity (*2.2.10*): maximum 100 mPa·s, determined using a rotating viscometer at 20 °C and a shear rate of 100 s^{-1}.

01/2008:0185
corrected 6.2

POTASSIUM CHLORIDE

Kalii chloridum

KCl M_r 74.6

[7447-40-7]

DEFINITION

Content: 99.0 per cent to 100.5 per cent of KCl (dried substance).

CHARACTERS

Appearance: white or almost white, crystalline powder or colourless crystals.

Solubility: freely soluble in water, practically insoluble in anhydrous ethanol.

IDENTIFICATION

A. It gives the reactions of chlorides (*2.3.1*).

B. Solution S (see Tests) gives the reactions of potassium (*2.3.1*).

TESTS

Solution S. Dissolve 10.0 g in *carbon dioxide-free water R* prepared from *distilled water R* and dilute to 100 ml with the same solvent.

Appearance of solution. Solution S is clear (*2.2.1*) and colourless (*2.2.2, Method II*).

Acidity or alkalinity. To 50 ml of solution S add 0.1 ml of *bromothymol blue solution R1*. Not more than 0.5 ml of *0.01 M hydrochloric acid* or *0.01 M sodium hydroxide* is required to change the colour of the indicator.

Bromides: maximum 0.1 per cent.

Dilute 1.0 ml of solution S to 50 ml with *water R*. To 5.0 ml of the solution add 2.0 ml of *phenol red solution R2* and 1.0 ml of *chloramine solution R1* and mix immediately. After exactly 2 min add 0.15 ml of *0.1 M sodium thiosulphate*, mix and dilute to 10.0 ml with *water R*. The absorbance (*2.2.25*) of the solution measured at 590 nm, using *water R* as the compensation liquid, is not greater than that of a standard prepared at the same time and in the same manner using 5 ml of a 3.0 mg/l solution of *potassium bromide R*.

Iodides. Moisten 5 g by the dropwise addition of a freshly prepared mixture of 0.15 ml of *sodium nitrite solution R*, 2 ml of *0.5 M sulphuric acid*, 25 ml of *iodide-free starch solution R* and 25 ml of *water R*. After 5 min, examine in daylight. The substance shows no blue colour.

Sulphates (*2.4.13*): maximum 300 ppm.

Dilute 5 ml of solution S to 15 ml with *distilled water R*.

Aluminium (*2.4.17*): maximum 1.0 ppm, if intended for use in the manufacture of haemodialysis solutions.

Prescribed solution. Dissolve 4 g in 100 ml of *water R* and add 10 ml of *acetate buffer solution pH 6.0 R*.

Reference solution. Mix 2 ml of *aluminium standard solution (2 ppm Al) R*, 10 ml of *acetate buffer solution pH 6.0 R* and 98 ml of *water R*.

Blank solution. Mix 10 ml of *acetate buffer solution pH 6.0 R* and 100 ml of *water R*.

Barium. To 5 ml of solution S add 5 ml of *distilled water R* and 1 ml of *dilute sulphuric acid R*. After 15 min, any opalescence in the solution is not more intense than that in a mixture of 5 ml of solution S and 6 ml of *distilled water R*.

Iron (*2.4.9*): maximum 20 ppm.

Dilute 5 ml of solution S to 10 ml with *water R*.

Magnesium and alkaline-earth metals (*2.4.7*): maximum 200 ppm, calculated as Ca, determined on 10.0 g using 0.15 g of *mordant black 11 triturate R*. The volume of *0.01 M sodium edetate* used does not exceed 5.0 ml.

Sodium: maximum 0.10 per cent, if intended for use in the manufacture of parenteral preparations or haemodialysis solutions.

Atomic emission spectrometry (*2.2.22, Method I*).

Test solution. Dissolve 1.00 g of the substance to be examined in *water R* and dilute to 100.0 ml with the same solvent.

Reference solutions. Prepare the reference solutions by diluting as required a solution containing 200 µg of Na per millilitre, prepared as follows: dissolve in *water R* 0.5084 g of *sodium chloride R,* previously dried at 100-105 °C for 3 h, and dilute to 1000.0 ml with the same solvent.

Wavelength: 589 nm.

Heavy metals (*2.4.8*): maximum 10 ppm.

12 ml of solution S complies with test A. Prepare the reference solution using *lead standard solution (1 ppm Pb) R.*

Loss on drying (*2.2.32*): maximum 1.0 per cent, determined on 1.000 g by drying in an oven at 105 °C for 3 h.

ASSAY

Dissolve 1.300 g in *water R* and dilute to 100.0 ml with the same solvent. To 10.0 ml of the solution add 50 ml of *water R,* 5 ml of *dilute nitric acid R,* 25.0 ml of *0.1 M silver nitrate* and 2 ml of *dibutyl phthalate R.* Shake. Titrate with *0.1 M ammonium thiocyanate,* using 2 ml of *ferric ammonium sulphate solution R2* as indicator and shaking vigorously towards the end-point.

1 ml of *0.1 M silver nitrate* is equivalent to 7.46 mg of KCl.

LABELLING

The label states:

– where applicable, that the substance is suitable for use in the manufacture of parenteral preparations;

– where applicable, that the substance is suitable for use in the manufacture of haemodialysis solutions.

07/2008:1367

PSEUDOEPHEDRINE HYDROCHLORIDE

Pseudoephedrini hydrochloridum

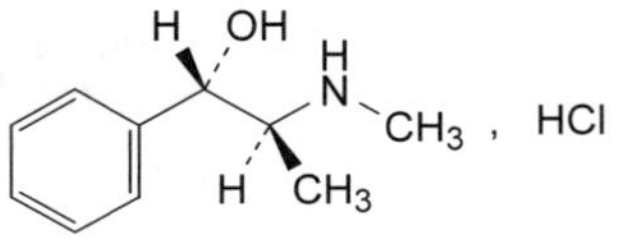

$C_{10}H_{16}ClNO$ M_r 201.7

[345-78-8]

DEFINITION

(1*S*,2*S*)-2-(Methylamino)-1-phenylpropan-1-ol hydrochloride.

Content: 99.0 per cent to 101.0 per cent (dried substance).

CHARACTERS

Appearance: white or almost white, crystalline powder or colourless crystals.

Solubility: freely soluble in water and in ethanol (96 per cent), sparingly soluble in methylene chloride.

mp: about 184 °C.

IDENTIFICATION

First identification: A, B, D.

Second identification: A, C, D.

A. Specific optical rotation (see Tests).

B. Infrared absorption spectrophotometry (*2.2.24*).

Comparison: *pseudoephedrine hydrochloride CRS.*

C. Thin-layer chromatography (*2.2.27*).

Test solution. Dissolve 20 mg of the substance to be examined in *methanol R* and dilute to 10 ml with the same solvent.

Reference solution (a). Dissolve 20 mg of *pseudoephedrine hydrochloride CRS* in *methanol R* and dilute to 10 ml with the same solvent.

Reference solution (b). Dissolve 10 mg of *ephedrine hydrochloride CRS* in reference solution (a) and dilute to 5 ml with reference solution (a).

Plate: *TLC silica gel plate R.*

Mobile phase: *methylene chloride R, concentrated ammonia R, 2-propanol R* (5:15:80 *V/V/V*).

Application: 10 µl.

Development: over 2/3 of the plate.

Drying: in air.

Detection: spray with *ninhydrin solution R* and heat at 110 °C for 5 min.

System suitability: reference solution (b):

– the chromatogram shows 2 clearly separated spots.

Results: the principal spot in the chromatogram obtained with the test solution is similar in position, colour and size to the principal spot in the chromatogram obtained with reference solution (a).

D. Solution S (see Tests) gives reaction (a) of chlorides (*2.3.1*).

TESTS

Solution S. Dissolve 1.25 g in *carbon dioxide-free water R* and dilute to 25.0 ml with the same solvent.

Appearance of solution. Solution S is clear (*2.2.1*) and colourless (*2.2.2, Method II*).

Acidity or alkalinity. Dilute 2 ml of solution S to 10 ml with *carbon dioxide-free water R.* Add 0.1 ml of *methyl red solution R* and 0.1 ml of *0.01 M sodium hydroxide*; the solution is yellow. Add 0.2 ml of *0.01 M hydrochloric acid*; the solution is red.

Specific optical rotation (*2.2.7*): + 61.0 to + 62.5 (dried substance), determined on solution S.

Related substances. Liquid chromatography (*2.2.29*).

Test solution. Dissolve 50.0 mg of the substance to be examined in the mobile phase and dilute to 25.0 ml with the mobile phase.

Reference solution (a). Dissolve 20.0 mg of *ephedrine hydrochloride CRS* (impurity A) in the mobile phase and dilute to 20.0 ml with the mobile phase. Dilute 1.0 ml of this solution to 50.0 ml with the mobile phase.

Reference solution (b). Dilute 1.0 ml of the test solution to 200.0 ml with the mobile phase.

Reference solution (c). Dissolve 10 mg of *ephedrine hydrochloride CRS* (impurity A) in 5 ml of the test solution and dilute to 100 ml with the mobile phase.

Column:

– *size*: l = 0.25 m, Ø = 4.6 mm;

– *stationary phase*: *phenylsilyl silica gel for chromatography R* (5 µm).

Mobile phase: mix 6 volumes of *methanol R* and 94 volumes of an 11.6 g/l solution of *ammonium acetate R* previously adjusted to pH 4.0 with *glacial acetic acid R.*

Flow rate: 1 ml/min.

Detection: spectrophotometer at 257 nm.

Monographs L-P

Injection: 20 μl.

Run time: 1.5 times the retention time of pseudoephedrine.

Relative retention with reference to pseudoephedrine (retention time = about 18 min): impurity A = about 0.9.

System suitability: reference solution (c):

– *resolution*: minimum 2.0 between the peaks due to impurity A and pseudoephedrine; if necessary, reduce the content of methanol in the mobile phase.

Limits:

– *impurity A*: not more than the area of the principal peak in the chromatogram obtained with reference solution (a) (1.0 per cent);
– *any other impurity*: for each impurity, not more than the area of the principal peak in the chromatogram obtained with reference solution (b) (0.5 per cent);
– *sum of impurities other than A*: not more than twice the area of the principal peak in the chromatogram obtained with reference solution (b) (1.0 per cent);
– *disregard limit*: 0.1 times the area of the principal peak in the chromatogram obtained with reference solution (b) (0.05 per cent).

Loss on drying (*2.2.32*): maximum 0.5 per cent, determined on 1.000 g by drying in an oven at 105 °C.

Sulphated ash (*2.4.14*): maximum 0.1 per cent, determined on 1.0 g.

ASSAY

Dissolve 0.170 g in 30 ml of *ethanol (96 per cent) R*. Add 5.0 ml of *0.01 M hydrochloric acid*. Carry out a potentiometric titration (*2.2.20*), using *0.1 M sodium hydroxide*. Read the volume added between the 2 points of inflexion.

1 ml of *0.1 M sodium hydroxide* is equivalent to 20.17 mg of $C_{10}H_{16}ClNO$.

STORAGE

Protected from light.

IMPURITIES

Specified impurities: *A*.

A. ephedrine.

Monographs L-P

R

07/2008:2171

RACECADOTRIL

Racecadotrilum

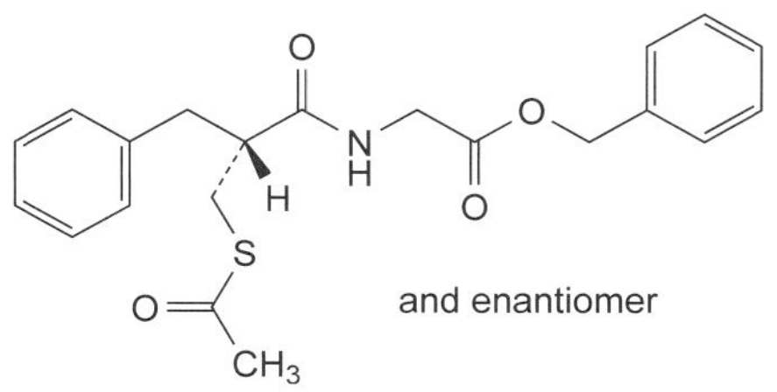

and enantiomer

$C_{21}H_{23}NO_4S$ M_r 385.5

[81110-73-8]

DEFINITION

Benzyl [[(2*RS*)-2-[(acetylsulfanyl)methyl]-3-phenylpropanoyl]amino]acetate.

Content: 98.0 per cent to 102.0 per cent (dried substance).

CHARACTERS

Appearance: white or almost white powder.

Solubility: practically insoluble in water, freely soluble in methanol and in methylene chloride.

IDENTIFICATION

A. Infrared absorption spectrophotometry (*2.2.24*).

Comparison: *racecadotril CRS*.

TESTS

Appearance of solution. The solution is clear (*2.2.1*) and not more intensely coloured than reference solution Y_6 (*2.2.2, Method II*).

Dissolve 5.0 g in 10 ml of *acetone R*.

Related substances. Liquid chromatography (*2.2.29*).

Solvent mixture: mobile phase A, mobile phase B (50:50 *V/V*).

Test solution (a). Dissolve 50.0 mg of the substance to be examined in the solvent mixture and dilute to 25.0 ml with the solvent mixture.

Test solution (b). Dilute 5.0 ml of test solution (a) to 25.0 ml with the solvent mixture.

Reference solution (a). Dilute 1.0 ml of test solution (a) to 100.0 ml with the solvent mixture. Dilute 1.0 ml of this solution to 10.0 ml with the solvent mixture.

Reference solution (b). Dilute 500 µl of *racecadotril impurity A CRS* in *acetonitrile R* and dilute to 250.0 ml with the same solvent. Dilute 1.0 ml of the solution to 10.0 ml with the solvent mixture. Dilute 1.0 ml of this solution to 100.0 ml with the solvent mixture.

Reference solution (c). Dissolve 5 mg of *racecadotril impurity G CRS* in the solvent mixture and dilute to 50 ml with the solvent mixture. To 5 ml of this solution add 1 ml of test solution (b) and dilute to 100 ml with the solvent mixture.

Reference solution (d). Dissolve 50.0 mg of *racecadotril CRS* in the solvent mixture and dilute to 25.0 ml with the solvent mixture. Dilute 5.0 ml of this solution to 25.0 ml with the solvent mixture.

Reference solution (e). Dissolve the contents of a vial of *racecadotril for peak identification CRS* (containing impurities C, E and F) in 1.0 ml of the solvent mixture.

Column:
- *size*: *l* = 0.25 m, Ø = 4.0 mm;
- *stationary phase*: *end-capped octadecylsilyl silica gel for chromatography R* (5 µm);
- *temperature*: 30 °C.

Mobile phase:
- *mobile phase A*: dissolve 1.0 g of *potassium dihydrogen phosphate R* in *water R*, adjust to pH 2.5 with *phosphoric acid R* and dilute to 1000 ml with *water R*;
- *mobile phase B*: *acetonitrile R1*;

Time (min)	Mobile phase A (per cent *V/V*)	Mobile phase B (per cent *V/V*)
0 - 5	60	40
5 - 25	60 → 20	40 → 80
25 - 35	20	80

Flow rate: 1.0 ml/min.

Detection: spectrophotometer at 210 nm.

Injection: 10 µl of the solvent mixture, test solution (a) and reference solutions (a), (b), (c) and (e).

Identification of impurities: use the chromatogram supplied with *racecadotril for peak identification CRS* and the chromatogram obtained with reference solution (e) to identify the peaks due to impurities C, E and F.

Relative retention with reference to racecadotril (retention time = about 16 min): impurity A = about 0.2; impurity C = about 0.3; impurity E = about 0.5; impurity F = about 0.9.

System suitability: reference solution (c):
- *resolution*: minimum 1.5 between the peaks due to impurity G and racecadotril.

Limits:
- *correction factors*: for the calculation of content, multiply the peak areas of the following impurities by the corresponding correction factor: impurity C = 1.4; impurity E = 0.6; impurity F = 0.7;
- *impurities C, E, F*: for each impurity, not more than twice the area of the principal peak in the chromatogram obtained with reference solution (a) (0.2 per cent);
- *impurity A*: not more than the area of the corresponding peak in the chromatogram obtained with reference solution (b) (0.1 per cent);
- *unspecified impurities*: for each impurity, not more than the area of the principal peak in the chromatogram obtained with reference solution (a) (0.10 per cent);
- *total*: not more than 5 times the area of the principal peak in the chromatogram obtained with reference solution (a) (0.5 per cent);
- *disregard limit*: 0.5 times the area of the principal peak in the chromatogram obtained with reference solution (a) (0.05 per cent).

Loss on drying (*2.2.32*): maximum 0.5 per cent, determined on 1.000 g by drying *in vacuo* at 60 °C for 4 h.

Sulphated ash (*2.4.14*): maximum 0.1 per cent, determined on 1.0 g.

ASSAY

Liquid chromatography (*2.2.29*) as described in the test for related substances with the following modification.

Injection: test solution (b) and reference solution (d).

Calculate the percentage content of $C_{21}H_{23}NO_4S$ from the declared content of *racecadotril CRS*.

IMPURITIES

Specified impurities: A, C, E, F.

Other detectable impurities (the following substances would, if present at a sufficient level, be detected by one or other of the tests in the monograph. They are limited by the general acceptance criterion for other/unspecified impurities and/or by the general monograph *Substances for pharmaceutical use (2034)*. It is therefore not necessary to identify these impurities for demonstration of compliance. See also *5.10. Control of impurities in substances for pharmaceutical use*): B, D, G, H.

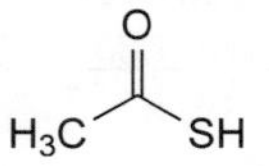

A. ethanethioic acid (thioacetic acid),

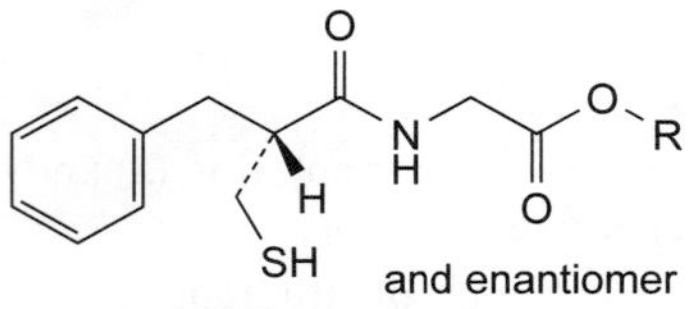

B. R = H: [[(2*RS*)-2-benzyl-3-sulfanylpropanoyl]amino]acetic acid,

G. R = CH_2-C_6H_5: benzyl [[(2*RS*)-2-benzyl-3-sulfanylpropanoyl]amino]acetate,

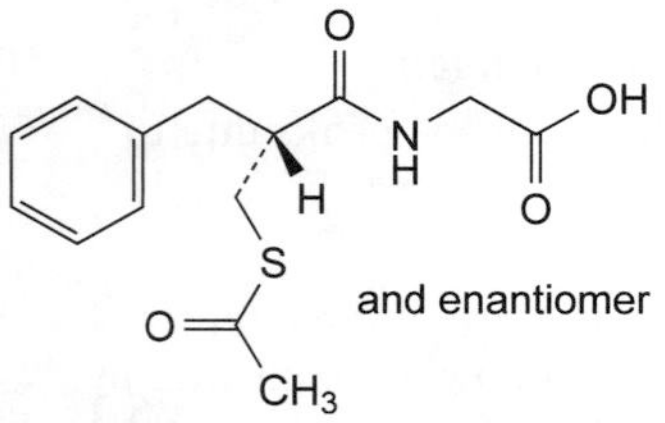

C. (2*RS*)-2-[(acetylsulfanyl)methyl]-3-phenylpropanoyl]-amino]acetic acid,

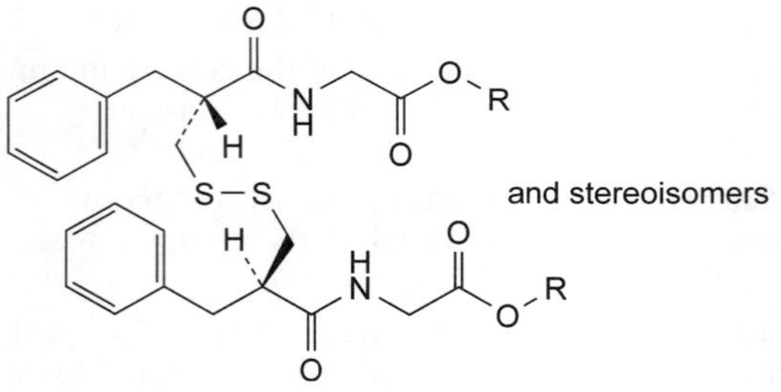

D. R = H: 5,10-dibenzyl-4,11-dioxo-7,8-dithia-3,12-diazatetradecanedioic acid,

H. R = CH_2-C_6H_5: dibenzyl 5,10-dibenzyl-4,11-dioxo-7,8-dithia-3,12-diazatetradecanedioate,

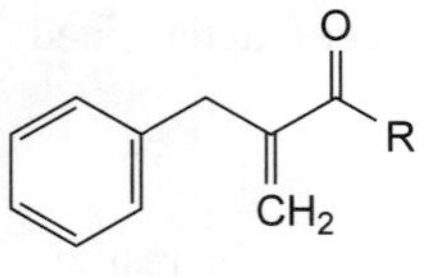

E. R = OH: 2-benzylprop-2-enoic acid (2-benzylacrylic acid),

F. R = NH-CH_2-CO-O-CH_2-C_6H_5: benzyl [(2-benzylprop-2-enoyl)amino]acetate.

07/2008:1368

RAMIPRIL

Ramiprilum

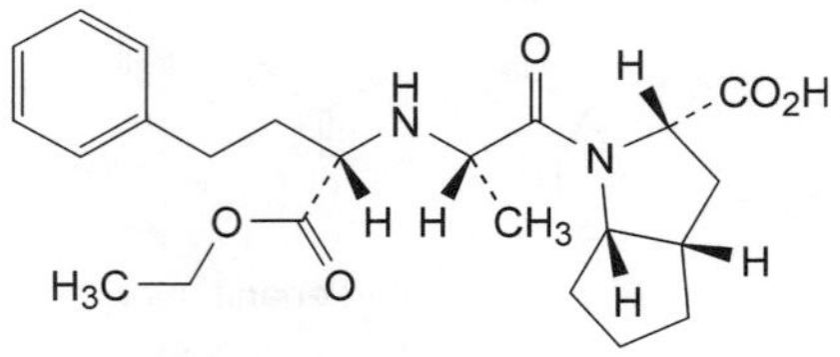

$C_{23}H_{32}N_2O_5$ M_r 416.5
[87333-19-5]

DEFINITION

(2*S*,3a*S*,6a*S*)-1-[(2*S*)-2-[[(1*S*)-1-(Ethoxycarbonyl)-3-phenylpropyl]amino]propanoyl]octahydrocyclopenta[*b*]pyrrole-2-carboxylic acid.

Content: 98.0 per cent to 101.0 per cent (dried substance).

CHARACTERS

Appearance: white or almost white, crystalline powder.

Solubility: sparingly soluble in water, freely soluble in methanol.

IDENTIFICATION

A. Specific optical rotation (see Tests).

B. Infrared absorption spectrophotometry (*2.2.24*).
Comparison: *ramipril CRS*.

TESTS

Appearance of solution. The solution is clear (*2.2.1*) and colourless (*2.2.2, Method II*).

Dissolve 0.1 g in *methanol R* and dilute to 10 ml with the same solvent.

Specific optical rotation (*2.2.7*): + 32.0 to + 38.0 (dried substance).

Dissolve 0.250 g in a mixture of 14 volumes of *hydrochloric acid R1* and 86 volumes of *methanol R* and dilute to 25.0 ml with the same mixture of solvents.

Related substances. Liquid chromatography (*2.2.29*).

Test solution. Dissolve 20.0 mg of the substance to be examined in mobile phase A and dilute to 20.0 ml with mobile phase A.

Reference solution (a). Dissolve 5 mg of *ramipril impurity A CRS*, 5 mg of *ramipril impurity B CRS*, 5 mg of *ramipril impurity C CRS* and 5 mg of *ramipril impurity D CRS* in 5 ml of the test solution, and dilute to 10 ml with mobile phase B.

Reference solution (b). Dilute 5.0 ml of the test solution to 100.0 ml with mobile phase B. Dilute 5.0 ml of this solution to 50.0 ml with mobile phase B.

Reference solution (c). Dilute 1.0 ml of reference solution (b) to 10.0 ml with mobile phase B.

Column:

– *size*: *l* = 0.25 m, Ø = 4.0 mm;
– *stationary phase*: *octadecylsilyl silica gel for chromatography R* (3 µm);
– *temperature*: 65 °C.

Mobile phase:

- *mobile phase A*: dissolve 2.0 g of *sodium perchlorate R* in a mixture of 0.5 ml of *triethylamine R* and 800 ml of *water R*; adjust to pH 3.6 with *phosphoric acid R* and add 200 ml of *acetonitrile R1*;
- *mobile phase B*: dissolve 2.0 g of *sodium perchlorate R* in a mixture of 0.5 ml of *triethylamine R* and 300 ml of *water R*; adjust to pH 2.6 with *phosphoric acid R* and add 700 ml of *acetonitrile R1*;

Time (min)	Mobile phase A (per cent *V/V*)	Mobile phase B (per cent *V/V*)
0 - 6	90	10
6 - 7	90 → 75	10 → 25
7 - 20	75 → 65	25 → 35
20 - 30	65 → 25	35 → 75
30 - 50	25	75

Flow rate: 1.0 ml/min.

Detection: spectrophotometer at 210 nm.

Equilibration: with the mobile phase at the initial composition for at least 35 min; if a suitable baseline cannot be obtained, use another grade of triethylamine.

Injection: 10 μl.

Relative retention with reference to ramipril (retention time = about 18 min): impurity A = about 0.8; impurity B = about 1.3; impurity G = about 1.4; impurity C = about 1.5; impurity D = about 1.7; impurity O = about 2.4.

System suitability:

- *resolution*: minimum 3.0 between the peaks due to impurity A and ramipril in the chromatogram obtained with reference solution (a);
- *signal-to-noise ratio*: minimum 3 for the principal peak in the chromatogram obtained with reference solution (c);
- *symmetry factor*: 0.8 to 2.0 for the peak due to ramipril in the chromatogram obtained with the test solution.

Limits:

- *correction factor*: for the calculation of content, multiply the peak area of impurity C by 2.4;
- *impurities A, B, C, D*: for each impurity, not more than the area of the principal peak in the chromatogram obtained with reference solution (b) (0.5 per cent);
- *unspecified impurities*: for each impurity, not more than 0.2 times the area of the principal peak in the chromatogram obtained with reference solution (b) (0.10 per cent);
- *total*: not more than twice the area of the principal peak in the chromatogram obtained with reference solution (b) (1.0 per cent);
- *disregard limit*: the area of the principal peak in the chromatogram obtained with reference solution (c) (0.05 per cent).

Palladium: maximum 20.0 ppm.

Atomic absorption spectrometry (*2.2.23, Method I*).

Test solution. Dissolve 0.200 g in a mixture of 0.3 volumes of *nitric acid R* and 99.7 volumes of *water R*, and dilute to 100.0 ml with the same mixture of solvents.

Reference solutions. Use solutions containing 0.02 μg, 0.03 μg and 0.05 μg of palladium per millilitre, freshly prepared by dilution of *palladium standard solution (0.5 ppm Pd) R* with a mixture of 0.3 volumes of *nitric acid R* and 99.7 volumes of *water R*.

Modifier solution. Dissolve 0.150 g of *magnesium nitrate R* in a mixture of 0.3 volumes of *nitric acid R* and 99.7 volumes of *water R*, and dilute to 100.0 ml with the same mixture of solvents.

Injection: 20 μl of the test solution and the reference solution, and 10 μl of the modifier solution.

Source: palladium hollow-cathode lamp using a transmission band preferably of 1 nm and a graphite tube.

Wavelength: 247.6 nm.

Loss on drying (*2.2.32*): maximum 0.2 per cent, determined on 1.000 g by drying in an oven under high vacuum at 60 °C for 4 h.

Sulphated ash (*2.4.14*): maximum 0.1 per cent, determined on 1.0 g.

ASSAY

Dissolve 0.300 g in 25 ml of *methanol R* and add 25 ml of *water R*. Titrate with *0.1 M sodium hydroxide*, determining the end-point potentiometrically (*2.2.20*). Carry out a blank titration.

1 ml of *0.1 M sodium hydroxide* is equivalent to 41.65 mg of $C_{23}H_{32}N_2O_5$.

STORAGE

Protected from light.

IMPURITIES

Specified impurities: *A, B, C, D*.

Other detectable impurities (the following substances would, if present at a sufficient level, be detected by one or other of the tests in the monograph. They are limited by the general acceptance criterion for other/unspecified impurities and/or by the general monograph *Substances for pharmaceutical use (2034)*. It is therefore not necessary to identify these impurities for demonstration of compliance. See also *5.10. Control of impurities in substances for pharmaceutical use*): *E, F, G, H, I, J, K, L, M, N, O*.

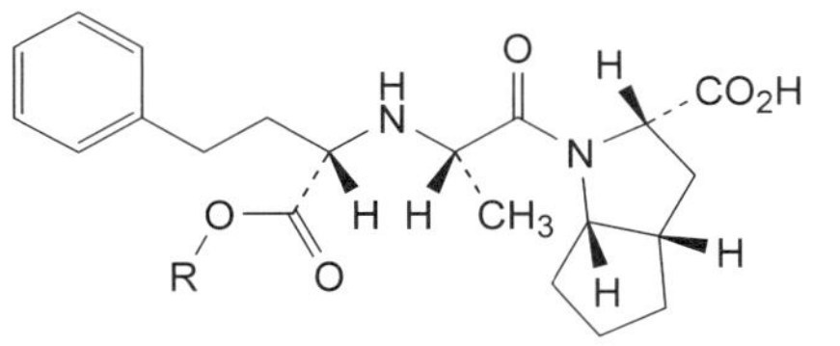

A. R = CH_3: (2*S*,3a*S*,6a*S*)-1-[(2*S*)-2-[[(1*S*)-1-(methoxy-carbonyl)-3-phenylpropyl]amino]propanoyl]octahydro-cyclopenta[*b*]pyrrole-2-carboxylic acid (ramipril methyl ester),

B. R = $CH(CH_3)_2$: (2*S*,3a*S*,6a*S*)-1-[(2*S*)-2-[[(1*S*)-1-[(1-methyl-ethoxy)carbonyl]-3-phenylpropyl]amino]propanoyl]-octahydrocyclopenta[*b*]pyrrole-2-carboxylic acid (ramipril isopropyl ester),

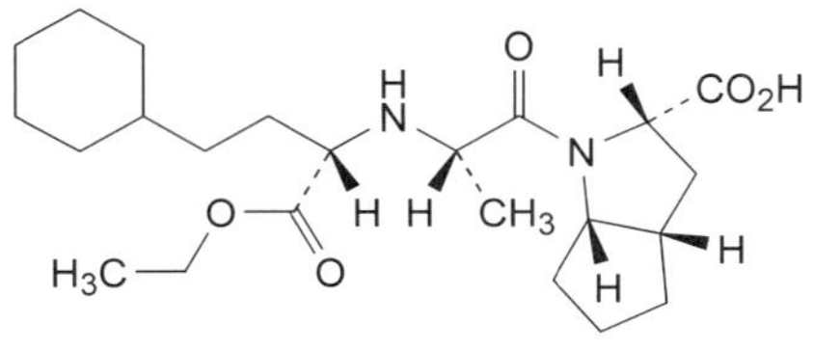

C. (2*S*,3a*S*,6a*S*)-1-[(2*S*)-2-[[(1*S*)-3-cyclohexyl-1-(ethoxy-carbonyl)-propyl]amino]propanoyl]octahydrocyclo-penta[*b*]pyrrole-2-carboxylic acid (hexahydroramipril),

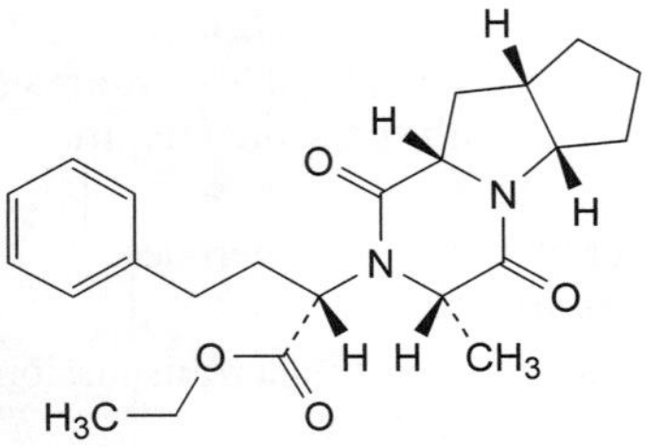

D. ethyl (2*S*)-2-[(3*S*,5a*S*,8a*S*,9a*S*)-3-methyl-1,4-dioxo-decahydro-2*H*-cyclopenta[4,5]pyrrolo[1,2-*a*]pyrazin-2-yl]-4-phenylbutanoate (ramipril diketopiperazine),

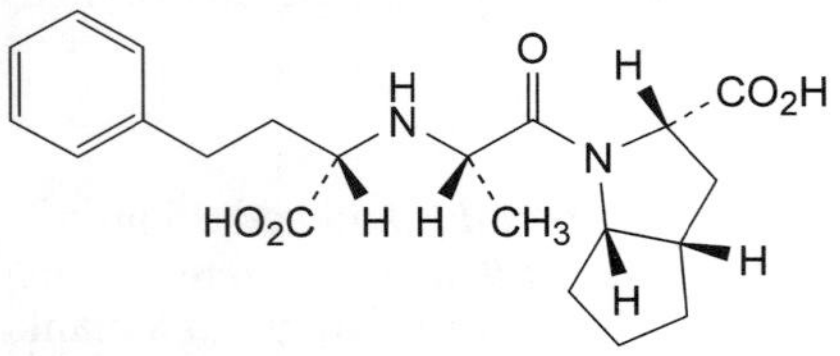

E. (2*S*,3a*S*,6a*S*)-1-[(2*S*)-2-[[(1*S*)-1-carboxy-3-phenylpropyl]-amino]propanoyl]octahydrocyclopenta[*b*]pyrrole-2-carboxylic acid (ramipril diacid),

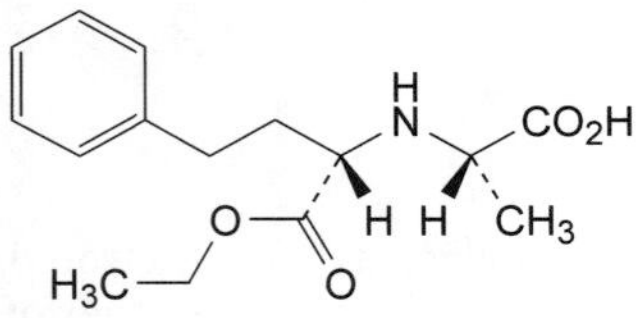

F. (2*S*)-2-[[(1*S*)-1-(ethoxycarbonyl)-3-phenylpropyl]amino]-propanoic acid,

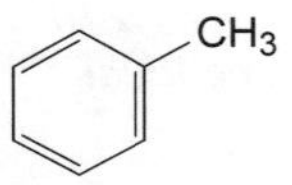

G. methylbenzene (toluene),

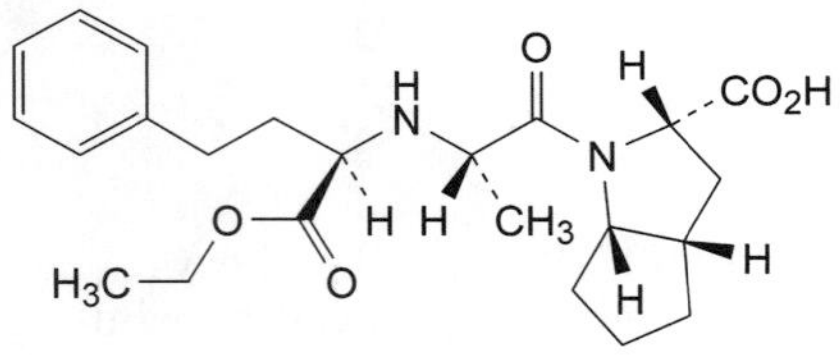

H. (2*S*,3a*S*,6a*S*)-1-[(2*S*)-2-[[(1*R*)-1-(ethoxycarbonyl)-3-phenyl-propyl]amino]propanoyl]octahydrocyclopenta-[*b*]pyrrole-2-carboxylic acid ((*R*,*S*,*S*,*S*,*S*)-epimer of ramipril),

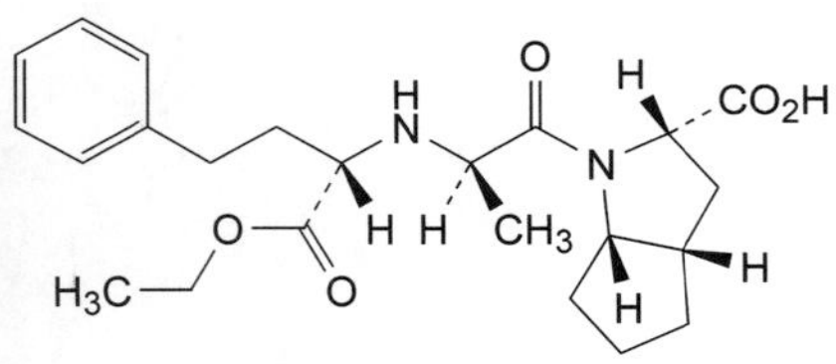

I. (2*S*,3a*S*,6a*S*)-1-[(2*R*)-2-[[(1*S*)-1-(ethoxycarbonyl)-3-phenyl-propyl]amino]propanoyl]octahydrocyclopenta-[*b*]pyrrole-2-carboxylic acid ((*S*,*R*,*S*,*S*,*S*)-epimer of ramipril),

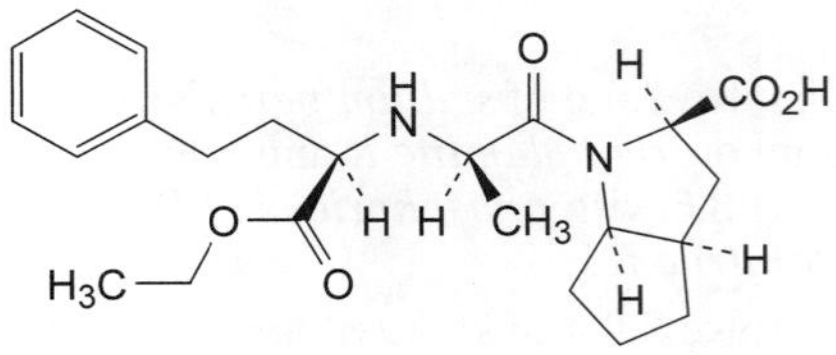

J. (2*R*,3a*R*,6a*R*)-1-[(2*R*)-2-[[(1*R*)-1-(ethoxycarbonyl)-3-phenyl-propyl]amino]propanoyl]octahydrocyclopenta-[*b*]pyrrole-2-carboxylic acid (enantiomer of ramipril),

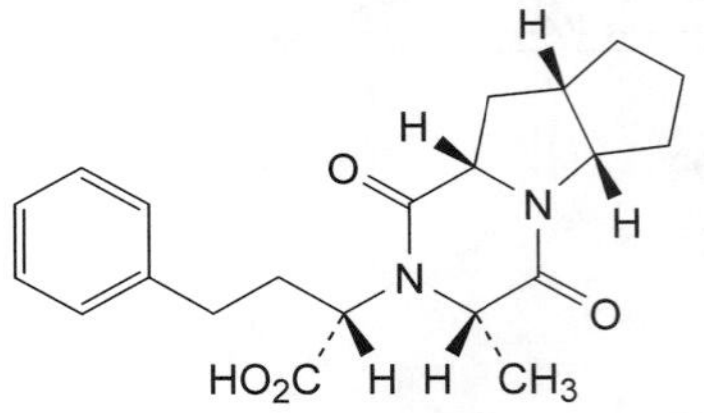

K. (2*S*)-2-[(3*S*,5a*S*,8a*S*,9a*S*)-3-methyl-1,4-dioxodecahydro-2*H*-cyclopenta[4,5]pyrrolo[1,2-*a*]pyrazin-2-yl]-4-phenyl-butanoic acid (ramipril diketopiperazine acid),

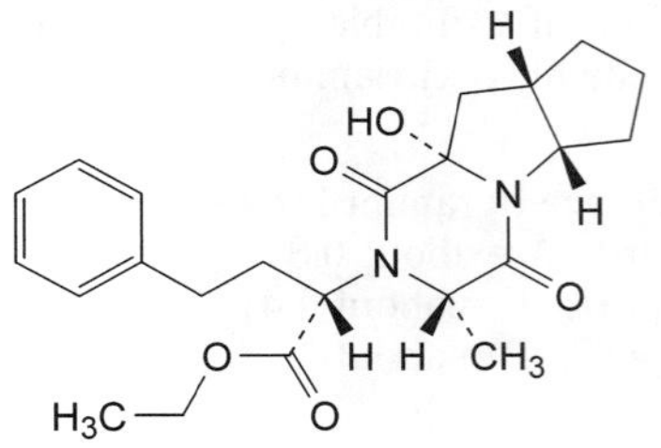

L. ethyl (2S)-2-[(3*S*,5a*S*,8a*S*,9a*S*)-9a-hydroxy-3-methyl-1,4-dioxodecahydro-2*H*-cyclopenta[4,5]pyrrolo[1,2-*a*]-pyrazin-2-yl]-4-phenylbutanoate (ramipril hydroxydiketopiperazine),

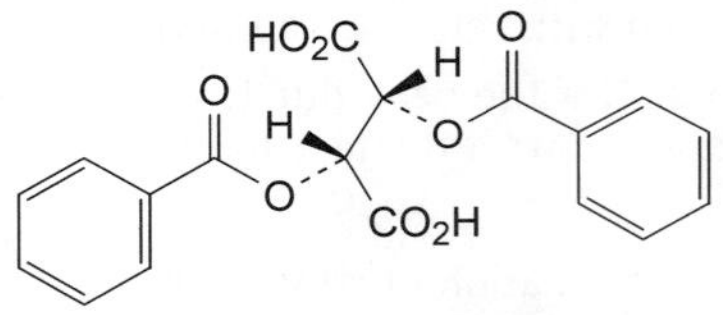

M. (2*R*,3*R*)-2,3-bis(benzoyloxy)butanedioic acid (dibenzoyltartric acid),

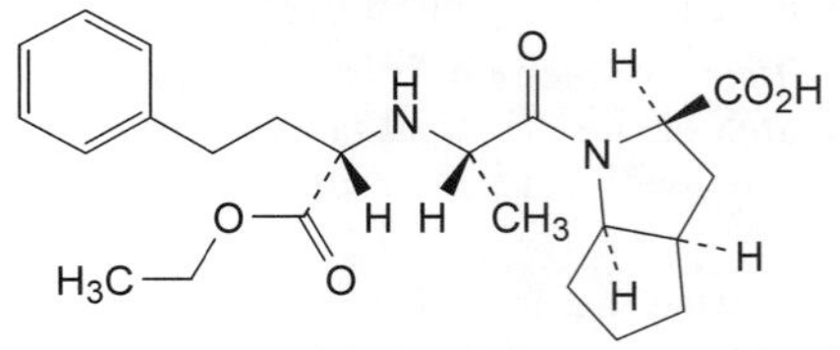

N. (2*R*,3a*R*,6a*R*)-1-[(2*S*)-2-[[(1*S*)-1-(ethoxycarbonyl)-3-phenyl-propyl]amino]propanoyl]octahydrocyclopenta-[*b*]pyrrole-2-carboxylic acid ((*S*,*S*,*R*,*R*,*R*)-isomer of ramipril),

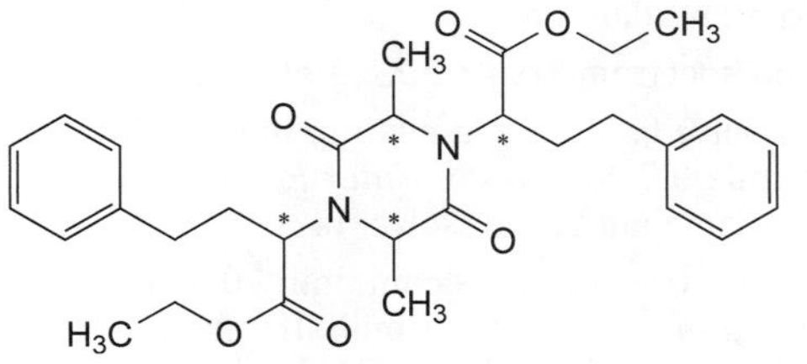

O. diethyl 2,2′-(2,5-dimethyl-3,6-dioxopiperazine-1,4-diyl)bis(4-phenylbutanoate).

01/2008:1369
corrected 6.2

RAPESEED OIL, REFINED

Rapae oleum raffinatum

DEFINITION

Fatty oil obtained from the seeds of *Brassica napus* L. and *Brassica campestris* L. by mechanical expression or by extraction. It is then refined. A suitable antioxidant may be added.

CHARACTERS

Appearance: clear, light yellow liquid.

Solubility: practically insoluble in water and in ethanol (96 per cent), miscible with light petroleum (bp: 40-60 °C).

Relative density: about 0.917.

Refractive index: about 1.473.

IDENTIFICATION

Identification of fatty oils by thin-layer chromatography (*2.3.2*).

Results: the chromatogram obtained is similar to the typical chromatogram for rapeseed oil.

TESTS

Acid value (*2.5.1*): maximum 0.5, determined on 10.0 g.

Peroxide value (*2.5.5, Method A*): maximum 10.0.

Unsaponifiable matter (*2.5.7*): maximum 1.5 per cent, determined on 5.0 g.

Alkaline impurities (*2.4.19*). It complies with the test.

Composition of fatty acids (*2.4.22, Method A*). Use the mixture of calibrating substances in Table 2.4.22.-3.

Composition of the fatty-acid fraction of the oil:

- *palmitic acid*: 2.5 per cent to 6.0 per cent;
- *stearic acid*: maximum 3.0 per cent;
- *oleic acid*: 50.0 per cent to 67.0 per cent;
- *linoleic acid*: 16.0 per cent to 30.0 per cent;
- *linolenic acid*: 6.0 per cent to 14.0 per cent;
- *eicosenoic acid*: maximum 5.0 per cent;
- *erucic acid*: maximum 2.0 per cent.

STORAGE

In an airtight, well-filled container, protected from light.

LABELLING

The label states whether the oil is obtained by mechanical expression or by extraction.

Monographs Q-Z

S

Monographs Q-Z

01/2008:1261

SENNA LEAF DRY EXTRACT, STANDARDISED

Sennae folii extractum siccum normatum

[8055-96-7]

DEFINITION

Standardised dry extract produced from *Senna leaf (0206)*.

Content: 5.5 per cent to 8.0 per cent of hydroxyanthracene glycosides, expressed as sennoside B ($C_{42}H_{38}O_{20}$; M_r 863) (dried extract). The measured content does not deviate from the value stated on the label by more than ± 10 per cent.

PRODUCTION

The extract is produced from the herbal drug by a suitable procedure using ethanol (50-80 per cent *V/V*).

CHARACTERS

Appearance: brownish or brown powder.

IDENTIFICATION

A. Thin-layer chromatography (*2.2.27*).

Solvent mixture: *ethanol (96 per cent) R, water R* (50:50 *V/V*).

Test solution. To 0.1 g of the extract to be examined add 5 ml of the solvent mixture and heat to boiling. Cool and centrifuge. Use the supernatant liquid.

Reference solution. Dissolve 10 mg of *senna extract CRS* in 1 ml of the solvent mixture (a slight residue remains).

Plate: *TLC silica gel plate R*.

Mobile phase: *glacial acetic acid R, water R, ethyl acetate R, 1-propanol R* (1:30:40:40 *V/V/V/V*).

Application: 10 µl as bands.

Development: over a path of 10 cm.

Drying: in air.

Detection: spray with a 20 per cent *V/V* solution of *nitric acid R* and heat at 120 °C for 10 min; allow to cool and spray with a 50 g/l solution of *potassium hydroxide R* in *ethanol (50 per cent V/V) R* until the zones appear.

Results: the principal zones in the chromatogram obtained with the test solution are similar in position, colour and size to the principal zones in the chromatogram obtained with the reference solution. The chromatograms show in the lower third a prominent brown zone due to sennoside B and above it a yellow zone followed by another prominent brown zone due to sennoside A. In the upper half of the chromatograms are visible, in order of increasing R_F value, a prominent reddish-brown zone and an orange-brown zone followed by a faint pink zone and 2 yellow zones. Close to the solvent front a dark pink zone appears, which may be followed by several faint zones.

B. Place about 25 mg of the extract to be examined in a conical flask and add 50 ml of *water R* and 2 ml of *hydrochloric acid R*. Heat in a water-bath for 15 min, cool and shake with 40 ml of *ether R*. Separate the ether layer, dry over *anhydrous sodium sulphate R*, evaporate 5 ml to dryness and to the cooled residue add 5 ml of *dilute ammonia R1*. A yellow or orange colour develops. Heat on a water-bath for 2 min. A reddish-violet colour develops.

TESTS

Loss on drying (*2.8.17*): maximum 5.0 per cent.

Microbial contamination. Total viable aerobic count (*2.6.12*) not more than 10^4 micro-organisms per gram, of which not more than 10^2 fungi per gram, determined by plate-count. It complies with the tests for *Escherichia coli* and *Salmonella* (*2.6.13*).

ASSAY

Carry out the assay protected from bright light.

Place 0.150 g of the extract to be examined in a 100 ml flask, dissolve in *water R* and dilute to 100.0 ml with the same solvent. Filter the solution, discard the first 10 ml of the filtrate. Transfer 20.0 ml of the filtrate to a 150 ml separating funnel. Add 0.1 ml of *dilute hydrochloric acid R* and shake with 3 quantities, each of 15 ml, of *ether R*. Allow the layers to separate and discard the ether layer. Add 0.10 g of *sodium hydrogen carbonate R* to the aqueous layer and shake for 3 min. Centrifuge and transfer 10.0 ml of the supernatant liquid to a 100 ml round-bottomed flask with a ground-glass neck. Add 20 ml of *ferric chloride solution R1* and mix. Heat for 20 min under a reflux condenser in a water-bath with the water level above that of the liquid in the flask; add 3 ml of *hydrochloric acid R* and heat for a further 30 min with frequent shaking to dissolve the precipitate. Cool, transfer the mixture to a separating funnel and shake with 3 quantities, each of 25 ml, of *ether R* previously used to rinse the flask. Combine the ether layers and wash with 2 quantities, each of 15 ml, of *water R*. Transfer the ether layers to a volumetric flask and dilute to 100.0 ml with *ether R*. Evaporate 10.0 ml carefully to dryness and dissolve the residue in 10.0 ml of a 5.0 g/l solution of *magnesium acetate R* in *methanol R*. Measure the absorbance (*2.2.25*) at 515 nm using *methanol R* as the compensation liquid.

Calculate the percentage content of hydroxyanthracene glycosides expressed as sennoside B using the following expression:

$$\frac{A \times 4.167}{m}$$

i.e. taking the specific absorbance of sennoside B to be 240.

A = absorbance at 515 nm;

m = mass of the herbal drug to be examined, in grams.

LABELLING

The label states the content of hydroxyanthracene glycosides.

01/2008:1149

SHELLAC

Lacca

DEFINITION

Purified material obtained from the resinous secretion of the female insect *Kerria lacca* (Kerr) Lindinger (*Laccifer lacca* Kerr). There are 4 types of shellac depending on the nature of the treatment of crude secretion (seedlac): wax-containing shellac, bleached shellac, dewaxed shellac and bleached, dewaxed shellac.

Wax-containing shellac is obtained from seedlac: it is purified by filtration of the molten substance and/or by hot extraction using a suitable solvent.

Bleached shellac is obtained from seedlac by treatment with sodium hypochlorite after dissolution in a suitable alkaline solution, precipitation by dilute acid and drying.

Dewaxed shellac is obtained from wax-containing shellac or seedlac by treatment with a suitable solvent and removal of the insoluble wax by filtering.

Bleached, dewaxed shellac is obtained from wax-containing shellac or seedlac by treatment with sodium hypochlorite after dissolution in a suitable alkaline solution; the insoluble wax is removed by filtration. It is precipitated by dilute acid and dried.

CHARACTERS

Appearance: brownish-orange or yellow, shining, translucent, hard or brittle, more or less thin flakes (wax-containing shellac and dewaxed shellac), or a creamy white or brownish-yellow powder (bleached shellac and bleached, dewaxed shellac).

Solubility: practically insoluble in water, gives a more or less opalescent solution (wax containing shellac and bleached shellac) or a clear solution (dewaxed shellac and bleached, dewaxed shellac) in anhydrous ethanol. When warmed it is sparingly soluble or soluble in alkaline solutions.

IDENTIFICATION

A. Thin-layer chromatography (*2.2.27*).

Test solution. Heat 0.25 g of the powdered substance (500) (*2.9.12*) on a water-bath with 2 ml of *dilute sodium hydroxide solution R* for 5 min. Cool, add 5 ml of *ethyl acetate R* and slowly, with stirring, 2 ml of *dilute acetic acid R*. Shake and filter the upper layer through *anhydrous sodium sulphate R*.

Reference solution. Dissolve 6.0 mg of *aleuritic acid R* in 1.0 ml of *methanol R*, heating slightly if necessary.

Plate: *TLC silica gel F_{254} plate R*.

Mobile phase: *acetic acid R, methanol R, methylene chloride R, ethyl acetate R* (1:8:32:60 *V/V/V/V*).

Application: 10 µl, as bands.

Development: twice over a path of 15 cm.

Drying: in air.

Detection: spray with *anisaldehyde solution R*, heat at 100-105 °C for 5-10 min and examine in daylight.

Results: the chromatogram obtained with the test solution shows several coloured zones, one of which is similar in position and colour to the zone in the chromatogram obtained with the reference solution. Above this zone the chromatogram obtained with the test solution shows a pink zone and below it several violet zones. Below the zone due to aleuritic acid, there is a light blue zone (shellolic acid) accompanied by zones of the same colour but of lower intensity. Other faint grey and violet zones may be visible.

B. Examine the chromatograms obtained in the test for colophony.

Results: for wax-containing shellac, in the chromatogram obtained with the test solution, a more or less strong bluish-grey zone is visible, just above the zone due to thymolphthalein in the chromatogram obtained with the reference solution; for dewaxed shellac, no such zone is visible just above the zone due to thymolphthalein in the chromatogram obtained with the reference solution.

TESTS

Acid value (*2.5.1*): 65 to 95 (dried substance).

Examine 1.00 g of the coarsely ground substance. Determine the end-point potentiometrically (*2.2.20*).

Colophony. Thin-layer chromatography (*2.2.27*) as described under identification test A with the following modifications.

Test solution. Dissolve 50 mg of the powdered substance (500) (*2.9.12*), with heating, in a mixture of 0.5 ml of *methylene chloride R* and 0.5 ml of *methanol R*.

Reference solution. Dissolve 2.0 mg of *thymolphthalein R* in 1.0 ml of *methanol R*.

Detection: examine in ultraviolet light at 254 nm; mark the quenching zones in the chromatogram obtained with the test solution that have similar R_F values to that of the quenching zone due to thymolphthalein in the chromatogram obtained with the reference solution; spray with *anisaldehyde solution R*, heat at 100-105 °C for 5-10 min and examine in daylight.

Results: the chromatogram obtained with the reference solution shows a principal zone with a reddish-violet colour (thymolphthalein). None of the quenching zones in the chromatogram obtained with the test solution that have an R_F value similar to the zone due to thymolphthalein in the reference solution show a more or less strong violet or brownish colour (colophony). Disregard any faint violet zone at this level that does not show quenching before spraying and heating.

Arsenic (*2.4.2, Method A*): maximum 3 ppm.

Introduce 0.33 g of the substance to be examined and 5 ml of *sulphuric acid R* into a combustion flask. Carefully add a few millilitres of *strong hydrogen peroxide solution R* and heat to boiling until a clear, colourless solution is obtained. Continue heating to eliminate the water and as much sulphuric acid as possible and dilute to 25 ml with *water R*.

Heavy metals (*2.4.8*): maximum 10 ppm.

2.0 g complies with test D. Prepare the reference solution using 2 ml of *lead standard solution (10 ppm Pb) R*.

Loss on drying (*2.2.32*): maximum 2.0 per cent for unbleached shellac and maximum 6.0 per cent for bleached shellac, determined on 1.000 g of the powdered substance (500) (*2.9.12*) by drying in an oven at 40-45 °C for 24 h.

STORAGE

Protected from light. Store bleached shellac and bleached, dewaxed shellac at a temperature not exceeding 15 °C.

LABELLING

The label indicates the type of shellac.

07/2008:1472

SODIUM HYALURONATE

Natrii hyaluronas

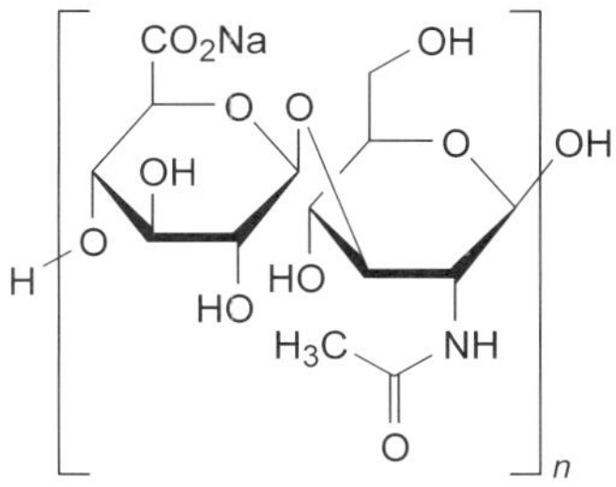

$(C_{14}H_{20}NNaO_{11})_n$
[9067-32-7]

DEFINITION

Sodium salt of hyaluronic acid, a glycosaminoglycan consisting of D-glucuronic acid and *N*-acetyl-D-glucosamine disaccharide units.

Content: 95.0 per cent to 105.0 per cent (dried substance).

Intrinsic viscosity: 90 per cent to 120 per cent of the value stated on the label.

PRODUCTION

It is extracted from cocks' combs or obtained by fermentation from *Streptococci,* Lancefield Groups A and C. When produced by fermentation of gram-positive bacteria, the process must be shown to reduce or eliminate pyrogenic or inflammatory components of the cell wall.

CHARACTERS

Appearance: white or almost white, very hygroscopic powder or fibrous aggregate.

Solubility: sparingly soluble or soluble in water, practically insoluble in acetone and in anhydrous ethanol.

IDENTIFICATION

A. Infrared absorption spectrophotometry (*2.2.24*).

Comparison: *Ph. Eur. reference spectrum of sodium hyaluronate.*

B. It gives reaction (a) of sodium (*2.3.1*).

TESTS

Solution S. Weigh a quantity of the substance to be examined equivalent to 0.10 g of the dried substance and add 30.0 ml of a 9 g/l solution of *sodium chloride R*. Mix gently on a shaker until dissolved (about 12 h).

Appearance of solution. Solution S is clear (*2.2.1*) and its absorbance (*2.2.25*) at 600 nm is not greater than 0.01.

pH (*2.2.3*): 5.0 to 8.5.

Dissolve the substance to be examined in *carbon dioxide-free water R* to obtain a solution containing a quantity equivalent to 5 mg of the dried substance per millilitre.

Intrinsic viscosity. *Sodium hyaluronate is very hygroscopic and must be protected from moisture during weighing.*

Buffer solution (0.15 M sodium chloride in 0.01 M phosphate buffer solution pH 7.0). Dissolve 0.78 g of *sodium dihydrogen phosphate R* and 4.50 g of *sodium chloride R* in *water R* and dilute to 500.0 ml with the same solvent (solution A). Dissolve 1.79 g of *disodium hydrogen phosphate R* and 4.50 g of *sodium chloride R* in *water R* and dilute to 500.0 ml with the same solvent (solution B). Mix solutions A and B until a pH of 7.0 is reached. Filter through a sintered-glass filter (4) (*2.1.2*).

Test solution (a). Weigh 0.200 g (m_{0p}) *(NOTE: this value is only indicative and should be adjusted after an initial measurement of the viscosity of test solution (a))* of the substance to be examined and dilute with 50.0 g (m_{0s}) of buffer solution at 4 °C. Mix the solution by shaking at 4 °C during 24 h. Weigh 5.00 g (m_{1p}) of the solution and dilute with 100.0 g (m_{1s}) of buffer solution at 25 °C. Mix this solution by shaking for 20 min. Filter the solution through a sintered-glass filter (100) (*2.1.2*), and discard the first 10 ml.

Test solution (b). Weigh 30.0 g (m_{2p}) of test solution (a) and dilute with 10.0 g (m_{2s}) of buffer solution at 25 °C. Mix this solution by shaking for 20 min. Filter the solution through a sintered-glass filter (100) (*2.1.2*) and discard the first 10 ml.

Test solution (c). Weigh 20.0 g (m_{3p}) of test solution (a) and dilute with 20.0 g (m_{3s}) of buffer solution at 25 °C. Mix this solution by shaking for 20 min. Filter the solution through a sintered-glass filter (100) (*2.1.2*) and discard the first 10 ml.

Test solution (d). Weigh 10.0 g (m_{4p}) of test solution (a) and dilute with 30.0 g (m_{4s}) of buffer solution at 25 °C. Mix this solution by shaking for 20 min. Filter the solution through a sintered-glass filter (100) (*2.1.2*) and discard the first 10 ml.

Determine the flow-times (*2.2.9*) for the buffer solution (t_0) and for the 4 test solutions (t_1, t_2, t_3 and t_4), at 25.00 ± 0.03 °C. Use an appropriate suspended level viscometer (specifications: viscometer constant about 0.005 mm^2/s^2, kinematic viscosity of 1-5 mm^2/s, internal diameter of tube *R* 0.53 mm, volume of bulb *C* 5.6 ml, internal diameter of tube *N* 2.8-3.2 mm) with a funnel-shaped lower capillary end. Use the same viscometer for all measurements; measure all outflow times in triplicate. The test is not valid unless the results do not differ by more than 0.35 per cent from the mean and if the flow time t_1 is not less than 1.6 and not more than 1.8 times t_0. If this is not the case, adjust the value of m_{0p} and repeat the procedure.

Calculation of the relative viscosities

Since the densities of the sodium hyaluronate solutions and of the solvent are almost equal, the relative viscosities η_{ri} (being η_{r1}, η_{r2}, η_{r3} and η_{r4}) can be calculated from the ratio of the flow times for the respective solutions t_i (being t_1, t_2, $t_3$and t_4) to the flow time of the solvent t_0, but taking into account the kinetic energy correction factor for the capillary (B = 30 800 s^3), using the following expression:

$$\frac{t_i - \frac{B}{t_i^2}}{t_0 - \frac{B}{t_0^2}}$$

Calculation of the concentrations

Calculate the concentration c_1 (expressed in kg/m^3) of sodium hyaluronate in test solution (a) using the following expression:

$$\frac{m_{0p} \times x \times (100 - h) \times m_{1p} \times \rho_{25}}{100 \times 100 \times (m_{0p} + m_{0s}) \times (m_{1p} + m_{1s})}$$

x = percentage content of sodium hyaluronate as determined under Assay;

h = percentage loss on drying;

ρ_{25} = 1005 kg/m^3 (density of the test solution at 25 °C).

Monographs Q-Z

Calculate the concentration c_2 (expressed in kg/m^3) of sodium hyaluronate in test solution (b) using the following expression:

$$c_1 \times \frac{m_{2p}}{m_{2s} + m_{2p}}$$

Calculate the concentration c_3 (expressed in kg/m^3) of sodium hyaluronate in test solution (c) using the following expression:

$$c_1 \times \frac{m_{3p}}{m_{3s} + m_{3p}}$$

Calculate the concentration c_4 (expressed in kg/m^3) of sodium hyaluronate in test solution (d) using the following expression:

$$c_1 \times \frac{m_{4p}}{m_{4s} + m_{4p}}$$

Calculation of the intrinsic viscosity

Calculate the intrinsic viscosity $[\eta]$ by linear least-squares regression analysis using the Martin equation:

$$\log\left(\frac{\eta_r - 1}{c}\right) = \log[\eta] + k[\eta]c$$

The decimal antilogarithm of the intercept is the intrinsic viscosity expressed in m^3/kg.

Sulphated glycosaminoglycans: maximum 1 per cent, if the product is extracted from cocks' combs.

Appropriate safety precautions are to be taken when handling perchloric acid at elevated temperature.

Test solution. Introduce a quantity of the substance to be examined equivalent to 50.0 mg of the dried substance into a test-tube 150 mm long and 16 mm in internal diameter and dissolve in 1.0 ml of *perchloric acid R.*

Reference solution. Dissolve 0.149 g of *anhydrous sodium sulphate R* in *water R* and dilute to 100.0 ml with the same solvent. Dilute 10.0 ml of this solution to 100.0 ml with *water R.* Evaporate 1.0 ml in a test-tube 150 mm long and 16 mm in internal diameter in a heating block at 90-95 °C, and dissolve the residue in 1.0 ml of *perchloric acid R.*

Plug each test-tube with a piece of glass wool. Place the test-tubes in a heating block or a silicone oil bath maintained at 180 °C and heat until clear, colourless solutions are obtained (about 12 h). Remove the test-tubes and cool to room temperature. Add to each test-tube 3.0 ml of a 33.3 g/l solution of *barium chloride R,* cap and shake vigorously. Allow the test-tubes to stand for 30 min. Shake each test-tube once again, and determine the absorbance (*2.2.25*) at 660 nm, using *water R* as a blank.

The absorbance obtained with the test solution is not greater than the absorbance obtained with the reference solution.

Nucleic acids. The absorbance (*2.2.25*) of solution S at 260 nm is maximum 0.5.

Protein: maximum 0.3 per cent; maximum 0.1 per cent, if intended for use in the manufacture of parenteral preparations.

Test solution (a). Dissolve the substance to be examined in *water R* to obtain a solution containing a quantity equivalent to about 10 mg of the dried substance per millilitre.

Test solution (b). Mix equal volumes of test solution (a) and *water R.*

Reference solutions. Prepare a 0.5 mg/ml stock solution of *bovine albumin R* in *water R.* Prepare 5 dilutions of the stock solution containing between 5 μg/ml and 50 μg/ml of *bovine albumin R.*

Add 2.5 ml of freshly prepared *cupri-tartaric solution R3* to test-tubes containing 2.5 ml of *water R* (blank), 2.5 ml of the test solutions (a) or (b) or 2.5 ml of the reference solutions. Mix after each addition. After about 10 min, add to each test-tube 0.50 ml of a mixture of equal volumes of *phosphomolybdotungstic reagent R* and *water R* prepared immediately before use. Mix after each addition. After 30 min, measure the absorbance (*2.2.25*) of each solution at 750 nm against the blank. From the calibration curve obtained with the 5 reference solutions determine the content of protein in the test solutions.

Chlorides (*2.4.4*): maximum 0.5 per cent.

Dissolve 67 mg in 100 ml of *water R.*

Iron: maximum 80.0 ppm.

Atomic absorption spectrometry (*2.2.23, Method II*).

Test solution. Dissolve a quantity of the substance to be examined equivalent to 0.25 g of the dried substance in 1 ml of *nitric acid R* by heating on a water-bath. Cool and dilute to 10.0 ml with *water R.*

Reference solutions. Prepare 2 reference solutions in the same manner as the test solution, adding 1.0 ml and 2.0 ml respectively of *iron standard solution (10 ppm Fe) R* to the dissolved substance to be examined.

Source: iron hollow-cathode lamp using a transmission band of 0.2 nm.

Wavelength: 248.3 nm.

Atomisation device: air-acetylene flame.

Heavy metals (*2.4.8*): maximum 20 ppm; maximum 10 ppm if intended for use in the manufacture of parenteral preparations.

1.0 g complies with test F. Prepare the reference solution using 2.0 ml of *lead standard solution (10 ppm Pb) R.*

Loss on drying (*2.2.32*): maximum 20.0 per cent, determined on 0.500 g by drying at 100-110 °C over *diphosphorus pentoxide R* for 6 h.

Microbial contamination. Total viable aerobic count (*2.6.12*) not more than 10^2 micro-organisms per gram. Use 1 g of the substance to be examined.

Bacterial endotoxins (*2.6.14*): less than 0.5 IU/mg, if intended for use in the manufacture of parenteral preparations without a further appropriate procedure for the removal of bacterial endotoxins; less than 0.05 IU/mg, if intended for use in the manufacture of intra-ocular preparations or intra-articular preparations without a further appropriate procedure for the removal of bacterial endotoxins.

Monographs Q-Z

ASSAY

Determine the glucuronic acid content by reaction with carbazole as described below.

Reagent A. Dissolve 0.95 g of *disodium tetraborate R* in 100.0 ml of *sulphuric acid R*.

Reagent B. Dissolve 0.125 g of *carbazole R* in 100.0 ml of *anhydrous ethanol R*.

Test solution. Prepare this solution in triplicate. Dissolve 0.170 g of the substance to be examined in *water R* and dilute to 100.0 g with the same solvent. Dilute 10.0 g of this solution to 200.0 g with *water R*.

Reference stock solution. Dissolve 0.100 g of *D-glucuronic acid R*, previously dried to constant mass in vacuum over *diphosphorus pentoxide R* (*2.2.32*), in *water R* and dilute to 100.0 g with the same solvent.

Reference solutions. Prepare 5 dilutions of the reference stock solution containing between 6.5 μg/g and 65 μg/g of *D-glucuronic acid R*.

Place 25 test-tubes, numbered 1 to 25, in iced water. Add 1.0 ml of the 5 reference solutions in triplicate to the test-tubes 1 to 15 (reference tubes), 1.0 ml of the 3 test solutions in triplicate to the test-tubes 16 to 24 (sample tubes), and 1.0 ml of *water R* to test-tube 25 (blank). Add to each test-tube 5.0 ml of freshly prepared reagent A, previously cooled in iced water. Tightly close the test-tubes with plastic caps, shake the contents, and place on a water bath for exactly 15 min. Cool in iced water, and add to each test tube 0.20 ml of reagent B. Recap the tubes, shake, and put them again on a water-bath for exactly 15 min. Cool to room temperature and measure the absorbance (*2.2.25*) of the solutions at 530 nm, against the blank.

From the calibration curve obtained with the mean absorbances read for each reference solution, determine the mean concentrations of D-glucuronic acid in the test solutions.

Calculate the percentage content of sodium hyaluronate using the following expression:

$$\frac{c_g}{c_s} \times Z \times \frac{100}{100-h} \times \frac{401.3}{194.1}$$

c_g = mean of concentrations of D-glucuronic acid in the test solutions, in milligrams per gram;

c_s = mean of concentrations of the substance to be examined in the test solutions, in milligrams per gram;

Z = determined percentage content of $C_6H_{10}O_7$ in *D-glucuronic acid R*;

h = percentage loss on drying;

401.3 = relative molecular mass of the disaccharide fragment;

194.1 = relative molecular mass of glucuronic acid.

STORAGE

In an airtight container, protected from light and humidity. If the substance is sterile, store in a sterile, airtight, tamper-proof container.

LABELLING

The label states:

- the intrinsic viscosity;
- the origin of the substance;
- the intended use of the substance;
- where applicable, that the substance is suitable for parenteral administration other than intra-articular administration;
- where applicable, that the substance is suitable for parenteral administration, including intra-articular administration;
- where applicable that the material is suitable for intra-ocular use.

01/2008:1265
corrected 6.2

SOYA-BEAN OIL, HYDROGENATED

Soiae oleum hydrogenatum

DEFINITION

Product obtained by refining, bleaching, hydrogenation and deodorisation of oil obtained from seeds of *Glycine soja* Sieb. and Zucc. and *Glycine max* (L.) Merr. (*G. hispida* (Moench) Maxim.). The product consists mainly of triglycerides of palmitic and stearic acids.

CHARACTERS

Appearance: white or almost white mass or powder which melts to a clear, pale yellow liquid when heated.

Solubility: practically insoluble in water, freely soluble in methylene chloride, in light petroleum (bp: 65-70 °C) after heating and in toluene, very slightly soluble in ethanol (96 per cent).

IDENTIFICATION

A. Melting point (see Tests).

B. Composition of fatty acids (see Tests).

TESTS

Melting point (*2.2.15*): 66 °C to 72 °C.

Acid value (*2.5.1*): maximum 0.5.

Dissolve 10.0 g in 50 ml of a hot mixture of equal volumes of *ethanol (96 per cent) R* and *toluene R*, previously neutralised with *0.1 M potassium hydroxide* using 0.5 ml of *phenolphthalein solution R1* as indicator. Titrate the solution immediately while still hot.

Peroxide value (*2.5.5, Method A*): maximum 5.0.

Unsaponifiable matter (*2.5.7*): maximum 1.0 per cent, determined on 5.0 g.

Alkaline impurities in fatty oils (*2.4.19*). Dissolve 2.0 g with gentle heating in a mixture of 1.5 ml of *ethanol (96 per cent) R* and 3 ml of *toluene R*. Add 0.05 ml of a 0.4 g/l solution of *bromophenol blue R* in *ethanol (96 per cent) R*. Not more than 0.4 ml of *0.01 M hydrochloric acid* is required to change the colour to yellow.

Composition of fatty acids (*2.4.22, Method A*). Use the mixture of calibrating substances in Table 2.4.22.-3.

Column:

- *material*: fused silica;
- *size*: l = 25 m, Ø = 0.25 mm;
- *stationary phase*: *poly(cyanopropyl)siloxane R* (film thickness 0.2 μm).

Carrier gas: *helium for chromatography R*.

Flow rate: 0.65 ml/min.

Split ratio: 1:100.

Temperature:
- *column*: 180 °C for 20 min;
- *injection port and detector*: 250 °C.

Detection: flame ionisation.

Composition of the fatty-acid fraction of the oil:
- *saturated fatty acids of chain length less than C_{14}*: maximum 0.1 per cent;
- *myristic acid*: maximum 0.5 per cent;
- *palmitic acid*: 9.0 per cent to 16.0 per cent;
- *stearic acid*: 79.0 per cent to 89.0 per cent;
- *oleic acid and isomers*: maximum 4.0 per cent;
- *linoleic acid and isomers*: maximum 1.0 per cent;
- *linolenic acid and isomers*: maximum 0.2 per cent;
- *arachidic acid*: maximum 1.0 per cent;
- *behenic acid*: maximum 1.0 per cent.

Nickel: maximum 1.0 ppm.

Atomic absorption spectrometry (*2.2.23, Method II*).

Test solution. Introduce 5.0 g into a platinum or silica crucible, previously tared after calcination. Cautiously heat and introduce into the substance a wick formed from twisted ashless filter paper. Light the wick. When the substance is alight stop heating. After combustion, ignite in a muffle furnace at about 600 ± 50 °C. Continue the ignition until white ash is obtained. After cooling, take up the residue with 2 quantities, each of 2 ml, of *dilute hydrochloric acid R* and transfer into a 25 ml graduated flask. Add 0.3 ml of *nitric acid R* and dilute to 25.0 ml with *water R*.

Reference solutions. Prepare 3 reference solutions by adding 1.0 ml, 2.0 ml and 4.0 ml of *nickel standard solution (0.2 ppm Ni) R* to 2.0 ml of the test solution and diluting to 10.0 ml with *water R*.

Source: nickel hollow-cathode lamp.

Wavelength: 232 nm.

Atomisation device: graphite furnace.

Carrier gas: *argon R*.

Water (*2.5.12*): maximum 0.3 per cent, determined on 1.000 g.

STORAGE

Protected from light.

07/2008:1473

SOYA-BEAN OIL, REFINED

Soiae oleum raffinatum

DEFINITION

Fatty oil obtained from seeds of *Glycine soja* Siebold et Zucc. and *Glycine max* (L.) Merr. (*Glycine hispida* (Moench) Maxim.) by extraction and subsequent refining. It may contain a suitable antioxidant.

CHARACTERS

Appearance: clear, pale yellow liquid.

Solubility: miscible with light petroleum (50-70 °C), practically insoluble in ethanol (96 per cent).

Relative density: about 0.922.

Refractive index: about 1.475.

IDENTIFICATION

Identification of fatty oils by thin-layer chromatography (*2.3.2*).

Results: the chromatogram obtained is similar to the typical chromatogram for soya-bean oil.

TESTS

Acid value (*2.5.1*): maximum 0.5, determined on 10.0 g.

Peroxide value (*2.5.5, Method A*): maximum 10.0, and maximum 5.0 if intended for use in the manufacture of parenteral preparations.

Unsaponifiable matter (*2.5.7*): maximum 1.5 per cent, determined on 5.0 g.

Alkaline impurities (*2.4.19*). It complies with the test.

Composition of fatty acids (*2.4.22, Method A*). Use the mixture of calibrating substances in Table 2.4.22.-3.

Composition of the fatty-acid fraction of the oil:
- *saturated fatty acids of chain length less than C_{14}*: maximum 0.1 per cent;
- *myristic acid*: maximum 0.2 per cent;
- *palmitic acid*: 9.0 per cent to 13.0 per cent;
- *palmitoleic acid*: maximum 0.3 per cent;
- *stearic acid*: 2.5 per cent to 5.0 per cent;
- *oleic acid*: 17.0 per cent to 30.0 per cent;
- *linoleic acid*: 48.0 per cent to 58.0 per cent;
- *linolenic acid*: 5.0 per cent to 11.0 per cent;
- *arachidic acid*: maximum 1.0 per cent;
- *eicosenoic acid*: maximum 1.0 per cent;
- *behenic acid*: maximum 1.0 per cent.

Brassicasterol (*2.4.23*): maximum 0.3 per cent in the sterol fraction of the oil.

Water (*2.5.32*): maximum 0.1 per cent, determined on 1.00 g, if intended for use in the manufacture of parenteral preparations. Use a mixture of equal volumes of *decanol R* and *anhydrous methanol R* as the solvent.

STORAGE

In a well-filled container, protected from light, at a temperature not exceeding 25 °C.

LABELLING

The label states, where applicable, that the substance is suitable for use in the manufacture of parenteral preparations.

07/2008:1849

SPANISH SAGE OIL

Salviae lavandulifoliae aetheroleum

DEFINITION

Essential oil obtained by steam distillation from the aerial parts of *Salvia lavandulifolia* Vahl, collected at the flowering stage.

CHARACTERS

Appearance: clear, colourless or pale yellow, mobile liquid.

Camphor-like odour.

IDENTIFICATION

First identification: B.

Second identification: A.

A. Thin-layer chromatography (*2.2.27*).

Test solution. Dissolve 0.1 ml of the oil to be examined in 10 ml of *toluene R*.

Reference solution. Dissolve 20 μl of *thujone R* and 30 μl of *cineole R* in 10 ml of *toluene R*.

Plate: *TLC silica gel plate R* (5-40 μm) [or *TLC silica gel plate R* (2-10 μm)].

Mobile phase: *ethyl acetate R, toluene R* (5:95 *V/V*).

Application: 10 μl [or 3 μl] as bands of 10 mm [or 6 mm].

Development: over a path of 15 cm [or 6 cm].

Drying: in air.

Detection: spray with a freshly prepared 200 g/l solution of *phosphomolybdic acid R* in *ethanol (96 per cent) R* and heat at 105 °C for 10 min; examine in daylight.

Results: see below the sequence of zones present in the chromatograms obtained with the reference solution and the test solution. Furthermore, other faint zones may be present in the chromatogram obtained with the test solution.

Top of the plate	
	A blue zone
———	———
Thujone: 2 pinkish-violet zones	
Cineole: a blue zone	A blue zone (cineole)
———	———
	3 blue zones
Reference solution	**Test solution**

B. Examine the chromatograms obtained in the test for chromatographic profile.

Results: the characteristic peaks in the chromatogram obtained with the test solution are similar in retention time to those in the chromatogram obtained with reference solution (a).

TESTS

Relative density (*2.2.5*): 0.907 to 0.932.

Refractive index (*2.2.6*): 1.465 to 1.473.

Optical rotation (*2.2.7*): + 7° to + 17°.

Acid value (*2.5.1*): maximum 2.0, determined on 5.00 g.

Solubility in alcohol (*2.8.10*): 1 volume is soluble in 2 volumes and more of *ethanol (80 per cent V/V) R*.

Chromatographic profile. Gas chromatography (*2.2.28*): use the normalisation procedure.

Test solution. Dissolve 0.200 g of the oil to be examined in *heptane R* and dilute to 10.0 ml with the same solvent.

Reference solution (a). Dissolve 0.200 g of *Spanish sage oil for peak identification CRS* in *heptane R* and dilute to 10.0 ml with the same solvent.

Reference solution (b). Dissolve 5 μl of *limonene R* in *heptane R* and dilute to 50.0 ml with the same solvent. Dilute 0.5 ml of this solution to 5.0 ml with *heptane R*.

Column:
- *material*: fused silica;
- *size*: l = 60 m, Ø = 0.25 mm;
- *stationary phase*: *macrogol 20 000 R* (film thickness 0.25 μm).

Carrier gas: *helium for chromatography R*.

Flow rate: 1.5 ml/min.

Split ratio: 1:50.

Temperature:

	Time (min)	**Temperature (°C)**
Column	0 - 43	60 → 232
Injection port		250
Detector		250

Detection: flame ionisation.

Injection: 1 μl.

System suitability: reference solution (a):
- the chromatogram obtained is similar to the chromatogram supplied with *Spanish sage oil for peak identification CRS*;
- *resolution*: minimum 1.5 between the peaks due to limonene and 1,8-cineole and minimum 1.5 between the peaks due to α-terpinyl acetate and borneol.

Use the chromatogram supplied with *Spanish sage oil for peak identification CRS* and the chromatogram obtained with reference solution (a) to locate the peaks due to α-pinene, sabinene, limonene, 1,8-cineole, thujone, camphor, linalol, linalyl acetate, terpinen-4-ol, sabinyl acetate, α-terpinyl acetate and borneol.

Determine the percentage content of each of these components. The percentages are within the following ranges:
- *α-pinene*: 4.0 per cent to 11.0 per cent;
- *sabinene*: 0.1 per cent to 3.5 per cent;
- *limonene*: 2.0 per cent to 6.5 per cent;
- *1,8-cineole*: 10.0 per cent to 30.5 per cent;
- *thujone*: less than 0.5 per cent;
- *camphor*: 11.0 per cent to 36.0 per cent;
- *linalol*: 0.3 per cent to 4.0 per cent;
- *linalyl acetate*: less than 5.0 per cent;
- *terpinen-4-ol*: less than 2.0 per cent;
- *sabinyl acetate*: 0.5 per cent to 9.0 per cent;
- *α-terpinyl acetate*: 0.5 per cent to 9.0 per cent;
- *borneol*: 1.0 per cent to 7.0 per cent;
- *disregard limit*: the area of the principal peak in the chromatogram obtained with reference solution (b) (0.05 per cent).

STORAGE

At a temperature not exceeding 25 °C.

07/2008:1438

ST. JOHN'S WORT

Hyperici herba

DEFINITION

Whole or cut, dried flowering tops of *Hypericum perforatum* L., harvested during flowering time.

Content: minimum 0.08 per cent of total hypericins, expressed as hypericin ($C_{30}H_{16}O_8$; M_r 504.4) (dried drug).

IDENTIFICATION

A. The branched and bare stem shows 2 more-or-less prominent longitudinal ridges. The leaves are opposite, sessile, exstipulate, oblong-oval and 15-30 mm long;

present on the leaf margins are glands which appear as black dots and over all the surface of the leaves many small, strongly translucent excretory glands which are visible in transmitted light. The flowers are regular and form corymbose clusters at the apex of the stem. They have 5 green, acute sepals, with black secretory glands on the margins; 5 orange-yellow petals, also with black secretory glands on the margins; 3 staminal blades, each divided into many orange-yellow stamens and 3 carpels surmounted by red styles.

The drug may also show the following: immature and ripe fruits and seeds. Immature fruits are green or yellowish, seeds are whitish. Occasional ripe fruits may be present; these are dry trilocular capsules containing numerous seeds, brown, broad or small-ovate, 5-10 mm long, with broad linear or punctiform glands, irregularly striated ducts, conducting secretions. Ripe seeds are 1-1.3 mm long, cylindrical or trigonous, shortly pointed at both ends, brown or almost black, minutely pitted longitudinally.

B. Reduce to a powder (355) (*2.9.12*). The powder is greenish-yellow. Examine under a microscope using *chloral hydrate solution R*. The powder shows the following diagnostic characters: fragments of polygonal cells of the epidermis with thickened and beaded walls and paracytic or anomocytic stomata (*2.8.3*); fragments of the leaf and sepal with large oil glands and red pigment cells; thin-walled, elongated cells of the petal epidermis with straight or wavy anticlinal walls; tracheids and tracheidal vessels with pitted walls and groups of thick-walled fibres; fragments of rectangular, lignified and pitted parenchyma; fibrous layer of the anther and elongated, thin-walled cells of the filament with a striated cuticle; numerous pollen grains with 3 pores and a smooth exine, occur singly or in dense groups, and calcium oxalate cluster crystals.

The powder may also show the following diagnostic characters: fragments of the fruit, exocarp solid with rounded polygonal-cells, endocarp with blunt, thick-walled fibres; fragments of the seed testa, whitish or brown with thick-walled hexagonal or rounded polygonal cells; fragments of the nutritive tissue and embryo, abundant oil droplets.

C. Thin-layer chromatography (*2.2.27*).

Test solution. Stir 0.5 g of the powdered drug (500) (*2.9.12*) in 10 ml of *methanol R* in a water-bath at 60 °C for 10 min and filter.

Reference solution. Dissolve 5 mg of *rutin R* and 5 mg of *hyperoside R* in *methanol R*, then dilute to 5 ml with the same solvent.

Plate: *TLC silica gel plate R.*

Mobile phase: *anhydrous formic acid R, water R, ethyl acetate R* (6:9:90 *V/V/V*).

Application: 10 µl of the test solution and 5 µl of the reference solution, as bands of 10 mm.

Development: over a path of 10 cm.

Drying: at 100-105 °C for 10 min.

Detection: spray with a 10 g/l solution of *diphenylboric acid aminoethyl ester R* in *methanol R* and then with a 50 g/l solution of *macrogol 400 R* in *methanol R*. After about 30 min, examine in ultraviolet light at 365 nm.

Results: the chromatogram obtained with the reference solution shows in the lower third the zone due to rutin and above it the zone due to hyperoside, both with yellow-orange fluorescence. The chromatogram obtained with the test solution shows in the lower third the reddish-orange fluorescent zones of rutin and hyperoside and in the lower part of the upper third the zone of pseudohypericin and above it the zone of hypericin, both with red fluorescence. Other yellow or blue fluorescent zones are visible.

TESTS

Foreign matter (*2.8.2*): maximum 3 per cent of stems with a diameter greater than 5 mm and maximum 2 per cent of other foreign matter.

Loss on drying (*2.2.32*): maximum 10.0 per cent, determined on 1.000 g of the powdered drug (500) (*2.9.12*) by drying in an oven at 105 °C for 2 h.

Total ash (*2.4.16*): maximum 7.0 per cent.

ASSAY

Test solution. In a 100 ml round-bottomed flask, introduce 0.800 g of the powdered drug (500) (*2.9.12*), 60 ml of a mixture of 20 volumes of *water R* and 80 volumes of *tetrahydrofuran R* and a magnetic stirrer. Boil the mixture in a water-bath at 70 °C under a reflux condenser for 30 min. Centrifuge (2 min at 700 *g*) and decant the supernatant into a 250 ml flask. Take up the residue with 60 ml of a mixture of 20 volumes of *water R* and 80 volumes of *tetrahydrofuran R*. Heat again under a reflux condenser for 30 min. Centrifuge (2 min at 700 *g*) and decant the supernatant. Combine the extracts and evaporate to dryness. Take up the residue with 15 ml of *methanol R* with the help of ultrasound and transfer to a 25 ml measuring flask. Rinse the 250 ml flask with *methanol R* and dilute to 25.0 ml with the same solvent. Centrifuge again, filter 10 ml through a syringe filter (0.2 µm). Discard the first 2 millilitres of the filtrate. Introduce 5.0 ml of the filtrate into a measuring flask and dilute to 25.0 ml with *methanol R*.

Compensation liquid. Methanol R.

Measure the absorbance (*2.2.25*) at 590 nm of the test solution, by comparison with the compensation liquid.

Calculate the percentage content of total hypericins, expressed as hypericin, using the following expression:

$$\frac{A \times 125}{m \times 870}$$

i.e. taking the specific absorbance of hypericin to be 870.

A = absorbance at 590 nm,

m = mass of the drug to be examined, in grams.

07/2008:1874

ST. JOHN'S WORT DRY EXTRACT, QUANTIFIED

Hyperici herbae extractum siccum quantificatum

DEFINITION

Quantified dry extract obtained from *St. John's wort (1438)*.

Content:

- *total hypericins, expressed as hypericin* ($C_{30}H_{16}O_8$; M_r 504.5): 0.10 per cent to 0.30 per cent (dried extract);
- *flavonoids, expressed as rutin* ($C_{27}H_{30}O_{16}$; M_r 610.5): minimum 6.0 per cent (dried extract);
- *hyperforin* ($C_{35}H_{52}O_4$; M_r 536.8): maximum 6.0 per cent (dried extract) and not more than the content stated on the label.

PRODUCTION

The extract is produced from the herbal drug by a suitable procedure using ethanol (50-80 per cent *V/V*) or methanol (50-80 per cent *V/V*).

CHARACTERS

Appearance: brownish-grey powder.

IDENTIFICATION

Thin-layer chromatography (*2.2.27*).

Test solution. Disperse 0.25 g of the extract to be examined in 5 ml of *methanol R*.

Reference solution. Dissolve 5 mg of *rutin R* and 5 mg of *hyperoside R* in *methanol R* and dilute to 10 ml with the same solvent.

Plate: *TLC silica gel plate R* (5-40 μm) [or *TLC silica gel plate R* (2-10 μm)].

Mobile phase: *anhydrous formic acid R, water R, ethyl acetate R* (6:9:90 *V/V/V*).

Application: 10 μl [or 5 μl] as bands of 10 mm [or 8 mm].

Development: over a path of 10 cm [or 7.5 cm] .

Drying: at 100-105 °C for 10 min.

Detection: spray with a 10 g/l solution of *diphenylboric acid aminoethyl ester R* in *methanol R* and then with a 50 g/l solution of *macrogol 400 R* in *methanol R*. Examine after about 30 min in ultraviolet light at 365 nm.

Results: see below the sequence of the zones present in the chromatograms obtained with the reference solution and the test solution. Furthermore, other fluorescent zones may be present in the chromatogram obtained with the test solution.

Top of the plate	
	A yellowish-orange fluorescent zone 2 red fluorescent zones (hypericin and pseudohypericin)
_______	_______
	3 yellowish-orange fluorescent zones
_______	_______
Hyperoside: a yellowish-orange fluorescent zone	A yellowish-orange fluorescent zone (hyperoside) Yellow and blue possibly superimposed fluorescent zones
Rutin: a yellowish-orange fluorescent zone	A yellowish-orange fluorescent zone (rutin)
Reference solution	**Test solution**

ASSAY

Total hypericins. Liquid chromatography (*2.2.29*).

Test solution. Dissolve 70.0 mg of the extract to be examined in 25.0 ml of *methanol R*. Sonicate and centrifuge the solution. Expose the solution to a xenon lamp at about 765 W/m^2 for 8 min.

Reference solution. Dissolve a quantity of *St. John's wort standardised dry extract CRS* corresponding to 0.15 mg of hypericin in 25.0 ml of *methanol R*. Sonicate and centrifuge. Expose the solution to a xenon lamp at about 765 W/m^2 for 8 min.

Column:

- *size*: *l* = 0.15 m, Ø = 4.6 mm;
- *stationary phase*: *octadecylsilyl silica gel for chromatography R* (5 μm);
- *temperature*: 40 °C.

Mobile phase: mix 39 volumes of *ethyl acetate R*, 41 volumes of a 15.6 g/l solution of *sodium dihydrogen phosphate R* adjusted to pH 2 with *phosphoric acid R* and 160 volumes of *methanol R*.

Flow rate: 1.0 ml/min.

Detection: spectrophotometer at 590 nm.

Injection: 20 μl.

Run time: 15 min.

Identification of peaks: use the chromatogram supplied with *St. John's wort standardised dry extract CRS* and the chromatogram obtained with the reference solution to identify the peaks due to pseudohypericin and hypericin.

System suitability: reference solution:

- the chromatogram obtained is similar to the chromatogram supplied with *St. John's wort standardised dry extract CRS*;
- *resolution*: minimum 2 between the peaks due to pseudohypericin and hypericin.

Calculate the percentage content of total hypericins, expressed as hypericin, using the following expression:

$$\frac{(A_1 + A_2) \times m_2 \times p}{A_3 \times m_1}$$

A_1 = area of the peak due to pseudohypericin in the chromatogram obtained with the test solution;

A_2 = area of the peak due to hypericin in the chromatogram obtained with the test solution;

A_3 = area of the peak due to hypericin in the chromatogram obtained with the reference solution;

m_1 = mass of the extract to be examined used to prepare the test solution, in grams;

m_2 = mass of *St. John's wort standardised dry extract CRS* used to prepare the reference solution, in grams;

p = percentage content of hypericin in *St. John's wort standardised dry extract CRS*.

Hyperforin and flavonoids. Liquid chromatography (*2.2.29*). *Carry out the assay protected from light.*

Solvent mixture: *water R, methanol R* (20:80 *V/V*).

Test solution. Dissolve 75.0 mg of the extract to be examined in 20.0 ml of the solvent mixture. Sonicate and centrifuge.

Reference solution (a). Dissolve 20.0 mg of *rutoside trihydrate CRS* in 200.0 ml of the solvent mixture.

Reference solution (b). Dissolve 75.0 mg of *St. John's wort standardised dry extract CRS* in 20.0 ml of the solvent mixture. Sonicate and centrifuge.

Column:

- *size*: *l* = 0.15 m, Ø = 4.6 mm;
- *stationary phase*: *octadecylsilyl silica gel for chromatography R* (3 μm).

Mobile phase:
- *mobile phase A*: *phosphoric acid R*, *water R* (3:1000 *V/V*);
- *mobile phase B*: *phosphoric acid R*, *acetonitrile R* (3:1000 *V/V*);

Time (min)	Mobile phase A (per cent *V/V*)	Mobile phase B (per cent *V/V*)
0 - 8	82	18
8 - 18	82 → 47	18 → 53
18 - 18.1	47 → 3	53 → 97
18.1 - 19	3	97
19 - 29	3	97
29 - 30	3 → 82	97 → 18

Detection: spectrophotometer at 360 nm, then at 275 nm after the elution of biapigenin (about 22 min).

Injection: 10 μl.

Identification of peaks: use the chromatogram supplied with *St. John's wort standardised dry extract CRS* and the chromatogram obtained with reference solution (b) to identify the peaks due to rutin, hyperoside, isoquercitroside, quercitroside, quercetin, biapigenin, hyperforin and adhyperforin.

System suitability: reference solution (b):
- the chromatogram obtained is similar to the chromatogram supplied with *St. John's wort standardised dry extract CRS*;
- *resolution*: minimum 2.0 between the peaks due to rutin and hyperoside, and minimum 2.0 between the peaks due to hyperforin and adhyperforin.

Calculate the percentage content of hyperforin using the following expression:

$$\frac{A_4 \times m_4 \times p \times 2.3}{A_5 \times m_3 \times 10}$$

A_4 = area of the peak due to hyperforin in the chromatogram obtained with the test solution;

A_5 = area of the peak due to rutin in the chromatogram obtained with reference solution (a);

m_3 = mass of the extract to be examined used to prepare the test solution, in grams;

m_4 = mass of *rutoside trihydrate CRS* used to prepare the reference solution, in grams;

2.3 = correction factor for hyperforin with respect to rutin;

p = percentage content of rutin in *rutoside trihydrate CRS*.

Calculate the percentage content of flavonoids, expressed as rutin, using the following expression:

$$\frac{m_4 \times p \times (A_6 + A_7 + A_8 + A_9 + A_{10} + A_{11})}{m_3 \times A_5 \times 10}$$

A_5 = area of the peak due to rutin in the chromatogram obtained with reference solution (a);

A_6 = area of the peak due to rutin in the chromatogram obtained with the test solution;

A_7 = area of the peak due to hyperoside in the chromatogram obtained with the test solution;

A_8 = area of the peak due to isoquercitroside in the chromatogram obtained with the test solution;

A_9 = area of the peak due to quercitroside in the chromatogram obtained with the test solution;

A_{10} = area of the peak due to quercetin in the chromatogram obtained with the test solution;

A_{11} = area of the peak due to biapigenin in the chromatogram obtained with the test solution;

m_3 = mass of the extract to be examined used to prepare the test solution, in grams;

m_4 = mass of *rutoside trihydrate CRS* used to prepare the reference solution, in grams;

p = percentage content of rutin in *rutoside trihydrate CRS*.

LABELLING

The label states the content of hyperforin.

01/2008:0247

STRAMONIUM, PREPARED

Stramonii pulvis normatus

DEFINITION

Stramonium leaf powder (180) (*2.9.12*) adjusted, if necessary, by the addition of powdered lactose or stramonium leaf of lower content of total alkaloids.

Content: 0.23 per cent to 0.27 per cent of total alkaloids, expressed as hyoscyamine ($C_{17}H_{23}NO_3$; M_r 289.4) (dried drug).

CHARACTERS

Appearance: greyish-green powder.

Unpleasant odour.

IDENTIFICATION

A. Examine under a microscope using *chloral hydrate solution R*. The powder shows the following diagnostic characters: fragments of leaf lamina showing epidermal cells with slightly wavy anticlinal walls and smooth cuticle; stomata are more frequent on the lower epidermis (anisocytic and anomocytic) (*2.8.3*); covering trichomes are conical, uniseriate with 3-5 cells and warty walls; glandular trichomes are short and clavate with heads formed by 2-7 cells; dorsiventral mesophyll, with a single layer of palisade cells and a spongy parenchyma containing cluster crystals of calcium oxalate; annularly and spirally thickened vessels. The powdered drug may also show the following diagnostic characters: fibres and reticulately thickened vessels from the stems; subspherical pollen grains usually about 60-80 μm in diameter with 3 germinal pores and nearly smooth exine; fragments of the corolla with papillose epidermis; seed fragments containing yellowish-brown, sinuous, thick-walled sclereids of testa; occasional prisms and microsphenoidal crystals of calcium oxalate. Examined in *glycerol (85 per cent) R*, it may be seen to contain lactose crystals.

B. Examine the chromatograms obtained in the Chromatography test.

Results: the principal zones in the chromatogram obtained with the test solution are similar in position, colour and size to the principal zones in the chromatogram obtained with the same volume of the reference solution.

C. Shake 1 g with 10 ml of *0.05 M sulphuric acid* for 2 min. Filter and add to the filtrate 1 ml of *concentrated ammonia R* and 5 ml of *water R*. Shake cautiously with 15 ml of *peroxide-free ether R*, avoiding the formation of an emulsion. Separate the ether layer and dry over *anhydrous sodium sulphate R*. Filter and evaporate the ether in a porcelain dish. Add 0.5 ml of *nitric acid R* and evaporate to dryness on a water-bath. Add 10 ml of *acetone R* and, dropwise, a 30 g/l solution of *potassium hydroxide R* in *ethanol (96 per cent) R*. A deep violet colour develops.

TESTS

Chromatography. Thin-layer chromatography (*2.2.27*).

Test solution. To 1.0 g of the drug to be examined add 10 ml of *0.05 M sulphuric acid*, shake for 15 min and filter. Wash the filter with *0.05 M sulphuric acid* until 25 ml of filtrate is obtained. To the filtrate add 1 ml of *concentrated ammonia R* and shake with 2 quantities, each of 10 ml, of *peroxide-free ether R*. If necessary, separate by centrifugation. Dry the combined ether layers over *anhydrous sodium sulphate R*, filter and evaporate to dryness on a water-bath. Dissolve the residue in 0.5 ml of *methanol R*.

Reference solution. Dissolve 50 mg of *hyoscyamine sulphate R* in 9 ml of *methanol R*. Dissolve 15 mg of *hyoscine hydrobromide R* in 10 ml of *methanol R*. Mix 3.8 ml of the hyoscyamine sulphate solution and 4.2 ml of the hyoscine hydrobromide solution and dilute to 10 ml with *methanol R*.

Plate: *TLC silica gel G plate R*.

Mobile phase: *concentrated ammonia R, water R, acetone R* (3:7:90 *V/V/V*).

Application: 10 µl and 20 µl of each solution as bands of 20 mm by 3 mm, leaving 1 cm between the bands.

Development: over a path of 10 cm.

Drying: at 100-105 °C for 15 min and allow to cool.

Detection A: spray with *potassium iodobismuthate solution R2*, using about 10 ml for a plate 200 mm square, until the orange or brown zones become visible against a yellow background.

Results A: the zones in the chromatograms obtained with the test solution are similar in position (hyoscyamine in the lower third, hyoscine in the upper third of the chromatogram) and colour to those in the chromatograms obtained with the reference solution. The zones in the chromatograms obtained with the test solution are at least equal in size to the corresponding zones in the chromatogram obtained with the same volume of the reference solution. Faint secondary zones may appear, particularly in the middle of the chromatogram obtained with 20 µl of the test solution or near the starting point in the chromatogram obtained with 10 µl of the test solution.

Detection B: spray with *sodium nitrite solution R* until the coating is transparent; examine after 15 min.

Results B: the zones due to hyoscyamine in the chromatograms obtained with the test solution and the reference solution change from brown to reddish-brown but not to greyish-blue (atropine) and any secondary zones disappear.

Loss on drying (*2.2.32*): maximum 5.0 per cent, determined on 1.000 g by drying in an oven at 105 °C.

Total ash (*2.4.16*): maximum 20.0 per cent.

Ash insoluble in hydrochloric acid (*2.8.1*): maximum 4.0 per cent.

ASSAY

a) Determine the loss on drying (*2.2.32*) on 2.000 g by drying in an oven at 105 °C.

b) Moisten 10.0 g with a mixture of 5 ml of *ammonia R*, 10 ml of *ethanol (96 per cent) R* and 30 ml of *peroxide-free ether R* and mix thoroughly. Transfer the mixture to a suitable percolator, if necessary with the aid of the extracting mixture. Allow to macerate for 4 h and percolate with a mixture of 1 volume of *chloroform R* and 3 volumes of *peroxide-free ether R* until the alkaloids are completely extracted. Evaporate to dryness a few millilitres of the liquid flowing from the percolator, dissolve the residue in *0.25 M sulphuric acid* and verify the absence of alkaloids using *potassium tetraiodomercurate solution R*. Concentrate the percolate to about 50 ml by distilling on a water-bath and transfer it to a separating funnel, rinsing with *peroxide-free ether R*. Add a quantity of *peroxide-free ether R* equal to at least 2.1 times the volume of the percolate to produce a liquid of a density well below that of water. Shake the solution with no fewer than 3 quantities, each of 20 ml, of *0.25 M sulphuric acid*, separate the 2 layers by centrifugation if necessary and transfer the acid layers to a 2nd separating funnel. Make the acid layer alkaline with *ammonia R* and shake with 3 quantities, each of 30 ml, of *chloroform R*. Combine the chloroform layers, add 4 g of *anhydrous sodium sulphate R* and allow to stand for 30 min with occasional shaking. Decant the chloroform and wash the sodium sulphate with 3 quantities, each of 10 ml, of *chloroform R*. Add the washings to the chloroform extract, evaporate to dryness on a water-bath and heat in an oven at 100-105 °C for 15 min. Dissolve the residue in a few millilitres of *chloroform R*, add 20.0 ml of *0.01 M sulphuric acid* and remove the chloroform by evaporation on a water-bath. Titrate the excess of acid with *0.02 M sodium hydroxide* using *methyl red mixed solution R* as indicator.

Calculate the percentage content of total alkaloids, expressed as hyoscyamine, using the following expression:

$$\frac{57.88\,(20 - n)}{(100 - d)\,m}$$

d = loss on drying, as a percentage;

n = volume of *0.02 M sodium hydroxide*, in millilitres;

m = mass of drug, in grams.

STORAGE

In an airtight container.

07/2008:0356

STREPTOKINASE CONCENTRATED SOLUTION

Streptokinasi solutio concentrata

DEFINITION

Streptokinase concentrated solution is a preparation of a protein obtained from culture filtrates of certain strains of haemolytic *Streptococcus* group C; it has the property of combining with human plasminogen to form plasminogen activator. It may contain buffer salts and other excipients. The potency is not less than 510 IU per microgram of nitrogen.

PRODUCTION

The method of manufacture is validated to demonstrate that the product, if tested, would comply with the following test.

Abnormal toxicity (*2.6.9*). Inject into each mouse a quantity of the preparation to be examined (if necessary, dilute with *water for injections R*) equivalent to 50 000 IU of streptokinase activity, the injection lasting 15-20 s.

CHARACTERS

Appearance: clear, colourless liquid.

IDENTIFICATION

A. Place 0.5 ml of citrated human plasma in a polystyrene tube maintained in a water-bath at 37 °C. Add 0.1 ml of a dilution of the preparation to be examined containing 10 000 IU of streptokinase activity per millilitre in *phosphate buffer solution pH 7.2 R* and 0.1 ml of a solution of *human thrombin R* containing 20 IU/ml in *phosphate buffer solution pH 7.2 R*. Mix immediately. A clot forms and lyses within 30 min. Repeat the procedure using citrated bovine plasma. The clot does not lyse within 60 min.

B. Perform an immunochemical test using double immunodiffusion techniques (*2.7.1*). Place in the central cavity about 80 µl of goat or rabbit antistreptokinase serum containing about 10 000 units of antistreptokinase activity per millilitre; place in each of the surrounding cavities about 80 µl of a dilution of the preparation to be examined containing 125 000 IU of streptokinase activity per millilitre. Allow the plates to stand in a humidified tank for 24 h. Only one precipitation arc appears and it is well defined.

TESTS

pH (*2.2.3*): 6.8 to 7.5.

Dilute the preparation to be examined in *carbon dioxide-free water R* to obtain a solution containing at least 1000 000 IU of streptokinase activity per millilitre.

Streptodornase: maximum 10 IU of streptodornase activity per 100 000 IU of streptokinase activity.

Test solution. Dilute the preparation to be examined in *imidazole buffer solution pH 6.5 R* to obtain a solution containing 150 000 IU of streptokinase activity per millilitre.

Reference solution. Dissolve in *imidazole buffer solution pH 6.5 R* a reference preparation of streptodornase, calibrated in International Units against the International Standard of streptodornase, to obtain a solution containing 20 IU of streptodornase activity per millilitre. The equivalence in International Units of the International Standard is stated by the World Health Organisation.

To each of 8 numbered centrifuge tubes, add 0.5 ml of a 1 g/l solution of *sodium deoxyribonucleate R* in *imidazole buffer solution pH 6.5 R*. To tube number 1 and tube number 2 add 0.25 ml of *imidazole buffer solution pH 6.5 R*, 0.25 ml of the test solution and, immediately, 3.0 ml of perchloric acid (25 g/l $HClO_4$). Mix, centrifuge at about 3000 *g* for 5 min and measure the absorbances (*2.2.25*) of the supernatant liquids at 260 nm, using as the compensation liquid a mixture of 1.0 ml of *imidazole buffer solution pH 6.5 R* and 3.0 ml of perchloric acid (25 g/l $HClO_4$) (absorbances A_1 and A_2). To the other 6 tubes (numbers 3 to 8) add 0.25 ml, 0.25 ml, 0.125 ml, 0.125 ml, 0 ml and 0 ml respectively of *imidazole buffer solution pH 6.5 R*; add to each tube 0.25 ml of the test solution and 0 ml, 0 ml, 0.125 ml, 0.125 ml, 0.25 ml and 0.25 ml respectively of the reference solution. Mix the contents of each tube and heat at 37 °C for 15 min. To each tube add 3.0 ml of perchloric acid (25 g/l $HClO_4$), mix and centrifuge. Measure the absorbances (*2.2.25*) of the supernatant liquids at 260 nm using the compensation liquid described above (absorbances A_3 to A_8). The absorbances comply with the following requirement:

$$(A_3 + A_4) - (A_1 + A_2) < \frac{(A_5 + A_6 + A_7 + A_8)}{2} - (A_3 + A_4)$$

Streptolysin. In a polystyrene tube, use a quantity of the preparation to be examined equivalent to 500 000 IU of streptokinase activity and dilute to 0.5 ml with a mixture of 1 volume of *phosphate buffer solution pH 7.2 R* and 9 volumes of a 9 g/l solution of *sodium chloride R*. Add 0.4 ml of a 23 g/l solution of *sodium thioglycollate R*. Heat in a water-bath at 37 °C for 10 min. Add 0.1 ml of a solution of a reference preparation of human antistreptolysin O containing 5 IU/ml. Heat at 37 °C for 5 min. Add 1 ml of *rabbit erythrocyte suspension R*. Heat at 37 °C for 30 min. Centrifuge at about 1000 *g*. In the same manner, prepare a polystyrene tube in which the solution of the preparation to be examined has been replaced by 0.5 ml of a mixture of 1 volume of *phosphate buffer solution pH 7.2 R* and 9 volumes of a 9 g/l solution of *sodium chloride R*. Measure the absorbances (*2.2.25*) of the supernatant liquids at 550 nm. The absorbance of the test solution is not more than 50 per cent greater than that of the reference solution.

Related substances. Liquid chromatography (*2.2.29*): use the normalisation procedure.

Test solution. Dilute the preparation to be examined with *water R* to obtain a concentration of about 0.5-1 g/l, depending on the chromatographic system used.

Reference solution. Dilute 1 volume of *streptokinase for system suitability CRS* with 49 volumes of *water R*.

Column:
- *size*: *l* = 0.10 m, Ø = 4.6 mm;
- *stationary phase*: *styrene-divinylbenzene copolymer R* (10 µm) with a pore size of 200 nm;
- *temperature*: 25 °C.

Mobile phase:
- *mobile phase A*: *trifluoroacetic acid R, water for injections R* (1:1000 *V/V*); degas;
- *mobile phase B*: *trifluoroacetic acid R, acetonitrile for chromatography R* (1:1000 *V/V*); degas;

Time (min)	Mobile phase A (per cent *V/V*)	Mobile phase B (per cent *V/V*)
0 - 1	68	32
1 - 4	68 → 52	32 → 48
4 - 5	52	48
5 - 7	0	100
7 - 10	68	32

The above conditions may be modified to improve the separation efficiency of the chromatographic system.

Flow rate: 5 ml/min.

Detection: spectrophotometer at 280 nm.

Injection: 20 µl.

Retention time: streptokinase = 2.3 min to 2.8 min.

System suitability: reference solution:
- *symmetry factor*: maximum 1.9 for the peak due to streptokinase;
- *peak-to-valley ratio*: minimum 2, where H_p = height above the baseline of the 1st peak eluting after the principal peak and H_v = height above the baseline of the lowest point of the curve separating this peak from the 2nd peak eluting after the principal peak;
- the chromatogram obtained with the reference solution is similar to the chromatogram supplied with *streptokinase for system suitability CRS*.

Limit:
– *total*: maximum 5 per cent.

Bacterial endotoxins (*2.6.14*): less than 0.02 IU per 100 IU of streptokinase activity, if intended for use without a further appropriate procedure for the removal of bacterial endotoxins.

ASSAY

Nitrogen (*2.5.9*).

Potency

The potency of streptokinase is determined by comparing its capacity to activate plasminogen to form plasmin with the same capacity of a reference preparation of streptokinase calibrated in International Units; the formation of plasmin is determined using a suitable chromogenic substrate.

The International Unit is the activity of a stated amount of the International Standard for streptokinase. The equivalence in International Units of the International Standard is stated by the World Health Organisation.

Reference and test solutions

Prepare 2 independent series of at least 3 dilutions of each of the preparation to be examined and of the reference preparation of streptokinase in *tris(hydroxymethyl)aminomethane sodium chloride buffer solution pH 7.4 R1*, in the linear range of the assay (a range of 0.5-4.0 IU/ml has been found suitable). Prepare and maintain all solutions at 37 °C.

Substrate solution

Mix 1.0 ml of *tris(hydroxymethyl)aminomethane buffer solution pH 7.4 R* with 1.0 ml of *chromophore substrate R3*. Add 5 µl of a 100 g/l solution of *polysorbate 20 R*. Keep at 37 °C in a water-bath. Immediately before commencing the activation assay, add 45 µl of a 1 mg/ml solution of *human plasminogen R*.

Method

Analyse each streptokinase dilution, maintained at 37 °C, in duplicate. Initiate the activation reaction by adding 60 µl of each dilution to 40 µl of substrate solution. For blank wells, use 60 µl of *tris(hydroxymethyl)aminomethane sodium chloride buffer solution pH 7.4 R1* instead of the reference and test solutions. Allow the reaction to proceed at 37 °C for 20 min and read the absorbance (*2.2.25*) at 405 nm. If a suitable thermostatted plate reader is available, this may be used to monitor the reaction. Alternatively, it may be necessary to stop the reaction after 20 min using 50 µl of a 50 per cent *V/V* solution of *glacial acetic acid R*. Best results are obtained when the absorbance for the highest streptokinase concentration is between 0.1 and 0.2 (after blank subtraction). If necessary, adjust the time of incubation in order to reach this range of absorbances.

Calculate the regression of the absorbance on log concentrations of the solutions of the preparation to be examined and of the reference preparation of streptokinase and calculate the potency of the preparation to be examined using a suitable statistical method, for example the parallel-line assay (*5.3*).

The estimated potency is not less than 90 per cent and not more than 111 per cent of the stated potency. The confidence limits (*P* = 0.95) are not less than 80 per cent and not more than 125 per cent of the estimated potency.

STORAGE

In an airtight container, protected from light and at a temperature of – 20 °C. If the preparation is sterile, store in a sterile, airtight, tamper-proof container.

LABELLING

The label states:
– the number of International Units of streptokinase activity per milligram, calculated with reference to the dried preparation;
– the name and quantity of any added substance;
– that the preparation is suitable for use in the manufacture of parenteral preparations.

01/2008:2209
corrected 6.2

SULBACTAM SODIUM

Sulbactamum natricum

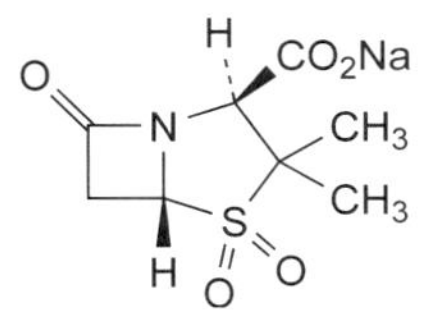

$C_8H_{10}NNaO_5S$ M_r 255.2
[69388-84-7]

DEFINITION

Sodium (2*S*,5*R*)-3,3-dimethyl-7-oxo-4-thia-1-azabicyclo[3.2.0]heptane-2-carboxylate 4,4-dioxide.

Semi-synthetic product derived from a fermentation product.

Content: 97.0 per cent to 102.0 per cent (anhydrous substance).

CHARACTERS

Appearance: white or almost white, hygroscopic, crystalline powder.

Solubility: freely soluble in water, sparingly soluble in ethyl acetate, very slightly soluble in ethanol (96 per cent). It is freely soluble in dilute acids.

IDENTIFICATION

A. Infrared absorption spectrophotometry (*2.2.24*).
Comparison: *sulbactam sodium CRS*.

B. It gives reaction (a) of sodium (*2.3.1*).

TESTS

Appearance of solution. The solution is clear (*2.2.1*).

Dissolve 2.0 g in *water R* and dilute to 20 ml with the same solvent.

Absorbance (*2.2.25*): maximum 0.10 at 430 nm.

Dissolve 1.0 g in *water R* and dilute to 100.0 ml with the same solvent.

pH (*2.2.3*): 4.5 to 7.2; if the substance is sterile: 5.2 to 7.2.

Dissolve 1.0 g in *carbon dioxide-free water R* and dilute to 20 ml with the same solvent.

Specific optical rotation (*2.2.7*): + 219 to + 233 (anhydrous substance).

Dissolve 0.500 g in *water R* and dilute to 50.0 ml with the same solvent.

Related substances. Liquid chromatography (*2.2.29*).

Solution A. 2.72 g/l solution of *potassium dihydrogen phosphate R* adjusted to pH 4.0 with *dilute phosphoric acid R*.

Solution B. Dilute 2 ml of *acetonitrile R1* to 100.0 ml with solution A.

Test solution. Suspend 77.0 mg of the substance to be examined in 2 ml of *acetonitrile R1* and sonicate for about 5 min. Dilute to 100.0 ml with solution A.

Reference solution (a). Suspend 70.0 mg of *sulbactam CRS* in 2 ml of *acetonitrile R1* and sonicate for about 5 min. Dilute to 100.0 ml with solution A.

Reference solution (b). Dilute 1.0 ml of reference solution (a) to 100.0 ml with solution B. Dilute 1.0 ml of this solution to 10.0 ml with solution B.

Reference solution (c). Dissolve 15.0 mg of *6-aminopenicillanic acid R* in solution A and dilute to 50.0 ml with solution A.

Reference solution (d). Mix 1 ml of reference solution (a) and 1 ml of reference solution (c) and dilute to 25.0 ml with solution B.

Reference solution (e). Dissolve 8 mg of *sulbactam for peak identification CRS* (containing impurities A, C, D, E and F) in 1 ml of *acetonitrile R1,* sonicate for about 5 min and dilute to 10 ml with solution B.

Column:

- *size*: *l* = 0.10 m, Ø = 4.0 mm;
- *stationary phase*: *octadecylsilyl silica gel for chromatography R* (3.0 μm);
- *temperature*: 40 °C.

Mobile phase:

- *mobile phase A*: 5.44 g/l solution of *potassium dihydrogen phosphate R* adjusted to pH 4.0 with *dilute phosphoric acid R;*
- *mobile phase B*: *acetonitrile R1;*

Time (min)	Mobile phase A (per cent *V/V*)	Mobile phase B (per cent *V/V*)
0 - 7.5	98 → 50	2 → 50
7.5 - 8.5	50	50
8.5 - 9.0	50 → 98	50 → 2
9.0 - 12.5	98	2

Flow rate: 1.0 ml/min.

Detection: spectrophotometer at 215 nm.

Injection: 20 μl of the test solution, solution B and reference solutions (b), (d) and (e).

Relative retention with reference to sulbactam (retention time = about 2.5 min): impurity A = about 0.4; impurity B = about 0.6; impurity C = about 1.6; impurity D = about 2.0; impurity E = about 2.1; impurity F = about 2.5.

Identification of impurities: use the chromatogram supplied with *sulbactam for peak identification CRS* and the chromatogram obtained with reference solution (e) to identify the peaks due to impurities A, C, D, E and F.

System suitability: reference solution (d):

- *resolution*: minimum 7.0 between the peaks due to impurity B and sulbactam.

Limits:

- *correction factors*: for the calculation of content, multiply the peak areas of the following impurities by the corresponding correction factor: impurity A = 0.6; impurity B = 0.5; impurity D = 0.5; impurity F = 0.6;
- *impurity A*: not more than 5 times the area of the principal peak in the chromatogram obtained with reference solution (b) (0.5 per cent);
- *impurities B, D, F*: for each impurity, not more than the area of the principal peak in the chromatogram obtained with reference solution (b) (0.1 per cent);
- *impurities C, E*: for each impurity, not more than twice the area of the principal peak in the chromatogram obtained with reference solution (b) (0.2 per cent);
- *unspecified impurities*: for each impurity, not more than the area of the principal peak in the chromatogram obtained with reference solution (b) (0.10 per cent);
- *total*: not more than 10 times the area of the principal peak in the chromatogram obtained with reference solution (b) (1.0 per cent);
- *disregard limit*: 0.5 times the area of the principal peak in the chromatogram obtained with reference solution (b) (0.05 per cent).

2-Ethylhexanoic acid (*2.4.28*): maximum 0.5 per cent *m/m*.

Heavy metals (*2.4.8*): maximum 20 ppm.

Dissolve 1.0 gin *water R* and dilute to 20 ml with the same solvent. 12 ml of the solution complies with test A. Prepare the reference solution using 10.0 ml of *lead standard solution (2 ppm Pb) R.*

Water (*2.5.12*): maximum 1.0 per cent, determined on 1.00 g.

Bacterial endotoxins (*2.6.14, Method A*): less than 0.17 IU/mg, if intended for use in the manufacture of parenteral preparations without a further appropriate procedure for the removal of bacterial endotoxins.

ASSAY

Liquid chromatography (*2.2.29*) as described in the test for related substances with the following modification.

Injection: test solution and reference solution (a).

Calculate the percentage content of sulbactam sodium by multiplying the percentage content of sulbactam by 1.094 and using the declared content of *sulbactam CRS.*

STORAGE

In an airtight container. If the substance is sterile, store in a sterile, airtight, tamper-proof container.

IMPURITIES

Specified impurities: A, B, C, D, E, F.

Other detectable impurities (the following substances would, if present at a sufficient level, be detected by one or other of the tests in the monograph. They are limited by the general acceptance criterion for other/unspecified impurities and/or by the general monograph *Substances for pharmaceutical use (2034).* It is therefore not necessary to identify these impurities for demonstration of compliance. See also *5.10. Control of impurities in substances for pharmaceutical use*): *G.*

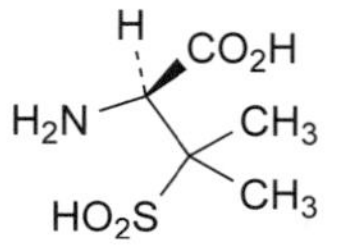

A. (2*S*)-2-amino-3-methyl-3-sulphinobutanoic acid,

Monographs Q-Z

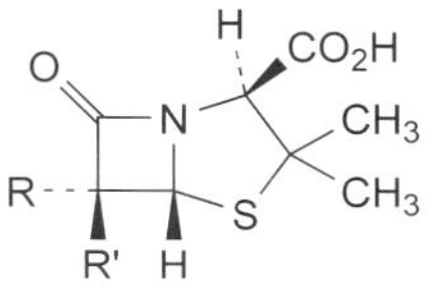

B. R = NH_2, R′ = H: (2*S*,5*R*,6*R*)-6-amino-3,3-dimethyl-7-oxo-4-thia-1-azabicyclo[3.2.0]heptane-2-carboxylic acid (6-aminopenicillanic acid),

D. R = Br, R′ = H: (2*S*,5*R*,6*R*)-6-bromo-3,3-dimethyl-7-oxo-4-thia-1-azabicyclo[3.2.0]heptane-2-carboxylic acid (6-bromopenicillanic acid),

F. R = R′ = Br: (2*S*,5*R*)-6,6-dibromo-3,3-dimethyl-7-oxo-4-thia-1-azabicyclo[3.2.0]heptane-2-carboxylic acid (6,6-dibromopenicillanic acid),

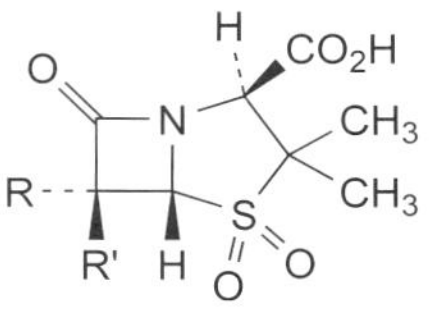

C. R = Br, R′ = H: (2*S*,5*R*,6*R*)-6-bromo-3,3-dimethyl-7-oxo-4-thia-1-azabicyclo[3.2.0]heptane-2-carboxylic acid 4,4-dioxide (6-bromopenicillanic acid sulphone),

E. R = R′ = Br: (2*S*,5*R*)-6,6-dibromo-3,3-dimethyl-7-oxo-4-thia-1-azabicyclo[3.2.0]heptane-2-carboxylic acid 4,4-dioxide (6,6-dibromopenicillanic acid sulphone),

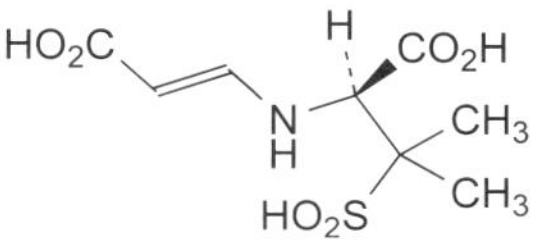

G. (2*E*)-3-[[(1*S*)-1-carboxy-2-methyl-2-sulphinopropyl]amino]prop-2-enoic acid.

07/2008:0107

SULFACETAMIDE SODIUM

Sulfacetamidum natricum

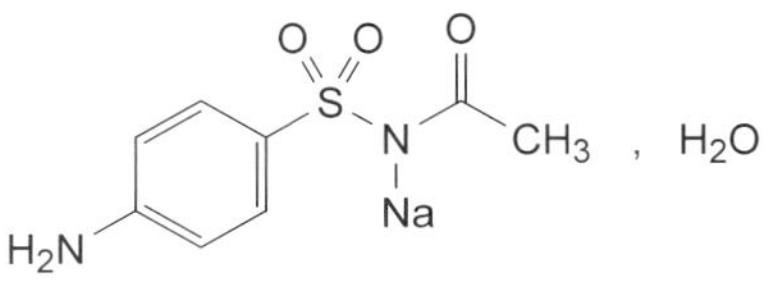

$C_8H_9N_2NaO_3S,H_2O$ M_r 254.2

DEFINITION

Sodium acetyl[(4-aminophenyl)sulphonyl]azanide.

Content: 99.0 per cent to 101.0 per cent (anhydrous substance).

CHARACTERS

Appearance: white or yellowish-white, crystalline powder.

Solubility: freely soluble in water, slightly soluble in anhydrous ethanol.

IDENTIFICATION

First identification: B, F.

Second identification: A, C, E, F.

A. Ultraviolet and visible absorption spectrophotometry (*2.2.25*).

Test solution. Dissolve 0.1 g in *phosphate buffer solution pH 7.0 R* and dilute to 100.0 ml with the same buffer solution. Dilute 1.0 ml of this solution to 100.0 ml with *phosphate buffer solution pH 7.0 R*.

Spectral range: 230-350 nm.

Absorption maximum: at 255 nm.

Specific absorbance at the absorption maximum: 660 to 720 (anhydrous substance).

B. Infrared absorption spectrophotometry (*2.2.24*).

Comparison: *sulfacetamide sodium CRS*.

C. Melting point (*2.2.14*): 181 °C to 185 °C.

Dissolve 1 g in 10 ml of *water R*, add 6 ml of *dilute acetic acid R* and filter. Wash the precipitate with a small quantity of *water R* and dry at 100-105 °C for 4 h.

E. Dissolve about 1 mg of the precipitate obtained in identification C, with heating, in 1 ml of *water R*. The solution gives the reaction of primary aromatic amines (*2.3.1*) with formation of an orange-red precipitate.

F. Solution S (see Tests) gives the reactions of sodium (*2.3.1*).

TESTS

Solution S. Dissolve 1.25 g in *carbon dioxide-free water R* and dilute to 25 ml with the same solvent.

Appearance of solution. Solution S is clear (*2.2.1*) and not more intensely coloured than reference solution GY_4 (*2.2.2, Method II*).

pH (*2.2.3*): 8.0 to 9.5 for solution S.

Related substances. Liquid chromatography (*2.2.29*). *Prepare the solutions immediately before use and carry out the test protected from light.*

Test solution. Dissolve 0.200 g of the substance to be examined in the mobile phase and dilute to 10.0 ml with the mobile phase.

Reference solution (a). Dissolve 5 mg of *sulfacetamide sodium CRS* and 5 mg of *sulfanilamide R* (impurity A) in 1.0 ml of the mobile phase.

Reference solution (b). Dilute 1.0 ml of the test solution to 100.0 ml with the mobile phase. Dilute 1.0 ml of this solution to 10.0 ml with the mobile phase.

Column:

– *size*: *l* = 0.125 m, Ø = 4 mm;

– *stationary phase*: *end-capped octadecylsilyl silica gel for chromatography R* (5 μm).

Mobile phase: *glacial acetic acid R, methanol R, water for chromatography R* (1:10:89 *V/V/V*).

Flow rate: 0.8 ml/min.

Detection: spectrophotometer at 254 nm.

Injection: 10 μl.

Run time: 7 times the retention time of sulfacetamide.

Relative retention with reference to sulfacetamide (retention time = about 5 min): impurity A = about 0.5.

System suitability: reference solution (a):

– *resolution*: minimum 5.0 between the peaks due to impurity A and sulfacetamide.

Limits:

– *correction factor*: for the calculation of the content, multiply the peak area of impurity A by 0.5;

- *impurity A*: not more than twice the area of the principal peak in the chromatogram obtained with reference solution (b) (0.2 per cent);
- *unspecified impurities*: for each impurity, not more than the area of the principal peak in the chromatogram obtained with reference solution (b) (0.10 per cent);
- *total*: not more than 5 times the area of the principal peak in the chromatogram obtained with reference solution (b) (0.5 per cent);
- *disregard limit*: 0.5 times the area of the principal peak in the chromatogram obtained with reference solution (b) (0.05 per cent).

Sulphates (*2.4.13*): maximum 200 ppm.

Dissolve 2.5 g in *distilled water R* and dilute to 25 ml with the same solvent. Add 25 ml of *dilute acetic acid R*, shake for 30 min and filter. 15 ml of the filtrate complies with the limit test for sulphates.

Heavy metals (*2.4.8*): maximum 20 ppm.

12 ml of the filtrate obtained in the test for sulphates complies with test A. Prepare the reference solution using *lead standard solution (1 ppm Pb) R*.

Water (*2.5.12*). 6.0 per cent to 8.0 per cent, determined on 0.200 g.

ASSAY

Dissolve 0.500 g in a mixture of 50 ml of *water R* and 20 ml of *dilute hydrochloric acid R*. Cool the solution in a bath of iced water and carry out the determination of primary aromatic amino-nitrogen (*2.5.8*), determining the end-point electrometrically.

1 ml of *0.1 M sodium nitrite* is equivalent to 23.62 mg of $C_8H_9N_2NaO_3S$.

STORAGE

Protected from light.

IMPURITIES

Specified impurities: A.

Other detectable impurities (the following substances would, if present at a sufficient level, be detected by one or other of the tests in the monograph. They are limited by the general acceptance criterion for other/unspecified impurities and/or by the general monograph *Substances for pharmaceutical use (2034)*. It is therefore not necessary to identify these impurities for demonstration of compliance. See also *5.10. Control of impurities in substances for pharmaceutical use*): *B, C, D*.

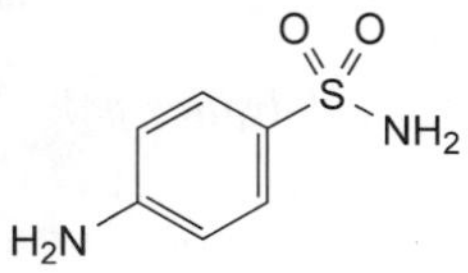

A. sulfanilamide,

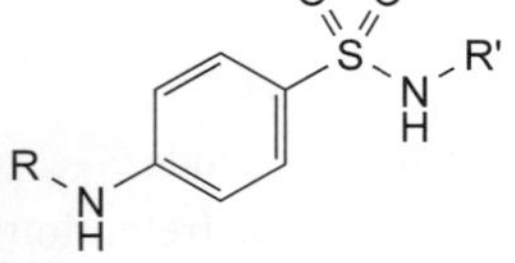

B. R = $CO\text{-}CH_3$, R′ = H: *N*-(4-sulphamoylphenyl)acetamide,

C. R = R′ = $CO\text{-}CH_3$: *N*-[[4-(acetylamino)phenyl]sulphonyl]-acetamide,

D. dapsone.

01/2008:1371
corrected 6.2

SUNFLOWER OIL, REFINED

Helianthi annui oleum raffinatum

DEFINITION

Fatty oil obtained from the seeds of *Helianthus annuus* L. by mechanical expression or by extraction. It is then refined. A suitable antioxidant may be added.

CHARACTERS

Appearance: clear, light yellow liquid.

Solubility: practically insoluble in water and in ethanol (96 per cent), miscible with light petroleum (bp: 40-60 °C).

Relative density: about 0.921.

Refractive index: about 1.474.

IDENTIFICATION

Identification of fatty oils by thin-layer chromatography (*2.3.2*).

Results: the chromatogram obtained is similar to the typical chromatogram for sunflower oil.

TESTS

Acid value (*2.5.1*): maximum 0.5, determined on 10.0 g.

Peroxide value (*2.5.5, Method A*): maximum 10.0.

Unsaponifiable matter (*2.5.7*): maximum 1.5 per cent, determined on 5.0 g.

Alkaline impurities (*2.4.19*). It complies with the test.

Composition of fatty acids (*2.4.22, Method A*). Use the mixture of calibrating substances in Table 2.4.22.-3.

Composition of the fatty-acid fraction of the oil:

- *palmitic acid*: 4.0 per cent to 9.0 per cent;
- *stearic acid*: 1.0 per cent to 7.0 per cent;
- *oleic acid*: 14.0 per cent to 40.0 per cent;
- *linoleic acid*: 48.0 per cent to 74.0 per cent.

STORAGE

In an airtight, well-filled container, protected from light.

LABELLING

The label states whether the oil is obtained by mechanical expression or by extraction.

T

07/2008:2154

TELMISARTAN

Telmisartanum

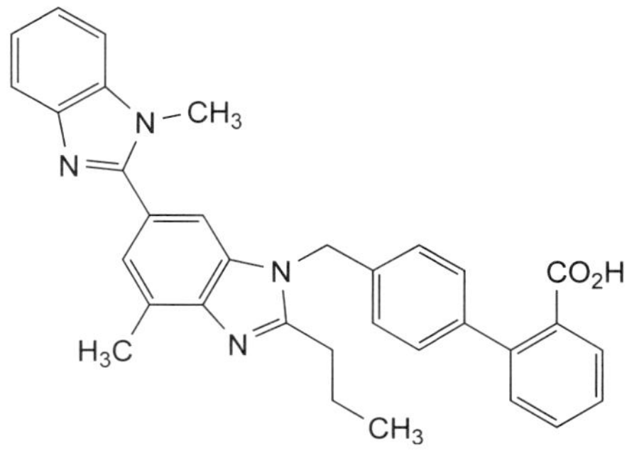

$C_{33}H_{30}N_4O_2$ M_r 514.6
[144701-48-4]

DEFINITION

4′-[[4-Methyl-6-(1-methyl-1*H*-benzimidazol-2-yl)-2-propyl-1*H*-benzimidazol-1-yl]methyl]biphenyl-2-carboxylic acid.

Content: 99.0 per cent to 101.0 per cent (dried substance).

CHARACTERS

Appearance: white or slightly yellowish, crystalline powder.

Solubility: practically insoluble in water, slightly soluble in methanol, sparingly soluble in methylene chloride. It dissolves in 1 M sodium hydroxide.

It shows polymorphism (*5.9*).

IDENTIFICATION

Infrared absorption spectrophotometry (*2.2.24*).

Comparison: *telmisartan CRS*.

If the spectra obtained in the solid state show differences, dissolve the substance to be examined and the reference substance separately in hot *anhydrous ethanol R*, evaporate to dryness and record new spectra using the residues.

TESTS

Appearance of solution. The solution is not more intensely coloured than reference solution Y_4 (*2.2.2, Method II*).

Dissolve 0.5 g in *1 M sodium hydroxide* and dilute to 10 ml with the same solvent.

Related substances. Liquid chromatography (*2.2.29*).

Test solution. To 25 mg of the substance to be examined add about 5 ml of *methanol R* and 100 µl of a 40 g/l solution of *sodium hydroxide R*. Dissolve with the aid of ultrasound and dilute to 50 ml with *methanol R*.

Reference solution (a). Dilute 1.0 ml of the test solution to 10.0 ml with *methanol R*. Dilute 1.0 ml of this solution to 100.0 ml with *methanol R*.

Reference solution (b). Dissolve the contents of a vial of *telmisartan for system suitability CRS* (containing impurities A, B, C, E and F) in 2 ml of *methanol R*.

Reference solution (c). To 5 mg of *telmisartan for peak identification CRS* (containing impurity D) add about 5 ml of *methanol R* and 100 µl of a 40 g/l solution of *sodium hydroxide R*. Dissolve with the aid of ultrasound and dilute to 10 ml with *methanol R*.

Column:
- *size*: *l* = 0.125 m, Ø = 4.0 mm;
- *stationary phase*: *octadecylsilyl silica gel for chromatography R* (5 µm) with a pore size of 10 nm;
- *temperature*: 40 °C.

Mobile phase:
- *mobile phase A*: dissolve 2.0 g of *potassium dihydrogen phosphate R* and 3.8 g of *sodium pentanesulphonate monohydrate R1* in *water R*, adjust to pH 3.0 with *dilute phosphoric acid R* and dilute to 1000 ml with *water R*;
- *mobile phase B*: *methanol R2, acetonitrile R1* (20:80 *V/V*);

Time (min)	Mobile phase A (per cent *V/V*)	Mobile phase B (per cent *V/V*)
0 - 3	70	30
3 - 28	70 → 20	30 → 80

Flow rate: 1 ml/min.

Detection: spectrophotometer at 230 nm.

Injection: 10 µl.

Identification of impurities: use the chromatogram supplied with *telmisartan for system suitability CRS* and the chromatogram obtained with reference solution (b) to identify the peaks due to impurities A, B, C, E and F; use the chromatogram supplied with *telmisartan for peak identification CRS* and the chromatogram obtained with reference solution (c) to identify the peak due to impurity D.

Relative retention with reference to telmisartan (retention time = about 12 min): impurity A = about 0.2; impurity E = about 0.6; impurity F = about 0.7; impurity B = about 0.9; impurity C = about 1.5; impurity D = about 1.6.

System suitability: reference solution (b):
- the chromatogram obtained with reference solution (b) is similar to the chromatogram supplied with *telmisartan for system suitability CRS*;
- *resolution*: minimum 3.0 between the peaks due to impurity B and telmisartan.

Limits:
- *impurities C, D*: for each impurity, not more than twice the area of the principal peak in the chromatogram obtained with reference solution (a) (0.2 per cent);
- *impurities A, B*: for each impurity, not more than 1.5 times the area of the principal peak in the chromatogram obtained with reference solution (a) (0.15 per cent);
- *unspecified impurities*: for each impurity, not more than the area of the principal peak in the chromatogram obtained with reference solution (a) (0.10 per cent);
- *total*: not more than 10 times the area of the principal peak in the chromatogram obtained with reference solution (a) (1.0 per cent);
- *disregard limit*: 0.5 times the area of the principal peak in the chromatogram obtained with reference solution (a) (0.05 per cent).

Loss on drying (*2.2.32*): maximum 0.5 per cent, determined on 1.000 g by drying in an oven at 105 °C.

Sulphated ash (*2.4.14*): maximum 0.1 per cent, determined on 1.0 g.

ASSAY

Dissolve 0.190 g in 5 ml of *anhydrous formic acid R*. Add 75 ml of *acetic anhydride R*. Titrate with *0.1 M perchloric acid*, determining the end-point potentiometrically (*2.2.20*).

1 ml of *0.1 M perchloric acid* is equivalent to 25.73 mg of $C_{33}H_{30}N_4O_2$.

IMPURITIES

Specified impurities: A, B, C, D.

Other detectable impurities (the following substances would, if present at a sufficient level, be detected by one or other of the tests in the monograph. They are limited by the general acceptance criterion for other/unspecified impurities and/or by the general monograph *Substances for pharmaceutical use (2034)*. It is therefore not necessary to identify these impurities for demonstration of compliance. See also *5.10. Control of impurities in substances for pharmaceutical use*): *E, F, G, H.*

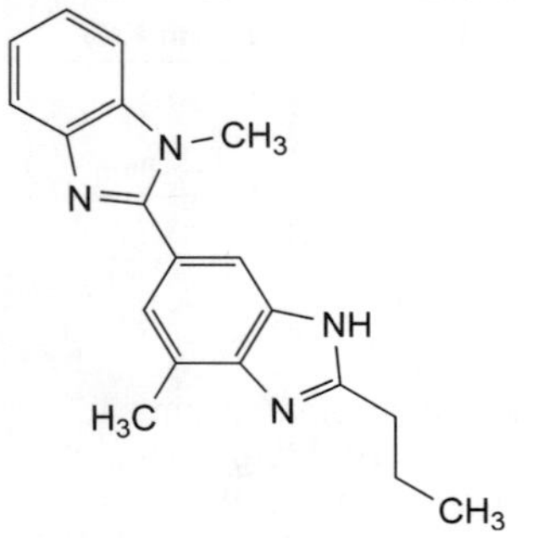

A. 4-methyl-6-(1-methyl-1*H*-benzimidazol-2-yl)-2-propyl-1*H*-benzimidazole,

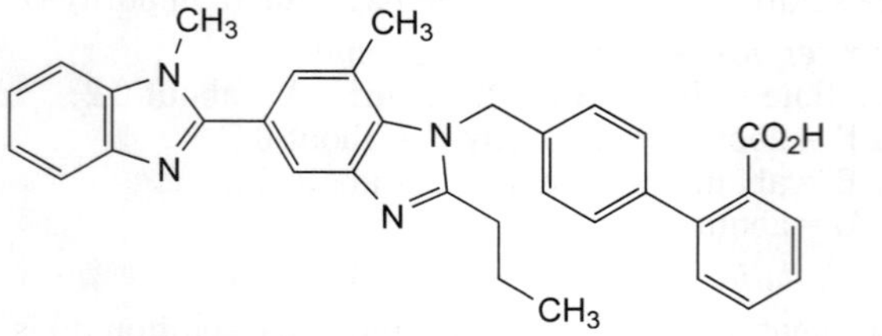

B. 4′-[[7-methyl-5-(1-methyl-1*H*-benzimidazol-2-yl)-2-propyl-1*H*-benzimidazol-1-yl]methyl]biphenyl-2-carboxylic acid,

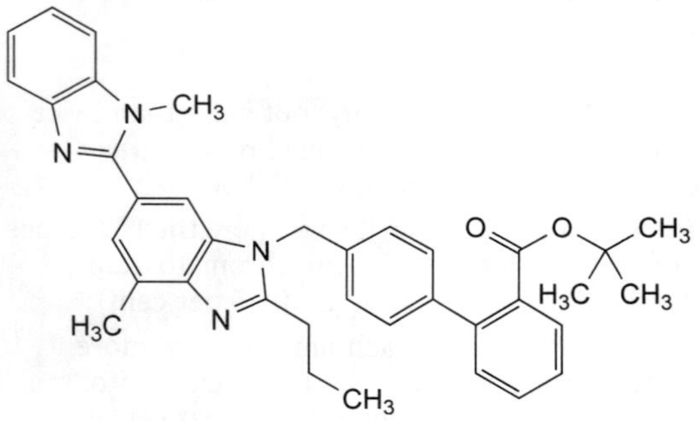

C. 1,1-dimethylethyl 4′-[[4-methyl-6-(1-methyl-1*H*-benzimidazol-2-yl)-2-propyl-1*H*-benzimidazol-1-yl]methyl]biphenyl-2-carboxylate,

D. unidentified impurity,

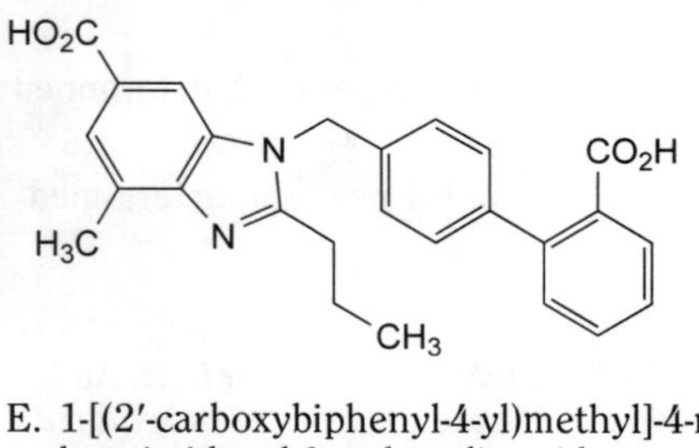

E. 1-[(2′-carboxybiphenyl-4-yl)methyl]-4-methyl-2-propyl-1*H*-benzimidazol-6-carboxylic acid,

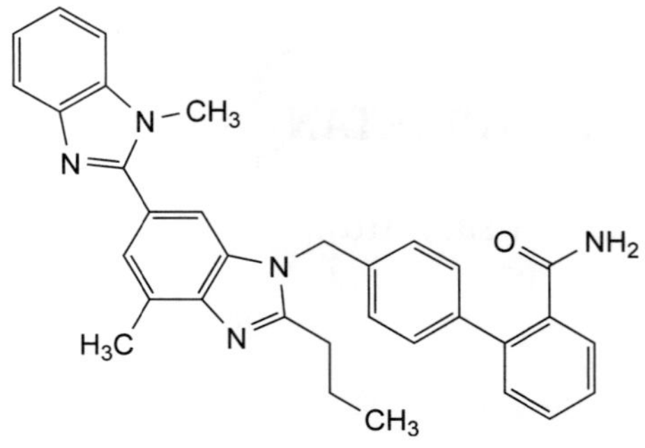

F. 4′-[[4-methyl-6-(1-methyl-1*H*-benzimidazol-2-yl)-2-propyl-1*H*-benzimidazol-1-yl]methyl]biphenyl-2-carboxamide,

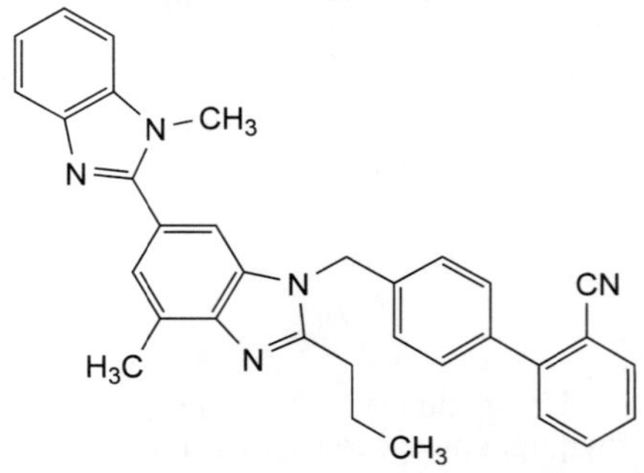

G. 4′-[[4-methyl-6-(1-methyl-1*H*-benzimidazol-2-yl)-2-propyl-1*H*-benzimidazol-1-yl]methyl]biphenyl-2-carbonitrile,

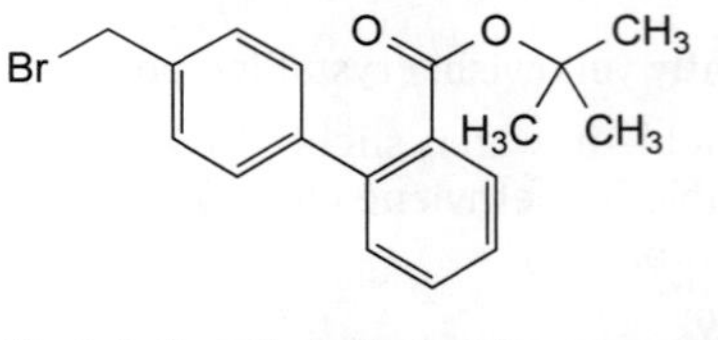

H. 1,1-dimethylethyl 4′-(bromomethyl)biphenyl-2-carboxylate.

07/2008:1051

TINIDAZOLE

Tinidazolum

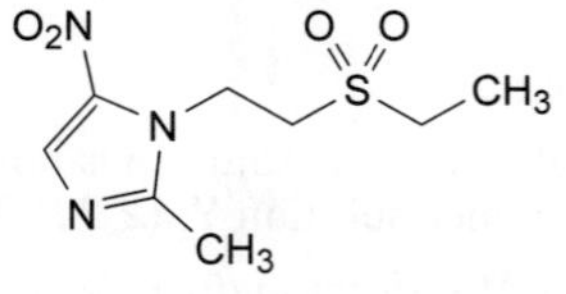

$C_8H_{13}N_3O_4S$ M_r 247.3

[19387-91-8]

DEFINITION

1-[2-(Ethylsulphonyl)ethyl]-2-methyl-5-nitro-1*H*-imidazole.

Content: 98.0 per cent to 101.0 per cent (dried substance).

CHARACTERS

Appearance: almost white or pale yellow, crystalline powder.

Solubility: practically insoluble in water, soluble in acetone and in methylene chloride, sparingly soluble in methanol.

IDENTIFICATION

First identification: A, C.

Second identification: A, B, D, E.

A. Melting point (*2.2.14*): 125 °C to 128 °C.

B. Ultraviolet and visible absorption spectrophotometry (*2.2.25*).

Test solution. Dissolve 10.0 mg in *methanol R* and dilute to 100.0 ml with the same solvent. Dilute 1.0 ml of this solution to 10.0 ml with *methanol R*.

Spectral range: 220-350 nm.

Absorption maximum: at 310 nm.

Specific absorbance at the absorption maximum: 340 to 360.

C. Infrared absorption spectrophotometry (*2.2.24*).

Comparison: *tinidazole CRS*.

D. Thin-layer chromatography (*2.2.27*).

Test solution. Dissolve 20 mg of the substance to be examined in *methanol R* and dilute to 10 ml with the same solvent.

Reference solution. Dissolve 20 mg of *tinidazole CRS* in *methanol R* and dilute to 10 ml with the same solvent.

Plate: *TLC silica gel GF_{254} plate R*.

Pretreatment: heat at 110 °C for 1 h and allow to cool.

Mobile phase: *butanol R, ethyl acetate R* (25:75 *V/V*).

Application: 10 µl.

Development: over 2/3 of the plate.

Drying: in air.

Detection: examine in ultraviolet light at 254 nm.

Results: the principal spot in the chromatogram obtained with the test solution is similar in position and size to the principal spot in the chromatogram obtained with the reference solution.

E. To about 10 mg add about 10 mg of *zinc powder R*, 0.3 ml of *hydrochloric acid R* and 1 ml of *water R*. Heat in a water-bath for 5 min and cool. The solution gives the reaction of primary aromatic amines (*2.3.1*).

TESTS

Appearance of solution. The solution is clear (*2.2.1*) and not more intensely coloured than reference solution Y_5 (*2.2.2, Method II*).

Dissolve 1.0 g in *acetone R* and dilute to 20 ml with the same solvent.

Related substances. Liquid chromatography (*2.2.29*). *Protect solutions from light.*

Test solution. Dissolve 10.0 mg of the substance to be examined in 10.0 ml of *methanol R* and dilute to 100.0 ml with the mobile phase.

Reference solution (a). Dilute 1.0 ml of the test solution to 100.0 ml with the mobile phase. Dilute 1.0 ml of this solution to 10.0 ml with the mobile phase.

Reference solution (b). Dissolve 5.0 mg of *tinidazole impurity A CRS* and 5.0 mg of *tinidazole impurity B CRS* in 10.0 ml of *methanol R* and dilute to 100.0 ml with the mobile phase. Dilute 2.0 ml of this solution to 10.0 ml with the mobile phase.

Reference solution (c). Dilute 1.0 ml of reference solution (b) to 50.0 ml with the mobile phase.

Column:

- *size*: *l* = 0.25 m, Ø = 3.0 mm;
- *stationary phase*: *octylsilyl silica gel for chromatography R* (5 µm).

Regular column conditioning by subsequent flushing with 50 ml of *water R*, 100 ml of *methanol R*, 25 ml of *water R* and 100 ml of the mobile phase is recommended.

Mobile phase: *acetonitrile R, methanol R, water R* (10:20:70 *V/V/V*).

Flow rate: 0.5 ml/min.

Detection: spectrophotometer at 320 nm.

Injection: 20 µl.

Run time: 1.5 times the retention time of tinidazole.

Relative retention with reference to tinidazole (retention time = about 6 min): impurity A = about 0.6; impurity B = about 0.7.

System suitability: reference solution (b):

- *resolution*: minimum 2.0 between the peaks due to impurities A and B.

Limits:

- *impurities A, B*: for each impurity, not more than the area of the corresponding peak in the chromatogram obtained with reference solution (c) (0.2 per cent);
- *unspecified impurities*: for each impurity, not more than the area of the principal peak in the chromatogram obtained with reference solution (a) (0.10 per cent);
- *total*: not more than 4 times the area of the principal peak in the chromatogram obtained with reference solution (a) (0.4 per cent);
- *disregard limit*: 0.5 times the area of the principal peak in the chromatogram obtained with reference solution (a) (0.05 per cent).

Heavy metals (*2.4.8*): maximum 20 ppm.

1.0 g complies with test D. Prepare the reference solution using 2 ml of *lead standard solution (10 ppm Pb) R*.

Loss on drying (*2.2.32*): maximum 0.5 per cent, determined on 1.000 g by drying in an oven at 105 °C.

Sulphated ash (*2.4.14*): maximum 0.1 per cent, determined on 1.0 g.

ASSAY

Dissolve 0.150 g in 25 ml of *anhydrous acetic acid R*. Titrate with *0.1 M perchloric acid*, determining the end-point potentiometrically (*2.2.20*).

1 ml of *0.1 M perchloric acid* is equivalent to 24.73 mg of $C_8H_{13}N_3O_4S$.

STORAGE

Protected from light.

IMPURITIES

Specified impurities: A, B.

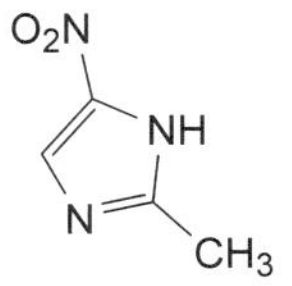

A. 2-methyl-5-nitro-1*H*-imidazole,

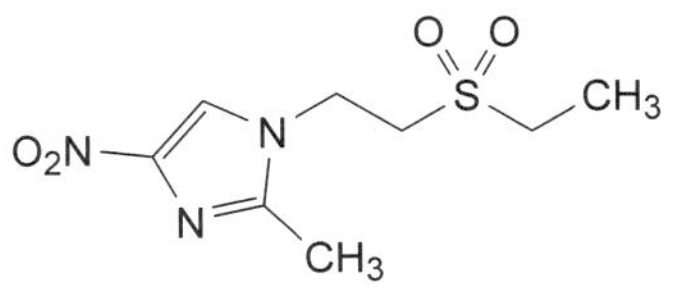

B. 1-[2-(ethylsulphonyl)ethyl]-2-methyl-4-nitro-1*H*-imidazole.

Monographs Q-Z

01/2008:0645
corrected 6.2

TOBRAMYCIN

Tobramycinum

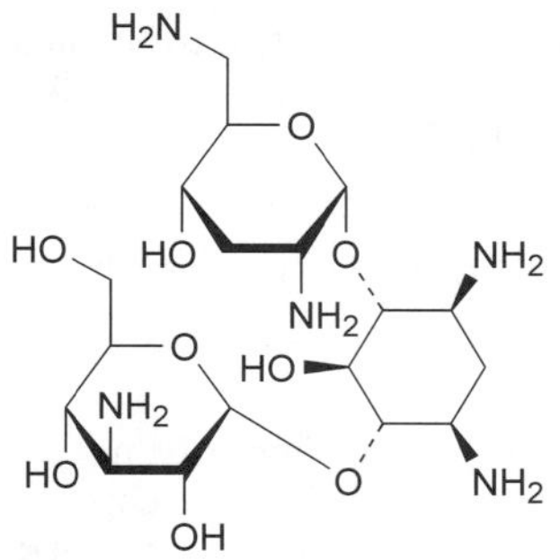

$C_{18}H_{37}N_5O_9$ M_r 467.5
[32986-56-4]

DEFINITION

4-*O*-(3-Amino-3-deoxy-α-D-glucopyranosyl)-2-deoxy-6-*O*-(2,6-diamino-2,3,6-trideoxy-α-D-*ribo*-hexopyranosyl)-L-streptamine.

Substance produced by *Streptomyces tenebrarius* or obtained by any other means.

Content: 97.0 per cent to 102.0 per cent (anhydrous substance).

PRODUCTION

It is produced by methods of manufacture designed to eliminate or minimise substances lowering blood pressure.

CHARACTERS

Appearance: white or almost white powder.

Solubility: freely soluble in water, very slightly soluble in ethanol (96 per cent).

IDENTIFICATION

First identification: A.

Second identification: B, C.

A. Nuclear magnetic resonance spectrometry (*2.2.33*).

Preparation: 100 g/l solution in *deuterium oxide R.*

Comparison: 100 g/l solution of *tobramycin CRS* in *deuterium oxide R.*

B. Thin-layer chromatography (*2.2.27*).

Test solution. Dissolve 20 mg of the substance to be examined in *water R* and dilute to 5 ml with the same solvent.

Reference solution (a). Dissolve 20 mg of *tobramycin CRS* in *water R* and dilute to 5 ml with the same solvent.

Reference solution (b). Dissolve 4 mg of *neomycin sulphate CRS* and 4 mg of *kanamycin monosulphate CRS* in 1 ml of reference solution (a).

Plate: *TLC silica gel plate R.*

Mobile phase: *methylene chloride R, concentrated ammonia R, methanol R* (17:33:50 *V/V/V*).

Application: 5 µl.

Development: over 2/3 of the plate.

Drying: in a current of warm air.

Detection: spray with a mixture of equal volumes of a 2 g/l solution of *1,3-dihydroxynaphthalene R* in *ethanol (96 per cent) R* and a 460 g/l solution of *sulphuric acid R*; heat at 105 °C for 5-10 min.

System suitability: the chromatogram obtained with reference solution (b) shows 3 major spots which are clearly separated.

Results: the principal spot in the chromatogram obtained with the test solution is similar in position, colour and size to the principal spot in the chromatogram obtained with reference solution (a).

C. Dissolve about 5 mg in 5 ml of *water R.* Add 5 ml of a 1 g/l solution of *ninhydrin R* in *ethanol (96 per cent) R* and heat in a water-bath for 3 min. A violet-blue colour develops.

TESTS

pH (*2.2.3*): 9.0 to 11.0.

Dissolve 1.0 g in 10 ml of *carbon dioxide-free water R.*

Specific optical rotation (*2.2.7*): + 138 to + 148 (anhydrous substance).

Dissolve 1.00 g in *water R* and dilute to 25.0 ml with the same solvent.

Related substances. Liquid chromatography (*2.2.29*).

Test solution (a). Dissolve 25.0 mg of the substance to be examined in the mobile phase and dilute to 25.0 ml with the mobile phase.

Test solution (b). Dilute 10.0 ml of test solution (a) to 100.0 ml with the mobile phase.

Reference solution (a). Dissolve 25.0 mg of *tobramycin CRS* in the mobile phase and dilute to 100.0 ml with the mobile phase.

Reference solution (b). Dilute 1.0 ml of reference solution (a) to 100.0 ml with the mobile phase.

Reference solution (c). Dilute 1.0 ml of reference solution (a) to 50.0 ml with the mobile phase.

Reference solution (d). Dissolve 10.0 mg of *kanamycin B sulphate CRS* in 20.0 ml of the mobile phase. To 1.0 ml of this solution, add 2.0 ml of reference solution (a) and dilute to 10.0 ml with the mobile phase.

Reference solution (e). Dilute 10.0 ml of reference solution (a) to 25.0 ml with the mobile phase.

Column:

- *size*: l = 0.25 m, Ø = 4.6 mm;
- *stationary phase*: *styrene-divinylbenzene copolymer R* (8 µm) with a pore size of 100 nm;
- *temperature*: 55 °C.

Mobile phase: mixture prepared with *carbon dioxide-free water R* containing 52 g/l of *anhydrous sodium sulphate R*, 1.5 g/l of *sodium octanesulphonate R*, 3 ml/l of *tetrahydrofuran R* stabilised with *butylhydroxytoluene R*, and 50 ml/l of *0.2 M potassium dihydrogen phosphate R* previously adjusted to pH 3.0 with *dilute phosphoric acid R*. Degas.

Flow rate: 1.0 ml/min.

Post-column solution: *carbonate-free sodium hydroxide solution R* diluted 25-fold with *carbon dioxide-free water R*, which is added pulselessly to the column effluent using a 375 µl polymeric mixing coil.

Flow rate: 0.3 ml/min.

Detection: pulsed amperometric detector or equivalent with a gold working electrode, a silver-silver chloride reference electrode and a stainless steel auxiliary electrode which is the cell body, held at respectively + 0.05 V detection, + 0.75 V oxidation and – 0.15 V reduction potentials, with pulse durations according to the instrument used. The temperature of the detector is set at 35 °C.

NOTE: to prevent problems due to salt precipitation, the electrochemical cell can be flushed with water R overnight.

Injection: 20 µl using a refrigerated injector (4-8 °C); inject test solution (a) and reference solutions (b), (c) and (d).

Run time: 1.5 times the retention time of tobramycin.

Relative retention with reference to tobramycin (retention time = about 18 min): impurity C = about 0.35; impurity B = about 0.40, impurity A = about 0.70.

System suitability:

- *resolution*: minimum 3.0 between the peaks due to impurity A and to tobramycin in the chromatogram obtained with reference solution (d); if necessary, adjust the concentration of sodium octanesulphonate in the mobile phase;
- *signal-to-noise ratio*: minimum 10 for the principal peak in the chromatogram obtained with reference solution (b).

Limits:

- *any impurity*: not more than twice the area of the principal peak in the chromatogram obtained with reference solution (c) (1.0 per cent) and not more than 1 such peak has an area greater than the area of the principal peak in the chromatogram obtained with reference solution (c) (0.5 per cent);
- *total*: not more than 3 times the area of the principal peak in the chromatogram obtained with reference solution (c) (1.5 per cent);
- *disregard limit*: the area of the principal peak in the chromatogram obtained with reference solution (b) (0.25 per cent).

2-Methyl-1-propanol (*2.4.24, System B*): maximum 1.0 per cent *m/m*.

Water (*2.5.12*): maximum 8.0 per cent, determined on 0.30 g.

Sulphated ash (*2.4.14*): maximum 0.3 per cent, determined on 1.0 g.

Bacterial endotoxins (*2.6.14*): less than 2.0 IU/mg, if intended for use in the manufacture of parenteral preparations without a further appropriate procedure for the removal of bacterial endotoxins.

ASSAY

Liquid chromatography (*2.2.29*) as described in the test for related substances with the following modifications.

Injection: test solution (b) and reference solution (e).

Calculate the percentage content of tobramycin.

STORAGE

If the substance is sterile, store in a sterile, airtight, tamper-proof container.

IMPURITIES

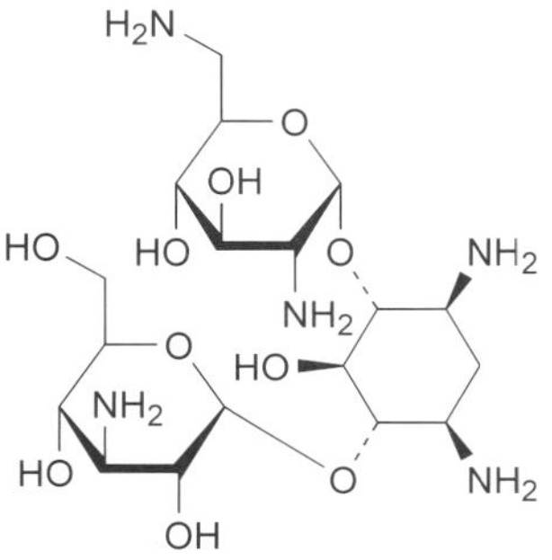

A. 4-*O*-(3-amino-3-deoxy-α-D-glucopyranosyl)-2-deoxy-6-*O*-(2,6-diamino-2,6-dideoxy-α-D-glucopyranosyl)-L-streptamine (kanamycin B),

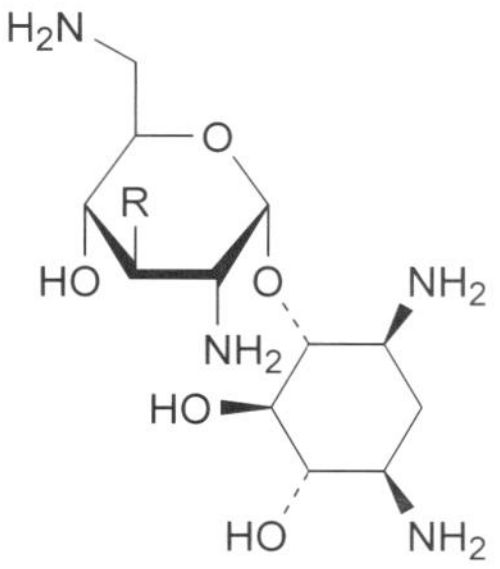

B. R = H: 2-deoxy-4-*O*-(2,6-diamino-2,3,6-trideoxy-α-D-ribo-hexopyranosyl)-D-streptamine (nebramine),

C. R = OH: 2-deoxy-4-*O*-(2,6-diamino-2,6-dideoxy-α-D-glucopyranosyl)-D-streptamine (neamine).

01/2008:0532

TRAGACANTH

Tragacantha

DEFINITION

Air-hardened, gummy exudate, flowing naturally or obtained by incision from the trunk and branches of *Astragalus gummifer* Labill. and certain other species of *Astragalus* from western Asia.

IDENTIFICATION

A. Tragacanth occurs in thin, flattened, ribbon-like, white or pale yellow, translucent strips, about 30 mm long and 10 mm wide and up to 1 mm thick, more or less curved, horny, with a short fracture; the surface is marked by fine longitudinal striae and concentric transverse ridges. It may also contain pieces similar in shape but somewhat thicker, more opaque and more difficult to fracture.

B. Reduce to a powder (355) (*2.9.12*). The powder is white or almost white and forms a mucilaginous gel with about 10 times its mass of *water R*. Examine under a microscope using a 50 per cent *V/V* solution of *glycerol R*. The powder shows in the gummy mass numerous stratified cellular membranes that turn slowly violet when treated with *iodinated zinc chloride solution R*. The gummy mass includes starch grains, isolated or in small groups, usually rounded in shape and sometimes deformed, with diameters varying between 4 µm and 10 µm, occasionally up to 20 µm, and a central hilum visible between crossed nicol prisms.

C. Examine the chromatograms obtained in the test for acacia.

Results: the chromatogram obtained with the test solution shows 3 zones due to galactose, arabinose and xylose. A faint yellowish zone at the solvent front and a greyish-green zone between the zones due to galactose and arabinose may be present.

D. Moisten 0.5 g of the powdered drug (355) (*2.9.12*) with 1 ml of *ethanol (96 per cent) R* and add gradually, while shaking, 50 ml of *water R* until a homogeneous mucilage is obtained. To 5 ml of the mucilage add 5 ml of *water R* and 2 ml of *barium hydroxide solution R*. A slight flocculent precipitate is formed. Heat on a water-bath for 10 min. An intense yellow colour develops.

TESTS

Acacia. Thin-layer chromatography (*2.2.27*).

Test solution. To 100 mg of the powdered drug (355) (*2.9.12*) in a thick-walled centrifuge test-tube, add 2 ml of a

100 g/l solution of *trifluoroacetic acid R*, shake vigorously to dissolve the forming gel, stopper the test-tube and heat the mixture at 120 °C for 1 h. Centrifuge the resulting hydrolysate, transfer the clear supernatant carefully into a 50 ml flask, add 10 ml of *water R* and evaporate the solution to dryness under reduced pressure. To the resulting clear film add 0.1 ml of *water R* and 0.9 ml of *methanol R*. Centrifuge to separate the amorphous precipitate, collect the supernatant and, if necessary, dilute to 1 ml with *methanol R*.

Reference solution. Dissolve 10 mg of *arabinose R*, 10 mg of *galactose R*, 10 mg of *rhamnose R* and 10 mg of *xylose R* in 1 ml of *water R* and dilute to 10 ml with *methanol R*.

Plate: *TLC silica gel plate R*.

Mobile phase: 16 g/l solution of *sodium dihydrogen phosphate R*, *butanol R*, *acetone R* (10:40:50 *V/V/V*).

Application: 10 µl as bands.

Development A: over a path of 10 cm.

Drying A: in a current of warm air for a few minutes.

Development B: over a path of 15 cm using the same mobile phase.

Drying B: at 110 °C for 10 min.

Detection: spray with *anisaldehyde solution R* and dry at 110 °C for 10 min.

Results: the chromatogram obtained with the reference solution shows 4 clearly separated coloured zones due to galactose (greyish-green or green), arabinose (yellowish-green), xylose (greenish-grey or yellowish-grey) and rhamnose (yellowish-green), in order of increasing R_F value; the chromatogram obtained with the test solution does not show a yellowish-green zone corresponding to the zone of rhamnose in the chromatogram obtained with the reference solution.

Methylcellulose. Examine the chromatograms obtained in the test for acacia.

Results: the chromatogram obtained with the test solution does not show a red zone near the solvent front.

Sterculia gum

A. Place 0.2 g of the powdered drug (355) (*2.9.12*) in a 10 ml ground-glass-stoppered cylinder graduated in 0.1 ml. Add 10 ml of *ethanol (60 per cent V/V) R* and shake. Any gel formed occupies not more than 1.5 ml.

B. To 1.0 g of the powdered drug (355) (*2.9.12*) add 100 ml of *water R* and shake. Add 0.1 ml of *methyl red solution R*. Not more than 5.0 ml of *0.01 M sodium hydroxide* is required to change the colour of the indicator.

Foreign matter: maximum 1.0 per cent.

Place 2.0 g of the powdered drug (355) (*2.9.12*) in a 250 ml round-bottomed flask and add 95 ml of *methanol R*. Swirl to moisten the powder and add 60 ml of *hydrochloric acid R1*. Add a few glass beads about 4 mm in diameter and heat on a water-bath under a reflux condenser for 3 h, shaking occasionally. Remove the glass beads and filter the hot suspension *in vacuo* through a sintered-glass filter (160) (*2.1.2*). Rinse the flask with a small quantity of *water R* and pass the rinsings through the filter. Wash the residue on the filter with about 40 ml of *methanol R* and dry to constant mass at 110 °C (about 1 h). Allow to cool in a desiccator and weigh. The residue weighs a maximum of 20 mg.

Flow time: minimum 10 s, or minimum 50 s if the substance to be examined is to be used for the preparation of emulsions.

Place 1.0 g of the powdered drug (125-250) (*2.9.12*) in a 1000 ml round-bottomed flask with a ground-glass stopper, add 8.0 ml of *ethanol (96 per cent) R* and close the flask. Disperse the suspension over the inner surface of the flask by shaking, taking care not to wet the stopper. Open the flask and add as a single portion 72.0 ml of *water R*. Stopper the flask and shake vigorously for 3 min. Allow to stand for 24 h and shake vigorously again for 3 min. Eliminate air bubbles by applying vacuum above the mucilage for 5 min. Transfer the mucilage to a 50 ml cylinder. Dip in the mucilage a piece of glass tubing 200 mm long and 6.0 mm in internal diameter and graduated at 20 mm and 120 mm from the lower end; the tubing must not be rinsed with surface-active substances. When the mucilage has reached the upper mark, close the tube with a finger. Withdraw the closed tube, remove the finger and measure with a stop-watch the time needed for the meniscus to reach the lower graduation. Carry out this operation 4 times and determine the average value of the last 3 determinations.

Total ash (*2.4.16*): maximum 4.0 per cent.

Microbial contamination. Total viable aerobic count (*2.6.12*) not more than 10^4 micro-organisms per gram, determined by plate count. It complies with the tests for *Escherichia coli* and *Salmonella* (*2.6.13*).

LABELLING

The label states whether or not the contents are suitable for preparing emulsions.

INDEX

To aid users the index includes a reference to the supplement where the latest version of a text can be found.

For example: Amikacin..**6.1**-3396

means the monograph Amikacin can be found on page 3396 of Supplement 6.1.

Note that where no reference to a supplement is made, the text can be found in the principal volume.

Monographs deleted from the 6th Edition are not included in the index; a list of deleted texts is found in the Contents of this supplement, page xxxv.

Numerics

1. General notices ... 3
2.1.1. Droppers ... 15
2.1.2. Comparative table of porosity of sintered-glass filters ... 15
2.1.3. Ultraviolet ray lamps for analytical purposes ... 15
2.1.4. Sieves ... 16
2.1.5. Tubes for comparative tests ... 17
2.1.6. Gas detector tubes ... 17
2.1. Apparatus ... 15
2.2.10. Viscosity - Rotating viscometer method ... 28
2.2.11. Distillation range ... 30
2.2.12. Boiling point ... 31
2.2.13. Determination of water by distillation ... 31
2.2.14. Melting point - capillary method ... 32
2.2.15. Melting point - open capillary method ... 32
2.2.16. Melting point - instantaneous method ... 33
2.2.17. Drop point ... 33
2.2.18. Freezing point ... 35
2.2.19. Amperometric titration ... 35
2.2.1. Clarity and degree of opalescence of liquids ... 21
2.2.20. Potentiometric titration ... 35
2.2.21. Fluorimetry ... 36
2.2.22. Atomic emission spectrometry ... 36
2.2.23. Atomic absorption spectrometry ... 37
2.2.24. Absorption spectrophotometry, infrared ... 39
2.2.25. Absorption spectrophotometry, ultraviolet and visible ... 41
2.2.26. Paper chromatography ... 43
2.2.27. Thin-layer chromatography ... 43
2.2.28. Gas chromatography ... 45
2.2.29. Liquid chromatography ... 46
2.2.2. Degree of coloration of liquids ... 22
2.2.30. Size-exclusion chromatography ... 47
2.2.31. Electrophoresis ... 48
2.2.32. Loss on drying ... 53
2.2.33. Nuclear magnetic resonance spectrometry ... 54
2.2.34. Thermal analysis ... **6.1**-3311
2.2.35. Osmolality ... 57
2.2.36. Potentiometric determination of ionic concentration using ion-selective electrodes ... 58
2.2.37. X-ray fluorescence spectrometry ... 59
2.2.38. Conductivity ... 59
2.2.39. Molecular mass distribution in dextrans ... 60
2.2.3. Potentiometric determination of pH ... 24
2.2.40. Near-infrared spectrophotometry ... 62
2.2.41. Circular dichroism ... 66
2.2.42. Density of solids ... 67
2.2.43. Mass spectrometry ... 68
2.2.44. Total organic carbon in water for pharmaceutical use ... 71
2.2.45. Supercritical fluid chromatography ... 71
2.2.46. Chromatographic separation techniques ... 72
2.2.47. Capillary electrophoresis ... 77
2.2.48. Raman spectrometry ... 82
2.2.49. Falling ball viscometer method ... 84
2.2.4. Relationship between reaction of solution, approximate pH and colour of certain indicators ... 25
2.2.54. Isoelectric focusing ... 84
2.2.55. Peptide mapping ... 86
2.2.56. Amino acid analysis ... 89
2.2.57. Inductively coupled plasma-atomic emission spectrometry ... 96
2.2.58. Inductively coupled plasma-mass spectrometry ... 98
2.2.5. Relative density ... 25
2.2.60. Melting point - instrumental method ... **6.1**-3313
2.2.6. Refractive index ... 26
2.2.7. Optical rotation ... 26
2.2.8. Viscosity ... 27
2.2.9. Capillary viscometer method ... 27
2.2. Physical and physicochemical methods ... 21
2.3.1. Identification reactions of ions and functional groups ... 103
2.3.2. Identification of fatty oils by thin-layer chromatography ... 106
2.3.3. Identification of phenothiazines by thin-layer chromatography ... 107
2.3.4. Odour ... 107
2.3. Identification ... 103
2.4.10. Lead in sugars ... 115
2.4.11. Phosphates ... 116
2.4.12. Potassium ... 116
2.4.13. Sulphates ... 116
2.4.14. Sulphated ash ... 116
2.4.15. Nickel in polyols ... 116
2.4.16. Total ash ... 116
2.4.17. Aluminium ... 117
2.4.18. Free formaldehyde ... 117
2.4.19. Alkaline impurities in fatty oils ... 117
2.4.1. Ammonium ... 111
2.4.21. Foreign oils in fatty oils by thin-layer chromatography ... 117
2.4.22. Composition of fatty acids by gas chromatography ... 118
2.4.23. Sterols in fatty oils ... 120
2.4.24. Identification and control of residual solvents ... 121
2.4.25. Ethylene oxide and dioxan ... 126
2.4.26. *N,N*-Dimethylaniline ... 127
2.4.27. Heavy metals in herbal drugs and fatty oils ... 128
2.4.28. 2-Ethylhexanoic acid ... 129
2.4.29. Composition of fatty acids in oils rich in omega-3 acids ... **6.2**-3623
2.4.2. Arsenic ... 111
2.4.30. Ethylene glycol and diethylene glycol in ethoxylated substances ... 131
2.4.31. Nickel in hydrogenated vegetable oils ... 131
2.4.32. Total cholesterol in oils rich in omega-3 acids ... 132
2.4.3. Calcium ... 111
2.4.4. Chlorides ... 112
2.4.5. Fluorides ... 112
2.4.6. Magnesium ... 112
2.4.7. Magnesium and alkaline-earth metals ... 112
2.4.8. Heavy metals ... 112
2.4.9. Iron ... 115
2.4. Limit tests ... 111
2.5.10. Oxygen-flask method ... 140
2.5.11. Complexometric titrations ... 140
2.5.12. Water: semi-micro determination ... 141
2.5.13. Aluminium in adsorbed vaccines ... 141
2.5.14. Calcium in adsorbed vaccines ... 142
2.5.15. Phenol in immunosera and vaccines ... 142
2.5.16. Protein in polysaccharide vaccines ... 142
2.5.17. Nucleic acids in polysaccharide vaccines ... 142
2.5.18. Phosphorus in polysaccharide vaccines ... 142
2.5.19. *O*-Acetyl in polysaccharide vaccines ... 143
2.5.1. Acid value ... 137
2.5.20. Hexosamines in polysaccharide vaccines ... 143
2.5.21. Methylpentoses in polysaccharide vaccines ... 143
2.5.22. Uronic acids in polysaccharide vaccines ... 144
2.5.23. Sialic acid in polysaccharide vaccines ... 144
2.5.24. Carbon dioxide in gases ... 144
2.5.25. Carbon monoxide in gases ... 145
2.5.26. Nitrogen monoxide and nitrogen dioxide in gases ... 146
2.5.27. Oxygen in gases ... 146
2.5.28. Water in gases ... 146
2.5.29. Sulphur dioxide ... 146
2.5.2. Ester value ... 137

2.5.30. Oxidising substances 147
2.5.31. Ribose in polysaccharide vaccines 147
2.5.32. Water: micro determination 147
2.5.33. Total protein 148
2.5.34. Acetic acid in synthetic peptides 151
2.5.35. Nitrous oxide in gases 152
2.5.36. Anisidine value 152
2.5.3. Hydroxyl value 137
2.5.4. Iodine value 137
2.5.5. Peroxide value 138
2.5.6. Saponification value 139
2.5.7. Unsaponifiable matter 139
2.5.8. Determination of primary aromatic amino-nitrogen 139
2.5.9. Determination of nitrogen by sulphuric acid digestion 139
2.5. Assays 137
2.6.10. Histamine 165
2.6.11. Depressor substances 166
2.6.12. Microbiological examination of non-sterile products: total viable aerobic count 166
2.6.13. Microbiological examination of non-sterile products: test for specified micro-organisms 173
2.6.14. Bacterial endotoxins 182
2.6.15. Prekallikrein activator 189
2.6.16. Tests for extraneous agents in viral vaccines for human use 190
2.6.17. Test for anticomplementary activity of immunoglobulin 191
2.6.18. Test for neurovirulence of live virus vaccines 193
2.6.19. Test for neurovirulence of poliomyelitis vaccine (oral) 193
2.6.1. Sterility 155
2.6.20. Anti-A and anti-B haemagglutinins (indirect method) 195
2.6.21. Nucleic acid amplification techniques 195
2.6.22. Activated coagulation factors 198
2.6.24. Avian viral vaccines: tests for extraneous agents in seed lots 198
2.6.25. Avian live virus vaccines: tests for extraneous agents in batches of finished product 202
2.6.26. Test for anti-D antibodies in human immunoglobulin for intravenous administration **6.2**-3627
2.6.27. Microbiological control of cellular products 205
2.6.2. Mycobacteria 159
2.6.7. Mycoplasmas **6.1**-3317
2.6.8. Pyrogens 164
2.6.9. Abnormal toxicity 165
2.6. Biological tests 155
2.7.10. Assay of human coagulation factor VII 228
2.7.11. Assay of human coagulation factor IX 229
2.7.12. Assay of heparin in coagulation factors 230
2.7.13. Assay of human anti-D immunoglobulin 230
2.7.14. Assay of hepatitis A vaccine 232
2.7.15. Assay of hepatitis B vaccine (rDNA) 233
2.7.16. Assay of pertussis vaccine (acellular) 233
2.7.17. Assay of human antithrombin III 234
2.7.18. Assay of human coagulation factor II 234
2.7.19. Assay of human coagulation factor X 235
2.7.19. Assay of human coagulation factor X (2.7.19.) 235
2.7.1. Immunochemical methods 209
2.7.20. *In vivo* assay of poliomyelitis vaccine (inactivated) 235
2.7.21. Assay of human von Willebrand factor 237
2.7.22. Assay of human coagulation factor XI 238
2.7.23. Numeration of CD34/CD45+ cells in haematopoietic products 238
2.7.24. Flow cytometry 240
2.7.25. Assay of human plasmin inhibitor **6.2**-3631
2.7.27. Flocculation value (Lf) of diphtheria and tetanus toxins and toxoids (Ramon assay) 241
2.7.28. Colony-forming cell assay for human haematopoietic progenitor cells 242
2.7.29. Nucleated cell count and viability 243
2.7.2. Microbiological assay of antibiotics 210
2.7.30. Assay of human protein C **6.2**-3631
2.7.31. Assay of human protein S **6.2**-3632
2.7.32. Assay of human α-1-proteinase inhibitor **6.2**-3633
2.7.4. Assay of human coagulation factor VIII 216
2.7.5. Assay of heparin 217
2.7.6. Assay of diphtheria vaccine (adsorbed) 217
2.7.7. Assay of pertussis vaccine 222
2.7.8. Assay of tetanus vaccine (adsorbed) 223
2.7.9. Test for Fc function of immunoglobulin 227
2.7. Biological assays 209
2.8.10. Solubility in alcohol of essential oils 250
2.8.11. Assay of 1,8-cineole in essential oils 250
2.8.12. Determination of essential oils in herbal drugs 251
2.8.13. Pesticide residues **6.2**-3637
2.8.14. Determination of tannins in herbal drugs 255
2.8.15. Bitterness value 255
2.8.16. Dry residue of extracts 256
2.8.17. Loss on drying of extracts 256
2.8.18. Determination of aflatoxin B_1 in herbal drugs 256
2.8.1. Ash insoluble in hydrochloric acid 249
2.8.20. Herbal drugs: sampling and sample preparation 258
2.8.2. Foreign matter 249
2.8.3. Stomata and stomatal index 249
2.8.4. Swelling index 249
2.8.5. Water in essential oils 249
2.8.6. Foreign esters in essential oils 250
2.8.7. Fatty oils and resinified essential oils in essential oils 250
2.8.8. Odour and taste of essential oils 250
2.8.9. Residue on evaporation of essential oils 250
2.8. Methods in pharmacognosy 249
2.9.10. Ethanol content and alcoholimetric tables 281
2.9.11. Test for methanol and 2-propanol 282
2.9.12. Sieve test 283
2.9.14. Specific surface area by air permeability 283
2.9.15. Apparent volume 285
2.9.16. Flowability 286
2.9.17. Test for extractable volume of parenteral preparations 287
2.9.18. Preparations for inhalation: aerodynamic assessment of fine particles 287
2.9.19. Particulate contamination: sub-visible particles 300
2.9.1. Disintegration of tablets and capsules 263
2.9.20. Particulate contamination: visible particles 302
2.9.22. Softening time determination of lipophilic suppositories 302
2.9.23. Gas pycnometric density of solids **6.2**-3642
2.9.25. Dissolution test for medicated chewing gums 304
2.9.26. Specific surface area by gas adsorption 306
2.9.27. Uniformity of mass of delivered doses from multidose containers 309
2.9.29. Intrinsic dissolution 309
2.9.2. Disintegration of suppositories and pessaries 265
2.9.31. Particle size analysis by laser light diffraction 311
2.9.32. Porosity and pore-size distribution of solids by mercury porosimetry **6.2**-3643
2.9.33. Characterisation of crystalline and partially crystalline solids by X-ray powder diffraction (XRPD) 314
2.9.34. Bulk density and tapped density of powders **6.2**-3646
2.9.35. Powder fineness **6.2**-3648
2.9.36. Powder flow 320
2.9.37. Optical microscopy 323

2.9.38. Particle-size distribution estimation by analytical sieving **6.2**-3649
2.9.3. Dissolution test for solid dosage forms 266
2.9.40. Uniformity of dosage units **6.1**-3325
2.9.41. Friability of granules and spheroids 330
2.9.42. Dissolution test for lipophilic solid dosage forms .. 332
2.9.43. Apparent dissolution **6.1**-3327
2.9.4. Dissolution test for transdermal patches 275
2.9.5. Uniformity of mass of single-dose preparations 278
2.9.6. Uniformity of content of single-dose preparations .. 278
2.9.7. Friability of uncoated tablets 278
2.9.8. Resistance to crushing of tablets 279
2.9.9. Measurement of consistency by penetrometry **6.2**-3641
2.9. Pharmaceutical technical procedures 263
3.1.10. Materials based on non-plasticised poly(vinyl chloride) for containers for non-injectable, aqueous solutions 360
3.1.11. Materials based on non-plasticised poly(vinyl chloride) for containers for dry dosage forms for oral administration 362
3.1.1.1. Materials based on plasticised poly(vinyl chloride) for containers for human blood and blood components 339
3.1.1.2. Materials based on plasticised poly(vinyl chloride) for tubing used in sets for the transfusion of blood and blood components 342
3.1.13. Plastic additives **6.2**-3655
3.1.14. Materials based on plasticised poly(vinyl chloride) for containers for aqueous solutions for intravenous infusion 366
3.1.15. Polyethylene terephthalate for containers for preparations not for parenteral use 369
3.1.1. Materials for containers for human blood and blood components 339
3.1.3. Polyolefines 344
3.1.4. Polyethylene without additives for containers for parenteral preparations and for ophthalmic preparations 348
3.1.5. Polyethylene with additives for containers for parenteral preparations and for ophthalmic preparations 349
3.1.6. Polypropylene for containers and closures for parenteral preparations and ophthalmic preparations ... 352
3.1.7. Poly(ethylene - vinyl acetate) for containers and tubing for total parenteral nutrition preparations 356
3.1.8. Silicone oil used as a lubricant 358
3.1.9. Silicone elastomer for closures and tubing 358
3.1. Materials used for the manufacture of containers 339
3.2.1. Glass containers for pharmaceutical use 373
3.2.2.1. Plastic containers for aqueous solutions for infusion 379
3.2.2. Plastic containers and closures for pharmaceutical use 378
3.2.3. Sterile plastic containers for human blood and blood components 379
3.2.4. Empty sterile containers of plasticised poly(vinyl chloride) for human blood and blood components 381
3.2.5. Sterile containers of plasticised poly(vinyl chloride) for human blood containing anticoagulant solution 382
3.2.6. Sets for the transfusion of blood and blood components 383
3.2.8. Sterile single-use plastic syringes 384
3.2.9. Rubber closures for containers for aqueous parenteral preparations, for powders and for freeze-dried powders 386
3.2. Containers 373
4.1.1. Reagents 391
4.1.1. Reagents **6.1**-3331
4.1.1. Reagents **6.2**-3661
4.1.2. Standard solutions for limit tests 504
4.1.3. Buffer solutions 508
4.1.3. Buffer solutions **6.1**-3331
4.1. Reagents, standard solutions, buffer solutions 391
4.2.1. Primary standards for volumetric solutions 514
4.2.2. Volumetric solutions 514
4.2. Volumetric analysis 514
4-Aminobenzoic acid 1164
4. Reagents 391
5.10. Control of impurities in substances for pharmaceutical use 653
5.11. Characters section in monographs 659
5.1.1. Methods of preparation of sterile products 525
5.1.2. Biological indicators of sterilisation 527
5.12. Reference standards 663
5.1.3. Efficacy of antimicrobial preservation 528
5.14. Gene transfer medicinal products for human use 669
5.1.4. Microbiological quality of pharmaceutical preparations 529
5.1.5. Application of the F_0 concept to steam sterilisation of aqueous preparations 531
5.15. Functionality-related characteristics of excipients **6.1**-3339
5.1.6. Alternative methods for control of microbiological quality 532
5.1.7. Viral safety 543
5.1. General texts on microbiology 525
5.2.1. Terminology used in monographs on biological products 547
5.2.2. Chicken flocks free from specified pathogens for the production and quality control of vaccines 547
5.2.3. Cell substrates for the production of vaccines for human use 550
5.2.4. Cell cultures for the production of veterinary vaccines 553
5.2.5. Substances of animal origin for the production of veterinary vaccines 555
5.2.6. Evaluation of safety of veterinary vaccines and immunosera 556
5.2.7. Evaluation of efficacy of veterinary vaccines and immunosera **6.1**-3335
5.2.8. Minimising the risk of transmitting animal spongiform encephalopathy agents via human and veterinary medicinal products 558
5.2.9. Evaluation of safety of each batch of veterinary vaccines and immunosera 567
5.2. General texts on biological products 547
5.3. Statistical analysis of results of biological assays and tests 571
5.4. Residual solvents 603
5.5. Alcoholimetric tables 613
5.6. Assay of interferons 627
5.7. Table of physical characteristics of radionuclides mentioned in the European Pharmacopoeia 633
5.8. Pharmacopoeial harmonisation 645
5.9. Polymorphism 649

A

Abbreviations and symbols (1.) 3
Abnormal toxicity (2.6.9.) 165
Absorption spectrophotometry, infrared (2.2.24.) 39
Absorption spectrophotometry, ultraviolet and visible (2.2.25.) 41
Acacia **6.2**-3683
Acacia, spray-dried **6.2**-3684
Acamprosate calcium 1088
Acarbose 1089
Acebutolol hydrochloride 1091
Aceclofenac **6.2**-3685
Acemetacin **6.1**-3393

Acesulfame potassium 1095
Acetazolamide 1096
Acetic acid, glacial 1097
Acetic acid in synthetic peptides (2.5.34.) 151
Acetone 1098
Acetylcholine chloride 1099
Acetylcysteine 1100
β-Acetyldigoxin 1101
Acetylsalicylic acid 1103
Acetyltryptophan, *N*- 1104
Acetyltyrosine, *N*- 1106
Aciclovir 1107
Acid value (2.5.1.) 137
Acitretin 1109
Actinobacillosis vaccine (inactivated), porcine 943
Activated charcoal 1488
Activated coagulation factors (2.6.22.) 198
Additives, plastic (3.1.13.) **6.2**-3655
Adenine 1110
Adenosine 1111
Adenovirus vectors for human use 670
Adipic acid 1113
Adrenaline **6.2**-3686
Adrenaline tartrate 1114
Aerodynamic assessment of fine particles in preparations for inhalation (2.9.18.) 287
Aflatoxin B_1 in herbal drugs, determination of (2.8.18.) 256
Agar **6.2**-3688
Agnus castus fruit **6.2**-3688
Agrimony 1117
Air, medicinal 1118
Air, synthetic medicinal 1121
Alanine 1121
Albendazole 1122
Albumin solution, human 2057
Alchemilla 1123
Alcoholimetric tables (2.9.10.) 281
Alcoholimetric tables (5.5.) 613
Alcuronium chloride 1124
Alexandrian senna pods 2870
Alfacalcidol 1126
Alfadex 1127
Alfentanil hydrochloride 1128
Alfuzosin hydrochloride **6.1**-3394
Alginic acid **6.2**-3690
Alkaline-earth metals and magnesium (2.4.7.) 112
Alkaline impurities in fatty oils (2.4.19.) 117
Allantoin 1131
Allergen products 679
Allopurinol 1132
all-*rac*-α-Tocopherol 3086
all-*rac*-α-Tocopheryl acetate 3089
Almagate 1134
Almond oil, refined 1136
Almond oil, virgin 1136
Aloes, Barbados 1137
Aloes, Cape 1138
Aloes dry extract, standardised **6.2**-3690
Alphacyclodextrin 1127
Alprazolam 1139
Alprenolol hydrochloride 1141
Alprostadil 1143
Alteplase for injection 1145
Alternative methods for control of microbiological quality (5.1.6.) 532
Altizide **6.2**-3691
Alum 1149
Aluminium (2.4.17.) 117
Aluminium chloride hexahydrate 1149
Aluminium hydroxide, hydrated, for adsorption **6.1**-3395
Aluminium in adsorbed vaccines (2.5.13.) 141
Aluminium magnesium silicate 1151
Aluminium oxide, hydrated 1152
Aluminium phosphate gel 1152
Aluminium phosphate, hydrated 1153
Aluminium sulphate 1154
Alverine citrate 1154
Amantadine hydrochloride 1156
Ambroxol hydrochloride 1156
Amfetamine sulphate 1158
Amidotrizoic acid dihydrate 1158
Amikacin **6.1**-3396
Amikacin sulphate **6.1**-3398
Amiloride hydrochloride 1163
Amino acid analysis (2.2.56.) 89
Aminobenzoic acid, 4- 1164
Aminocaproic acid 1166
Aminoglutethimide 1167
Amiodarone hydrochloride 1168
Amisulpride 1170
Amitriptyline hydrochloride 1172
Amlodipine besilate 1173
Ammonia (^{13}N) injection 981
Ammonia solution, concentrated 1175
Ammonio methacrylate copolymer (type A) 1175
Ammonio methacrylate copolymer (type B) 1176
Ammonium (2.4.1.) 111
Ammonium bromide 1177
Ammonium chloride 1178
Ammonium glycyrrhizate 1179
Ammonium hydrogen carbonate 1180
Amobarbital 1180
Amobarbital sodium 1181
Amoxicillin sodium 1182
Amoxicillin trihydrate 1184
Amperometric titration (2.2.19.) 35
Amphotericin B 1187
Ampicillin, anhydrous 1188
Ampicillin sodium 1190
Ampicillin trihydrate 1193
Anaesthetic ether 1834
Analysis, thermal (2.2.34.) **6.1**-3311
Analytical sieving, particle-size distribution estimation by (2.9.38.) **6.2**-3649
Angelica root 1196
Animal anti-T lymphocyte immunoglobulin for human use 1203
Animal immunosera for human use 685
Animal spongiform encephalopathies, products with risk of transmitting agents of 694
Animal spongiform encephalopathy agents, minimising the risk of transmitting via human and veterinary medicinal products (5.2.8.) 558
Aniseed 1199
Anise oil 1197
Anisidine value (2.5.36.) 152
Antazoline hydrochloride 1199
Anthrax spore vaccine (live) for veterinary use 859
Anthrax vaccine for human use (adsorbed, prepared from culture filtrates) 757
Anti-A and anti-B haemagglutinins (indirect method) (2.6.20.) 195
Antibiotics, microbiological assay of (2.7.2.) 210
Antibodies (anti-D) in human immunoglobulin for intravenous administration, test for (2.6.26.) **6.2**-3627
Antibodies for human use, monoclonal 690
Anticoagulant and preservative solutions for human blood 1200

Anticomplementary activity of immunoglobulin (2.6.17.) ..191
Anti-D antibodies in human immunoglobulin for intravenous administration, test for (2.6.26.) **6.2**-3627
Anti-D immunoglobulin for intravenous administration, human 2059
Anti-D immunoglobulin, human **6.2**-3757
Anti-D immunoglobulin, human, assay of (2.7.13.) 230
Antimicrobial preservation, efficacy of (5.1.3.) 528
Antiserum, European viper venom 970
Antithrombin III concentrate, human 2060
Antithrombin III, human, assay of (2.7.17.) 234
Anti-T lymphocyte immunoglobulin for human use, animal 1203
Apomorphine hydrochloride 1207
Apparatus (2.1.) 15
Apparent dissolution (2.9.43.) **6.1**-3327
Apparent volume (2.9.15.) 285
Application of the F_0 concept to steam sterilisation of aqueous preparations (5.1.5.) 531
Aprotinin 1208
Aprotinin concentrated solution **6.2**-3692
Arachis oil, hydrogenated **6.2**-3694
Arachis oil, refined 1211
Arginine 1212
Arginine aspartate 1213
Arginine hydrochloride 1214
Arnica flower **6.1**-3400
Arnica tincture 1216
Arsenic (2.4.2.) 111
Arsenious trioxide for homoeopathic preparations 1073
Articaine hydrochloride 1217
Artichoke leaf 1219
Ascorbic acid 1221
Ascorbyl palmitate 1222
Ash insoluble in hydrochloric acid (2.8.1.) 249
Ash leaf 1222
Asparagine monohydrate 1223
Aspartame 1224
Aspartic acid 1225
Assay of 1,8-cineole in essential oils (2.8.11.) 250
Assay of diphtheria vaccine (adsorbed) (2.7.6.) 217
Assay of heparin (2.7.5.) 217
Assay of heparin in coagulation factors (2.7.12.) 230
Assay of hepatitis A vaccine (2.7.14.) 232
Assay of hepatitis B vaccine (rDNA) (2.7.15.) 233
Assay of human anti-D immunoglobulin (2.7.13.) 230
Assay of human antithrombin III (2.7.17.) 234
Assay of human coagulation factor II (2.7.18.) 234
Assay of human coagulation factor IX (2.7.11.) 229
Assay of human coagulation factor VII (2.7.10.) 228
Assay of human coagulation factor VIII (2.7.4.) 216
Assay of human coagulation factor X (2.7.19.) 235
Assay of human coagulation factor XI (2.7.22.) 238
Assay of human plasmin inhibitor (2.7.25.) **6.2**-3631
Assay of human protein C (2.7.30.) **6.2**-3631
Assay of human protein S (2.7.31.) **6.2**-3632
Assay of human von Willebrand factor (2.7.21.) 237
Assay of interferons (5.6.) 627
Assay of pertussis vaccine (2.7.7.) 222
Assay of pertussis vaccine (acellular) (2.7.16.) 233
Assay of poliomyelitis vaccine (inactivated), *in vivo* (2.7.20.) 235
Assay of tetanus vaccine (adsorbed) (2.7.8.) 223
Assays (2.5.) 137
Astemizole 1226
Atenolol 1228
Atomic absorption spectrometry (2.2.23.) 37
Atomic emission spectrometry (2.2.22.) 36
Atomic emission spectrometry, inductively coupled plasma- (2.2.57.) 96
Atracurium besilate 1230
Atropine **6.1**-3403
Atropine sulphate **6.1**-3404
Aujeszky's disease vaccine (inactivated) for pigs 859
Aujeszky's disease vaccine (live) for pigs for parenteral administration 861
Avian infectious bronchitis vaccine (inactivated) 864
Avian infectious bronchitis vaccine (live) **6.1**-3371
Avian infectious bursal disease vaccine (inactivated) 867
Avian infectious bursal disease vaccine (live) 869
Avian infectious encephalomyelitis vaccine (live) 871
Avian infectious laryngotracheitis vaccine (live) 872
Avian live virus vaccines: tests for extraneous agents in batches of finished product (2.6.25.) 202
Avian paramyxovirus 1 (Newcastle disease) vaccine (inactivated) 937
Avian paramyxovirus 3 vaccine (inactivated) 874
Avian tuberculin purified protein derivative 3146
Avian viral tenosynovitis vaccine (live) 875
Avian viral vaccines: tests for extraneous agents in seed lots (2.6.24.) 198
Azaperone for veterinary use 1234
Azathioprine 1236
Azelastine hydrochloride 1236
Azithromycin 1238

B

Bacampicillin hydrochloride **6.1**-3409
Bacitracin 1245
Bacitracin zinc 1247
Baclofen 1250
Bacterial cells used for the manufacture of plasmid vectors for human use 676
Bacterial endotoxins (2.6.14.) 182
Bambuterol hydrochloride 1251
Barbados aloes 1137
Barbital 1252
Barium chloride dihydrate for homoeopathic preparations 1073
Barium sulphate 1253
Basic butylated methacrylate copolymer 1254
BCG for immunotherapy 758
BCG vaccine, freeze-dried 759
Bearberry leaf **6.1**-3410
Beclometasone dipropionate, anhydrous 1256
Beclometasone dipropionate monohydrate 1258
Bee for homoeopathic preparations, honey 1079
Beeswax, white 1260
Beeswax, yellow 1261
Belladonna leaf 1261
Belladonna leaf dry extract, standardised **6.2**-3697
Belladonna leaf tincture, standardised 1264
Belladonna, prepared **6.2**-3698
Bendroflumethiazide 1266
Benfluorex hydrochloride 1267
Benperidol 1269
Benserazide hydrochloride 1270
Bentonite 1271
Benzalkonium chloride 1272
Benzalkonium chloride solution 1273
Benzathine benzylpenicillin 1283
Benzbromarone 1273
Benzethonium chloride 1275
Benzocaine 1276
Benzoic acid 1276
Benzoin, Siam 1277
Benzoin, Sumatra 1278

Benzoin tincture, Siam 1278
Benzoin tincture, Sumatra 1279
Benzoyl peroxide, hydrous 1280
Benzyl alcohol 1281
Benzyl benzoate 1283
Benzylpenicillin, benzathine 1283
Benzylpenicillin potassium 1285
Benzylpenicillin, procaine 1287
Benzylpenicillin sodium 1288
Betacarotene 1290
Betacyclodextrin 1291
Betacyclodextrin, poly(hydroxypropyl) ether **6.2**-3763
Betadex 1291
Betahistine dihydrochloride 1292
Betahistine mesilate 1293
Betamethasone 1295
Betamethasone acetate 1297
Betamethasone dipropionate 1298
Betamethasone sodium phosphate 1300
Betamethasone valerate 1301
Betaxolol hydrochloride 1303
Bezafibrate 1304
Bifonazole 1306
Bilberry fruit, dried 1307
Bilberry fruit dry extract, fresh, refined and standardised **6.2**-3745
Bilberry fruit, fresh **6.1**-3412
Biological assays (2.7.) 209
Biological assays and tests, statistical analysis of results of (5.3.) 571
Biological indicators of sterilisation (5.1.2.) 527
Biological products, general texts on (5.2.) 547
Biological products, terminology used in monographs on (5.2.1.) 547
Biological tests (2.6.) 155
Biotin 1308
Biperiden hydrochloride 1309
Biphasic insulin injection 2140
Biphasic isophane insulin injection 2140
Birch leaf **6.2**-3699
Bisacodyl 1312
Bismuth subcarbonate 1313
Bismuth subgallate 1314
Bismuth subnitrate, heavy 1315
Bismuth subsalicylate 1316
Bisoprolol fumarate **6.1**-3412
Bistort rhizome 1317
Bitter fennel 1873
Bitter-fennel fruit oil 1318
Bitterness value (2.8.15.) 255
Bitter-orange epicarp and mesocarp 1319
Bitter-orange-epicarp and mesocarp tincture 1320
Bitter-orange flower 1320
Bitter-orange-flower oil 2490
Black horehound 1321
Bleomycin sulphate 1322
Blood and blood components, empty sterile containers of plasticised poly(vinyl chloride) for (3.2.4.) 381
Blood and blood components, materials for containers for (3.1.1.) 339
Blood and blood components, sets for the transfusion of (3.2.6.) 383
Blood and blood components, sterile plastic containers for (3.2.3.) 379
Blood, anticoagulant and preservative solutions for 1200
Blood, sterile containers of plasticised poly(vinyl chloride) containing anticoagulant solution (3.2.5.) 382
Bogbean leaf 1323
Boiling point (2.2.12.) 31
Boldo leaf 1324
Boldo leaf dry extract **6.1**-3415
Borage (starflower) oil, refined 1326
Borax 1326
Boric acid 1327
Botulinum antitoxin 965
Botulinum toxin type A for injection 1327
Bovine infectious rhinotracheitis vaccine (live) 924
Bovine insulin 2135
Bovine leptospirosis vaccine (inactivated) 876
Bovine parainfluenza virus vaccine (live) 878
Bovine respiratory syncytial virus vaccine (live) 879
Bovine serum 1329
Bovine tuberculin purified protein derivative 3147
Bovine viral diarrhoea vaccine (inactivated) 880
Bromazepam 1331
Bromhexine hydrochloride 1332
Bromocriptine mesilate 1333
Bromperidol 1335
Bromperidol decanoate 1337
Brompheniramine maleate 1339
Brotizolam 1340
Brucellosis vaccine (live) (Brucella melitensis Rev. 1 strain) for veterinary use 881
Buccal tablets and sublingual tablets 734
Buckwheat herb 1341
Budesonide 1342
Bufexamac 1344
Buffer solutions (4.1.3.) 508
Buffer solutions (4.1.3.) **6.1**-3331
Buflomedil hydrochloride 1345
Bulk density and tapped density of powders (2.9.34.) **6.2**-3646
Bumetanide 1346
Bupivacaine hydrochloride 1347
Buprenorphine 1349
Buprenorphine hydrochloride 1350
Buserelin 1351
Buspirone hydrochloride 1353
Busulfan 1355
Butcher's broom **6.1**-3416
Butylated methacrylate copolymer, basic 1254
Butylhydroxyanisole 1357
Butylhydroxytoluene 1357
Butyl parahydroxybenzoate 1358

C

Cabergoline 1363
Cachets 719
Cadmium sulphate hydrate for homoeopathic preparations 1074
Caffeine **6.1**-3421
Caffeine monohydrate 1365
Calcifediol 1366
Calcipotriol, anhydrous 1367
Calcipotriol monohydrate 1370
Calcitonin (salmon) 1372
Calcitriol 1375
Calcium (2.4.3.) 111
Calcium acetate 1376
Calcium ascorbate 1377
Calcium carbonate **6.2**-3703
Calcium carboxymethylcellulose 1422
Calcium chloride dihydrate 1378
Calcium chloride hexahydrate 1379
Calcium dobesilate monohydrate **6.2**-3703
Calcium folinate 1380
Calcium glucoheptonate 1383
Calcium gluconate 1384

Calcium gluconate for injection.. 1385
Calcium glycerophosphate.. 1386
Calcium hydrogen phosphate, anhydrous........................ 1387
Calcium hydrogen phosphate dihydrate.......................... 1388
Calcium hydroxide... 1389
Calcium in adsorbed vaccines (2.5.14.)............................. 142
Calcium iodide tetrahydrate for homoeopathic preparations... 1074
Calcium lactate, anhydrous.. 1389
Calcium lactate monohydrate... 1390
Calcium lactate pentahydrate... 1390
Calcium lactate trihydrate... 1391
Calcium levofolinate pentahydrate.................................. 1392
Calcium levulinate dihydrate.. 1394
Calcium pantothenate.. 1395
Calcium phosphate... 1396
Calcium stearate... 1397
Calcium sulphate dihydrate.. 1398
Calendula flower... 1398
Calf coronavirus diarrhoea vaccine (inactivated).............. 882
Calf rotavirus diarrhoea vaccine (inactivated).................. 884
Calicivirosis vaccine (inactivated), feline........................... 909
Calicivirosis vaccine (live), feline.. 910
Camphor, D-... 1400
Camphor, racemic... 1401
Canine adenovirus vaccine (inactivated)............................ 885
Canine adenovirus vaccine (live)... 886
Canine distemper vaccine (live)... 887
Canine leptospirosis vaccine (inactivated)......................... 888
Canine parainfluenza virus vaccine (live)........................... 890
Canine parvovirosis vaccine (inactivated).......................... 891
Canine parvovirosis vaccine (live)....................................... 892
Cape aloes.. 1138
Capillary electrophoresis (2.2.47.)... 77
Capillary viscometer method (2.2.9.)..................................... 27
Caprylic acid.. 1402
Caprylocaproyl macrogolglycerides................................... 1403
Capsicum...**6.2**-3704
Capsicum oleoresin, refined and quantified..................... 1405
Capsicum tincture, standardised.. 1406
Capsules... 717
Capsules and tablets, disintegration of (2.9.1.).................. 263
Capsules, gastro-resistant... 718
Capsules, hard... 718
Capsules, intrauterine... 726
Capsules, modified-release... 718
Capsules, oromucosal... 734
Capsules, rectal... 745
Capsules, soft.. 718
Capsules, vaginal.. 752
Captopril.. 1407
Caraway fruit... 1408
Caraway oil.. 1408
Carbachol... 1410
Carbamazepine.. 1411
Carbasalate calcium.. 1412
Carbidopa... 1413
Carbimazole... 1414
Carbocisteine... 1415
Carbomers...**6.1**-3422
Carbon dioxide.. 1417
Carbon dioxide in gases (2.5.24.)... 144
Carbon monoxide (^{15}O).. 982
Carbon monoxide in gases (2.5.25.)..................................... 145
Carboplatin.. 1419
Carboprost trometamol... 1420
Carboxymethylcellulose calcium.. 1422
Carboxymethylcellulose sodium... 1423
Carboxymethylcellulose sodium, cross-linked.................. 1626
Carboxymethylcellulose sodium, low-substituted............ 1424
Carisoprodol... 1421
Carmellose calcium.. 1422
Carmellose sodium... 1423
Carmellose sodium and microcrystalline cellulose.......... 2422
Carmellose sodium, low-substituted.................................. 1424
Carmustine... 1425
Carnauba wax... 1425
Carprofen for veterinary use....................................**6.2**-3706
Carteolol hydrochloride.. 1426
Carvedilol... 1427
Cascara... 1429
Cascara dry extract, standardised..................................... 1430
Cassia oil...**6.2**-3707
Castor oil, hydrogenated... 1432
Castor oil, polyoxyl.. 2304
Castor oil, polyoxyl hydrogenated..................................... 2303
Castor oil, refined.. 1433
Castor oil, virgin.. 1434
Catgut, sterile... 1045
Catgut, sterile, in distributor for veterinary use............... 1057
CD34/CD45+ cells in haematopoietic products, numeration of (2.7.23.)... 238
Cefaclor.. 1435
Cefadroxil monohydrate...**6.1**-3423
Cefalexin monohydrate...**6.1**-3425
Cefalotin sodium.. 1440
Cefamandole nafate... 1441
Cefapirin sodium.. 1443
Cefatrizine propylene glycol.. 1444
Cefazolin sodium.. 1445
Cefepime dihydrochloride monohydrate........................... 1448
Cefixime.. 1450
Cefoperazone sodium.. 1451
Cefotaxime sodium.. 1453
Cefoxitin sodium.. 1455
Cefradine.. 1457
Ceftazidime... 1459
Ceftriaxone sodium.. 1461
Cefuroxime axetil... 1462
Cefuroxime sodium.. 1464
Celiprolol hydrochloride.. 1465
Cell count and viability, nucleated (2.7.29.)........................ 243
Cell cultures for the production of veterinary vaccines (5.2.4.)... 553
Cell substrates for the production of vaccines for human use (5.2.3.)... 550
Cellular products, microbiological control of (2.6.27.)...... 205
Cellulose acetate.. 1467
Cellulose acetate butyrate... 1468
Cellulose acetate phthalate... 1468
Cellulose, microcrystalline...**6.2**-3708
Cellulose (microcrystalline) and carmellose sodium........ 2422
Cellulose, powdered...**6.2**-3712
Centaury... 1477
Centella... 1477
Cetirizine dihydrochloride..**6.2**-3715
Cetostearyl alcohol.. 1480
Cetostearyl alcohol (type A), emulsifying..................**6.2**-3717
Cetostearyl alcohol (type B), emulsifying..................**6.2**-3718
Cetostearyl isononanoate.. 1484
Cetrimide.. 1484
Cetyl alcohol... 1485
Cetyl palmitate... 1486
Cetylpyridinium chloride... 1486
Ceylon cinnamon bark oil...**6.2**-3721
Ceylon cinnamon leaf oil... 1544
CFC assay for human haematopoietic progenitor cells (2.7.28.)... 242

Chamomile flower, Roman 1487
Characterisation of crystalline and partially crystalline solids by X-ray powder diffraction (XRPD) (2.9.33.) 314
Characters section in monographs (5.11.) 659
Charcoal, activated 1488
Chenodeoxycholic acid 1489
Chewing gum, medicated (2.9.25.) 304
Chewing gums, medicated 719
Chicken flocks free from specified pathogens for the production and quality control of vaccines (5.2.2.) 547
Chicken infectious anaemia vaccine (live) 925
Chitosan hydrochloride 1490
Chlamydiosis vaccine (inactivated), feline 911
Chloral hydrate 1491
Chlorambucil 1492
Chloramine 3103
Chloramphenicol 1492
Chloramphenicol palmitate 1493
Chloramphenicol sodium succinate 1495
Chlorcyclizine hydrochloride 1496
Chlordiazepoxide 1497
Chlordiazepoxide hydrochloride 1498
Chlorhexidine diacetate 1499
Chlorhexidine digluconate solution 1500
Chlorhexidine dihydrochloride 1502
Chlorides (2.4.4.) 112
Chlorobutanol, anhydrous 1503
Chlorobutanol hemihydrate 1504
Chlorocresol 1504
Chloroquine phosphate 1505
Chloroquine sulphate 1506
Chlorothiazide 1507
Chlorphenamine maleate **6.1**-3427
Chlorpromazine hydrochloride 1509
Chlorpropamide 1510
Chlorprothixene hydrochloride 1511
Chlortalidone 1513
Chlortetracycline hydrochloride 1514
Cholecalciferol 1516
Cholecalciferol concentrate (oily form) 1517
Cholecalciferol concentrate (powder form) 1519
Cholecalciferol concentrate (water-dispersible form) 1521
Cholera vaccine 761
Cholera vaccine, freeze-dried 761
Cholera vaccine (inactivated, oral) 762
Cholesterol 1524
Cholesterol in oils rich in omega-3 acids, total (2.4.32.) 132
Chondroitin sulphate sodium 1525
Chromatographic separation techniques (2.2.46.) 72
Chromatography, gas (2.2.28.) 45
Chromatography, liquid (2.2.29.) 46
Chromatography, paper (2.2.26.) 43
Chromatography, size-exclusion (2.2.30.) 47
Chromatography, supercritical fluid (2.2.45.) 71
Chromatography, thin-layer (2.2.27.) 43
Chromium (^{51}Cr) edetate injection **6.2**-3677
Chymotrypsin 1527
Ciclopirox 1528
Ciclopirox olamine 1530
Ciclosporin 1531
Cilastatin sodium **6.1**-3428
Cilazapril 1534
Cimetidine 1536
Cimetidine hydrochloride 1537
Cinchocaine hydrochloride 1538
Cinchona bark **6.2**-3720
Cinchona liquid extract, standardised 1540
Cineole 1541
Cineole in essential oils, 1,8-, assay of (2.8.11.) 250
Cinnamon 1542
Cinnamon bark oil, Ceylon **6.2**-3721
Cinnamon leaf oil, Ceylon 1544
Cinnamon tincture 1545
Cinnarizine 1545
Ciprofibrate 1547
Ciprofloxacin 1548
Ciprofloxacin hydrochloride 1550
Circular dichroism (2.2.41.) 66
Cisapride monohydrate 1551
Cisapride tartrate 1552
Cisplatin 1554
Citric acid, anhydrous 1554
Citric acid monohydrate 1555
Citronella oil 1556
Cladribine 1557
Clarithromycin 1559
Clarity and degree of opalescence of liquids (2.2.1.) 21
Clary sage oil 1561
Classical swine-fever vaccine (live, prepared in cell cultures) **6.2**-3669
Clazuril for veterinary use 1562
Clebopride malate 1564
Clemastine fumarate **6.1**-3430
Clenbuterol hydrochloride 1567
Clindamycin hydrochloride 1568
Clindamycin phosphate 1570
Clioquinol 1571
Clobazam 1572
Clobetasol propionate 1573
Clobetasone butyrate 1575
Clodronate disodium tetrahydrate **6.2**-3722
Clofazimine 1577
Clofibrate 1578
Clomifene citrate 1579
Clomipramine hydrochloride 1580
Clonazepam 1582
Clonidine hydrochloride 1583
Clopamide **6.1**-3431
Closantel sodium dihydrate for veterinary use 1584
Clostridium botulinum vaccine for veterinary use 894
Clostridium chauvoei vaccine for veterinary use 894
Clostridium novyi alpha antitoxin for veterinary use 973
Clostridium novyi (type b) vaccine for veterinary use 895
Clostridium perfringens beta antitoxin for veterinary use 974
Clostridium perfringens epsilon antitoxin for veterinary use 975
Clostridium perfringens vaccine for veterinary use 897
Clostridium septicum vaccine for veterinary use 899
Closures and containers for parenteral preparations and ophthalmic preparations, polypropylene for (3.1.6.) 352
Closures and containers for pharmaceutical use, plastic (3.2.2.) 378
Closures and tubing, silicone elastomer for (3.1.9.) 358
Closures for containers for aqueous parenteral preparations, for powders and for freeze-dried powders, rubber (3.2.9.) 386
Clotrimazole **6.1**-3433
Clove 1587
Clove oil 1588
Cloxacillin sodium 1589
Clozapine 1590
Coagulation factor II, assay of (2.7.18.) 234
Coagulation factor IX, human 2064
Coagulation factor IX, human, assay of (2.7.11.) 229
Coagulation factors, activated (2.6.22.) 198
Coagulation factors, assay of heparin (2.7.12.) 230
Coagulation factor VII, human 2061

Coagulation factor VII, human, assay of (2.7.10.) ... 228
Coagulation factor VIII, human ... 2062
Coagulation factor VIII, human, assay of (2.7.4.) ... 216
Coagulation factor VIII (rDNA), human ... 2063
Coagulation factor X, assay of (2.7.19.) ... 235
Coagulation factor XI, human ... 2065
Coagulation factor XI, human, assay of (2.7.22.) ... 238
Coated granules ... 724
Coated tablets ... 749
Cocaine hydrochloride ... 1592
Coccidiosis vaccine (live) for chickens ... **6.2**-3665
Coconut oil, refined ... **6.2**-3723
Cocoyl caprylocaprate ... 1594
Codeine ... **6.1**-3434
Codeine hydrochloride dihydrate ... 1596
Codeine phosphate hemihydrate ... 1598
Codeine phosphate sesquihydrate ... 1599
Codergocrine mesilate ... 1601
Cod-liver oil (type A) ... 1603
Cod-liver oil (type B) ... 1607
Cola ... 1611
Colchicine ... 1612
Cold-water vibriosis vaccine (inactivated) for salmonids ... **6.2**-3671
Colestyramine ... 1613
Colibacillosis vaccine (inactivated), neonatal piglet ... 934
Colibacillosis vaccine (inactivated), neonatal ruminant ... 936
Colistimethate sodium ... 1614
Colistin sulphate ... 1615
Colloidal anhydrous silica ... 2877
Colloidal hydrated silica ... 2877
Colloidal silica, hydrophobic ... 2878
Colloidal silver, for external use ... 2879
Colony-forming cell assay for human haematopoietic progenitor cells (2.7.28.) ... 242
Colophony ... 1617
Coloration of liquids (2.2.2.) ... 22
Common stinging nettle for homoeopathic preparations ... 1075
Comparative table of porosity of sintered-glass filters (2.1.2.) ... 15
Complexometric titrations (2.5.11.) ... 140
Composition of fatty acids by gas chromatography (2.4.22.) ... 118
Composition of fatty acids in oils rich in omega-3 acids (2.4.29.) ... **6.2**-3623
Compressed lozenges ... 734
Concentrated solutions for haemodialysis ... 2022
Concentrates for injections or infusions ... 736
Concentrates for intrauterine solutions ... 726
Conductivity (2.2.38.) ... 59
Coneflower herb, purple ... 2785
Coneflower root, narrow-leaved ... 2483
Coneflower root, pale ... 2602
Coneflower root, purple ... 2787
Conjugated estrogens ... 1824
Consistency by penetrometry, measurement of (2.9.9.) ... **6.2**-3641
Containers (3.2.) ... 373
Containers and closures for parenteral preparations and ophthalmic preparations, polypropylene for (3.1.6.) ... 352
Containers and closures for pharmaceutical use, plastic (3.2.2.) ... 378
Containers and tubing for total parenteral nutrition preparations, poly(ethylene - vinyl acetate) for (3.1.7.) ... 356
Containers for aqueous solutions for infusion, plastic (3.2.2.1.) ... 379
Containers for aqueous solutions for intravenous infusion, materials based on plasticised poly(vinyl chloride) for (3.1.14.) ... 366
Containers for dry dosage forms for oral administration, materials based on non-plasticised poly(vinyl chloride) for (3.1.11.) ... 362
Containers for human blood and blood components, materials based on plasticised poly(vinyl chloride) for (3.1.1.1.) ... 339
Containers for human blood and blood components, materials for (3.1.1.) ... 339
Containers for human blood and blood components, plastic, sterile (3.2.3.) ... 379
Containers for non-injectable aqueous solutions, materials based on non-plasticised poly(vinyl chloride) for (3.1.10.) ... 360
Containers for parenteral preparations and for ophthalmic preparations, polyethylene with additives for (3.1.5.) ... 349
Containers for parenteral preparations and for ophthalmic preparations, polyethylene without additives for (3.1.4.) ... 348
Containers for pharmaceutical use, glass (3.2.1.) ... 373
Containers for preparations not for parenteral use, polyethylene terephthalate for (3.1.15) ... 369
Containers of plasticised poly(vinyl chloride) for human blood and blood components, empty sterile (3.2.4.) ... 381
Containers of plasticised poly(vinyl chloride) for human blood containing anticoagulant solution, sterile (3.2.5.) ... 382
Contamination, microbial: test for specified micro-organisms (2.6.13.) ... 173
Contamination, microbial: total viable aerobic count (2.6.12.) ... 166
Content uniformity of single-dose preparations (2.9.6.) ... 278
Control of impurities in substances for pharmaceutical use (5.10.) ... 653
Control of microbiological quality, alternative methods for (5.1.6.) ... 532
Copolymer, basic butylated methacrylate ... 1254
Copolymer, methacrylic acid - ethyl acrylate (1:1) ... **6.2**-3781
Copolymer (type A), ammonio methacrylate ... 1175
Copolymer (type B), ammonio methacrylate ... 1176
Copovidone ... 1617
Copper acetate monohydrate for homoeopathic preparations ... 1075
Copper for homoeopathic preparations ... 1076
Copper sulphate, anhydrous ... 1619
Copper sulphate pentahydrate ... 1620
Coriander ... 1620
Coriander oil ... 1621
Cortisone acetate ... 1622
Cotton, absorbent ... 1624
Cottonseed oil, hydrogenated ... **6.2**-3724
Couch grass rhizome ... 1625
Creams ... 747
Cresol, crude ... 1626
Croscarmellose sodium ... 1626
Crospovidone ... 1628
Crotamiton ... 1629
Crystalline and partially crystalline solids, characterisation by X-ray powder diffraction (XRPD) of (2.9.33.) ... 314
Cutaneous application, liquid preparations for ... 728
Cutaneous application, powders for ... 738
Cutaneous application, semi-solid preparations for ... 746
Cutaneous application, veterinary liquid preparations for ... 752
Cutaneous foams ... 728
Cyanocobalamin ... 1630
Cyanocobalamin (^{57}Co) capsules ... 983
Cyanocobalamin (^{57}Co) solution ... 984

Cyanocobalamin (^{58}Co) capsules ... 985
Cyanocobalamin (^{58}Co) solution ... 986
Cyclizine hydrochloride ... **6.2**-3725
Cyclopentolate hydrochloride ... 1632
Cyclophosphamide ... 1633
Cyproheptadine hydrochloride ... 1634
Cyproterone acetate ... 1635
Cysteine hydrochloride monohydrate ... 1636
Cystine ... 1637
Cytarabine ... 1638

D

Dacarbazine ... 1641
Dalteparin sodium ... 1642
Danaparoid sodium ... 1644
Dapsone ... 1646
Daunorubicin hydrochloride ... 1647
D-Camphor ... 1400
Decyl oleate ... 1648
Deferoxamine mesilate ... 1649
Degree of coloration of liquids (2.2.2.) ... 22
Dembrexine hydrochloride monohydrate for veterinary use ... 1650
Demeclocycline hydrochloride ... 1651
Density of powders, bulk density and tapped (2.9.34.) ... **6.2**-3646
Density of solids (2.2.42.) ... 67
Density of solids, gas pycnometric (2.9.23.) ... **6.2**-3642
Density, relative (2.2.5.) ... 25
Dental type silica ... 2878
Depressor substances (2.6.11.) ... 166
Deptropine citrate ... 1653
Dequalinium chloride ... 1654
Desflurane ... **6.1**-3439
Desipramine hydrochloride ... 1655
Deslanoside ... 1656
Desmopressin ... 1657
Desogestrel ... 1658
Desoxycortone acetate ... 1659
Detector tubes, gas (2.1.6.) ... 17
Determination of aflatoxin B_1 in herbal drugs (2.8.18.) ... 256
Determination of essential oils in herbal drugs (2.8.12.) .. 251
Determination of nitrogen by sulphuric acid digestion (2.5.9.) ... 139
Determination of primary aromatic amino-nitrogen (2.5.8.) ... 139
Determination of tannins in herbal drugs (2.8.14.) ... 255
Determination of water by distillation (2.2.13.) ... 31
Detomidine hydrochloride for veterinary use ... 1660
Devil's claw dry extract ... 1662
Devil's claw root ... **6.2**-3729
Dexamethasone ... 1663
Dexamethasone acetate ... 1665
Dexamethasone isonicotinate ... 1666
Dexamethasone sodium phosphate ... 1667
Dexchlorpheniramine maleate ... 1669
Dexpanthenol ... 1670
Dextran 1 for injection ... 1671
Dextran 40 for injection ... 1672
Dextran 60 for injection ... 1673
Dextran 70 for injection ... 1674
Dextranomer ... 1675
Dextrans, molecular mass distribution in (2.2.39.) ... 60
Dextrin ... 1675
Dextromethorphan hydrobromide ... 1676
Dextromoramide tartrate ... 1677
Dextropropoxyphene hydrochloride ... 1678
Diazepam ... 1679
Diazoxide ... 1680
Dibrompropamidine diisetionate ... 1681
Dibutyl phthalate ... 1682
Dichloromethane ... 2387
Diclazuril for veterinary use ... 1683
Diclofenac potassium ... 1685
Diclofenac sodium ... 1686
Dicloxacillin sodium ... 1687
Dicycloverine hydrochloride ... 1689
Didanosine ... 1689
Dienestrol ... 1691
Diethylcarbamazine citrate ... 1693
Diethylene glycol and ethylene glycol in ethoxylated substances (2.4.30.) ... 131
Diethylene glycol monoethyl ether ... 1694
Diethylene glycol palmitostearate ... 1695
Diethyl phthalate ... **6.1**-3441
Diethylstilbestrol ... 1696
Diffraction, laser light, particle size analysis by (2.9.31.) ..311
Diflunisal ... 1697
Digitalis leaf ... 1698
Digitoxin ... 1700
Digoxin ... 1701
Dihydralazine sulphate, hydrated ... **6.1**-3442
Dihydrocodeine hydrogen tartrate ... 1704
Dihydroergocristine mesilate ... 1705
Dihydroergotamine mesilate ... **6.1**-3444
Dihydroergotamine tartrate ... 1709
Dihydrostreptomycin sulphate for veterinary use ... **6.2**-3730
Dihydrotachysterol ... 1712
Diltiazem hydrochloride ... **6.1**-3446
Dimenhydrinate ... 1715
Dimercaprol ... 1716
Dimethylacetamide ... 1717
Dimethylaniline, *N,N*- (2.4.26.) ... 127
Dimethyl sulfoxide ... 1716
Dimeticone ... **6.2**-3732
Dimetindene maleate ... 1719
Dinoprostone ... 1722
Dinoprost trometamol ... 1720
Diosmin ... 1723
Dioxan and ethylene oxide (2.4.25.) ... 126
Dip concentrates ... 753
Diphenhydramine hydrochloride ... 1725
Diphenoxylate hydrochloride ... 1726
Diphtheria and tetanus toxins and toxoids, flocculation value (Lf) of, (Ramon assay) (2.7.27.) ... 241
Diphtheria and tetanus vaccine (adsorbed) ... 763
Diphtheria and tetanus vaccine (adsorbed, reduced antigen(s) content) ... 764
Diphtheria antitoxin ... 965
Diphtheria, tetanus and hepatitis B (rDNA) vaccine (adsorbed) ... 765
Diphtheria, tetanus and pertussis (acellular, component) vaccine (adsorbed) ... 767
Diphtheria, tetanus and pertussis vaccine (adsorbed) ... 768
Diphtheria, tetanus and poliomyelitis (inactivated) vaccine (adsorbed, reduced antigen(s) content) ... 770
Diphtheria, tetanus, pertussis (acellular, component) and haemophilus type b conjugate vaccine (adsorbed) ... 771
Diphtheria, tetanus, pertussis (acellular, component) and hepatitis B (rDNA) vaccine (adsorbed) ... 774
Diphtheria, tetanus, pertussis (acellular, component) and poliomyelitis (inactivated) vaccine (adsorbed) ... 775
Diphtheria, tetanus, pertussis (acellular, component) and poliomyelitis (inactivated) vaccine (adsorbed, reduced antigen(s) content) ... 778
Diphtheria, tetanus, pertussis (acellular, component), hepatitis B (rDNA), poliomyelitis (inactivated) and haemophilus type b conjugate vaccine (adsorbed) ... 780

Diphtheria, tetanus, pertussis (acellular, component), poliomyelitis (inactivated) and haemophilus type b conjugate vaccine (adsorbed)........ 783
Diphtheria, tetanus, pertussis and poliomyelitis (inactivated) vaccine (adsorbed)........ 785
Diphtheria, tetanus, pertussis, poliomyelitis (inactivated) and haemophilus type b conjugate vaccine (adsorbed)........ 787
Diphtheria vaccine (adsorbed)........ 789
Diphtheria vaccine (adsorbed), assay of (2.7.6.)........ 217
Diphtheria vaccine (adsorbed, reduced antigen content).. 791
Dipivefrine hydrochloride........ 1727
Dipotassium clorazepate........ 1728
Dipotassium phosphate........ 1729
Diprophylline........ 1730
Dipyridamole........ 1731
Dirithromycin........ **6.1**-3447
Disintegration of suppositories and pessaries (2.9.2.)........ 265
Disintegration of tablets and capsules (2.9.1.)........ 263
Disodium edetate........ 1734
Disodium phosphate, anhydrous........ 1735
Disodium phosphate dihydrate........ 1735
Disodium phosphate dodecahydrate........ **6.1**-3449
Disopyramide........ 1737
Disopyramide phosphate........ 1738
Dispersible tablets........ 750
Dissolution, apparent (2.9.43.)........ **6.1**-3327
Dissolution, intrinsic (2.9.29.)........ 309
Dissolution test for lipophilic solid dosage forms (2.9.42.)........ 332
Dissolution test for solid dosage forms (2.9.3.)........ 266
Dissolution test for transdermal patches (2.9.4.)........ 275
Distemper vaccine (live), canine........ 887
Distemper vaccine (live) for mustelids........ 900
Distillation range (2.2.11.)........ 30
Distribution estimation by analytical sieving, particle-size (2.9.38.)........ **6.2**-3649
Disulfiram........ 1739
Dithranol........ 1740
DL-Methionine........ 2380
DL-α-Tocopheryl hydrogen succinate........ 3093
Dobutamine hydrochloride........ 1741
Docusate sodium........ 1743
Dodecyl gallate........ 1744
Dog rose........ 1744
Domperidone........ 1745
Domperidone maleate........ 1747
Dopamine hydrochloride........ 1749
Dopexamine dihydrochloride........ 1750
Dorzolamide hydrochloride........ 1752
Dosage units, uniformity of (2.9.40.)........ **6.1**-3325
Dosulepin hydrochloride........ 1753
Doxapram hydrochloride........ 1754
Doxazosin mesilate........ 1756
Doxepin hydrochloride........ **6.1**-3449
Doxorubicin hydrochloride........ 1759
Doxycycline hyclate........ 1760
Doxycycline monohydrate........ 1762
Doxylamine hydrogen succinate........ **6.1**-3451
Droperidol........ 1765
Droppers (2.1.1.)........ 15
Drop point (2.2.17.)........ 33
Drops (nasal) and sprays (liquid nasal)........ 731
Drops, oral........ 730
Dry extracts........ **6.1**-3344
Dry residue of extracts (2.8.16.)........ 256
Duck plague vaccine (live)........ 901
Duck viral hepatitis type I vaccine (live)........ 902
Dwarf pine oil........ 1766

E

Ear drops and ear sprays........ 720
Ear powders........ 720
Ear preparations........ 719
Ear preparations, semi-solid........ 720
Ear sprays and ear drops........ 720
Ear tampons........ 720
Ear washes........ 720
Ebastine........ 1771
Econazole........ 1772
Econazole nitrate........ 1773
Edetic acid........ 1774
Edrophonium chloride........ 1775
Effervescent granules........ 724
Effervescent powders........ 739
Effervescent tablets........ 749
Efficacy of antimicrobial preservation (5.1.3.)........ 528
Efficacy of veterinary vaccines and immunosera, evaluation of (5.2.7.)........ **6.1**-3335
Egg drop syndrome '76 vaccine (inactivated)........ 904
Elder flower........ 1776
Electrophoresis (2.2.31.)........ 48
Electrophoresis, capillary (2.2.47.)........ 77
Eleutherococcus........ 1777
Emedastine difumarate........ 1779
Emetine hydrochloride heptahydrate........ 1780
Emetine hydrochloride pentahydrate........ 1781
Empty sterile containers of plasticised poly(vinyl chloride) for human blood and blood components (3.2.4.)........ 381
Emulsifying cetostearyl alcohol (type A)........ **6.2**-3717
Emulsifying cetostearyl alcohol (type B)........ **6.2**-3718
Emulsions, solutions and suspensions, oral........ 729
Enalaprilat dihydrate........ 1784
Enalapril maleate........ 1782
Encephalitis vaccine (inactivated), tick-borne........ 845
Endotoxins, bacterial (2.6.14.)........ 182
Enilconazole for veterinary use........ 1785
Enoxaparin sodium........ 1787
Enoxolone........ 1788
Ephedrine, anhydrous........ 1789
Ephedrine hemihydrate........ 1790
Ephedrine hydrochloride........ 1791
Ephedrine hydrochloride, racemic........ 1792
Epinephrine........ **6.2**-3686
Epinephrine tartrate........ 1114
Epirubicin hydrochloride........ 1793
Equine herpesvirus vaccine (inactivated)........ 905
Equine influenza vaccine (inactivated)........ 907
Equisetum stem........ 1794
Ergocalciferol........ 1795
Ergometrine maleate........ 1797
Ergotamine tartrate........ 1798
Erysipelas vaccine (inactivated), swine........ 955
Erythritol........ 1800
Erythromycin........ 1801
Erythromycin estolate........ 1803
Erythromycin ethylsuccinate........ 1806
Erythromycin lactobionate........ 1808
Erythromycin stearate........ 1810
Erythropoietin concentrated solution........ 1813
Eserine salicylate........ 2677
Eserine sulphate........ 2678
Esketamine hydrochloride........ 1817
Essential oils........ 680
Essential oils, assay of 1,8-cineole in (2.8.11.)........ 250
Essential oils, fatty oils and resinified essential oils in (2.8.7.)........ 250
Essential oils, foreign esters in (2.8.6.)........ 250
Essential oils in herbal drugs, determination of (2.8.12.).. 251

Essential oils, odour and taste (2.8.8.) ... 250
Essential oils, residue on evaporation (2.8.9.) ... 250
Essential oils, solubility in alcohol (2.8.10.) ... 250
Essential oils, water in (2.8.5.) ... 249
Ester value (2.5.2.) ... 137
Estradiol benzoate ... **6.1**-3455
Estradiol hemihydrate ... 1819
Estradiol valerate ... 1821
Estriol ... 1822
Estrogens, conjugated ... 1824
Etacrynic acid ... 1826
Etamsylate ... **6.2**-3737
Ethacridine lactate monohydrate ... 1828
Ethambutol hydrochloride ... **6.1**-3456
Ethanol (96 per cent) ... 1829
Ethanol, anhydrous ... 1831
Ethanol content and alcoholimetric tables (2.9.10.) ... 281
Ether ... 1833
Ether, anaesthetic ... 1834
Ethinylestradiol ... 1834
Ethionamide ... 1835
Ethosuximide ... 1836
Ethoxylated substances, ethylene glycol and diethylene glycol in (2.4.30.) ... 131
Ethyl acetate ... 1838
Ethyl acrylate - methacrylic acid copolymer (1:1) ... **6.2**-3781
Ethylcellulose ... 1841
Ethylenediamine ... 1843
Ethylene glycol and diethylene glycol in ethoxylated substances (2.4.30.) ... 131
Ethylene glycol monopalmitostearate ... 1842
Ethylene glycol monostearate ... 1842
Ethylene oxide and dioxan (2.4.25.) ... 126
Ethylhexanoic acid, 2- (2.4.28.) ... 129
Ethylmorphine hydrochloride ... 1843
Ethyl oleate ... 1838
Ethyl parahydroxybenzoate ... 1839
Ethyl parahydroxybenzoate sodium ... 1840
Etidronate disodium ... 1844
Etilefrine hydrochloride ... 1845
Etodolac ... 1847
Etofenamate ... 1849
Etofylline ... 1850
Etomidate ... 1851
Etoposide ... 1852
Eucalyptus leaf ... 1857
Eucalyptus oil ... **6.2**-3738
Eugenol ... 1859
European goldenrod ... 2000
European viper venom antiserum ... 970
Evaluation of efficacy of veterinary vaccines and immunosera (5.2.7.) ... **6.1**-3335
Evaluation of safety of each batch of veterinary vaccines and immunosera (5.2.9.) ... 567
Evaluation of safety of veterinary vaccines and immunosera (5.2.6.) ... 556
Evening primrose oil, refined ... 1860
Extractable volume of parenteral preparations, test for (2.9.17.) ... 287
Extracts ... **6.1**-3343
Extracts, dry ... **6.1**-3344
Extracts, dry residue of (2.8.16.) ... 256
Extracts, liquid ... **6.1**-3343
Extracts, loss on drying of (2.8.17.) ... 256
Extracts, soft ... **6.1**-3344
Extraneous agents in viral vaccines for human use, tests for (2.6.16.) ... 190
Extraneous agents: tests in batches of finished product of avian live virus vaccines (2.6.25.) ... 202
Extraneous agents: tests in seed lots of avian viral vaccines (2.6.24.) ... 198
Eye drops ... 721
Eye lotions ... 721
Eye preparations ... 721
Eye preparations, semi-solid ... 722

F

F_0 concept to steam sterilisation of aqueous preparations, application of (5.1.5.) ... 531
Factor II, human coagulation, assay of (2.7.18.) ... 234
Factor IX, human coagulation ... 2064
Factor IX, human coagulation, assay of (2.7.11.) ... 229
Factor VII, human coagulation ... 2061
Factor VII, human coagulation, assay of (2.7.10.) ... 228
Factor VIII, human coagulation ... 2062
Factor VIII, human coagulation, assay of (2.7.4.) ... 216
Factor VIII (rDNA), human coagulation ... 2063
Factor X, human coagulation, assay of (2.7.19.) ... 235
Factor XI, human coagulation ... 2065
Factor XI, human coagulation, assay of (2.7.22.) ... 238
Falling ball viscometer method (2.2.49.) ... 84
Famotidine ... 1865
Fatty acids, composition by gas chromatography (2.4.22.) ... 118
Fatty acids in oils rich in omega-3 acids, composition of (2.4.29.) ... **6.2**-3623
Fatty oils, alkaline impurities in (2.4.19.) ... 117
Fatty oils and herbal drugs, heavy metals in (2.4.27.) ... 128
Fatty oils and resinified essential oils in essential oils (2.8.7.) ... 250
Fatty oils, foreign oils in, by thin-layer chromatography (2.4.21.) ... 117
Fatty oils, identification by thin-layer chromatography (2.3.2.) ... 106
Fatty oils, sterols in (2.4.23.) ... 120
Fatty oils, vegetable ... 712
Fc function of immunoglobulin, test for (2.7.9.) ... 227
Febantel for veterinary use ... 1870
Felbinac ... 1866
Feline calicivirosis vaccine (inactivated) ... 909
Feline calicivirosis vaccine (live) ... 910
Feline chlamydiosis vaccine (inactivated) ... 911
Feline infectious enteritis (feline panleucopenia) vaccine (inactivated) ... 912
Feline infectious enteritis (feline panleucopenia) vaccine (live) ... 913
Feline leukaemia vaccine (inactivated) ... 914
Feline panleucopenia vaccine (inactivated) ... 912
Feline panleucopenia vaccine (live) ... 913
Feline viral rhinotracheitis vaccine (inactivated) ... 916
Feline viral rhinotracheitis vaccine (live) ... 917
Felodipine ... 1867
Felypressin ... 1869
Fenbendazole for veterinary use ... 1871
Fenbufen ... 1872
Fennel, bitter ... 1873
Fennel, sweet ... 1874
Fenofibrate ... 1875
Fenoterol hydrobromide ... 1876
Fentanyl ... 1878
Fentanyl citrate ... 1879
Fenticonazole nitrate ... 1880
Fenugreek ... 1882
Fermentation, products of ... 693
Ferric chloride hexahydrate ... 1882
Ferrous fumarate ... 1883
Ferrous gluconate ... 1884
Ferrous sulphate, dried ... 1885

Ferrous sulphate heptahydrate....1886
Feverfew....1887
Fexofenadine hydrochloride....1888
Fibrinogen, human....2066
Fibrin sealant kit....1890
Finasteride....1891
Fineness, powder (2.9.35.)....**6.2**-3648
Fish oil, rich in omega-3 acids....1893
Flavoxate hydrochloride....1895
Flecainide acetate....1896
Flocculation value (Lf) of diphtheria and tetanus toxins and toxoids (Ramon assay) (2.7.27.)....241
Flowability (2.9.16.)....286
Flow cytometry (2.7.24.)....240
Flubendazole....1898
Flucloxacillin magnesium octahydrate....**6.2**-3741
Flucloxacillin sodium....1899
Fluconazole....1900
Flucytosine....1902
Fludarabine phosphate....1903
Fludeoxyglucose (^{18}F) injection....**6.2**-3678
Fludrocortisone acetate....1906
Flumazenil....1908
Flumazenil (*N*-[^{11}C]methyl) injection....989
Flumequine....1909
Flumetasone pivalate....1910
Flunarizine dihydrochloride....1911
Flunitrazepam....1913
Flunixin meglumine for veterinary use....1914
Fluocinolone acetonide....1915
Fluocortolone pivalate....1916
Fluorescein....1918
Fluorescein sodium....1919
Fluorides (2.4.5.)....112
Fluorimetry (2.2.21.)....36
Fluorodopa (^{18}F) (prepared by electrophilic substitution) injection....990
Fluorouracil....1920
Fluoxetine hydrochloride....1922
Flupentixol dihydrochloride....1924
Fluphenazine decanoate....1926
Fluphenazine dihydrochloride....1928
Fluphenazine enantate....1927
Flurazepam monohydrochloride....1930
Flurbiprofen....1931
Fluspirilene....1932
Flutamide....1933
Fluticasone propionate....1934
Flutrimazole....1936
Fluvoxamine maleate....**6.2**-3742
Foams, cutaneous....728
Foams, intrauterine....726
Foams, medicated....723
Foams, rectal....746
Foams, vaginal....752
Folic acid....1938
Foot-and-mouth disease (ruminants) vaccine (inactivated)....918
Foreign esters in essential oils (2.8.6.)....250
Foreign matter (2.8.2.)....249
Foreign oils in fatty oils by thin-layer chromatography (2.4.21.)....117
Formaldehyde, free (2.4.18.)....117
Formaldehyde solution (35 per cent)....1939
Formoterol fumarate dihydrate....1940
Foscarnet sodium hexahydrate....1942
Fosfomycin calcium....1943
Fosfomycin sodium....1945
Fosfomycin trometamol....1946
Fowl cholera vaccine (inactivated)....920
Fowl-pox vaccine (live)....921
Framycetin sulphate....1947
Frangula bark....1949
Frangula bark dry extract, standardised....**6.2**-3744
Frankincense, Indian....2128
Free formaldehyde (2.4.18.)....117
Freezing point (2.2.18.)....35
Fresh bilberry fruit dry extract, refined and standardised....**6.2**-3745
Friability of granules and spheroids (2.9.41.)....330
Friability of uncoated tablets (2.9.7.)....278
Fructose....1951
Fucus....2213
Fumitory....1952
Functional groups and ions, identification reactions of (2.3.1.)....103
Furosemide....1953
Furunculosis vaccine (inactivated, oil-adjuvanted, injectable) for salmonids....**6.2**-3668
Fusidic acid....1954

G

Galactose....1959
Gallamine triethiodide....1959
Gallium (^{67}Ga) citrate injection....992
Gargles....733
Garlic for homoeopathic preparations....1077
Garlic powder....1961
Gas chromatography (2.2.28.)....45
Gas detector tubes (2.1.6.)....17
Gases, carbon dioxide in (2.5.24.)....144
Gases, carbon monoxide in (2.5.25.)....145
Gases, nitrogen monoxide and nitrogen dioxide in (2.5.26.)....146
Gases, nitrous oxide in (2.5.35.)....152
Gases, oxygen in (2.5.27.)....146
Gases, water in (2.5.28.)....146
Gas-gangrene antitoxin, mixed....966
Gas-gangrene antitoxin (novyi)....966
Gas-gangrene antitoxin (perfringens)....967
Gas-gangrene antitoxin (septicum)....968
Gas pycnometric density of solids (2.9.23.)....**6.2**-3642
Gastro-resistant capsules....718
Gastro-resistant granules....724
Gastro-resistant tablets....750
Gelatin....1961
Gels....747
Gels for injections....737
Gemcitabine hydrochloride....1963
Gemfibrozil....1964
General notices (1.)....3
General texts on biological products (5.2.)....547
General texts on microbiology (5.1.)....525
Gene transfer medicinal products for human use (5.14.)....669
Gentamicin sulphate....1965
Gentian root....1967
Gentian tincture....1968
Ginger....**6.2**-3751
Gingival solutions....733
Ginkgo dry extract, refined and quantified....**6.1**-3461
Ginkgo leaf....1969
Ginseng....1971
Glass containers for pharmaceutical use (3.2.1.)....373
Glibenclamide....1972
Gliclazide....1974
Glimepiride....1975
Glipizide....1977
Glossary....717

Glossary (dosage forms) 717
Glucagon, human 1979
Glucose, anhydrous 1981
Glucose, liquid **6.2**-3752
Glucose, liquid, spray-dried 1982
Glucose monohydrate 1983
Glutamic acid 1984
Glutathione **6.1**-3463
Glycerol 1987
Glycerol (85 per cent) 1988
Glycerol dibehenate 1990
Glycerol distearate 1991
Glycerol monocaprylate 1992
Glycerol monocaprylocaprate 1993
Glycerol monolinoleate 1994
Glycerol mono-oleate 1995
Glycerol monostearate 40-55 1996
Glycerol triacetate 3112
Glyceryl trinitrate solution **6.1**-3465
Glycine 1998
Glycyrrhizate ammonium 1179
Goldenrod 1999
Goldenrod, European 2000
Goldenseal rhizome **6.1**-3467
Gonadorelin acetate 2003
Gonadotrophin, chorionic 2004
Gonadotrophin, equine serum, for veterinary use 2005
Goserelin 2005
Gramicidin 2007
Granisetron hydrochloride 2009
Granules 723
Granules and powders for oral solutions and suspensions 729
Granules and powders for syrups 730
Granules and spheroids, friability of (2.9.41.) 330
Granules, coated 724
Granules, effervescent 724
Granules, gastro-resistant 724
Granules, modified-release 724
Greater celandine 2010
Griseofulvin 2011
Guaiacol 2012
Guaifenesin 2014
Guanethidine monosulphate 2015
Guar **6.2**-3752
Guar galactomannan **6.2**-3753

H

Haematopoietic products, numeration of CD34/CD45+ cells in (2.7.23.) 238
Haematopoietic progenitor cells, human, colony-forming cell assay for (2.7.28.) 242
Haematopoietic stem cells, human 2067
Haemodiafiltration and for haemofiltration, solutions for 2025
Haemodialysis, concentrated solutions for 2022
Haemodialysis solutions, concentrated, water for diluting 2021
Haemodialysis, solutions for 2022
Haemofiltration and for haemodiafiltration, solutions for 2025
Haemophilus type b (conjugate), diphtheria, tetanus and pertussis (acellular, component) vaccine (adsorbed) 771
Haemophilus type b (conjugate), diphtheria, tetanus, pertussis (acellular, component) and poliomyelitis (inactivated) vaccine (adsorbed) 783
Haemophilus type b (conjugate), diphtheria, tetanus, pertussis (acellular, component), hepatitis B (rDNA) and poliomyelitis (inactivated) vaccine (adsorbed) 780
Haemophilus type b (conjugate), diphtheria, tetanus, pertussis and poliomyelitis (inactivated) vaccine (adsorbed) 787
Haemophilus type b conjugate vaccine 792
Haemorrhagic disease vaccine (inactivated), rabbit 949
Halofantrine hydrochloride 2027
Haloperidol 2028
Haloperidol decanoate 2030
Halothane 2031
Hamamelis leaf **6.1**-3471
Hard capsules 718
Hard fat 2034
Hard paraffin 2612
Hawthorn berries 2034
Hawthorn leaf and flower 2035
Hawthorn leaf and flower dry extract 2036
Hawthorn leaf and flower liquid extract, quantified 2037
Heavy bismuth subnitrate 1315
Heavy kaolin 2213
Heavy magnesium carbonate **6.2**-3779
Heavy magnesium oxide 2320
Heavy metals (2.4.8.) 112
Heavy metals in herbal drugs and fatty oils (2.4.27.) 128
Hedera helix for homoeopathic preparations 1078
Helium 2038
Heparin, assay of (2.7.5.) 217
Heparin calcium 2039
Heparin in coagulation factors, assay of (2.7.12.) 230
Heparins, low-molecular-mass 2041
Heparin sodium 2040
Hepatitis A immunoglobulin, human 2068
Hepatitis A (inactivated) and hepatitis B (rDNA) vaccine (adsorbed) 794
Hepatitis A vaccine, assay of (2.7.14.) 232
Hepatitis A vaccine (inactivated, adsorbed) 795
Hepatitis A vaccine (inactivated, virosome) 797
Hepatitis B immunoglobulin for intravenous administration, human 2069
Hepatitis B immunoglobulin, human 2069
Hepatitis B (rDNA), diphtheria and tetanus vaccine (adsorbed) 765
Hepatitis B (rDNA), diphtheria, tetanus and pertussis (acellular, component) vaccine (adsorbed) 774
Hepatitis B (rDNA), diphtheria, tetanus, pertussis (acellular, component), poliomyelitis (inactivated) and haemophilus type b conjugate vaccine (adsorbed) 780
Hepatitis B vaccine (rDNA) 800
Hepatitis B vaccine (rDNA), assay of (2.7.15.) 233
Hepatitis C virus (HCV), validation of nucleic acid amplification techniques for the detection of HCV RNA in plasma pools: Guidelines 195
Heptaminol hydrochloride 2043
Herbal drug preparations 684
Herbal drugs 684
Herbal drugs and fatty oils, heavy metals in (2.4.27.) 128
Herbal drugs, determination of aflatoxin B_1 in (2.8.18.) 256
Herbal drugs, determination of essential oils in herbal drugs (2.8.12.) 251
Herbal drugs, determination of tannins (2.8.14.) 255
Herbal drugs for homoeopathic preparations 1065
Herbal teas 685
Hexamidine diisetionate 2044
Hexetidine 2045
Hexobarbital 2047
Hexosamines in polysaccharide vaccines (2.5.20.) 143
Hexylresorcinol 2047
Highly purified water 3212
Histamine (2.6.10.) 165
Histamine dihydrochloride 2049

Histamine phosphate ... 2049
Histidine ... 2050
Histidine hydrochloride monohydrate ... 2051
Homatropine hydrobromide ... 2052
Homatropine methylbromide ... 2053
Homoeopathic preparations ... 1065
Homoeopathic preparations, arsenious trioxide for ... 1073
Homoeopathic preparations, calcium iodide tetrahydrate for ... 1074
Homoeopathic preparations, common stinging nettle for ... 1075
Homoeopathic preparations, copper acetate monohydrate for ... 1075
Homoeopathic preparations, copper for ... 1076
Homoeopathic preparations, garlic for ... 1077
Homoeopathic preparations, hedera helix for ... 1078
Homoeopathic preparations, herbal drugs for ... 1065
Homoeopathic preparations, honey bee for ... 1079
Homoeopathic preparations, hyoscyamus for ... 1079
Homoeopathic preparations, hypericum for ... 1080
Homoeopathic preparations, iron for ... 1081
Homoeopathic preparations, mother tinctures for ... 1072
Homoeopathic preparations, oriental cashew for ... 1082
Homoeopathic preparations, saffron for ... 1084
Homoeopathic stocks (methods of preparation of) and potentisation ... **6.1**-3385
Honey ... 2055
Honey bee for homoeopathic preparations ... 1079
Hop strobile ... **6.1**-3472
Human α-1-proteinase inhibitor ... **6.2**-3762
Human albumin injection, iodinated (^{125}I) ... 993
Human albumin solution ... 2057
Human anti-D immunoglobulin ... **6.2**-3757
Human anti-D immunoglobulin, assay of (2.7.13.) ... 230
Human anti-D immunoglobulin for intravenous administration ... 2059
Human antithrombin III, assay of (2.7.17.) ... 234
Human antithrombin III concentrate ... 2060
Human coagulation factor II, assay of (2.7.18.) ... 234
Human coagulation factor IX ... 2064
Human coagulation factor IX, assay of (2.7.11.) ... 229
Human coagulation factor VII ... 2061
Human coagulation factor VII, assay of (2.7.10.) ... 228
Human coagulation factor VIII ... 2062
Human coagulation factor VIII, assay of (2.7.4.) ... 216
Human coagulation factor VIII (rDNA) ... 2063
Human coagulation factor X, assay of (2.7.19.) ... 235
Human coagulation factor XI ... 2065
Human coagulation factor XI, assay of (2.7.22.) ... 238
Human fibrinogen ... 2066
Human haematopoietic progenitor cells, colony-forming cell assay for (2.7.28.) ... 242
Human haematopoietic stem cells ... 2067
Human hepatitis A immunoglobulin ... 2068
Human hepatitis B immunoglobulin ... 2069
Human hepatitis B immunoglobulin for intravenous administration ... 2069
Human insulin ... 2137
Human measles immunoglobulin ... 2069
Human normal immunoglobulin ... **6.2**-3757
Human normal immunoglobulin for intravenous administration ... 2072
Human plasma for fractionation ... **6.2**-3759
Human plasma (pooled and treated for virus inactivation) ... **6.2**-3760
Human plasmine inhibitor, assay of (2.7.25.) ... **6.2**-3631
Human protein C, assay of (2.7.30.) ... **6.2**-3631
Human protein S, assay of (2.7.31.) ... **6.2**-3632
Human prothrombin complex ... 2076
Human rabies immunoglobulin ... 2078
Human rubella immunoglobulin ... 2079
Human tetanus immunoglobulin ... 2079
Human varicella immunoglobulin ... 2080
Human varicella immunoglobulin for intravenous administration ... 2081
Human von Willebrand factor ... 2081
Human von Willebrand factor, assay of (2.7.21.) ... 237
Hyaluronidase ... 2082
Hydralazine hydrochloride ... 2083
Hydrochloric acid, concentrated ... 2085
Hydrochloric acid, dilute ... 2085
Hydrochlorothiazide ... 2086
Hydrocodone hydrogen tartrate 2.5-hydrate ... 2087
Hydrocortisone ... 2089
Hydrocortisone acetate ... 2091
Hydrocortisone hydrogen succinate ... 2092
Hydrogenated arachis oil ... **6.2**-3694
Hydrogenated castor oil ... 1432
Hydrogenated cottonseed oil ... **6.2**-3724
Hydrogenated soya-bean oil ... **6.2**-3837
Hydrogenated vegetable oils, nickel in (2.4.31.) ... 131
Hydrogenated wool fat ... 3226
Hydrogen peroxide solution (30 per cent) ... 2094
Hydrogen peroxide solution (3 per cent) ... 2094
Hydromorphone hydrochloride ... 2095
Hydrophobic colloidal silica ... 2878
Hydrous wool fat ... 3227
Hydroxocobalamin acetate ... 2096
Hydroxocobalamin chloride ... 2098
Hydroxocobalamin sulphate ... 2099
Hydroxycarbamide ... 2100
Hydroxyethylcellulose ... 2102
Hydroxyethylmethylcellulose ... 2390
Hydroxyethyl salicylate ... 2101
Hydroxyl value (2.5.3.) ... 137
Hydroxypropylbetadex ... **6.2**-3763
Hydroxypropylcellulose ... 2105
Hydroxypropylmethylcellulose ... **6.1**-3473
Hydroxypropylmethylcellulose phthalate ... **6.1**-3475
Hydroxyzine hydrochloride ... 2106
Hymecromone ... 2107
Hyoscine ... 2108
Hyoscine butylbromide ... 2109
Hyoscine hydrobromide ... 2110
Hyoscyamine sulphate ... 2112
Hyoscyamus for homoeopathic preparations ... 1079
Hypericum ... **6.2**-3839
Hypericum for homoeopathic preparations ... 1080
Hypromellose ... **6.1**-3473
Hypromellose phthalate ... **6.1**-3475

I

Ibuprofen ... **6.1**-3479
Iceland moss ... 2121
ICH (5.8.) ... 645
Ichthammol ... 2122
Identification (2.3.) ... 103
Identification and control of residual solvents (2.4.24.) ... 121
Identification of fatty oils by thin-layer chromatography (2.3.2.) ... 106
Identification of phenothiazines by thin-layer chromatography (2.3.3.) ... 107
Identification reactions of ions and functional groups (2.3.1.) ... 103
Idoxuridine ... 2122
Ifosfamide ... 2123
Imipenem ... 2125
Imipramine hydrochloride ... **6.2**-3769

Immunochemical methods (2.7.1.) ... 209
Immunoglobulin for human use, anti-T lymphocyte, animal ... 1203
Immunoglobulin for intravenous administration, human anti-D ... 2059
Immunoglobulin for intravenous administration, human hepatitis B ... 2069
Immunoglobulin for intravenous administration, human normal ... 2072
Immunoglobulin for intravenous administration, human varicella ... 2081
Immunoglobulin, human anti-D ... **6.2**-3757
Immunoglobulin, human anti-D, assay of (2.7.13.) ... 230
Immunoglobulin, human hepatitis A ... 2068
Immunoglobulin, human hepatitis B ... 2069
Immunoglobulin, human measles ... 2069
Immunoglobulin, human normal ... **6.2**-3757
Immunoglobulin, human rabies ... 2078
Immunoglobulin, human rubella ... 2079
Immunoglobulin, human tetanus ... 2079
Immunoglobulin, human varicella ... 2080
Immunoglobulin, test for anticomplementary activity of (2.6.17.) ... 191
Immunoglobulin, test for Fc function of (2.7.9.) ... 227
Immunosera and vaccines, phenol in (2.5.15.) ... 142
Immunosera and vaccines, veterinary, evaluation of efficacy of (5.2.7.) ... **6.1**-3335
Immunosera and vaccines, veterinary, evaluation of safety (5.2.6.) ... 556
Immunosera and vaccines, veterinary, evaluation of the safety of each batch (5.2.9.) ... 567
Immunosera for human use, animal ... 685
Immunosera for veterinary use ... 687
Implants ... 737
Impurities in substances for pharmaceutical use, control of (5.10.) ... 653
Indapamide ... 2127
Indian frankincense ... 2128
Indicators, relationship between approximate pH and colour (2.2.4.) ... 25
Indinavir sulphate ... 2130
Indium (^{111}In) chloride solution ... 994
Indium (^{111}In) oxine solution ... 995
Indium (^{111}In) pentetate injection ... 996
Indometacin ... 2132
Inductively coupled plasma-atomic emission spectrometry (2.2.57.) ... 96
Inductively coupled plasma-mass spectrometry (2.2.58.) ... 98
Infectious bovine rhinotracheitis vaccine (live) ... 924
Infectious bronchitis vaccine (inactivated), avian ... 864
Infectious bronchitis vaccine (live), avian ... **6.1**-3371
Infectious bursal disease vaccine (inactivated), avian ... 867
Infectious bursal disease vaccine (live), avian ... 869
Infectious chicken anaemia vaccine (live) ... 925
Infectious encephalomyelitis vaccine (live), avian ... 871
Infectious laryngotracheitis vaccine (live), avian ... 872
Influenza vaccine (split virion, inactivated) ... 801
Influenza vaccine (surface antigen, inactivated) ... 803
Influenza vaccine (surface antigen, inactivated, prepared in cell cultures) ... 804
Influenza vaccine (surface antigen, inactivated, virosome) ... 806
Influenza vaccine (whole virion, inactivated) ... 808
Influenza vaccine (whole virion, inactivated, prepared in cell cultures) ... 810
Infrared absorption spectrophotometry (2.2.24.) ... 39
Infusions ... 736
Inhalation gas, krypton (^{81M}Kr) ... 1000
Inhalation, preparations for ... 739
Inhalation, preparations for: aerodynamic assessment of fine particles (2.9.18.) ... 287
Injectable insulin preparations ... 2146
Injections ... 736
Injections, gels for ... 737
Injections or infusions, concentrates for ... 736
Injections or infusions, powders for ... 736
Inositol, *myo-* ... 2460
Inserts, ophthalmic ... 722
Insulin aspart ... 2133
Insulin, bovine ... 2135
Insulin, human ... 2137
Insulin injection, biphasic ... 2140
Insulin injection, biphasic isophane ... 2140
Insulin injection, isophane ... 2141
Insulin injection, soluble ... 2141
Insulin lispro ... 2141
Insulin, porcine ... 2144
Insulin preparations, injectable ... 2146
Insulin zinc injectable suspension ... 2148
Insulin zinc injectable suspension (amorphous) ... 2149
Insulin zinc injectable suspension (crystalline) ... 2149
Interferon alfa-2 concentrated solution ... 2150
Interferon gamma-1b concentrated solution ... 2153
Interferons, assay of (5.6.) ... 627
International System (SI) units (1.) ... 3
Intramammary preparations for veterinary use ... 725
Intraruminal devices ... 725
Intrauterine capsules ... 726
Intrauterine foams ... 726
Intrauterine preparations for veterinary use ... 726
Intrauterine solutions, suspensions ... 726
Intrauterine sticks ... 726
Intrauterine tablets ... 726
Intrinsic dissolution (2.9.29.) ... 309
In vivo assay of poliomyelitis vaccine (inactivated) (2.7.20.) ... 235
Iobenguane (^{123}I) injection ... 997
Iobenguane (^{131}I) injection for diagnostic use ... 998
Iobenguane (^{131}I) injection for therapeutic use ... 999
Iobenguane sulphate for radiopharmaceutical preparations ... **6.1**-3381
Iodinated (^{125}I) human albumin injection ... 993
Iodinated povidone ... 2734
Iodine ... 2156
Iodine value (2.5.4.) ... 137
Iohexol ... 2157
Ionic concentration, potentiometric determination of using ion-selective electrodes (2.2.36.) ... 58
Ions and functional groups, identification reactions of (2.3.1.) ... 103
Ion-selective electrodes, potentiometric determination of ionic concentration (2.2.36.) ... 58
Iopamidol ... 2160
Iopanoic acid ... 2162
Iotalamic acid ... 2163
Iotrolan ... 2164
Ioxaglic acid ... 2167
Ipecacuanha liquid extract, standardised ... 2168
Ipecacuanha, prepared ... **6.2**-3770
Ipecacuanha root ... 2170
Ipecacuanha tincture, standardised ... 2171
Ipratropium bromide ... **6.2**-3771
Iron (2.4.9.) ... 115
Iron for homoeopathic preparations ... 1081
Irrigation, preparations for ... 743
Isoconazole ... 2173
Isoconazole nitrate ... 2175
Isoelectric focusing (2.2.54.) ... 84

Isoflurane....2176
Isoleucine....2177
Isomalt....2178
Isoniazid....2180
Isophane insulin injection....2141
Isoprenaline hydrochloride....2181
Isoprenaline sulphate....2182
Isopropyl alcohol....2182
Isopropyl myristate....2183
Isopropyl palmitate....2184
Isosorbide dinitrate, diluted....2185
Isosorbide mononitrate, diluted....2186
Isotretinoin....2188
Isoxsuprine hydrochloride....2189
Ispaghula husk....2191
Ispaghula seed....2192
Isradipine....2192
Itraconazole....2194
Ivermectin....2196
Ivy leaf....2198

J

Javanese turmeric....3150
Java tea....2203
Josamycin....2204
Josamycin propionate....2205
Juniper....2206
Juniper oil....2207

K

Kanamycin acid sulphate....2211
Kanamycin monosulphate....2212
Kaolin, heavy....2213
Kelp....2213
Ketamine hydrochloride....2214
Ketobemidone hydrochloride....2215
Ketoconazole....2216
Ketoprofen....2218
Ketorolac trometamol....2220
Ketotifen hydrogen fumarate....2221
Knotgrass....2223
Krypton (^{81m}Kr) inhalation gas....1000

L

Labetalol hydrochloride....2227
Lactic acid....2228
Lactic acid, (*S*)-....2229
Lactitol monohydrate....2229
Lactobionic acid....2231
Lactose, anhydrous....2232
Lactose monohydrate....2233
Lactulose....2234
Lactulose, liquid....2236
Lamivudine....2238
Lansoprazole....2240
Laser light diffraction, particle size analysis by (2.9.31.)....311
Lauroyl macrogolglycerides....2242
Lavender flower....2243
Lavender oil....2244
Lead in sugars (2.4.10.)....115
Leflunomide....2245
Lemon oil....2246
Lemon verbena leaf....2248
Leptospirosis vaccine (inactivated), bovine....876
Leptospirosis vaccine (inactivated), canine....888
Letrozole....2249
Leucine....2250
Leuprorelin....2251
Levamisole for veterinary use....2253
Levamisole hydrochloride....2254
Levocabastine hydrochloride....2255
Levocarnitine....2257
Levodopa....2258
Levodropropizine....2260
Levomenthol....2261
Levomepromazine hydrochloride....2262
Levomepromazine maleate....2263
Levomethadone hydrochloride....2264
Levonorgestrel....2266
Levothyroxine sodium....2267
Lidocaine....**6.1**-3485
Lidocaine hydrochloride....2269
Light liquid paraffin....2612
Light magnesium carbonate....2316
Light magnesium oxide....2321
Lime flower....2270
Limit tests (2.4.)....111
Limit tests, standard solutions for (4.1.2.)....504
Lincomycin hydrochloride....2271
Lindane....2272
Linen thread, sterile, in distributor for veterinary use....1058
Linoleoyl macrogolglycerides....2273
Linseed....2273
Linseed oil, virgin....2274
Liothyronine sodium....**6.1**-3486
Lipophilic solid dosage forms, dissolution test for (2.9.42.)....332
Liquid chromatography (2.2.29.)....46
Liquid extracts....**6.1**-3343
Liquid glucose....**6.2**-3752
Liquid glucose, spray-dried....1982
Liquid lactulose....2236
Liquid maltitol....2332
Liquid paraffin....2613
Liquid preparations for cutaneous application....728
Liquid preparations for cutaneous application, veterinary....752
Liquid preparations for inhalation....740
Liquid preparations for oral use....728
Liquids, clarity and degree of opalescence of (2.2.1.)....21
Liquid sorbitol (crystallising)....2942
Liquid sorbitol (non-crystallising)....2943
Liquid sorbitol, partially dehydrated....2944
Liquorice dry extract for flavouring purposes....**6.1**-3488
Liquorice ethanolic liquid extract, standardised....**6.2**-3775
Liquorice root....2276
Lisinopril dihydrate....2277
Lithium carbonate....2279
Lithium citrate....2279
L-Methionine ([^{11}C]methyl) injection....1001
Lobeline hydrochloride....2280
Lomustine....2281
Loosestrife....2283
Loperamide hydrochloride....2283
Loperamide oxide monohydrate....2285
Loratadine....2286
Lorazepam....2288
Loss on drying (2.2.32.)....53
Loss on drying of extracts (2.8.17.)....256
Lovage root....2290
Lovastatin....2291
Low-molecular-mass heparins....2041
Lozenges and pastilles....734
Lozenges, compressed....734
Lubricant, silicone oil (3.1.8.)....358
Lymecycline....**6.1**-3489
Lynestrenol....2294

Lyophilisates, oral 748
Lysine acetate 2295
Lysine hydrochloride 2296

M

Macrogol 15 hydroxystearate 2305
Macrogol 20 glycerol monostearate 2304
Macrogol 40 sorbitol heptaoleate 2310
Macrogol 6 glycerol caprylocaprate 2302
Macrogol cetostearyl ether 2301
Macrogolglycerol cocoates 2302
Macrogolglycerol hydroxystearate 2303
Macrogolglycerol ricinoleate 2304
Macrogol lauryl ether 2306
Macrogol oleate 2307
Macrogol oleyl ether 2308
Macrogols 2308
Macrogol stearate 2311
Macrogol stearyl ether 2312
Magaldrate 2312
Magnesium (2.4.6.) 112
Magnesium acetate tetrahydrate 2313
Magnesium and alkaline-earth metals (2.4.7.) 112
Magnesium aspartate dihydrate 2314
Magnesium carbonate, heavy **6.2**-3779
Magnesium carbonate, light 2316
Magnesium chloride 4.5-hydrate 2317
Magnesium chloride hexahydrate 2316
Magnesium citrate, anhydrous 2318
Magnesium gluconate **6.1**-3495
Magnesium glycerophosphate 2318
Magnesium hydroxide 2319
Magnesium lactate dihydrate 2320
Magnesium oxide, heavy 2320
Magnesium oxide, light 2321
Magnesium peroxide 2321
Magnesium pidolate 2322
Magnesium stearate 2323
Magnesium sulphate heptahydrate 2325
Magnesium trisilicate 2325
Maize oil, refined **6.2**-3779
Maize starch 2326
Malathion 2327
Maleic acid 2328
Malic acid 2329
Mallow flower 2330
Maltitol 2330
Maltitol, liquid 2332
Maltodextrin 2333
Mandarin oil 2333
Manganese gluconate **6.1**-3495
Manganese glycerophosphate, hydrated 2334
Manganese sulphate monohydrate 2335
Mannheimia vaccine (inactivated) for cattle 927
Mannheimia vaccine (inactivated) for sheep 928
Mannitol 2336
Maprotiline hydrochloride 2337
Marbofloxacin for veterinary use **6.1**-3496
Marek's disease vaccine (live) 930
Marshmallow leaf 2338
Marshmallow root 2339
Mass spectrometry (2.2.43.) 68
Mass spectrometry, inductively coupled plasma- (2.2.58.) .. 98
Mass uniformity of delivered doses from multidose containers (2.9.27.) 309
Mass uniformity of single-dose preparations (2.9.5.) 278
Mastic 2340
Materials based on non-plasticised poly(vinyl chloride) for containers for dry dosage forms for oral administration (3.1.11.) 362
Materials based on non-plasticised poly(vinyl chloride) for containers for non-injectable, aqueous solutions (3.1.10.) 360
Materials based on plasticised poly(vinyl chloride) for containers for aqueous solutions for intravenous infusion (3.1.14.) 366
Materials based on plasticised poly(vinyl chloride) for containers for human blood and blood components (3.1.1.1.) 339
Materials based on plasticised poly(vinyl chloride) for tubing used in sets for the transfusion of blood and blood components (3.1.1.2.) 342
Materials for containers for human blood and blood components (3.1.1.) 339
Materials used for the manufacture of containers (3.1.) ... 339
Matricaria flower 2340
Matricaria liquid extract **6.2**-3780
Matricaria oil 2342
Meadowsweet 2344
Measles immunoglobulin, human 2069
Measles, mumps and rubella vaccine (live) **6.1**-3347
Measles vaccine (live) **6.1**-3348
Measurement of consistency by penetrometry (2.9.9.) **6.2**-3641
Mebendazole 2345
Meclozine hydrochloride 2346
Medicated chewing gum (2.9.25.) 304
Medicated chewing gums 719
Medicated feeding stuffs for veterinary use, premixes for .. 739
Medicated foams 723
Medicated plasters 747
Medicated tampons 751
Medicated vaginal tampons 752
Medicinal air 1118
Medicinal air, synthetic 1121
Medium-chain triglycerides 3122
Medroxyprogesterone acetate 2347
Mefenamic acid 2349
Mefloquine hydrochloride 2350
Megestrol acetate 2352
Meglumine 2353
Melilot 2354
Melissa leaf 2355
Melting point - capillary method (2.2.14.) 32
Melting point - instantaneous method (2.2.16.) 33
Melting point - open capillary method (2.2.15.) 32
Menadione 2356
Meningococcal group C conjugate vaccine 814
Meningococcal polysaccharide vaccine 816
Menthol, racemic 2356
Mepivacaine hydrochloride 2357
Meprobamate 2359
Mepyramine maleate 2360
Mercaptopurine 2361
Mercuric chloride 2361
Mercury porosimetry, porosity and pore-size distribution of solids by (2.9.32.) **6.2**-3643
Mesalazine 2362
Mesna 2364
Mesterolone 2366
Mestranol 2367
Metacresol 2368
Metamizole sodium 2369
Metformin hydrochloride 2370
Methacrylate copolymer, basic butylated 1254
Methacrylic acid - ethyl acrylate copolymer (1:1) **6.2**-3781

Methacrylic acid - ethyl acrylate copolymer (1:1) dispersion 30 per cent 2372
Methacrylic acid - methyl methacrylate copolymer (1:1) ..2373
Methacrylic acid - methyl methacrylate copolymer (1:2) ..2374
Methadone hydrochloride 2374
Methanol 2376
Methanol and 2-propanol, test for (2.9.11.) 282
Methaqualone 2377
Methenamine 2378
Methionine 2379
Methionine ([^{11}C]methyl) injection, L- 1001
Methionine, DL- 2380
Methods in pharmacognosy (2.8.) 249
Methods of preparation of homoeopathic stocks and potentisation **6.1**-3385
Methods of preparation of sterile products (5.1.1.) 525
Methotrexate 2380
Methylatropine bromide 2383
Methylatropine nitrate 2383
Methylcellulose **6.1**-3497
Methyldopa 2386
Methylene blue 2402
Methylene chloride 2387
Methylergometrine maleate 2388
Methylhydroxyethylcellulose 2390
Methyl nicotinate 2390
Methyl parahydroxybenzoate 2391
Methylpentoses in polysaccharide vaccines (2.5.21.) 143
Methylphenobarbital 2392
Methylprednisolone 2393
Methylprednisolone acetate 2395
Methylprednisolone hydrogen succinate 2397
Methylpyrrolidone, *N*- 2399
Methylrosanilinium chloride 2400
Methyl salicylate 2401
Methyltestosterone **6.2**-3782
Methylthioninium chloride 2402
Metixene hydrochloride 2404
Metoclopramide **6.2**-3783
Metoclopramide hydrochloride 2407
Metolazone 2407
Metoprolol succinate 2409
Metoprolol tartrate 2410
Metrifonate 2412
Metronidazole 2414
Metronidazole benzoate 2415
Mexiletine hydrochloride 2416
Mianserin hydrochloride 2417
Miconazole 2418
Miconazole nitrate 2420
Microbial enumeration tests (microbiological examination of non-sterile products) (2.6.12.) 166
Microbiological assay of antibiotics (2.7.2.) 210
Microbiological control of cellular products (2.6.27.) 205
Microbiological examination of non-sterile products: test for specified micro-organisms (2.6.13.) 173
Microbiological examination of non-sterile products: total viable aerobic count (2.6.12.) 166
Microbiological quality, alternative methods for control of (5.1.6.) 532
Microbiological quality of pharmaceutical preparations (5.1.4.) 529
Microbiology, general texts on (5.1.) 525
Microcrystalline cellulose **6.2**-3708
Microcrystalline cellulose and carmellose sodium 2422
Micro determination of water (2.5.32.) 147
Microscopy, optical (2.9.37.) 323
Midazolam 2422
Milk thistle dry extract, refined and standardised 2426
Milk-thistle fruit 2425
Minimising the risk of transmitting animal spongiform encephalopathy agents via human and veterinary medicinal products (5.2.8.) 558
Minocycline hydrochloride dihydrate 2427
Minoxidil 2429
Mint oil, partly dementholised 2430
Mirtazapine 2431
Misoprostol 2433
Mitomycin 2434
Mitoxantrone hydrochloride 2436
Modafinil 2437
Modified-release capsules 718
Modified-release granules 724
Modified-release tablets 750
Molecular mass distribution in dextrans (2.2.39.) 60
Molgramostim concentrated solution 2438
Molsidomine **6.1**-3499
Mometasone furoate 2441
Monoclonal antibodies for human use 690
Morantel hydrogen tartrate for veterinary use 2443
Morphine hydrochloride **6.1**-3501
Morphine sulphate **6.2**-3785
Moss, Iceland 2121
Mother tinctures for homoeopathic preparations 1072
Motherwort 2447
Mouthwashes 733
Moxidectin for veterinary use 2448
Moxifloxacin hydrochloride **6.2**-3786
Moxonidine 2453
Mucoadhesive preparations 735
Mullein flower 2454
Multidose containers, uniformity of mass of delivered doses (2.9.27.) 309
Mumps, measles and rubella vaccine (live) **6.1**-3347
Mumps vaccine (live) **6.1**-3349
Mupirocin 2454
Mupirocin calcium 2456
Mycobacteria (2.6.2.) 159
Mycophenolate mofetil 2458
Mycoplasma gallisepticum vaccine (inactivated) 932
Mycoplasmas (2.6.7.) **6.1**-3317
myo-Inositol 2460
Myrrh 2461
Myrrh tincture 2461
Myxomatosis vaccine (live) for rabbits 933

N

Nabumetone 2465
N-Acetyltryptophan 1104
N-Acetyltyrosine 1106
Nadolol 2466
Nadroparin calcium 2467
Naftidrofuryl hydrogen oxalate 2470
Nalidixic acid 2472
Naloxone hydrochloride dihydrate 2473
Naltrexone hydrochloride 2474
Nandrolone decanoate 2476
Naphazoline hydrochloride 2478
Naphazoline nitrate 2479
Naproxen **6.2**-3791
Naproxen sodium **6.1**-3507
Narrow-leaved coneflower root 2483
Nasal drops and liquid nasal sprays 731
Nasal powders 732
Nasal preparations 730
Nasal preparations, semi-solid 732
Nasal sprays (liquid) and nasal drops 730
Nasal sticks 732

Nasal washes 732
Near-infrared spectrophotometry (2.2.40.) 62
Neohesperidin-dihydrochalcone 2485
Neomycin sulphate 2487
Neonatal piglet colibacillosis vaccine (inactivated) 934
Neonatal ruminant colibacillosis vaccine (inactivated) 936
Neostigmine bromide 2489
Neostigmine metilsulfate 2490
Neroli oil 2490
Netilmicin sulphate 2492
Nettle leaf 2493
Neurovirulence test for poliomyelitis vaccine (oral) (2.6.19.) 193
Neurovirulence test of live viral vaccines (2.6.18.) 193
Nevirapine, anhydrous 2495
Newcastle disease vaccine (inactivated) 937
Newcastle disease vaccine (live) 939
Nicergoline 2496
Nickel in hydrogenated vegetable oils (2.4.31.) 131
Nickel in polyols (2.4.15.) 116
Niclosamide, anhydrous 2497
Niclosamide monohydrate 2498
Nicotinamide 2499
Nicotine 2500
Nicotine resinate 2501
Nicotinic acid 2502
Nifedipine 2503
Niflumic acid **6.1**-3508
Nifuroxazide **6.1**-3510
Nikethamide 2505
Nilutamide **6.2**-3792
Nimesulide 2506
Nimodipine 2507
Nitrazepam 2508
Nitrendipine 2509
Nitric acid 2510
Nitric oxide **6.2**-3794
Nitrofural 2512
Nitrofurantoin 2513
Nitrogen **6.2**-3795
Nitrogen determination by sulphuric acid digestion (2.5.9.) 139
Nitrogen determination, primary aromatic amino (2.5.8.) 139
Nitrogen, low-oxygen 2514
Nitrogen monoxide and nitrogen dioxide in gases (2.5.26.) 146
Nitrous oxide 2515
Nitrous oxide in gases (2.5.35.) 152
Nizatidine 2516
N-Methylpyrrolidone 2399
N,N-Dimethylaniline (2.4.26.) 127
Nomegestrol acetate 2518
Nonoxinol 9 2519
Non-sterile products, microbiological examination of (test for specified micro-organisms) (2.6.13.) 173
Non-sterile products, microbiological examination of (total viable aerobic count) (2.6.12.) 166
Noradrenaline hydrochloride 2520
Noradrenaline tartrate 2521
Norcholesterol injection, iodinated (^{131}I) 1003
Norepinephrine hydrochloride 2520
Norepinephrine tartrate 2521
Norethisterone 2523
Norethisterone acetate 2524
Norfloxacin **6.2**-3796
Norgestimate 2526
Norgestrel 2527
Normal immunoglobulin for intravenous administration, human 2072
Normal immunoglobulin, human **6.2**-3757
Nortriptyline hydrochloride 2528
Noscapine 2529
Noscapine hydrochloride 2530
Notoginseng root 2531
Nuclear magnetic resonance spectrometry (2.2.33.) 54
Nucleated cell count and viability (2.7.29.) 243
Nucleic acid amplification techniques (2.6.21.) 195
Nucleic acids in polysaccharide vaccines (2.5.17.) 142
Numeration of CD34/CD45+ cells in haematopoietic products (2.7.23.) 238
Nutmeg oil **6.2**-3797
Nystatin 2534

O

O-Acetyl in polysaccharide vaccines (2.5.19.) 143
Oak bark 2539
Octoxinol 10 2539
Octyldodecanol 2540
Octyl gallate 2539
Odour (2.3.4.) 107
Odour and taste of essential oils (2.8.8.) 250
Ofloxacin **6.2**-3801
Oils, essential 680
Oils, fatty, vegetable 712
Oils rich in omega-3 acids, composition of fatty acids in (2.4.29.) **6.2**-3623
Oils rich in omega-3 acids, total cholesterol in (2.4.32.) 132
Ointments 747
Oleic acid 2543
Oleoresins **6.1**-3344
Oleoyl macrogolglycerides 2543
Oleyl alcohol 2544
Olive leaf 2545
Olive oil, refined **6.2**-3802
Olive oil, virgin **6.2**-3803
Olsalazine sodium 2548
Omega-3 acid ethyl esters 60 2550
Omega-3-acid ethyl esters 90 2552
Omega-3 acids, composition of fatty acids in oils rich in (2.4.29.) **6.2**-3623
Omega-3 acids, fish oil rich in 1893
Omega-3 acids, total cholesterol in oils rich in (2.4.32.) 132
Omega-3 acid triglycerides 2554
Omeprazole 2557
Omeprazole sodium 2558
Ondansetron hydrochloride dihydrate 2560
Opalescence of liquids, clarity and degree of (2.2.1.) 21
Ophthalmic inserts 722
Opium dry extract, standardised 2562
Opium, prepared 2563
Opium, raw 2564
Opium tincture, standardised 2565
Optical microscopy (2.9.37.) 323
Optical rotation (2.2.7.) 26
Oral drops 730
Oral lyophilisates 748
Oral powders 738
Oral solutions, emulsions and suspensions 729
Oral use, liquid preparations for 728
Orciprenaline sulphate **6.2**-3804
Oregano 2568
Organ preservation, solutions for 2929
Oriental cashew for homoeopathic preparations 1082
Orodispersible tablets 750
Oromucosal capsules 734

Oromucosal drops, oromucosal sprays and sublingual sprays 733
Oromucosal preparations 732
Oromucosal preparations, semi-solid 733
Oromucosal solutions and oromucosal suspensions 733
Oromucosal sprays, oromucosal drops and sublingual sprays 732
Oromucosal suspensions and oromucosal solutions 732
Orphenadrine citrate 2569
Orphenadrine hydrochloride 2570
Osmolality (2.2.35.) 57
Ouabain 2571
Oxacillin sodium monohydrate **6.2**-3806
Oxaliplatin 2574
Oxazepam 2577
Oxeladin hydrogen citrate 2578
Oxfendazole for veterinary use **6.2**-3808
Oxidising substances (2.5.30.) 147
Oxitropium bromide 2581
Oxolinic acid 2582
Oxprenolol hydrochloride 2583
Oxybuprocaine hydrochloride 2584
Oxybutynin hydrochloride 2585
Oxycodone hydrochloride 2587
Oxygen (^{15}O) 1004
Oxygen **6.2**-3809
Oxygen-flask method (2.5.10.) 140
Oxygen in gases (2.5.27.) 146
Oxymetazoline hydrochloride 2589
Oxytetracycline dihydrate 2590
Oxytetracycline hydrochloride 2591
Oxytocin 2593
Oxytocin concentrated solution 2594

P

Paclitaxel **6.1**-3515
Pale coneflower root 2602
Palmitic acid 2604
Pamidronate disodium pentahydrate 2604
Pancreas powder **6.2**-3813
Pancuronium bromide 2608
Pansy, wild (flowering aerial parts) 3217
Pantoprazole sodium sesquihydrate **6.1**-3518
Papaverine hydrochloride 2609
Paper chromatography (2.2.26.) 43
Paracetamol 2611
Paraffin, hard 2612
Paraffin, light liquid 2612
Paraffin, liquid 2613
Paraffin, white soft **6.2**-3815
Paraffin, yellow soft **6.2**-3816
Parainfluenza virus vaccine (live), bovine 878
Parainfluenza virus vaccine (live), canine 890
Paraldehyde 2615
Paramyxovirus 1 (Newcastle disease) vaccine (inactivated), avian 937
Parenteral preparations 735
Parenteral preparations, test for extractable volume of (2.9.17.) 287
Parnaparin sodium 2616
Paroxetine hydrochloride, anhydrous 2616
Paroxetine hydrochloride hemihydrate 2619
Particles, fine, aerodynamic assessment of in preparations for inhalation (2.9.18.) 287
Particle size analysis by laser light diffraction (2.9.31.) 311
Particle-size distribution estimation by analytical sieving (2.9.38.) **6.2**-3649
Particulate contamination: sub-visible particles (2.9.19.) 300
Particulate contamination: visible particles (2.9.20.) 302
Parvovirosis vaccine (inactivated), canine 891
Parvovirosis vaccine (inactivated), porcine 946
Parvovirosis vaccine (live), canine 892
Passion flower 2621
Passion flower dry extract 2622
Pastes 747
Pasteurella vaccine (inactivated) for sheep 941
Pastilles and lozenges 734
Patches, transdermal 737
Patches, transdermal, dissolution test for (2.9.4.) 275
Pefloxacin mesilate dihydrate 2623
Pelargonium root 2625
Penbutolol sulphate 2625
Penetrometry, measurement of consistency by (2.9.9.) **6.2**-3641
Penicillamine 2626
Pentaerythrityl tetranitrate, diluted 2628
Pentamidine diisetionate 2630
Pentazocine 2631
Pentazocine hydrochloride 2632
Pentazocine lactate 2632
Pentobarbital 2633
Pentobarbital sodium 2634
Pentoxifylline 2635
Pentoxyverine hydrogen citrate 2637
Peppermint leaf 2638
Peppermint oil 2639
Pepsin powder 2640
Peptide mapping (2.2.55.) 86
Peptides, synthetic, acetic acid in (2.5.34.) 151
Pergolide mesilate 2641
Perindopril *tert*-butylamine 2643
Peritoneal dialysis, solutions for 2646
Peroxide value (2.5.5.) 138
Perphenazine 2648
Pertussis (acellular, component), diphtheria and tetanus vaccine (adsorbed) 767
Pertussis (acellular, component), diphtheria, tetanus and haemophilus type b conjugate vaccine (adsorbed) 771
Pertussis (acellular, component), diphtheria, tetanus and hepatitis B (rDNA) vaccine (adsorbed) 774
Pertussis (acellular, component), diphtheria, tetanus and poliomyelitis (inactivated) vaccine (adsorbed) 775
Pertussis (acellular, component), diphtheria, tetanus and poliomyelitis (inactivated) vaccine (adsorbed, reduced antigen(s) content) 778
Pertussis (acellular, component), diphtheria, tetanus, hepatitis B (rDNA), poliomyelitis (inactivated) and haemophilus type b conjugate vaccine (adsorbed) 780
Pertussis (acellular, component), diphtheria, tetanus, poliomyelitis (inactivated) and haemophilus type b conjugate vaccine (adsorbed) 783
Pertussis, diphtheria, tetanus and poliomyelitis (inactivated) vaccine (adsorbed) 785
Pertussis, diphtheria, tetanus, poliomyelitis (inactivated) and haemophilus type b conjugate vaccine (adsorbed) 787
Pertussis vaccine (acellular), assay of (2.7.16.) 233
Pertussis vaccine (acellular, component, adsorbed) 820
Pertussis vaccine (acellular, co-purified, adsorbed) 822
Pertussis vaccine (adsorbed) 824
Pertussis vaccine, assay of (2.7.7.) 222
Peru balsam **6.2**-3817
Pessaries 751
Pessaries and suppositories, disintegration of (2.9.2.) 265
Pesticide residues (2.8.13.) **6.2**-3637
Pethidine hydrochloride 2650
Pharmaceutical technical procedures (2.9.) 263
Pharmacognosy, methods in (2.8.) 249

Pharmacopoeial harmonisation (5.8.) 645
Phenazone 2651
Pheniramine maleate 2652
Phenobarbital 2653
Phenobarbital sodium 2654
Phenol 2655
Phenol in immunosera and vaccines (2.5.15.) 142
Phenolphthalein 2656
Phenolsulfonphthalein 2657
Phenothiazines, identification by thin-layer chromatography (2.3.3.) 107
Phenoxyethanol 2657
Phenoxymethylpenicillin **6.1**-3520
Phenoxymethylpenicillin potassium **6.1**-3521
Phentolamine mesilate 2662
Phenylalanine 2663
Phenylbutazone 2664
Phenylephrine 2665
Phenylephrine hydrochloride 2667
Phenylmercuric acetate 2668
Phenylmercuric borate 2669
Phenylmercuric nitrate 2669
Phenylpropanolamine hydrochloride 2670
Phenytoin 2671
Phenytoin sodium 2672
Phloroglucinol, anhydrous 2672
Phloroglucinol dihydrate 2673
Pholcodine 2674
Phosphates (2.4.11.) 116
Phosphoric acid, concentrated 2675
Phosphoric acid, dilute 2676
Phosphorus in polysaccharide vaccines (2.5.18.) 142
pH, potentiometric determination of (2.2.3.) 24
Phthalylsulfathiazole 2676
Physical and physicochemical methods (2.2.) 21
Physostigmine salicylate 2677
Physostigmine sulphate 2678
Phytomenadione 2679
Phytosterol 2680
Picotamide monohydrate 2682
Pilocarpine hydrochloride 2682
Pilocarpine nitrate 2684
Pimobendan 2685
Pimozide 2686
Pindolol 2688
Pine (dwarf) oil 1766
Pine sylvestris oil 2689
Pinus pinaster type turpentine oil 3151
Pipemidic acid trihydrate 2690
Piperacillin 2691
Piperacillin sodium 2692
Piperazine adipate 2694
Piperazine citrate 2695
Piperazine hydrate 2696
Piracetam 2697
Pirenzepine dihydrochloride monohydrate 2698
Piretanide 2699
Piroxicam 2700
Pivampicillin 2702
Pivmecillinam hydrochloride 2704
Plasma for fractionation, human **6.2**-3759
Plasma (pooled and treated for virus inactivation), human **6.2**-3760
Plasmid vectors for human use 674
Plasmid vectors for human use, bacterial cells used for the manufacture of 676
Plasmin inhibitor, assay of human (2.7.25.) **6.2**-3631
Plasters, medicated 746
Plastic additives (3.1.13.) **6.2**-3655
Plastic containers and closures for pharmaceutical use (3.2.2.) 378
Plastic containers for aqueous solutions for infusion (3.2.2.1.) 379
Plastic containers for human blood and blood components, sterile (3.2.3.) 379
Plastic syringes, single-use, sterile (3.2.8.) 384
Pneumococcal polysaccharide conjugate vaccine (adsorbed) 825
Pneumococcal polysaccharide vaccine 827
Poliomyelitis (inactivated), diphtheria and tetanus vaccine (adsorbed, reduced antigen(s) content) 770
Poliomyelitis (inactivated), diphtheria, tetanus and pertussis (acellular, component) vaccine (adsorbed) 775
Poliomyelitis (inactivated), diphtheria, tetanus and pertussis (acellular, component) vaccine (adsorbed, reduced antigen(s) content) 778
Poliomyelitis (inactivated), diphtheria, tetanus and pertussis vaccine (adsorbed) 785
Poliomyelitis (inactivated), diphtheria, tetanus, pertussis (acellular, component) and haemophilus type b conjugate vaccine (adsorbed) 783
Poliomyelitis (inactivated), diphtheria, tetanus, pertussis (acellular, component), hepatitis B (rDNA) and haemophilus type b conjugate vaccine (adsorbed) 780
Poliomyelitis (inactivated), diphtheria, tetanus, pertussis and haemophilus type b conjugate vaccine (adsorbed) 787
Poliomyelitis vaccine (inactivated) 829
Poliomyelitis vaccine (inactivated), *in vivo* assay of (2.7.20.) 235
Poliomyelitis vaccine (oral) **6.1**-3351
Poliomyelitis vaccine (oral), test for neurovirulence (2.6.19.) 193
Poloxamers 2705
Polyacrylate dispersion 30 per cent 2706
Polyamide 6/6 suture, sterile, in distributor for veterinary use 1059
Polyamide 6 suture, sterile, in distributor for veterinary use 1058
Polyethyleneglycols 2308
Polyethylene terephthalate for containers for preparations not for parenteral use (3.1.15.) 369
Poly(ethylene terephthalate) suture, sterile, in distributor for veterinary use 1059
Poly(ethylene - vinyl acetate) for containers and tubing for total parenteral nutrition preparations (3.1.7.) 356
Polyethylene with additives for containers for parenteral preparations and for ophthalmic preparations (3.1.5.) 349
Polyethylene without additives for containers for parenteral preparations and for ophthalmic preparations (3.1.4.) 348
Polymorphism (5.9.) 649
Polymyxin B sulphate 2707
Polyolefines (3.1.3.) 344
Polyoxyl castor oil 2304
Polyoxyl hydrogenated castor oil 2303
Polypropylene for containers and closures for parenteral preparations and ophthalmic preparations (3.1.6.) 352
Polysaccharide vaccines, hexosamines in (2.5.20.) 143
Polysaccharide vaccines, methylpentoses in (2.5.21.) 143
Polysaccharide vaccines, nucleic acids in (2.5.17.) 142
Polysaccharide vaccines, *O*-acetyl in (2.5.19.) 143
Polysaccharide vaccines, phosphorus in (2.5.18.) 142
Polysaccharide vaccines, protein in (2.5.16.) 142
Polysaccharide vaccines, ribose in (2.5.31.) 147
Polysaccharide vaccines, sialic acid in (2.5.23.) 144
Polysaccharide vaccines, uronic acids in (2.5.22.) 144
Polysorbate 20 2709
Polysorbate 40 2710
Polysorbate 60 2710

Polysorbate 80 ... 2711
Poly(vinyl acetate) ... 2712
Poly(vinyl acetate) dispersion 30 per cent ... **6.2**-3818
Poly(vinyl alcohol) ... 2715
Poly(vinyl chloride), non-plasticised, materials based on for containers for dry dosage forms for oral administration (3.1.11.) ... 362
Poly(vinyl chloride), non-plasticised, materials based on for containers for non-injectable aqueous solutions (3.1.10.) ... 360
Poly(vinyl chloride), plasticised, empty sterile containers of for human blood and blood components (3.2.4.) ... 381
Poly(vinyl chloride), plasticised, materials based on for containers for aqueous solutions for intravenous infusion (3.1.14.) ... 366
Poly(vinyl chloride), plasticised, materials based on for containers for human blood and blood components (3.1.1.1.) ... 339
Poly(vinyl chloride), plasticised, materials based on for tubing used in sets for the transfusion of blood and blood components (3.1.1.2.) ... 342
Poly(vinyl chloride), plasticised, sterile containers of for human blood containing anticoagulant solution (3.2.5.) ... 382
Poppy petals, red ... 2811
Porcine actinobacillosis vaccine (inactivated) ... 943
Porcine influenza vaccine (inactivated) ... 944
Porcine insulin ... 2144
Porcine parvovirosis vaccine (inactivated) ... 946
Porcine progressive atrophic rhinitis vaccine (inactivated) ... **6.1**-3373
Pore-size distribution of solids by mercury porosimetry, porosity and (2.9.32.) ... **6.2**-3643
Porosimetry, mercury, porosity and pore-size distribution of solids by (2.9.32.) ... **6.2**-3643
Porosity and pore-size distribution of solids by mercury porosimetry (2.9.32.) ... **6.2**-3643
Porosity of sintered-glass filters (2.1.2.) ... 15
Potassium (2.4.12.) ... 116
Potassium acetate ... 2716
Potassium bromide ... 2716
Potassium carbonate ... 2717
Potassium chloride ... **6.2**-3819
Potassium citrate ... 2718
Potassium clavulanate ... 2719
Potassium clavulanate, diluted ... 2721
Potassium dihydrogen phosphate ... 2723
Potassium hydrogen aspartate hemihydrate ... 2723
Potassium hydrogen carbonate ... 2724
Potassium hydrogen tartrate ... 2725
Potassium hydroxide ... 2726
Potassium iodide ... 2726
Potassium metabisulphite ... 2727
Potassium nitrate ... 2728
Potassium perchlorate ... 2728
Potassium permanganate ... 2729
Potassium sodium tartrate tetrahydrate ... 2729
Potassium sorbate ... 2730
Potassium sulphate ... 2731
Potato starch ... 2731
Potentiometric determination of ionic concentration using ion-selective electrodes (2.2.36.) ... 58
Potentiometric determination of pH (2.2.3.) ... 24
Potentiometric titration (2.2.20.) ... 35
Potentisation, methods of preparation of homoeopathic stocks and ... **6.1**-3385
Poultices ... 747
Pour-on preparations ... 753
Povidone ... **6.1**-3523
Povidone, iodinated ... 2734
Powdered cellulose ... **6.2**-3712
Powder fineness (2.9.35.) ... **6.2**-3648
Powder flow (2.9.36.) ... 320
Powders and granules for oral solutions and suspensions ... 729
Powders and granules for syrups ... 730
Powders and tablets for rectal solutions and suspensions .. 746
Powders, bulk density and tapped density of (2.9.34.) ... **6.2**-3646
Powders, ear ... 720
Powders, effervescent ... 739
Powders for cutaneous application ... 738
Powders for eye drops and powders for eye lotions ... 722
Powders for inhalation ... 742
Powders for injections or infusions ... 736
Powders for oral drops ... 730
Powders, nasal ... 732
Powders, oral ... 738
Poxvirus vectors for human use ... 672
Pravastatin sodium ... 2735
Prazepam ... 2736
Praziquantel ... 2737
Prazosin hydrochloride ... 2738
Prednicarbate ... 2740
Prednisolone ... 2741
Prednisolone acetate ... 2742
Prednisolone pivalate ... 2744
Prednisolone sodium phosphate ... 2745
Prednisone ... 2746
Prekallikrein activator (2.6.15.) ... 189
Premixes for medicated feeding stuffs for veterinary use .. 739
Preparations for inhalation ... 739
Preparations for inhalation: aerodynamic assessment of fine particles (2.9.18.) ... 287
Preparations for irrigation ... 743
Pressurised pharmaceutical preparations ... 744
Prilocaine ... 2748
Prilocaine hydrochloride ... 2750
Primaquine diphosphate ... 2751
Primary aromatic amino-nitrogen, determination of (2.5.8.) ... 139
Primary standards for volumetric solutions (4.2.1.) ... 514
Primidone ... 2752
Primula root ... 2753
Probenecid ... 2754
Procainamide hydrochloride ... 2755
Procaine benzylpenicillin ... 1287
Procaine hydrochloride ... 2756
Prochlorperazine maleate ... 2756
Products of fermentation ... 693
Products of recombinant DNA technology ... 701
Products with risk of transmitting agents of animal spongiform encephalopathies ... 694
Progenitor cells, human haematopoietic, colony-forming cell assay for (2.7.28.) ... 242
Progesterone ... 2757
Progressive atrophic rhinitis vaccine (inactivated), porcine ... **6.1**-3373
Proguanil hydrochloride ... 2758
Proline ... 2760
Promazine hydrochloride ... 2761
Promethazine hydrochloride ... 2761
Propacetamol hydrochloride ... 2763
Propafenone hydrochloride ... 2764
Propanol ... 2766
Propanol and methanol, 2-, test for (2.9.11.) ... 282
Propantheline bromide ... 2767
Propofol ... 2768

Propranolol hydrochloride....2770
Propylene glycol....2773
Propylene glycol dicaprylocaprate....2774
Propylene glycol dilaurate....2774
Propylene glycol monolaurate....2775
Propylene glycol monopalmitostearate....2776
Propylene glycol monostearate....2776
Propyl gallate....2771
Propyl parahydroxybenzoate....2772
Propylthiouracil....2777
Propyphenazone....2778
Protamine hydrochloride....2779
Protamine sulphate....2780
Protein C, human, assay of (2.7.30.)....**6.2**-3631
Protein in polysaccharide vaccines (2.5.16.)....142
Protein S, human, assay of (2.7.31.)....**6.2**-3632
Protein, total (2.5.33.)....148
Prothrombin complex, human....2076
Protirelin....2781
Proxyphylline....2783
Pseudoephedrine hydrochloride....**6.2**-3820
Psyllium seed....2785
Purified water....3213
Purified water, highly....3212
Purple coneflower herb....2785
Purple coneflower root....2787
Pycnometric density of solids, gas (2.9.23.)....**6.2**-3642
Pygeum africanum bark....2789
Pyrantel embonate....2790
Pyrazinamide....2791
Pyridostigmine bromide....2792
Pyridoxine hydrochloride....2793
Pyrimethamine....2794
Pyrogens (2.6.8.)....164
Pyrrolidone....2794

Q

Quality of pharmaceutical preparations, microbiological (5.1.4.)....529
Quantified hawthorn leaf and flower liquid extract....2037
Quinidine sulphate....2799
Quinine hydrochloride....2800
Quinine sulphate....2802

R

Rabbit haemorrhagic disease vaccine (inactivated)....949
Rabies immunoglobulin, human....2078
Rabies vaccine for human use prepared in cell cultures....**6.1**-3355
Rabies vaccine (inactivated) for veterinary use....**6.1**-3375
Rabies vaccine (live, oral) for foxes....952
Racecadotril....**6.2**-3825
Racemic camphor....1401
Racemic ephedrine hydrochloride....1792
Racemic menthol....2356
Raclopride ([^{11}C]methoxy) injection....1005
Radionuclides, table of physical characteristics (5.7.)....633
Radiopharmaceutical preparations....695
Radiopharmaceutical preparations, iobenguane sulphate for....**6.1**-3381
Raman spectrometry (2.2.48.)....82
Ramipril....**6.2**-3826
Ramon assay, flocculation value (Lf) of diphtheria and tetanus toxins and toxoids (2.7.27.)....241
Ranitidine hydrochloride....2809
Rapeseed oil, refined....**6.2**-3829
Reagents (4.)....391
Reagents (4.1.1.)....391
Reagents (4.1.1.)....**6.1**-3331
Reagents (4.1.1.)....**6.2**-3661
Reagents, standard solutions, buffer solutions (4.1.)....391
Recombinant DNA technology, products of....701
Rectal capsules....745
Rectal foams....746
Rectal preparations....744
Rectal preparations, semi-solid....746
Rectal solutions and suspensions, powders and tablets for....744
Rectal solutions, emulsions and suspensions....745
Rectal tampons....746
Red poppy petals....2811
Reference standards (5.12.)....663
Refractive index (2.2.6.)....26
Relationship between reaction of solution, approximate pH and colour of certain indicators (2.2.4.)....25
Relative density (2.2.5.)....25
Repaglinide....2812
Reserpine....2814
Residual solvents (5.4.)....603
Residual solvents, identification and control (2.4.24.)....121
Residue on evaporation of essential oils (2.8.9.)....250
Resistance to crushing of tablets (2.9.8.)....279
Resorcinol....2815
Restharrow root....2815
Rhatany root....2816
Rhatany tincture....2817
Rhinotracheitis vaccine (inactivated), viral, feline....916
Rhinotracheitis vaccine (live), viral, feline....917
Rhubarb....2817
Ribavirin....2818
Riboflavin....2820
Riboflavin sodium phosphate....2821
Ribose in polysaccharide vaccines (2.5.31.)....147
Ribwort plantain....2823
Rice starch....2824
Rifabutin....2825
Rifampicin....2826
Rifamycin sodium....2827
Rilmenidine dihydrogen phosphate....2829
Risperidone....2830
Ritonavir....2832
Rocuronium bromide....2835
Roman chamomile flower....1487
Ropivacaine hydrochloride monohydrate....2837
Roselle....**6.1**-3529
Rosemary leaf....2839
Rosemary oil....2840
Rotating viscometer method - viscosity (2.2.10.)....28
Rotation, optical (2.2.7.)....26
Roxithromycin....2842
RRR-α-Tocopherol....3088
RRR-α-Tocopheryl acetate....3090
RRR-α-Tocopheryl hydrogen succinate....3095
Rubber closures for containers for aqueous parenteral preparations, for powders and for freeze-dried powders (3.2.9.)....386
Rubella immunoglobulin, human....2079
Rubella, measles and mumps vaccine (live)....**6.1**-3347
Rubella vaccine (live)....**6.1**-3358
Rutoside trihydrate....2844

S

Saccharin....2849
Saccharin sodium....2850
Safety, viral (5.1.7.)....543
Safflower flower....2851
Safflower oil, refined....2852

Saffron for homoeopathic preparations....1084
Sage leaf (salvia officinalis)....2853
Sage leaf, three-lobed....2854
Sage oil, Spanish....**6.2**-3838
Sage tincture....2854
Salbutamol....2855
Salbutamol sulphate....2857
Salicylic acid....2859
Salmeterol xinafoate....2860
Salmonella Enteritidis vaccine (inactivated) for chickens..953
Salmonella Typhimurium vaccine (inactivated) for chickens....954
Salmon oil, farmed....2862
Sanguisorba root....**6.1**-3533
Saponification value (2.5.6.)....139
Saw palmetto fruit....2864
Scopolamine....2108
Scopolamine butylbromide....2109
Scopolamine hydrobromide....2110
Selamectin for veterinary use....**6.1**-3534
Selegiline hydrochloride....2866
Selenium disulphide....2867
Semi-micro determination of water (2.5.12.)....141
Semi-solid ear preparations....720
Semi-solid eye preparations....722
Semi-solid intrauterine preparations....726
Semi-solid nasal preparations....732
Semi-solid oromucosal preparations....733
Semi-solid preparations for cutaneous application....746
Semi-solid rectal preparations....746
Semi-solid vaginal preparations....752
Senega root....2867
Senna leaf....2868
Senna leaf dry extract, standardised....**6.2**-3833
Senna pods, Alexandrian....2870
Senna pods, Tinnevelly....2871
Separation techniques, chromatographic (2.2.46.)....72
Serine....2872
Sertaconazole nitrate....**6.1**-3535
Sertraline hydrochloride....**6.1**-3537
Sesame oil, refined....2874
Sets for the transfusion of blood and blood components (3.2.6.)....383
Shampoos....728
Shellac....**6.2**-3833
Sialic acid in polysaccharide vaccines (2.5.23.)....144
Siam benzoin tincture....1278
Sieves (2.1.4.)....16
Sieve test (2.9.12.)....283
Sieving, analytical, particle-size distribution estimation by (2.9.38.)....**6.2**-3649
SI (International System) units (1.)....3
Silica, colloidal anhydrous....2877
Silica, colloidal hydrated....2877
Silica, dental type....2878
Silica, hydrophobic colloidal....2878
Silicone elastomer for closures and tubing (3.1.9.)....358
Silicone oil used as a lubricant (3.1.8.)....358
Silk suture, sterile, braided, in distributor for veterinary use....1059
Silver, colloidal, for external use....2879
Silver nitrate....2880
Simeticone....2880
Simvastatin....2881
Single-dose preparations, uniformity of content (2.9.6.)...278
Single-dose preparations, uniformity of mass (2.9.5.)....278
Sintered-glass filters (2.1.2.)....15
Size-exclusion chromatography (2.2.30.)....47
(*S*)-Lactic acid....2229
Smallpox vaccine (live)....**6.1**-3359
Sodium acetate ([1-^{11}C]) injection....1006
Sodium acetate trihydrate....2883
Sodium alendronate....2884
Sodium alginate....2885
Sodium amidotrizoate....2886
Sodium aminosalicylate dihydrate....2887
Sodium ascorbate....2888
Sodium aurothiomalate....2889
Sodium benzoate....2890
Sodium bromide....2891
Sodium calcium edetate....2892
Sodium caprylate....2893
Sodium carbonate, anhydrous....2894
Sodium carbonate decahydrate....2894
Sodium carbonate monohydrate....2895
Sodium carboxymethylcellulose....1423
Sodium carboxymethylcellulose, cross-linked....1626
Sodium carboxymethylcellulose, low-substituted....1424
Sodium cetostearyl sulphate....2895
Sodium chloride....2897
Sodium chromate (^{51}Cr) sterile solution....1007
Sodium citrate....2898
Sodium cromoglicate....2899
Sodium cyclamate....2900
Sodium dihydrogen phosphate dihydrate....2901
Sodium fluoride....2902
Sodium fluoride (^{18}F) injection....1008
Sodium fusidate....2902
Sodium glycerophosphate, hydrated....2903
Sodium hyaluronate....**6.2**-3835
Sodium hydrogen carbonate....2906
Sodium hydroxide....2907
Sodium iodide....2907
Sodium iodide (^{123}I) injection....1009
Sodium iodide (^{123}I) solution for radiolabelling....1010
Sodium iodide (^{131}I) capsules for diagnostic use....1011
Sodium iodide (^{131}I) capsules for therapeutic use....1012
Sodium iodide (^{131}I) solution....1013
Sodium iodide (^{131}I) solution for radiolabelling....1014
Sodium iodohippurate (^{123}I) injection....1014
Sodium iodohippurate (^{131}I) injection....1015
Sodium lactate solution....2908
Sodium laurilsulfate....2910
Sodium metabisulphite....2911
Sodium methyl parahydroxybenzoate....2911
Sodium molybdate (^{99}Mo) solution (fission)....1016
Sodium molybdate dihydrate....2912
Sodium nitrite....2913
Sodium nitroprusside....2913
Sodium perborate, hydrated....2914
Sodium pertechnetate (^{99m}Tc) injection (fission)....1018
Sodium pertechnetate (^{99m}Tc) injection (non-fission)....1020
Sodium phenylbutyrate....**6.1**-3539
Sodium phosphate (^{32}P) injection....1020
Sodium picosulfate....2915
Sodium polystyrene sulphonate....2916
Sodium propionate....2917
Sodium propyl parahydroxybenzoate....2918
Sodium salicylate....2919
Sodium selenite pentahydrate....2919
Sodium (*S*)-lactate solution....2909
Sodium starch glycolate (type A)....2920
Sodium starch glycolate (type B)....2921
Sodium starch glycolate (type C)....2922
Sodium stearate....2923
Sodium stearyl fumarate....2924
Sodium sulphate, anhydrous....2924
Sodium sulphate decahydrate....2925

Sodium sulphite, anhydrous....2926
Sodium sulphite heptahydrate....2926
Sodium thiosulphate....2927
Sodium valproate....2927
Soft capsules....718
Softening time determination of lipophilic suppositories (2.9.22.)....302
Soft extracts....**6.1**-3344
Solid dosage forms, dissolution test for (2.9.3.)....266
Solids by mercury porosimetry, porosity and pore-size distribution of (2.9.32.)....**6.2**-3643
Solids, density of (2.2.42.)....67
Solids, gas pycnometric density of (2.9.23.)....**6.2**-3642
Solubility in alcohol of essential oils (2.8.10.)....250
Soluble tablets....750
Solutions, emulsions and suspensions, oral....729
Solutions for haemodialysis....2022
Solutions for haemodialysis, concentrated, water for diluting....2021
Solutions for haemofiltration and for haemodiafiltration....2025
Solutions for organ preservation....2929
Solutions for peritoneal dialysis....2646
Solutions, suspensions, intrauterine....726
Solvents, residual (5.4.)....603
Solvents, residual, identification and control (2.4.24.)....121
Somatostatin....2930
Somatropin....2931
Somatropin concentrated solution....2933
Somatropin for injection....2935
Sorbic acid....2937
Sorbitan laurate....2938
Sorbitan oleate....2938
Sorbitan palmitate....2939
Sorbitan sesquioleate....2939
Sorbitan stearate....2940
Sorbitan trioleate....2940
Sorbitol....2941
Sorbitol, liquid (crystallising)....2942
Sorbitol, liquid (non-crystallising)....2943
Sorbitol, liquid, partially dehydrated....2944
Sotalol hydrochloride....2944
Soya-bean oil, hydrogenated....**6.2**-3837
Soya-bean oil, refined....**6.2**-3838
Spanish sage oil....**6.2**-3838
Specific surface area by air permeability (2.9.14.)....283
Specific surface area by gas adsorption (2.9.26.)....306
Spectinomycin dihydrochloride pentahydrate....2947
Spectinomycin sulphate tetrahydrate for veterinary use....2949
Spectrometry, atomic absorption (2.2.23.)....37
Spectrometry, atomic emission (2.2.22.)....36
Spectrometry, mass (2.2.43.)....68
Spectrometry, nuclear magnetic resonance (2.2.33.)....54
Spectrometry, Raman (2.2.48.)....82
Spectrometry, X-ray fluorescence (2.2.37.)....59
Spectrophotometry, infrared absorption (2.2.24.)....39
Spectrophotometry, near-infrared (2.2.40.)....62
Spectrophotometry, ultraviolet and visible absorption (2.2.25.)....41
SPF chicken flocks for the production and quality control of vaccines (5.2.2.)....547
Spheroids and granules, friability of (2.9.41.)....330
Spiramycin....**6.1**-3540
Spirapril hydrochloride monohydrate....2954
Spironolactone....2955
Spot-on preparations....753
Sprays....753
Sprays (liquid nasal) and drops (nasal)....731
Squalane....2956
Standard solutions for limit tests (4.1.2.)....504
Standards, reference (5.12.)....663
Stannous chloride dihydrate....2959
Star anise....2960
Star anise oil....2962
Starch glycolate (type A), sodium....2920
Starch glycolate (type B), sodium....2921
Starch glycolate (type C), sodium....2922
Starch, maize....2326
Starch, potato....2731
Starch, pregelatinised....2964
Starch, rice....2824
Starch, wheat....3215
Starflower (borage) oil, refined....1326
Statistical analysis of results of biological assays and tests (5.3.)....571
Stavudine....2964
Steam sterilisation of aqueous preparations, application of the F_0 concept (5.1.5.)....531
Stearic acid....2966
Stearoyl macrogolglycerides....2967
Stearyl alcohol....2968
Stem cells, human haematopoietic....2067
Sterile braided silk suture in distributor for veterinary use....1059
Sterile catgut....1045
Sterile catgut in distributor for veterinary use....1057
Sterile containers of plasticised poly(vinyl chloride) for human blood containing anticoagulant solution (3.2.5.)....382
Sterile linen thread in distributor for veterinary use....1058
Sterile non-absorbable strands in distributor for veterinary use....1060
Sterile non-absorbable sutures....1046
Sterile plastic containers for human blood and blood components (3.2.3.)....379
Sterile polyamide 6/6 suture in distributor for veterinary use....1059
Sterile polyamide 6 suture in distributor for veterinary use....1058
Sterile poly(ethylene terephthalate) suture in distributor for veterinary use....1059
Sterile products, methods of preparation (5.1.1.)....525
Sterile single-use plastic syringes (3.2.8.)....384
Sterile synthetic absorbable braided sutures....1050
Sterile synthetic absorbable monofilament sutures....1052
Sterilisation procedures, biological indicators (5.1.2.)....527
Sterility (2.6.1.)....155
Sterols in fatty oils (2.4.23.)....120
Sticks....748
Sticks, intrauterine....726
Sticks, nasal....732
St. John's wort....**6.2**-3839
St. John's wort dry extract, quantified....**6.2**-3840
Stomata and stomatal index (2.8.3.)....249
Stramonium leaf....2968
Stramonium, prepared....**6.2**-3842
Strands, sterile non-absorbable, in distributor for veterinary use....1060
Streptokinase concentrated solution....**6.2**-3843
Streptomycin sulphate....2972
Strontium (^{89}Sr) chloride injection....1021
Subdivision of tablets....748
Sublingual sprays, oromucosal drops and oromucosal sprays....732
Sublingual tablets and buccal tablets....734
Substances for pharmaceutical use....703
Substances for pharmaceutical use, control of impurities in (5.10.)....653

Substances of animal origin for the production of veterinary vaccines (5.2.5.) 555
Sub-visible particles, particulate contamination (2.9.19.) .. 300
Succinylsulfathiazole 2974
Sucrose 2975
Sucrose monopalmitate **6.1**-3543
Sucrose stearate **6.1**-3544
Sufentanil 2977
Sufentanil citrate 2978
Sugars, lead in (2.4.10.) 115
Sugar spheres 2979
Sulbactam sodium **6.2**-3845
Sulfacetamide sodium **6.2**-3847
Sulfadiazine 2983
Sulfadimidine 2984
Sulfadoxine 2984
Sulfafurazole 2985
Sulfaguanidine 2986
Sulfamerazine 2987
Sulfamethizole 2988
Sulfamethoxazole 2989
Sulfamethoxypyridazine for veterinary use 2990
Sulfanilamide 2991
Sulfasalazine 2992
Sulfathiazole 2994
Sulfinpyrazone 2995
Sulfisomidine 2996
Sulindac 2996
Sulphated ash (2.4.14.) 116
Sulphates (2.4.13.) 116
Sulphur dioxide (2.5.29.) 146
Sulphur for external use 2998
Sulphuric acid 2998
Sulpiride 2999
Sultamicillin **6.1**-3545
Sultamicillin tosilate dihydrate **6.1**-3548
Sumatra benzoin 1278
Sumatra benzoin tincture 1279
Sumatriptan succinate 3005
Sunflower oil, refined **6.2**-3848
Supercritical fluid chromatography (2.2.45.) 71
Suppositories 745
Suppositories and pessaries, disintegration of (2.9.2.) 265
Suppositories, lipophilic, softening time determination (2.9.22.) 302
Suspensions, solutions and emulsions, oral 729
Suspensions, solutions, intrauterine 726
Sutures, sterile non-absorbable 1046
Sutures, sterile synthetic absorbable braided 1050
Sutures, sterile synthetic absorbable monofilament 1052
Suxamethonium chloride 3007
Suxibuzone 3008
Sweet fennel 1874
Sweet orange oil 3009
Swelling index (2.8.4.) 249
Swine erysipelas vaccine (inactivated) 955
Swine-fever vaccine (live, prepared in cell cultures), classical **6.2**-3669
Symbols and abbreviations (1.) 3
Synthetic absorbable braided sutures, sterile 1050
Synthetic absorbable monofilament sutures, sterile 1052
Syringes, plastic, sterile single-use (3.2.8.) 384
Syrups 730

T

Table of physical characteristics of radionuclides mentioned in the European Pharmacopoeia (5.7.) 633
Tablets 748
Tablets and capsules, disintegration of (2.9.1.) 263
Tablets, buccal 734
Tablets, coated 749
Tablets, dispersible 750
Tablets, effervescent 749
Tablets for intrauterine solutions and suspensions 726
Tablets for use in the mouth 750
Tablets for vaginal solutions and suspensions 752
Tablets, gastro-resistant 750
Tablets, intrauterine 726
Tablets, modified-release 750
Tablets, orodispersible 750
Tablets, resistance to crushing (2.9.8.) 279
Tablets, soluble 750
Tablets, subdivision of 748
Tablets, sublingual 734
Tablets, uncoated 749
Tablets, uncoated, friability of (2.9.7.) 278
Tablets, vaginal 752
Talc 3013
Tamoxifen citrate 3014
Tampons, ear 720
Tampons, medicated 751
Tampons, rectal 746
Tampons, vaginal, medicated 752
Tamsulosin hydrochloride 3016
Tannic acid 3018
Tannins in herbal drugs, determination of (2.8.14.) 255
Tapped density of powders, bulk density and (2.9.34.) **6.2**-3646
Tartaric acid 3018
Teat dips 753
Tea tree oil 3019
Teat sprays 753
Technetium (^{99m}Tc) bicisate injection 1022
Technetium (^{99m}Tc) colloidal rhenium sulphide injection 1023
Technetium (^{99m}Tc) colloidal sulphur injection 1024
Technetium (^{99m}Tc) colloidal tin injection 1025
Technetium (^{99m}Tc) etifenin injection 1026
Technetium (^{99m}Tc) exametazime injection 1027
Technetium (^{99m}Tc) gluconate injection 1028
Technetium (^{99m}Tc) human albumin injection 1029
Technetium (^{99m}Tc) macrosalb injection 1030
Technetium (^{99m}Tc) medronate injection 1031
Technetium (^{99m}Tc) mertiatide injection 1033
Technetium (^{99m}Tc) microspheres injection 1034
Technetium (^{99m}Tc) pentetate injection 1035
Technetium (^{99m}Tc) sestamibi injection 1036
Technetium (^{99m}Tc) succimer injection 1037
Technetium (^{99m}Tc) tin pyrophosphate injection 1038
Telmisartan **6.2**-3851
Temazepam 3020
Tenosynovitis avian viral vaccine (live) 875
Tenoxicam 3021
Terazosin hydrochloride dihydrate 3022
Terbinafine hydrochloride 3024
Terbutaline sulphate 3025
Terconazole **6.1**-3553
Terfenadine **6.1**-3554
Terminology used in monographs on biological products (5.2.1.) 547
Test for anticomplementary activity of immunoglobulin (2.6.17.) 191
Test for anti-D antibodies in human immunoglobulin for intravenous administration (2.6.26.) **6.2**-3627
Test for extractable volume of parenteral preparations (2.9.17.) 287
Test for Fc function of immunoglobulin (2.7.9.) 227
Test for methanol and 2-propanol (2.9.11.) 282

Test for neurovirulence of live virus vaccines (2.6.18.) 193
Test for neurovirulence of poliomyelitis vaccine (oral) (2.6.19.) 193
Test for specified micro-organisms (microbiological examination of non-sterile products) (2.6.13.) 173
Testosterone 3030
Testosterone decanoate 3031
Testosterone enantate 3033
Testosterone isocaproate 3034
Testosterone propionate 3035
Tests for extraneous agents in viral vaccines for human use (2.6.16.) 190
Tetanus and diphtheria toxins and toxoids, flocculation value (Lf) of, (Ramon assay) (2.7.27.) 241
Tetanus and diphtheria vaccine (adsorbed, reduced antigen(s) content) 764
Tetanus antitoxin for human use 969
Tetanus antitoxin for veterinary use 976
Tetanus, diphtheria and hepatitis B (rDNA) vaccine (adsorbed) 765
Tetanus, diphtheria and pertussis (acellular, component) vaccine (adsorbed) 767
Tetanus, diphtheria and poliomyelitis (inactivated) vaccine (adsorbed, reduced antigen(s) content) 770
Tetanus, diphtheria, pertussis (acellular, component) and haemophilus type b conjugate vaccine (adsorbed) 771
Tetanus, diphtheria, pertussis (acellular, component) and hepatitis B (rDNA) vaccine (adsorbed) 774
Tetanus, diphtheria, pertussis (acellular, component) and poliomyelitis (inactivated) vaccine (adsorbed) 775
Tetanus, diphtheria, pertussis (acellular, component) and poliomyelitis (inactivated) vaccine (adsorbed, reduced antigen(s) content) 778
Tetanus, diphtheria, pertussis (acellular, component), hepatitis B (rDNA), poliomyelitis (inactivated) and haemophilus type b conjugate vaccine (adsorbed) 780
Tetanus, diphtheria, pertussis (acellular, component), poliomyelitis (inactivated) and haemophilus type b conjugate vaccine (adsorbed) 783
Tetanus, diphtheria, pertussis and poliomyelitis (inactivated) vaccine (adsorbed) 785
Tetanus, diphtheria, pertussis, poliomyelitis (inactivated) and haemophilus type b conjugate vaccine (adsorbed) 787
Tetanus immunoglobulin, human 2079
Tetanus vaccine (adsorbed) 844
Tetanus vaccine (adsorbed), assay of (2.7.8.) 223
Tetanus vaccine for veterinary use 957
Tetracaine hydrochloride **6.1**-3556
Tetracosactide 3037
Tetracycline 3040
Tetracycline hydrochloride 3041
Tetrazepam 3043
Tetryzoline hydrochloride 3044
Thallous (^{201}Tl) chloride injection 1039
Theobromine 3045
Theophylline 3046
Theophylline-ethylenediamine 3048
Theophylline-ethylenediamine hydrate 3049
Theophylline monohydrate 3047
Thermal analysis (2.2.34.) **6.1**-3311
Thermogravimetry (2.2.34.) **6.1**-3311
Thiamazole 3050
Thiamine hydrochloride 3051
Thiamine nitrate 3053
Thiamphenicol 3054
Thin-layer chromatography (2.2.27.) 43
Thioctic acid 3055
Thiomersal 3056
Thiopental sodium and sodium carbonate 3057
Thioridazine 3058
Thioridazine hydrochloride 3059
Three-lobed sage leaf 2854
Threonine 3060
Thyme 3061
Thyme oil 3063
Thyme, wild 3219
Thymol 3064
Tiabendazole 3064
Tiamulin for veterinary use 3065
Tiamulin hydrogen fumarate for veterinary use 3068
Tianeptine sodium 3070
Tiapride hydrochloride 3071
Tiaprofenic acid 3072
Tibolone 3074
Ticarcillin sodium 3075
Tick-borne encephalitis vaccine (inactivated) 845
Ticlopidine hydrochloride 3077
Tilidine hydrochloride hemihydrate 3079
Timolol maleate 3080
Tinctures **6.1**-3344
Tinidazole **6.2**-3852
Tinnevelly senna pods 2871
Tinzaparin sodium 3082
Tioconazole 3083
Titanium dioxide 3084
Titration, amperometric (2.2.19.) 35
Titration, potentiometric (2.2.20.) 35
Titrations, complexometric (2.5.11.) 140
Tobramycin **6.2**-3854
Tocopherol, all-*rac*-α- 3086
Tocopherol, *RRR*-α- 3088
Tocopheryl acetate, all-*rac*-α- 3089
α-Tocopheryl acetate concentrate (powder form) 3091
Tocopheryl acetate, *RRR*-α- 3090
Tocopheryl hydrogen succinate, DL-α- 3093
Tocopheryl hydrogen succinate, *RRR*-α- 3095
Tolbutamide 3097
Tolfenamic acid 3097
Tolnaftate 3099
Tolu balsam 3099
Torasemide, anhydrous 3100
Tormentil 3101
Tormentil tincture 3102
Tosylchloramide sodium 3103
Total ash (2.4.16.) 116
Total cholesterol in oils rich in omega-3 acids (2.4.32.) 132
Total organic carbon in water for pharmaceutical use (2.2.44.) 71
Total protein (2.5.33.) 148
Total viable aerobic count (microbiological examination of non-sterile products) (2.6.12.) 166
Toxicity, abnormal (2.6.9.) 165
Toxin, botulinum type A for injection 1327
Tragacanth **6.2**-3855
Tramadol hydrochloride 3104
Tramazoline hydrochloride monohydrate 3106
Trandolapril 3107
Tranexamic acid 3108
Transdermal patches 737
Transdermal patches, dissolution test for (2.9.4.) 275
Trapidil 3110
Tretinoin 3111
Triacetin 3112
Triamcinolone 3112
Triamcinolone acetonide 3114
Triamcinolone hexacetonide 3115
Triamterene **6.1**-3557
Tribenoside 3117

Tributyl acetylcitrate ... 3118
Trichloroacetic acid ... 3119
Triethanolamine ... 3133
Triethyl citrate ... 3120
Trifluoperazine hydrochloride ... 3121
Triflusal ... 3121
Triglycerides, medium-chain ... 3122
Triglycerides, omega-3 acid ... 2554
Triglycerol diisostearate ... **6.1**-3558
Trihexyphenidyl hydrochloride ... 3125
Trimetazidine dihydrochloride ... 3126
Trimethadione ... 3127
Trimethoprim ... 3128
Trimipramine maleate ... 3130
Tri-*n*-butyl phosphate ... 3132
Tritiated (^{3}H) water injection ... 1040
Trolamine ... 3133
Trometamol ... 3135
Tropicamide ... 3135
Tropisetron hydrochloride ... 3136
Trospium chloride ... 3138
Troxerutin ... 3139
Trypsin ... 3141
Tryptophan ... 3142
TSE, animal, minimising the risk of transmitting via human and veterinary medicinal products (5.2.8.) ... 558
TSE, animal, products with risk of transmitting agents of ... 694
Tuberculin for human use, old ... 3144
Tuberculin purified protein derivative, avian ... 3146
Tuberculin purified protein derivative, bovine ... 3147
Tuberculin purified protein derivative for human use ... 3147
Tubes for comparative tests (2.1.5.) ... 17
Tubing and closures, silicone elastomer for (3.1.9.) ... 358
Tubing and containers for total parenteral nutrition preparations, poly(ethylene - vinyl acetate) for (3.1.7.) ... 356
Tubing used in sets for the transfusion of blood and blood components, materials based on plasticised poly(vinyl chloride) for (3.1.1.2.) ... 342
Tubocurarine chloride ... 3150
Turmeric, Javanese ... 3150
Turpentine oil, Pinus pinaster type ... 3151
Tylosin for veterinary use ... 3152
Tylosin phosphate bulk solution for veterinary use ... 3154
Tylosin tartrate for veterinary use ... 3156
Typhoid polysaccharide vaccine ... 847
Typhoid vaccine ... 849
Typhoid vaccine, freeze-dried ... 849
Typhoid vaccine (live, oral, strain Ty 21a) ... 849
Tyrosine ... 3157
Tyrothricin ... 3158

U

Ubidecarenone ... 3163
Udder-washes ... 753
Ultraviolet and visible absorption spectrophotometry (2.2.25.) ... 41
Ultraviolet ray lamps for analytical purposes (2.1.3.) ... 15
Uncoated tablets ... 749
Undecylenic acid ... 3164
Uniformity of content of single-dose preparations (2.9.6.) ... 278
Uniformity of dosage units (2.9.40.) ... **6.1**-3325
Uniformity of mass of delivered doses from multidose containers (2.9.27.) ... 309
Uniformity of mass of single-dose preparations (2.9.5.) ... 278
Units of the International System (SI) used in the Pharmacopoeia and equivalence with other units (1.) ... 3
Unsaponifiable matter (2.5.7.) ... 139
Urea ... 3165
Urofollitropin ... 3166
Urokinase ... 3167
Uronic acids in polysaccharide vaccines (2.5.22.) ... 144
Ursodeoxycholic acid ... 3168

V

Vaccines, adsorbed, aluminium in (2.5.13.) ... 141
Vaccines, adsorbed, calcium in (2.5.14.) ... 142
Vaccines and immunosera, phenol in (2.5.15.) ... 142
Vaccines and immunosera, veterinary, evaluation of efficacy of (5.2.7.) ... **6.1**-3335
Vaccines and immunosera, veterinary, evaluation of safety (5.2.6.) ... 556
Vaccines and immunosera, veterinary, evaluation of the safety of each batch (5.2.9.) ... 567
Vaccines for human use ... 705
Vaccines for human use, cell substrates for the production of (5.2.3.) ... 550
Vaccines for human use, viral, extraneous agents in (2.6.16.) ... 190
Vaccines for veterinary use ... 707
Vaccines, polysaccharide, hexosamines in (2.5.20.) ... 143
Vaccines, polysaccharide, methylpentoses in (2.5.21.) ... 143
Vaccines, polysaccharide, nucleic acids in (2.5.17.) ... 142
Vaccines, polysaccharide, *O*-acetyl in (2.5.19.) ... 143
Vaccines, polysaccharide, phosphorus in (2.5.18.) ... 142
Vaccines, polysaccharide, protein in (2.5.16.) ... 142
Vaccines, polysaccharide, ribose in (2.5.31.) ... 147
Vaccines, polysaccharide, sialic acid in (2.5.23.) ... 144
Vaccines, polysaccharide, uronic acids in (2.5.22.) ... 144
Vaccines, SPF chicken flocks for the production and quality control of (5.2.2.) ... 547
Vaccines, veterinary, cell cultures for the production of (5.2.4.) ... 553
Vaccines, veterinary, substances of animal origin for the production of (5.2.5.) ... 555
Vaccines, viral live, test for neurovirulence (2.6.18.) ... 193
Vaginal capsules ... 752
Vaginal foams ... 752
Vaginal preparations ... 751
Vaginal preparations, semi-solid ... 752
Vaginal solutions and suspensions, tablets for ... 752
Vaginal solutions, emulsions and suspensions ... 752
Vaginal tablets ... 752
Vaginal tampons, medicated ... 752
Valerian dry hydroalcoholic extract ... 3173
Valerian root ... 3174
Valerian tincture ... 3175
Valine ... 3176
Valnemulin hydrochloride for veterinary use ... 3177
Valproic acid ... 3178
Vancomycin hydrochloride ... 3180
Vanillin ... 3182
Varicella immunoglobulin for intravenous administration, human ... 2081
Varicella immunoglobulin, human ... 2080
Varicella vaccine (live) ... **6.1**-3364
Vectors for human use, adenovirus ... 670
Vectors for human use, plasmid ... 674
Vectors for human use, plasmid, bacterial cells used for the manufacture of ... 676
Vectors for human use, poxvirus ... 672
Vecuronium bromide ... 3183
Vegetable fatty oils ... 712
Venlafaxine hydrochloride ... 3184
Verapamil hydrochloride ... 3186
Verbena herb ... 3188
Veterinary liquid preparations for cutaneous application ... 752

Veterinary vaccines and immunosera, evaluation of efficacy of (5.2.7.) **6.1**-3335
Viability, nucleated cell count and (2.7.29.) 243
Vibriosis (cold-water) vaccine (inactivated) for salmonids **6.2**-3671
Vibriosis vaccine (inactivated) for salmonids **6.2**-3672
VICH (5.8.) 645
Vinblastine sulphate 3189
Vincristine sulphate 3190
Vindesine sulphate 3192
Vinorelbine tartrate 3194
Vinpocetine 3196
Viper venom antiserum, European 970
Viral rhinotracheitis vaccine (inactivated), feline 916
Viral rhinotracheitis vaccine (live), feline 917
Viral safety (5.1.7.) 543
Viscometer method, capillary (2.2.9.) 27
Viscometer method, falling ball (2.2.49.) 84
Viscose wadding, absorbent 3197
Viscosity (2.2.8.) 27
Viscosity - rotating viscometer method (2.2.10.) 28
Visible and ultraviolet absorption spectrophotometry (2.2.25.) 41
Visible particles, particulate contamination (2.9.20.) 302
Vitamin A 3199
Vitamin A concentrate (oily form), synthetic 3200
Vitamin A concentrate (powder form), synthetic 3201
Vitamin A concentrate (solubilisate/emulsion), synthetic 3203
Volumetric analysis (4.2.) 514
Volumetric solutions (4.2.2.) 514
Volumetric solutions, primary standards for (4.2.1.) 514
von Willebrand factor, human 2081
von Willebrand factor, human, assay of (2.7.21.) 237

W

Warfarin sodium 3207
Warfarin sodium clathrate 3208
Washes, nasal 732
Water (^{15}O) injection 1040
Water, determination by distillation (2.2.13.) 31
Water for diluting concentrated haemodialysis solutions 2021
Water for injections 3209
Water for pharmaceutical use, total organic carbon in (2.2.44.) 71
Water, highly purified 3212
Water in essential oils (2.8.5.) 249
Water in gases (2.5.28.) 146
Water: micro determination (2.5.32.) 147
Water, purified 3213
Water: semi-micro determination (2.5.12.) 141
Wheat-germ oil, refined 3215
Wheat-germ oil, virgin 3216
Wheat starch 3215
White beeswax 1260
White horehound 3216
White soft paraffin **6.2**-3815
Wild pansy (flowering aerial parts) 3217
Wild thyme 3219
Willow bark **6.1**-3563
Willow bark dry extract **6.1**-3564
Wool alcohols 3221
Wool fat 3222
Wool fat, hydrogenated 3226
Wool fat, hydrous 3227
Wormwood 3228

X

Xanthan gum **6.1**-3569
Xenon (^{133}Xe) injection 1042
X-ray fluorescence spectrometry (2.2.37.) 59
X-ray powder diffraction (XRPD), characterisation of crystalline and partially crystalline solids by (2.9.33.) 314
Xylazine hydrochloride for veterinary use 3234
Xylitol 3235
Xylometazoline hydrochloride 3237
Xylose 3238

Y

Yarrow 3243
Yellow beeswax 1261
Yellow fever vaccine (live) **6.1**-3365
Yellow soft paraffin **6.2**-3816
Yohimbine hydrochloride 3244

Z

Zidovudine 3249
Zinc acetate dihydrate 3250
Zinc acexamate 3251
Zinc chloride 3253
Zinc oxide 3253
Zinc stearate 3254
Zinc sulphate heptahydrate 3254
Zinc sulphate hexahydrate 3255
Zinc sulphate monohydrate 3255
Zinc undecylenate 3256
Zolpidem tartrate 3256
Zopiclone 3257
Zuclopenthixol decanoate 3259

Numerics

α-1-Proteinasi inhibitor humanum **6.2**-3762

A

Absinthii herba 3228
Acaciae gummi **6.2**-3683
Acaciae gummi dispersione desiccatum **6.2**-3684
Acamprosatum calcicum 1088
Acarbosum 1089
Acebutololi hydrochloridum 1091
Aceclofenacum **6.2**-3685
Acemetacinum **6.1**-3393
Acesulfamum kalicum 1095
Acetazolamidum 1096
Acetonum 1098
Acetylcholini chloridum 1099
Acetylcysteinum 1100
β-Acetyldigoxinum 1101
Aciclovirum 1107
Acidi methacrylici et ethylis acrylatis polymerisati 1:1 dispersio 30 per centum 2372
Acidi methacrylici et ethylis acrylatis polymerisatum 1:1 .... **6.2**-3781
Acidi methacrylici et methylis methacrylatis polymerisatum 1:1 2373
Acidi methacrylici et methylis methacrylatis polymerisatum 1:2 2374
Acidum 4-aminobenzoicum 1164
Acidum aceticum glaciale 1097
Acidum acetylsalicylicum 1103
Acidum adipicum 1113
Acidum alginicum **6.2**-3690
Acidum amidotrizoicum dihydricum 1158
Acidum aminocaproicum 1166
Acidum ascorbicum 1221
Acidum asparticum 1225
Acidum benzoicum 1276
Acidum boricum 1327
Acidum caprylicum 1402
Acidum chenodeoxycholicum 1489
Acidum citricum anhydricum 1554
Acidum citricum monohydricum 1555
Acidum edeticum 1774
Acidum etacrynicum 1826
Acidum folicum 1938
Acidum fusidicum 1954
Acidum glutamicum 1984
Acidum hydrochloridum concentratum 2085
Acidum hydrochloridum dilutum 2085
Acidum iopanoicum 2162
Acidum iotalamicum 2163
Acidum ioxaglicum 2167
Acidum lacticum 2228
Acidum lactobionicum 2231
Acidum maleicum 2328
Acidum malicum 2329
Acidum mefenamicum 2349
Acidum nalidixicum 2472
Acidum nicotinicum 2502
Acidum niflumicum **6.1**-3508
Acidum nitricum 2510
Acidum oleicum 2543
Acidum oxolinicum 2582
Acidum palmiticum 2604
Acidum phosphoricum concentratum 2675
Acidum phosphoricum dilutum 2676
Acidum pipemidicum trihydricum 2690
Acidum salicylicum 2859
Acidum (S)-lacticum 2229
Acidum sorbicum 2937
Acidum stearicum 2966
Acidum sulfuricum 2998
Acidum tartaricum 3018
Acidum thiocticum 3055
Acidum tiaprofenicum 3072
Acidum tolfenamicum 3097
Acidum tranexamicum 3108
Acidum trichloraceticum 3119
Acidum undecylenicum 3164
Acidum ursodeoxycholicum 3168
Acidum valproicum 3178
Acitretinum 1109
Adeninum 1110
Adenosinum 1111
Adeps lanae 3222
Adeps lanae cum aqua 3227
Adeps lanae hydrogenatus 3226
Adeps solidus 2034
Adrenalini tartras 1114
Adrenalinum **6.2**-3686
Aer medicinalis 1118
Aer medicinalis artificiosus 1121
Aether 1833
Aether anaestheticus 1834
Aetherolea 680
Agar **6.2**-3688
Agni casti fructus **6.2**-3688
Agrimoniae herba 1117
Alaninum 1121
Albendazolum 1122
Albumini humani solutio 2057
Alchemillae herba 1123
Alcohol benzylicus 1281
Alcohol cetylicus 1485
Alcohol cetylicus et stearylicus 1480
Alcohol cetylicus et stearylicus emulsificans A **6.2**-3717
Alcohol cetylicus et stearylicus emulsificans B **6.2**-3718
Alcoholes adipis lanae 3221
Alcohol isopropylicus 2182
Alcohol oleicus 2544
Alcohol stearylicus 2968
Alcuronii chloridum 1124
Alfacalcidolum 1126
Alfadexum 1127
Alfentanili hydrochloridum 1128
Alfuzosini hydrochloridum **6.1**-3394
Allantoinum 1131
Allii sativi bulbi pulvis 1961
Allium sativum ad praeparationes homoeopathicas 1077
Allopurinolum 1132
Almagatum 1134
Aloe barbadensis 1137
Aloe capensis 1138
Aloes extractum siccum normatum **6.2**-3690
Alprazolamum 1139
Alprenololi hydrochloridum 1141
Alprostadilum 1143
Alteplasum ad iniectabile 1145
Althaeae folium 2338
Althaeae radix 2339
Altizidum **6.2**-3691
Alumen 1149
Aluminii chloridum hexahydricum 1149
Aluminii hydroxidum hydricum ad adsorptionem **6.1**-3395
Aluminii magnesii silicas 1151
Aluminii oxidum hydricum 1152
Aluminii phosphas hydricus 1153

Aluminii phosphatis liquamen 1152
Aluminii sulfas 1154
Alverini citras 1154
Amantadini hydrochloridum 1156
Ambroxoli hydrochloridum 1156
Amfetamini sulfas 1158
Amikacini sulfas **6.1**-3398
Amikacinum **6.1**-3396
Amiloridi hydrochloridum 1163
Aminoglutethimidum 1167
Amiodaroni hydrochloridum 1168
Amisulpridum 1170
Amitriptylini hydrochloridum 1172
Amlodipini besilas 1173
Ammoniae (^{13}N) solutio iniectabilis 981
Ammoniae solutio concentrata 1175
Ammonii bromidum 1177
Ammonii chloridum 1178
Ammonii glycyrrhizas 1179
Ammonii hydrogenocarbonas 1180
Ammonio methacrylatis copolymerum A 1175
Ammonio methacrylatis copolymerum B 1176
Amobarbitalum 1180
Amobarbitalum natricum 1181
Amoxicillinum natricum 1182
Amoxicillinum trihydricum 1184
Amphotericinum B 1187
Ampicillinum anhydricum 1188
Ampicillinum natricum 1190
Ampicillinum trihydricum 1193
Amygdalae oleum raffinatum 1136
Amygdalae oleum virginale 1136
Amylum pregelificatum 2964
Angelicae radix 1196
Anisi aetheroleum 1197
Anisi fructus 1199
Anisi stellati aetheroleum 2962
Anisi stellati fructus 2960
Antazolini hydrochloridum 1199
Anticorpora monoclonalia ad usum humanum 690
Antithrombinum III humanum densatum 2060
Apis mellifera ad praeparationes homoeopathicas 1079
Apomorphini hydrochloridum 1207
Aprotinini solutio concentrata **6.2**-3692
Aprotininum 1208
Aqua ad dilutionem solutionum concentratarum ad haemodialysim 2021
Aqua ad iniectabilia 3209
Aquae (^{15}O) solutio iniectabilis 1040
Aquae tritiatae (^{3}H) solutio iniectabilis 1040
Aqua purificata 3213
Aqua valde purificata 3212
Arachidis oleum hydrogenatum **6.2**-3694
Arachidis oleum raffinatum 1211
Argenti nitras 2880
Argentum colloidale ad usum externum 2879
Arginini aspartas 1213
Arginini hydrochloridum 1214
Argininum 1212
Arnicae flos **6.1**-3400
Arnicae tinctura 1216
Arsenii trioxidum ad praeparationes homoeopathicas 1073
Articaini hydrochloridum 1217
Ascorbylis palmitas 1222
Asparaginum monohydricum 1223
Aspartamum 1224
Astemizolum 1226
Atenololum 1228
Atracurii besilas 1230
Atropini sulfas **6.1**-3404
Atropinum **6.1**-3403
Aurantii amari epicarpii et mesocarpii tinctura 1320
Aurantii amari epicarpium et mesocarpium 1319
Aurantii amari flos 1320
Aurantii dulcis aetheroleum 3009
Auricularia 719
Azaperonum ad usum veterinarium 1234
Azathioprinum 1236
Azelastini hydrochloridum 1236
Azithromycinum 1238

B

Bacampicillini hydrochloridum **6.1**-3409
Bacitracinum 1245
Bacitracinum zincum 1247
Baclofenum 1250
Ballotae nigrae herba 1321
Balsamum peruvianum **6.2**-3817
Balsamum tolutanum 3099
Bambuteroli hydrochloridum 1251
Barbitalum 1252
Barii chloridum dihydricum ad praeparationes homoeopathicas 1073
Barii sulfas 1253
BCG ad immunocurationem 758
Beclometasoni dipropionas anhydricus 1256
Beclometasoni dipropionas monohydricus 1258
Belladonnae folii extractum siccum normatum **6.2**-3697
Belladonnae folii tinctura normata 1264
Belladonnae folium 1261
Belladonnae pulvis normatus **6.2**-3698
Bendroflumethiazidum 1266
Benfluorexi hydrochloridum 1267
Benperidolum 1269
Benserazidi hydrochloridum 1270
Bentonitum 1271
Benzalkonii chloridi solutio 1273
Benzalkonii chloridum 1272
Benzbromaronum 1273
Benzethonii chloridum 1275
Benzocainum 1276
Benzoe sumatranus 1278
Benzoe tonkinensis 1277
Benzois sumatrani tinctura 1279
Benzois tonkinensis tinctura 1278
Benzoylis peroxidum cum aqua 1280
Benzylis benzoas 1283
Benzylpenicillinum benzathinum 1283
Benzylpenicillinum kalicum 1285
Benzylpenicillinum natricum 1288
Benzylpenicillinum procainum 1287
Betacarotenum 1290
Betadexum 1291
Betahistini dihydrochloridum 1292
Betahistini mesilas 1293
Betamethasoni acetas 1297
Betamethasoni dipropionas 1298
Betamethasoni natrii phosphas 1300
Betamethasoni valeras 1301
Betamethasonum 1295
Betaxololi hydrochloridum 1303
Betulae folium **6.2**-3699
Bezafibratum 1304
Bifonazolum 1306
Biotinum 1308
Biperideni hydrochloridum 1309
Bisacodylum 1312
Bismuthi subcarbonas 1313

Bismuthi subgallas 1314
Bismuthi subnitras ponderosus 1315
Bismuthi subsalicylas 1316
Bisoprololi fumaras **6.1**-3412
Bistortae rhizoma 1317
Bleomycini sulfas 1322
Boldi folii extractum siccum **6.1**-3415
Boldi folium 1324
Boragonis officinalis oleum raffinatum 1326
Borax 1326
Bromazepamum 1331
Bromhexini hydrochloridum 1332
Bromocriptini mesilas 1333
Bromperidoli decanoas 1337
Bromperidolum 1335
Brompheniramini maleas 1339
Brotizolamum 1340
Budesonidum 1342
Bufexamacum 1344
Buflomedili hydrochloridum 1345
Bumetanidum 1346
Bupivacaini hydrochloridum 1347
Buprenorphini hydrochloridum 1350
Buprenorphinum 1349
Buserelinum 1351
Buspironi hydrochloridum 1353
Busulfanum 1355
Butylhydroxyanisolum 1357
Butylhydroxytoluenum 1357
Butylis parahydroxybenzoas 1358

C

Cabergolinum 1363
Cadmii sulfas hydricus ad praeparationes homoeopathicas 1074
Calcifediolum 1366
Calcii acetas 1376
Calcii ascorbas 1377
Calcii carbonas **6.2**-3703
Calcii chloridum dihydricum 1378
Calcii chloridum hexahydricum 1379
Calcii dobesilas monohydricus **6.2**-3703
Calcii folinas 1380
Calcii glucoheptonas 1383
Calcii gluconas 1384
Calcii gluconas ad iniectabile 1385
Calcii glycerophosphas 1386
Calcii hydrogenophosphas anhydricus 1387
Calcii hydrogenophosphas dihydricus 1388
Calcii hydroxidum 1389
Calcii iodidum tetrahydricum ad praeparationes homoeopathicas 1074
Calcii lactas anhydricus 1389
Calcii lactas monohydricus 1390
Calcii lactas pentahydricus 1390
Calcii lactas trihydricus 1391
Calcii laevulinas dihydricus 1394
Calcii levofolinas pentahydricus 1392
Calcii pantothenas 1395
Calcii stearas 1397
Calcii sulfas dihydricus 1398
Calcipotriolum anhydricum 1367
Calcipotriolum monohydricum 1370
Calcitoninum salmonis 1372
Calcitriolum 1375
Calendulae flos 1398
Camphora racemica 1401
Capsici fructus **6.2**-3704
Capsici oleoresina raffinata et quantificata 1405
Capsici tinctura normata 1406
Capsulae 717
Captoprilum 1407
Carbacholum 1410
Carbamazepinum 1411
Carbasalatum calcicum 1412
Carbidopum 1413
Carbimazolum 1414
Carbo activatus 1488
Carbocisteinum 1415
Carbomera **6.1**-3422
Carbonei dioxidum 1417
Carbonei monoxidum (^{15}O) 982
Carboplatinum 1419
Carboprostum trometamolum 1420
Carboxymethylamylum natricum A 2920
Carboxymethylamylum natricum B 2921
Carboxymethylamylum natricum C 2922
Carisoprodolum 1421
Carmellosum calcicum 1422
Carmellosum natricum 1423
Carmellosum natricum conexum 1626
Carmellosum natricum, substitutum humile 1424
Carmustinum 1425
Carprofenum ad usum veterinarium **6.2**-3706
Carteololi hydrochloridum 1426
Carthami flos 2851
Carthami oleum raffinatum 2852
Carvedilolum 1427
Carvi aetheroleum 1408
Carvi fructus 1408
Caryophylli floris aetheroleum 1588
Caryophylli flos 1587
Cefaclorum 1435
Cefadroxilum monohydricum **6.1**-3423
Cefalexinum monohydricum **6.1**-3425
Cefalotinum natricum 1440
Cefamandoli nafas 1441
Cefapirinum natricum 1443
Cefatrizinum propylen glycolum 1444
Cefazolinum natricum 1445
Cefepimi dihydrochloridum monohydricum 1448
Cefiximum 1450
Cefoperazonum natricum 1451
Cefotaximum natricum 1453
Cefoxitinum natricum 1455
Cefradinum 1457
Ceftazidimum 1459
Ceftriaxonum natricum 1461
Cefuroximum axetili 1462
Cefuroximum natricum 1464
Celiprololi hydrochloridum 1465
Cellulae stirpes haematopoieticae humanae 2067
Cellulosi acetas 1467
Cellulosi acetas butyras 1468
Cellulosi acetas phthalas 1468
Cellulosi pulvis **6.2**-3712
Cellulosum microcristallinum **6.2**-3708
Cellulosum microcristallinum et carmellosum natricum 2422
Centaurii herba 1477
Centellae asiaticae herba 1477
Cera alba 1260
Cera carnauba 1425
Cera flava 1261
Cetirizini dihydrochloridum **6.2**-3715
Cetobemidoni hydrochloridum 2215
Cetostearylis isononanoas 1484
Cetrimidum 1484

Cetylis palmitas 1486
Cetylpyridinii chloridum 1486
Chamomillae romanae flos 1487
Chelidonii herba 2010
Chinidini sulfas 2799
Chinini hydrochloridum 2800
Chinini sulfas 2802
Chitosani hydrochloridum 1490
Chlorali hydras 1491
Chlorambucilum 1492
Chloramphenicoli natrii succinas 1495
Chloramphenicoli palmitas 1493
Chloramphenicolum 1492
Chlorcyclizini hydrochloridum 1496
Chlordiazepoxidi hydrochloridum 1498
Chlordiazepoxidum 1497
Chlorhexidini diacetas 1499
Chlorhexidini digluconatis solutio 1500
Chlorhexidini dihydrochloridum 1502
Chlorobutanolum anhydricum 1503
Chlorobutanolum hemihydricum 1504
Chlorocresolum 1504
Chloroquini phosphas 1505
Chloroquini sulfas 1506
Chlorothiazidum 1507
Chlorphenamini maleas **6.1**-3427
Chlorpromazini hydrochloridum 1509
Chlorpropamidum 1510
Chlorprothixeni hydrochloridum 1511
Chlortalidonum 1513
Chlortetracyclini hydrochloridum 1514
Cholecalciferoli pulvis 1519
Cholecalciferolum 1516
Cholecalciferolum densatum oleosum 1517
Cholecalciferolum in aqua dispergibile 1521
Cholesterolum 1524
Chondroitini natrii sulfas 1525
Chorda resorbilis sterilis 1045
Chorda resorbilis sterilis in fuso ad usum veterinarium 1057
Chromii (^{51}Cr) edetatis solutio iniectabilis **6.2**-3677
Chymotrypsinum 1527
Ciclopirox olaminum 1530
Ciclopiroxum 1528
Ciclosporinum 1531
Cilastatinum natricum **6.1**-3428
Cilazaprilum 1534
Cimetidini hydrochloridum 1537
Cimetidinum 1536
Cinchocaini hydrochloridum 1538
Cinchonae cortex **6.2**-3720
Cinchonae extractum fluidum normatum 1540
Cineolum 1541
Cinnamomi cassiae aetheroleum **6.2**-3707
Cinnamomi cortex 1542
Cinnamomi corticis tinctura 1545
Cinnamomi zeylanici folii aetheroleum 1544
Cinnamomi zeylanicii corticis aetheroleum **6.2**-3721
Cinnarizinum 1545
Ciprofibratum 1547
Ciprofloxacini hydrochloridum 1550
Ciprofloxacinum 1548
Cisapridi tartras 1552
Cisapridum monohydricum 1551
Cisplatinum 1554
Citri reticulatae aetheroleum 2333
Citronellae aetheroleum 1556
Cladribinum 1557
Clarithromycinum 1559
Clazurilum ad usum veterinarium 1562
Clebopridi malas 1564
Clemastini fumaras **6.1**-3430
Clenbuteroli hydrochloridum 1567
Clindamycini hydrochloridum 1568
Clindamycini phosphas 1570
Clioquinolum 1571
Clobazamum 1572
Clobetasoli propionas 1573
Clobetasoni butyras 1575
Clofaziminum 1577
Clofibratum 1578
Clomifeni citras 1579
Clomipramini hydrochloridum 1580
Clonazepamum 1582
Clonidini hydrochloridum 1583
Clopamidum **6.1**-3431
Closantelum natricum dihydricum ad usum veterinarium 1584
Clotrimazolum **6.1**-3433
Cloxacillinum natricum 1589
Clozapinum 1590
Cocaini hydrochloridum 1592
Cocois oleum raffinatum **6.2**-3723
Cocoylis caprylocapras 1594
Codeini hydrochloridum dihydricum 1596
Codeini phosphas hemihydricus 1598
Codeini phosphas sesquihydricus 1599
Codeinum **6.1**-3434
Codergocrini mesilas 1601
Coffeinum **6.1**-3421
Coffeinum monohydricum 1365
Colae semen 1611
Colchicinum 1612
Colestyraminum 1613
Colistimethatum natricum 1614
Colistini sulfas 1615
Colophonium 1617
Compressi 748
Copolymerum methacrylatis butylati basicum 1254
Copovidonum 1617
Coriandri aetheroleum 1621
Coriandri fructus 1620
Corpora ad usum pharmaceuticum 703
Cortisoni acetas 1622
Crataegi folii cum flore extractum fluidum quantificatum 2037
Crataegi folii cum flore extractum siccum 2036
Crataegi folium cum flore 2035
Crataegi fructus 2034
Cresolum crudum 1626
Croci stigma ad praeparationes homoeopathicas 1084
Crospovidonum 1628
Crotamitonum 1629
Cupri acetas monohydricus ad praeparationes homoeopathicas 1075
Cupri sulfas anhydricus 1619
Cupri sulfas pentahydricus 1620
Cuprum ad praeparationes homoeopathicas 1076
Curcumae xanthorrhizae rhizoma 3150
Cyamopsidis seminis pulvis **6.2**-3752
Cyanocobalamini (^{57}Co) capsulae 983
Cyanocobalamini (^{57}Co) solutio 984
Cyanocobalamini (^{58}Co) capsulae 985
Cyanocobalamini (^{58}Co) solutio 986
Cyanocobalaminum 1630
Cyclizini hydrochloridum **6.2**-3725
Cyclopentolati hydrochloridum 1632
Cyclophosphamidum 1633

Cynarae folium 1219
Cyproheptadini hydrochloridum 1634
Cyproteroni acetas 1635
Cysteini hydrochloridum monohydricum 1636
Cystinum 1637
Cytarabinum 1638

D

Dacarbazinum 1641
Dalteparinum natricum 1642
Danaparoidum natricum 1644
Dapsonum 1646
Daunorubicini hydrochloridum 1647
D-Camphora 1400
Decylis oleas 1648
Deferoxamini mesilas 1649
Dembrexini hydrochloridum monohydricum ad usum veterinarium 1650
Demeclocyclini hydrochloridum 1651
Deptropini citras 1653
Dequalinii chloridum 1654
Desfluranum **6.1**-3439
Desipramini hydrochloridum 1655
Deslanosidum 1656
Desmopressinum 1657
Desogestrelum 1658
Desoxycortoni acetas 1659
Detomidini hydrochloridum ad usum veterinarium 1660
Dexamethasoni acetas 1665
Dexamethasoni isonicotinas 1666
Dexamethasoni natrii phosphas 1667
Dexamethasonum 1663
Dexchlorpheniramini maleas 1669
Dexpanthenolum 1670
Dextranomerum 1675
Dextranum 1 ad iniectabile 1671
Dextranum 40 ad iniectabile 1672
Dextranum 60 ad iniectabile 1673
Dextranum 70 ad iniectabile 1674
Dextrinum 1675
Dextromethorphani hydrobromidum 1676
Dextromoramidi tartras 1677
Dextropropoxypheni hydrochloridum 1678
Diazepamum 1679
Diazoxidum 1680
Dibrompropamidini diisetionas 1681
Dibutylis phthalas 1682
Diclazurilum ad usum veterinarium 1683
Diclofenacum kalicum 1685
Diclofenacum natricum 1686
Dicloxacillinum natricum 1687
Dicycloverini hydrochloridum 1689
Didanosinum 1689
Dienestrolum 1691
Diethylcarbamazini citras 1693
Diethylenglycoli aether monoethilicus 1694
Diethylenglycoli palmitostearas 1695
Diethylis phthalas **6.1**-3441
Diethylstilbestrolum 1696
Diflunisalum 1697
Digitalis purpureae folium 1698
Digitoxinum 1700
Digoxinum 1701
Dihydralazini sulfas hydricus **6.1**-3442
Dihydrocodeini hydrogenotartras 1704
Dihydroergocristini mesilas 1705
Dihydroergotamini mesilas **6.1**-3444
Dihydroergotamini tartras 1709
Dihydrostreptomycini sulfas ad usum veterinarium 1710
Dihydrostreptomycini sulfas ad usum veterinarium **6.2**-3730
Dihydrotachysterolum 1712
Dikalii clorazepas 1728
Dikalii phosphas 1729
Diltiazemi hydrochloridum **6.1**-3446
Dimenhydrinatum 1715
Dimercaprolum 1716
Dimethylacetamidum 1717
Dimethylis sulfoxidum 1716
Dimeticonum **6.2**-3732
Dimetindeni maleas 1719
Dinatrii clodronas tetrahydricus **6.2**-3722
Dinatrii edetas 1734
Dinatrii etidronas 1844
Dinatrii pamidronas pentahydricus 2604
Dinatrii phosphas anhydricus 1735
Dinatrii phosphas dihydricus 1735
Dinatrii phosphas dodecahydricus **6.1**-3449
Dinitrogenii oxidum 2515
Dinoprostonum 1722
Dinoprostum trometamolum 1720
Diosminum 1723
Diphenhydramini hydrochloridum 1725
Diphenoxylati hydrochloridum 1726
Dipivefrini hydrochloridum 1727
Diprophyllinum 1730
Dipyridamolum 1731
Dirithromycinum **6.1**-3447
Disopyramidi phosphas 1738
Disopyramidum 1737
Disulfiramum 1739
Dithranolum 1740
DL-Methioninum 2380
DL-α-Tocopherylis hydrogenosuccinas 3093
Dobutamini hydrochloridum 1741
Dodecylis gallas 1744
Domperidoni maleas 1747
Domperidonum 1745
Dopamini hydrochloridum 1749
Dopexamini dihydrochloridum 1750
Dorzolamidi hydrochloridum 1752
Dosulepini hydrochloridum 1753
Doxaprami hydrochloridum 1754
Doxazosini mesilas 1756
Doxepini hydrochloridum **6.1**-3449
Doxorubicini hydrochloridum 1759
Doxycyclini hyclas 1760
Doxycyclinum monohydricum 1762
Doxylamini hydrogenosuccinas **6.1**-3451
Droperidolum 1765

E

Ebastinum 1771
Echinaceae angustifoliae radix 2483
Echinaceae pallidae radix 2602
Echinaceae purpureae herba 2785
Echinaceae purpureae radix 2787
Econazoli nitras 1773
Econazolum 1772
Edrophonii chloridum 1775
Eleutherococci radix 1777
Emedastini difumaras 1779
Emetini hydrochloridum heptahydricum 1780
Emetini hydrochloridum pentahydricum 1781
Emplastra transcutanea 737
Enalaprilatum dihydricum 1784
Enalaprili maleas 1782
Enilconazolum ad usum veterinarium 1785

Enoxaparinum natricum ... 1787
Enoxolonum ... 1788
Ephedrini hydrochloridum ... 1791
Ephedrini racemici hydrochloridum ... 1792
Ephedrinum anhydricum ... 1789
Ephedrinum hemihydricum ... 1790
Epirubicini hydrochloridum ... 1793
Equiseti herba ... 1794
Ergocalciferolum ... 1795
Ergometrini maleas ... 1797
Ergotamini tartras ... 1798
Erythritolum ... 1800
Erythromycini estolas ... 1803
Erythromycini ethylsuccinas ... 1806
Erythromycini lactobionas ... 1808
Erythromycini stearas ... 1810
Erythromycinum ... 1801
Erythropoietini solutio concentrata ... 1813
Eserini salicylas ... 2677
Eserini sulfas ... 2678
Esketamini hydrochloridum ... 1817
Estradioli benzoas ... **6.1**-3455
Estradioli valeras ... 1821
Estradiolum hemihydricum ... 1819
Estriolum ... 1822
Estrogeni coniuncti ... 1824
Etamsylatum ... **6.2**-3737
Ethacridini lactas monohydricus ... 1828
Ethambutoli hydrochloridum ... **6.1**-3456
Ethanolum (96 per centum) ... 1829
Ethanolum anhydricum ... 1831
Ethinylestradiolum ... 1834
Ethionamidum ... 1835
Ethosuximidum ... 1836
Ethylcellulosum ... 1841
Ethylendiaminum ... 1843
Ethylenglycoli monopalmitostearas ... 1842
Ethylis acetas ... 1838
Ethylis oleas ... 1838
Ethylis parahydroxybenzoas ... 1839
Ethylis parahydroxybenzoas natricus ... 1840
Ethylmorphini hydrochloridum ... 1843
Etilefrini hydrochloridum ... 1845
Etodolacum ... 1847
Etofenamatum ... 1849
Etofyllinum ... 1850
Etomidatum ... 1851
Etoposidum ... 1852
Eucalypti aetheroleum ... **6.2**-3738
Eucalypti folium ... 1857
Eugenolum ... 1859
Extracta ... **6.1**-3343

F

Factor humanus von Willebrandi ... 2081
Factor IX coagulationis humanus ... 2064
Factor VII coagulationis humanus ... 2061
Factor VIII coagulationis humanus ... 2062
Factor VIII coagulationis humanus (ADNr) ... 2063
Factor XI coagulationis humanus ... 2065
Fagopyri herba ... 1341
Famotidinum ... 1865
Febantelum ad usum veterinarium ... 1870
Felbinacum ... 1866
Felodipinum ... 1867
Felypressinum ... 1869
Fenbendazolum ad usum veterinarium ... 1871
Fenbufenum ... 1872
Fenofibratum ... 1875
Fenoteroli hydrobromidum ... 1876
Fentanyli citras ... 1879
Fentanylum ... 1878
Fenticonazoli nitras ... 1880
Ferri chloridum hexahydricum ... 1882
Ferrosi fumaras ... 1883
Ferrosi gluconas ... 1884
Ferrosi sulfas desiccatus ... 1885
Ferrosi sulfas heptahydricus ... 1886
Ferrum ad praeparationes homoeopathicas ... 1081
Fexofenadini hydrochloridum ... 1888
Fibrini glutinum ... 1890
Fibrinogenum humanum ... 2066
Fila non resorbilia sterilia ... 1046
Fila non resorbilia sterilia in fuso ad usum veterinarium ... 1060
Fila resorbilia synthetica monofilamenta sterilia ... 1052
Fila resorbilia synthetica torta sterilia ... 1050
Filipendulae ulmariae herba ... 2344
Filum bombycis tortum sterile in fuso ad usum veterinarium ... 1059
Filum ethyleni polyterephthalici sterile in fuso ad usum veterinarium ... 1059
Filum lini sterile in fuso ad usum veterinarium ... 1058
Filum polyamidicum-6/6 sterile in fuso ad usum veterinarium ... 1059
Filum polyamidicum-6 sterile in fuso ad usum veterinarium ... 1058
Finasteridum ... 1891
Flavoxati hydrochloridum ... 1895
Flecainidi acetas ... 1896
Flubendazolum ... 1898
Flucloxacillinum magnesicum octahydricum ... **6.2**-3741
Flucloxacillinum natricum ... 1899
Fluconazolum ... 1900
Flucytosinum ... 1902
Fludarabini phosphas ... 1903
Fludeoxyglucosi (^{18}F) solutio iniectabilis ... **6.2**-3678
Fludrocortisoni acetas ... 1906
Flumazenili (N-[^{11}C]methyl) solutio iniectabilis ... 989
Flumazenilum ... 1908
Flumequinum ... 1909
Flumetasoni pivalas ... 1910
Flunarizini dihydrochloridum ... 1911
Flunitrazepamum ... 1913
Flunixini megluminum ad usum veterinarium ... 1914
Fluocinoloni acetonidum ... 1915
Fluocortoloni pivalas ... 1916
Fluoresceinum ... 1918
Fluoresceinum natricum ... 1919
Fluorodopae (^{18}F) ab electrophila substitutione solutio iniectabilis ... 990
Fluorouracilum ... 1920
Fluoxetini hydrochloridum ... 1922
Flupentixoli dihydrochloridum ... 1924
Fluphenazini decanoas ... 1926
Fluphenazini dihydrochloridum ... 1928
Fluphenazini enantas ... 1927
Flurazepami monohydrochloridum ... 1930
Flurbiprofenum ... 1931
Fluspirilenum ... 1932
Flutamidum ... 1933
Fluticasoni propionas ... 1934
Flutrimazolum ... 1936
Fluvoxamini maleas ... **6.2**-3742
Foeniculi amari fructus ... 1873
Foeniculi amari fructus aetheroleum ... 1318
Foeniculi dulcis fructus ... 1874
Formaldehydi solutio (35 per centum) ... 1939

Formoterololi fumaras dihydricus ... 1940
Foscarnetum natricum hexahydricum ... 1942
Fosfomycinum calcicum ... 1943
Fosfomycinum natricum ... 1945
Fosfomycinum trometamolum ... 1946
Framycetini sulfas ... 1947
Frangulae cortex ... 1949
Frangulae corticis extractum siccum normatum ... **6.2**-3744
Fraxini folium ... 1222
Fructosum ... 1951
Fucus vel Ascophyllum ... 2213
Fumariae herba ... 1952
Furosemidum ... 1953

G

Galactosum ... 1959
Gallamini triethiodidum ... 1959
Gallii (^{67}Ga) citratis solutio iniectabilis ... 992
Gelatina ... 1961
Gemcitabini hydrochloridum ... 1963
Gemfibrozilum ... 1964
Gentamicini sulfas ... 1965
Gentianae radix ... 1967
Gentianae tinctura ... 1968
Ginkgonis extractum siccum raffinatum et quantificatum ... **6.1**-3461
Ginkgonis folium ... 1969
Ginseng radix ... 1971
Glibenclamidum ... 1972
Gliclazidum ... 1974
Glimepiridum ... 1975
Glipizidum ... 1977
Glucagonum humanum ... 1979
Glucosum anhydricum ... 1981
Glucosum liquidum ... **6.2**-3752
Glucosum liquidum dispersione desiccatum ... 1982
Glucosum monohydricum ... 1983
Glutathionum ... **6.1**-3463
Glyceroli dibehenas ... 1990
Glyceroli distearas ... 1991
Glyceroli monocaprylas ... 1992
Glyceroli monocaprylocapras ... 1993
Glyceroli monolinoleas ... 1994
Glyceroli mono-oleas ... 1995
Glyceroli monostearas 40-55 ... 1996
Glyceroli trinitratis solutio ... **6.1**-3465
Glycerolum ... 1987
Glycerolum (85 per centum) ... 1988
Glycinum ... 1998
Gonadorelini acetas ... 2003
Gonadotropinum chorionicum ... 2004
Gonadotropinum sericum equinum ad usum veterinarium ... 2005
Goserelinum ... 2005
Gossypii oleum hydrogenatum ... **6.2**-3724
Gramicidinum ... 2007
Graminis rhizoma ... 1625
Granisetroni hydrochloridum ... 2009
Granulata ... 723
Griseofulvinum ... 2011
Guaiacolum ... 2012
Guaifenesinum ... 2014
Guanethidini monosulfas ... 2015
Guar galactomannanum ... **6.2**-3753

H

Halofantrini hydrochloridum ... 2027
Haloperidoli decanoas ... 2030
Haloperidolum ... 2028
Halothanum ... 2031
Hamamelidis folium ... **6.1**-3471
Harpagophyti extractum siccum ... 1662
Harpagophyti radix ... **6.2**-3729
Hederae folium ... 2198
Hedera helix ad praeparationes homoeopathicas ... 1078
Helianthi annui oleum raffinatum ... **6.2**-3848
Helium ... 2038
Heparina massae molecularis minoris ... 2041
Heparinum calcicum ... 2039
Heparinum natricum ... 2040
Heptaminoli hydrochloridum ... 2043
Hexamidini diisetionas ... 2044
Hexetidinum ... 2045
Hexobarbitalum ... 2047
Hexylresorcinolum ... 2047
Hibisci sabdariffae flos ... **6.1**-3529
Histamini dihydrochloridum ... 2049
Histamini phosphas ... 2049
Histidini hydrochloridum monohydricum ... 2051
Histidinum ... 2050
Homatropini hydrobromidum ... 2052
Homatropini methylbromidum ... 2053
Hyaluronidasum ... 2082
Hydralazini hydrochloridum ... 2083
Hydrargyri dichloridum ... 2361
Hydrastis rhizoma ... **6.1**-3467
Hydrochlorothiazidum ... 2086
Hydrocodoni hydrogenotartras 2.5-hydricus ... 2087
Hydrocortisoni acetas ... 2091
Hydrocortisoni hydrogenosuccinas ... 2092
Hydrocortisonum ... 2089
Hydrogenii peroxidum 30 per centum ... 2094
Hydrogenii peroxidum 3 per centum ... 2094
Hydromorphoni hydrochloridum ... 2095
Hydroxocobalamini acetas ... 2096
Hydroxocobalamini chloridum ... 2098
Hydroxocobalamini sulfas ... 2099
Hydroxycarbamidum ... 2100
Hydroxyethylcellulosum ... 2102
Hydroxyethylis salicylas ... 2101
Hydroxypropylbetadexum ... **6.2**-3763
Hydroxypropylcellulosum ... 2105
Hydroxyzini hydrochloridum ... 2106
Hymecromonum ... 2107
Hyoscini butylbromidum ... 2109
Hyoscini hydrobromidum ... 2110
Hyoscinum ... 2108
Hyoscyamini sulfas ... 2112
Hyoscyamus niger ad praeparationes homoeopathicas ... 1079
Hyperici herba ... **6.2**-3839
Hyperici herbae extractum siccum quantificatum ... **6.2**-3840
Hypericum perforatum ad praeparationes homoeopathicas ... 1080
Hypromellosi phthalas ... **6.1**-3475
Hypromellosum ... **6.1**-3473

I

Ibuprofenum ... **6.1**-3479
Ichthammolum ... 2122
Idoxuridinum ... 2122
Iecoris aselli oleum A ... 1603
Iecoris aselli oleum B ... 1607
Ifosfamidum ... 2123
Imipenemum ... 2125
Imipramini hydrochloridum ... **6.2**-3769

Immunoglobulinum anti-T lymphocytorum ex animale ad usum humanum 1203
Immunoglobulinum humanum anti-D **6.2**-3757
Immunoglobulinum humanum anti-D ad usum intravenosum 2059
Immunoglobulinum humanum hepatitidis A 2068
Immunoglobulinum humanum hepatitidis B 2069
Immunoglobulinum humanum hepatitidis B ad usum intravenosum 2069
Immunoglobulinum humanum morbillicum 2069
Immunoglobulinum humanum normale **6.2**-3757
Immunoglobulinum humanum normale ad usum intravenosum 2072
Immunoglobulinum humanum rabicum 2078
Immunoglobulinum humanum rubellae 2079
Immunoglobulinum humanum tetanicum 2079
Immunoglobulinum humanum varicellae 2080
Immunoglobulinum humanum varicellae ad usum intravenosum 2081
Immunosera ad usum veterinarium 687
Immunosera ex animali ad usum humanum 685
Immunoserum botulinicum 965
Immunoserum Clostridii novyi alpha ad usum veterinarium 973
Immunoserum Clostridii perfringentis beta ad usum veterinarium 974
Immunoserum Clostridii perfringentis epsilon ad usum veterinarium 975
Immunoserum contra venena viperarum europaearum 970
Immunoserum diphthericum 965
Immunoserum gangraenicum (Clostridium novyi) 966
Immunoserum gangraenicum (Clostridium perfringens) 967
Immunoserum gangraenicum (Clostridium septicum) 968
Immunoserum gangraenicum mixtum 966
Immunoserum tetanicum ad usum humanum 969
Immunoserum tetanicum ad usum veterinarium 976
Indapamidum 2127
Indii (^{111}In) chloridi solutio 994
Indii (^{111}In) oxini solutio 995
Indii (^{111}In) pentetatis solutio iniectabilis 996
Indinaviri sulfas 2130
Indometacinum 2132
Inhalanda 739
Insulini zinci amorphi suspensio iniectabilis 2149
Insulini zinci cristallini suspensio iniectabilis 2149
Insulini zinci suspensio iniectabilis 2148
Insulinum aspartum 2133
Insulinum biphasicum iniectabile 2140
Insulinum bovinum 2135
Insulinum humanum 2137
Insulinum isophanum biphasicum iniectabile 2140
Insulinum isophanum iniectabile 2141
Insulinum lisprum 2141
Insulinum porcinum 2144
Insulinum solubile iniectabile 2141
Interferoni alfa-2 solutio concentrata 2150
Interferoni gamma-1b solutio concentrata 2153
int-rac-α-Tocopherolum 3086
int-rac-α-Tocopherylis acetas 3089
Iobenguani (^{123}I) solutio iniectabilis 997
Iobenguani (^{131}I) solutio iniectabilis ad usum diagnosticum 998
Iobenguani (^{131}I) solutio iniectabilis ad usum therapeuticum 999
Iobenguani sulfas ad radiopharmaceutica **6.1**-3381
Iodinati (^{125}I) humani albumini solutio iniectabilis 993
Iodum 2156
Iohexolum 2157
Iopamidolum 2160
Iotrolanum 2164
Ipecacuanhae extractum fluidum normatum 2168
Ipecacuanhae pulvis normatus **6.2**-3770
Ipecacuanhae radix 2170
Ipecacuanhae tinctura normata 2171
Ipratropii bromidum **6.2**-3771
Isoconazoli nitras 2175
Isoconazolum 2173
Isofluranum 2176
Isoleucinum 2177
Isomaltum 2178
Isoniazidum 2180
Isoprenalini hydrochloridum 2181
Isoprenalini sulfas 2182
Isopropylis myristas 2183
Isopropylis palmitas 2184
Isosorbidi dinitras dilutus 2185
Isosorbidi mononitras dilutus 2186
Isotretinoinum 2188
Isoxsuprini hydrochloridum 2189
Isradipinum 2192
Itraconazolum 2194
Iuniperi aetheroleum 2207
Iuniperi pseudo-fructus 2206
Ivermectinum 2196

J

Josamycini propionas 2205
Josamycinum 2204

K

Kalii acetas 2716
Kalii bromidum 2716
Kalii carbonas 2717
Kalii chloridum **6.2**-3819
Kalii citras 2718
Kalii clavulanas 2719
Kalii clavulanas dilutus 2721
Kalii dihydrogenophosphas 2723
Kalii hydrogenoaspartas hemihydricus 2723
Kalii hydrogenocarbonas 2724
Kalii hydrogenotartras 2725
Kalii hydroxidum 2726
Kalii iodidum 2726
Kalii metabisulfis 2727
Kalii natrii tartras tetrahydricus 2729
Kalii nitras 2728
Kalii perchloras 2728
Kalii permanganas 2729
Kalii sorbas 2730
Kalii sulfas 2731
Kanamycini monosulfas 2212
Kanamycini sulfas acidus 2211
Kaolinum ponderosum 2213
Ketamini hydrochloridum 2214
Ketoconazolum 2216
Ketoprofenum 2218
Ketorolacum trometamolum 2220
Ketotifeni hydrogenofumaras 2221
Kryptonum (^{81m}Kr) ad inhalationem 1000

L

Labetaloli hydrochloridum 2227
Lacca **6.2**-3833
Lactitolum monohydricum 2229
Lactosum anhydricum 2232

Lactosum monohydricum 2233
Lactulosum 2234
Lactulosum liquidum 2236
Lamivudinum 2238
Lansoprazolum 2240
Lanugo cellulosi absorbens 3197
Lanugo gossypii absorbens 1624
Lavandulae aetheroleum 2244
Lavandulae flos 2243
Leflunomidum 2245
Leonuri cardiacae herba 2447
Letrozolum 2249
Leucinum 2250
Leuprorelinum 2251
Levamisoli hydrochloridum 2254
Levamisolum ad usum veterinarium 2253
Levistici radix 2290
Levocabastini hydrochloridum 2255
Levocarnitinum 2257
Levodopum 2258
Levodropropizinum 2260
Levomentholum 2261
Levomepromazini hydrochloridum 2262
Levomepromazini maleas 2263
Levomethadoni hydrochloridum 2264
Levonorgestrelum 2266
Levothyroxinum natricum 2267
Lichen islandicus 2121
Lidocaini hydrochloridum 2269
Lidocainum **6.1**-3485
Limonis aetheroleum 2246
Lincomycini hydrochloridum 2271
Lindanum 2272
Lini oleum virginale 2274
Lini semen 2273
Liothyroninum natricum **6.1**-3486
Liquiritiae extractum fluidum ethanolicum normatum **6.2**-3775
Liquiritiae extractum siccum ad saporandum **6.1**-3488
Liquiritiae radix 2276
Lisinoprilum dihydricum 2277
Lithii carbonas 2279
Lithii citras 2279
L-Methionini ([^{11}C]methyl) solutio iniectabilis 1001
Lobelini hydrochloridum 2280
Lomustinum 2281
Loperamidi hydrochloridum 2283
Loperamidi oxidum monohydricum 2285
Loratadinum 2286
Lorazepamum 2288
Lovastatinum 2291
Lupuli flos **6.1**-3472
Lymecyclinum **6.1**-3489
Lynestrenolum 2294
Lysini acetas 2295
Lysini hydrochloridum 2296
Lythri herba 2283

M

Macrogol 20 glyceroli monostearas 2304
Macrogol 40 sorbitoli heptaoleas 2310
Macrogol 6 glyceroli caprylocapras 2302
Macrogola 2308
Macrogolglyceridorum caprylocaprates 1403
Macrogolglyceridorum laurates 2242
Macrogolglyceridorum linoleates 2273
Macrogolglyceridorum oleates 2543
Macrogolglyceridorum stearates 2967
Macrogolglyceroli cocoates 2302
Macrogolglyceroli hydroxystearas 2303
Macrogolglyceroli ricinoleas 2304
Macrogoli 15 hydroxystearas 2305
Macrogoli aether cetostearylicus 2301
Macrogoli aether laurilicus 2306
Macrogoli aether oleicus 2308
Macrogoli aether stearylicus 2312
Macrogoli oleas 2307
Macrogoli stearas 2311
Magaldratum 2312
Magnesii acetas tetrahydricus 2313
Magnesii aspartas dihydricus 2314
Magnesii chloridum 4.5-hydricum 2317
Magnesii chloridum hexahydricum 2316
Magnesii citras anhydricus 2318
Magnesii gluconas **6.1**-3495
Magnesii glycerophosphas 2318
Magnesii hydroxidum 2319
Magnesii lactas dihydricus 2320
Magnesii oxidum leve 2321
Magnesii oxidum ponderosum 2320
Magnesii peroxidum 2321
Magnesii pidolas 2322
Magnesii stearas 2323
Magnesii subcarbonas levis 2316
Magnesii subcarbonas ponderosus **6.2**-3779
Magnesii sulfas heptahydricus 2325
Magnesii trisilicas 2325
Malathionum 2327
Maltitolum 2330
Maltitolum liquidum 2332
Maltodextrinum 2333
Malvae sylvestris flos 2330
Mangani gluconas **6.1**-3495
Mangani glycerophosphas hydricus 2334
Mangani sulfas monohydricus 2335
Mannitolum 2336
Maprotilini hydrochloridum 2337
Marbofloxacinum ad usum veterinarium **6.1**-3496
Marrubii herba 3216
Masticabilia gummis medicata 719
Mastix 2340
Matricariae aetheroleum 2342
Matricariae extractum fluidum **6.2**-3780
Matricariae flos 2340
Maydis amylum 2326
Maydis oleum raffinatum **6.2**-3779
Mebendazolum 2345
Meclozini hydrochloridum 2346
Medroxyprogesteroni acetas 2347
Mefloquini hydrochloridum 2350
Megestroli acetas 2352
Megluminum 2353
Mel 2055
Melaleucae aetheroleum 3019
Meliloti herba 2354
Melissae folium 2355
Menadionum 2356
Menthae arvensis aetheroleum partim mentholum depletum 2430
Menthae piperitae aetheroleum 2639
Menthae piperitae folium 2638
Mentholum racemicum 2356
Menyanthidis trifoliatae folium 1323
Mepivacaini hydrochloridum 2357
Meprobamatum 2359
Mepyramini maleas 2360
Mercaptopurinum 2361
Mesalazinum 2362

Mesnum 2364
Mesterolonum 2366
Mestranolum 2367
Metacresolum 2368
Metamizolum natricum 2369
Metformini hydrochloridum 2370
Methadoni hydrochloridum 2374
Methanolum 2376
Methaqualonum 2377
Methenaminum 2378
Methioninum 2379
Methotrexatum 2380
Methylatropini bromidum 2383
Methylatropini nitras 2383
Methylcellulosum **6.1**-3497
Methyldopum 2386
Methyleni chloridum 2387
Methylergometrini maleas 2388
Methylhydroxyethylcellulosum 2390
Methylis nicotinas 2390
Methylis parahydroxybenzoas 2391
Methylis parahydroxybenzoas natricus 2911
Methylis salicylas 2401
Methylphenobarbitalum 2392
Methylprednisoloni acetas 2395
Methylprednisoloni hydrogenosuccinas 2397
Methylprednisolonum 2393
Methylrosanilinii chloridum 2400
Methyltestosteronum **6.2**-3782
Methylthioninii chloridum 2402
Metixeni hydrochloridum 2404
Metoclopramidi hydrochloridum 2407
Metoclopramidum **6.2**-3783
Metolazonum 2407
Metoprololi succinas 2409
Metoprololi tartras 2410
Metrifonatum 2412
Metronidazoli benzoas 2415
Metronidazolum 2414
Mexiletini hydrochloridum 2416
Mianserini hydrochloridum 2417
Miconazoli nitras 2420
Miconazolum 2418
Midazolamum 2422
Millefolii herba 3243
Minocyclini hydrochloridum dihydricum 2427
Minoxidilum 2429
Mirtazapinum 2431
Misoprostolum 2433
Mitomycinum 2434
Mitoxantroni hydrochloridum 2436
Modafinilum 2437
Molgramostimi solutio concentrata 2438
Molsidominum **6.1**-3499
Mometasoni furoas 2441
Moranteli hydrogenotartras ad usum veterinarium 2443
Morphini hydrochloridum **6.1**-3501
Morphini sulfas **6.2**-3785
Moxidectinum ad usum veterinarium 2448
Moxifloxacini hydrochloridum **6.2**-3786
Moxonidinum 2453
Mupirocinum 2454
Mupirocinum calcicum 2456
Musci medicati 723
Mycophenolas mofetil 2458
myo-Inositolum 2460
Myristicae fragrantis aetheroleum **6.2**-3797
Myrrha 2461
Myrrhae tinctura 2461
Myrtilli fructus recens **6.1**-3412
Myrtilli fructus recentis extractum siccum raffinatum et normatum **6.2**-3745
Myrtilli fructus siccus 1307

N

Nabumetonum 2465
N-Acetyltryptophanum 1104
N-Acetyltyrosinum 1106
Nadololum 2466
Nadroparinum calcicum 2467
Naftidrofuryli hydrogenooxalas 2470
Naloxoni hydrochloridum dihydricum 2473
Naltrexoni hydrochloridum 2474
Nandroloni decanoas 2476
Naphazolini hydrochloridum 2478
Naphazolini nitras 2479
Naproxenum **6.2**-3791
Naproxenum natricum **6.1**-3507
Nasalia 730
Natrii acetas trihydricus 2883
Natrii acetatis ([1-^{11}C]) solutio iniectabilis 1006
Natrii alendronas 2884
Natrii alginas 2885
Natrii amidotrizoas 2886
Natrii aminosalicylas dihydricus 2887
Natrii ascorbas 2888
Natrii aurothiomalas 2889
Natrii benzoas 2890
Natrii bromidum 2891
Natrii calcii edetas 2892
Natrii caprylas 2893
Natrii carbonas anhydricus 2894
Natrii carbonas decahydricus 2894
Natrii carbonas monohydricus 2895
Natrii cetylo- et stearylosulfas. 2895
Natrii chloridum 2897
Natrii chromatis (^{51}Cr) solutio sterilis 1007
Natrii citras 2898
Natrii cromoglicas 2899
Natrii cyclamas 2900
Natrii dihydrogenophosphas dihydricus 2901
Natrii docusas 1743
Natrii fluoridi (^{18}F) solutio iniectabilis 1008
Natrii fluoridum 2902
Natrii fusidas 2902
Natrii glycerophosphas hydricus 2903
Natrii hyaluronas **6.2**-3835
Natrii hydrogenocarbonas 2906
Natrii hydroxidum 2907
Natrii iodidi (^{123}I) solutioad radio-signandum 1010
Natrii iodidi (^{123}I) solutio iniectabilis 1009
Natrii iodidi (^{131}I) capsulae ad usum diagnosticum 1011
Natrii iodidi (^{131}I) capsulae ad usum therapeuticum 1012
Natrii iodidi (^{131}I) solutio 1013
Natrii iodidi (^{131}I) solutio ad radio-signandum 1014
Natrii iodidum 2907
Natrii iodohippurati (^{123}I) solutio iniectabilis 1014
Natrii iodohippurati (^{131}I) solutio iniectabilis 1015
Natrii lactatis solutio 2908
Natrii laurilsulfas 2910
Natrii metabisulfis 2911
Natrii molybdas dihydricus 2912
Natrii molybdatis (^{99}Mo) fissione formati solutio 1016
Natrii nitris 2913
Natrii nitroprussias 2913
Natrii perboras hydricus 2914
Natrii pertechnetatis (^{99m}Tc) fissione formati solutio iniectabilis 1018

Natrii pertechnetatis (^{99m}Tc) sine fissione formati solutio iniectabilis 1020
Natrii phenylbutyras **6.1**-3539
Natrii phosphatis (^{32}P) solutio iniectabilis 1020
Natrii picosulfas 2915
Natrii polystyrenesulfonas 2916
Natrii propionas 2917
Natrii salicylas 2919
Natrii selenis pentahydricus 2919
Natrii (S)-lactatis solutio 2909
Natrii stearas 2923
Natrii stearylis fumaras 2924
Natrii sulfas anhydricus 2924
Natrii sulfas decahydricus 2925
Natrii sulfis anhydricus 2926
Natrii sulfis heptahydricus 2926
Natrii thiosulfas 2927
Natrii valproas 2927
Neohesperidin-dihydrochalconum 2485
Neomycini sulfas 2487
Neostigmini bromidum 2489
Neostigmini metilsulfas 2490
Neroli aetheroleum 2490
Netilmicini sulfas 2492
Nevirapinum anhydricum 2495
Nicergolinum 2496
Nicethamidum 2505
Niclosamidum anhydricum 2497
Niclosamidum monohydricum 2498
Nicotinamidum 2499
Nicotini resinas 2501
Nicotinum 2500
Nifedipinum 2503
Nifuroxazidum **6.1**-3510
Nilutamidum **6.2**-3792
Nimesulidum 2506
Nimodipinum 2507
Nitrazepamum 2508
Nitrendipinum 2509
Nitrofuralum 2512
Nitrofurantoinum 2513
Nitrogenii oxidum **6.2**-3794
Nitrogenium **6.2**-3795
Nitrogenium oxygenio depletum 2514
Nizatidinum 2516
N-Methylpyrrolidonum 2399
Nomegestroli acetas 2518
Nonoxinolum 9 2519
Noradrenalini hydrochloridum 2520
Noradrenalini tartras 2521
Norcholesteroli iodinati (^{131}I) solutio iniectabilis 1003
Norethisteroni acetas 2524
Norethisteronum 2523
Norfloxacinum **6.2**-3796
Norgestimatum 2526
Norgestrelum 2527
Nortriptylini hydrochloridum 2528
Noscapini hydrochloridum 2530
Noscapinum 2529
Notoginseng radix 2531
Nystatinum 2534

O

Octoxinolum 10 2539
Octyldodecanolum 2540
Octylis gallas 2539
Oenotherae oleum raffinatum 1860
Ofloxacinum **6.2**-3801
Oleae folium 2545
Olea herbaria 712
Olibanum indicum 2128
Olivae oleum raffinatum **6.2**-3802
Olivae oleum virginale **6.2**-3803
Olsalazinum natricum 2548
Omega-3 acidorum esteri ethylici 60 2550
Omega-3 acidorum esteri ethylici 90 2552
Omega-3 acidorum triglycerida 2554
Omeprazolum 2557
Omeprazolum natricum 2558
Ondansetroni hydrochloridum dihydricum 2560
Ononidis radix 2815
Ophthalmica 721
Opii extractum siccum normatum 2562
Opii pulvis normatus 2563
Opii tinctura normata 2565
Opium crudum 2564
Orciprenalini sulfas **6.2**-3804
Origani herba 2568
Orphenadrini citras 2569
Orphenadrini hydrochloridum 2570
Orthosiphonis folium 2203
Oryzae amylum 2824
Ouabainum 2571
Oxacillinum natricum monohydricum **6.2**-3806
Oxaliplatinum 2574
Oxazepamum 2577
Oxeladini hydrogenocitras 2578
Oxfendazolum ad usum veterinarium **6.2**-3808
Oxitropii bromidum 2581
Oxprenololi hydrochloridum 2583
Oxybuprocaini hydrochloridum 2584
Oxybutynini hydrochloridum 2585
Oxycodoni hydrochloridum 2587
Oxygenium (^{15}O) 1004
Oxygenium **6.2**-3809
Oxymetazolini hydrochloridum 2589
Oxytetracyclini hydrochloridum 2591
Oxytetracyclinum dihydricum 2590
Oxytocini solutio concentrata 2594
Oxytocinum 2593

P

Paclitaxelum **6.1**-3515
Pancreatis pulvis **6.2**-3813
Pancuronii bromidum 2608
Pantoprazolum natricum sesquihydricum **6.1**-3518
Papaverini hydrochloridum 2609
Papaveris rhoeados flos 2811
Paracetamolum 2611
Paraffinum liquidum 2613
Paraffinum perliquidum 2612
Paraffinum solidum 2612
Paraldehydum 2615
Parenteralia 735
Parnaparinum natricum 2616
Paroxetini hydrochloridum anhydricum 2616
Paroxetini hydrochloridum hemihydricum 2619
Passiflorae herba 2621
Passiflorae herbae extractum siccum 2622
Pefloxacini mesilas dihydricus 2623
Pelargonii radix 2625
Penbutololi sulfas 2625
Penicillaminum 2626
Pentaerythrityli tetranitras dilutus 2628
Pentamidini diisetionas 2630
Pentazocini hydrochloridum 2632
Pentazocini lactas 2632
Pentazocinum 2631

Pentobarbitalum 2633
Pentobarbitalum natricum 2634
Pentoxifyllinum 2635
Pentoxyverini hydrogenocitras 2637
Pepsini pulvis 2640
Pergolidi mesilas 2641
Perphenazinum 2648
Pethidini hydrochloridum 2650
Phenazonum 2651
Pheniramini maleas 2652
Phenobarbitalum 2653
Phenobarbitalum natricum 2654
Phenolphthaleinum 2656
Phenolsulfonphthaleinum 2657
Phenolum 2655
Phenoxyethanolum 2657
Phenoxymethylpenicillinum **6.1**-3520
Phenoxymethylpenicillinum kalicum **6.1**-3521
Phentolamini mesilas 2662
Phenylalaninum 2663
Phenylbutazonum 2664
Phenylephrini hydrochloridum 2667
Phenylephrinum 2665
Phenylhydrargyri acetas 2668
Phenylhydrargyri boras 2669
Phenylhydrargyri nitras 2669
Phenylpropanolamini hydrochloridum 2670
Phenytoinum 2671
Phenytoinum natricum 2672
Phloroglucinolum anhydricum 2672
Phloroglucinolum dihydricum 2673
Pholcodinum 2674
Phthalylsulfathiazolum 2676
Physostigmini salicylas 2677
Physostigmini sulfas 2678
Phytomenadionum 2679
Phytosterolum 2680
Picotamidum monohydricum 2682
Pilocarpini hydrochloridum 2682
Pilocarpini nitras 2684
Pimobendanum 2685
Pimozidum 2686
Pindololum 2688
Pini pumilionis aetheroleum 1766
Pini sylvestris aetheroleum 2689
Piperacillinum 2691
Piperacillinum natricum 2692
Piperazini adipas 2694
Piperazini citras 2695
Piperazinum hydricum 2696
Piracetamum 2697
Pirenzepini dihydrochloridum monohydricum 2698
Piretanidum 2699
Piroxicamum 2700
Piscis oleum omega-3 acidis abundans 1893
Pivampicillinum 2702
Pivmecillinami hydrochloridum 2704
Plantae ad ptisanam 685
Plantae medicinales 684
Plantae medicinales ad praeparationes homoeopathicas 1065
Plantae medicinales praeparatae 684
Plantaginis lanceolatae folium 2823
Plantaginis ovatae semen 2192
Plantaginis ovatae seminis tegumentum 2191
Plasma humanum ad separationem **6.2**-3759
Plasma humanum coagmentatum conditumque ad exstinguendum virum **6.2**-3760
Poloxamera 2705
Polyacrylatis dispersio 30 per centum 2706
Poly(alcohol vinylicus) 2715
Polygalae radix 2867
Polygoni avicularis herba 2223
Polymyxini B sulfas 2707
Polysorbatum 20 2709
Polysorbatum 40 2710
Polysorbatum 60 2710
Polysorbatum 80 2711
Poly(vinylis acetas) 2712
Poly(vinylis acetas) dispersio 30 per centum **6.2**-3818
Povidonum **6.1**-3523
Povidonum iodinatum 2734
Praeadmixta ad alimenta medicata ad usum veterinarium 739
Praeparationes ad irrigationem 743
Praeparationes buccales 732
Praeparationes homoeopathicas 1065
Praeparationes insulini iniectabiles 2146
Praeparationes intramammariae ad usum veterinarium 725
Praeparationes intraruminales 725
Praeparationes intra-uterinae ad usum veterinarium 726
Praeparationes liquidae ad usum dermicum 728
Praeparationes liquidae peroraliae 728
Praeparationes liquidae veterinariae ad usum dermicum 752
Praeparationes molles ad usum dermicum 746
Praeparationes pharmaceuticae in vasis cum pressu 744
Pravastatinum natricum 2735
Prazepamum 2736
Praziquantelum 2737
Prazosini hydrochloridum 2738
Prednicarbatum 2740
Prednisoloni acetas 2742
Prednisoloni natrii phosphas 2745
Prednisoloni pivalas 2744
Prednisolonum 2741
Prednisonum 2746
Prilocaini hydrochloridum 2750
Prilocainum 2748
Primaquini diphosphas 2751
Primidonum 2752
Primulae radix 2753
Probenecidum 2754
Procainamidi hydrochloridum 2755
Procaini hydrochloridum 2756
Prochlorperazini maleas 2756
Producta ab arte ADN recombinandorum 701
Producta ab fermentatione 693
Producta allergenica 679
Producta cum possibili transmissione vectorium enkephalopathiarum spongiformium animalium 694
Progesteronum 2757
Proguanili hydrochloridum 2758
Prolinum 2760
Promazini hydrochloridum 2761
Promethazini hydrochloridum 2761
Propacetamoli hydrochloridum 2763
Propafenoni hydrochloridum 2764
Propanolum 2766
Propanthelini bromidum 2767
Propofolum 2768
Propranololi hydrochloridum 2770
Propylenglycoli dicaprylocapras 2774
Propylenglycoli dilauras 2774
Propylenglycoli monolauras 2775
Propylenglycoli monopalmitostearas 2776
Propylenglycolum 2773

Propylis gallas 2771
Propylis parahydroxybenzoas 2772
Propylis parahydroxybenzoas natricus 2918
Propylthiouracilum 2777
Propyphenazonum 2778
Protamini hydrochloridum 2779
Protamini sulfas 2780
Prothrombinum multiplex humanum 2076
Protirelinum 2781
Proxyphyllinum 2783
Pruni africanae cortex 2789
Pseudoephedrini hydrochloridum **6.2**-3820
Psyllii semen 2785
Pulveres ad usum dermicum 738
Pulveres perorales 738
Pyranteli embonas 2790
Pyrazinamidum 2791
Pyridostigmini bromidum 2792
Pyridoxini hydrochloridum 2793
Pyrimethaminum 2794
Pyrrolidonum 2794

Q

Quercus cortex 2539

R

Racecadotrilum **6.2**-3825
Raclopridi ([^{11}C]methoxy) solutio iniectabilis 1005
Radiopharmaceutica 695
Ramiprilum **6.2**-3826
Ranitidini hydrochloridum 2809
Rapae oleum raffinatum **6.2**-3829
Ratanhiae radix 2816
Ratanhiae tinctura 2817
Rectalia 744
Repaglinidum 2812
Reserpinum 2814
Resorcinolum 2815
Rhamni purshianae cortex 1429
Rhamni purshianae extractum siccum normatum 1430
Rhei radix 2817
Rhenii sulfidi colloidalis et technetii (^{99m}Tc) solutio iniectabilis 1023
Ribavirinum 2818
Riboflavini natrii phosphas 2821
Riboflavinum 2820
Ricini oleum hydrogenatum 1432
Ricini oleum raffinatum 1433
Ricini oleum virginale 1434
Rifabutinum 2825
Rifampicinum 2826
Rifamycinum natricum 2827
Rilmenidini dihydrogenophosphas 2829
Risperidonum 2830
Ritonavirum 2832
Rocuronii bromidum 2835
Ropivacaini hydrochloridum monohydricum 2837
Rosae pseudo-fructus 1744
Rosmarini aetheroleum 2840
Rosmarini folium 2839
Roxithromycinum 2842
RRR-α-Tocopherolum 3088
RRR-α-Tocopherylis acetas 3090
RRR-α-Tocopherylis hydrogenosuccinas 3095
Rusci rhizoma **6.1**-3416
Rutosidum trihydricum 2844

S

Sabalis serrulatae fructus 2864
Sacchari monopalmitas **6.1**-3543
Saccharinum 2849
Saccharinum natricum 2850
Sacchari sphaerae 2979
Sacchari stearas **6.1**-3544
Saccharum 2975
Salbutamoli sulfas 2857
Salbutamolum 2855
Salicis cortex **6.1**-3563
Salicis corticis extractum siccum **6.1**-3564
Salmeteroli xinafoas 2860
Salmonis domestici oleum 2862
Salviae lavandulifoliae aetheroleum **6.2**-3838
Salviae officinalis folium 2853
Salviae sclareae aetheroleum 1561
Salviae tinctura 2854
Salviae trilobae folium 2854
Sambuci flos 1776
Sanguisorbae radix **6.1**-3533
Scopolamini butylbromidum 2109
Scopolamini hydrobromidum 2110
Scopolaminum 2108
Selamectinum ad usum veterinarium **6.1**-3534
Selegilini hydrochloridum 2866
Selenii disulfidum 2867
Semecarpus anacardium ad praeparationes homoeopathicas 1082
Sennae folii extractum siccum normatum **6.2**-3833
Sennae folium 2868
Sennae fructus acutifoliae 2870
Sennae fructus angustifoliae 2871
Serinum 2872
Serpylli herba 3219
Sertaconazoli nitras **6.1**-3535
Sertralini hydrochloridum **6.1**-3537
Serum bovinum 1329
Sesami oleum raffinatum 2874
Silica ad usum dentalem 2878
Silica colloidalis anhydrica 2877
Silica colloidalis hydrica 2877
Silica hydrophobica colloidalis 2878
Silybi mariani extractum siccum raffinatum et normatum 2426
Silybi mariani fructus 2425
Simeticonum 2880
Simvastatinum 2881
Soiae oleum hydrogenatum **6.2**-3837
Soiae oleum raffinatum **6.2**-3838
Solani amylum 2731
Solidaginis herba 1999
Solidaginis virgaureae herba 2000
Solutiones ad conservationem partium corporis 2929
Solutiones ad haemocolaturam haemodiacolaturamque 2025
Solutiones ad haemodialysim 2022
Solutiones ad peritonealem dialysim 2646
Solutiones anticoagulantes et sanguinem humanum conservantes 1200
Somatostatinum 2930
Somatropini solutio concentrata 2933
Somatropinum 2931
Somatropinum iniectabile 2935
Sorbitani lauras 2938
Sorbitani oleas 2938
Sorbitani palmitas 2939
Sorbitani sesquioleas 2939
Sorbitani stearas 2940

T

U

V

Vitamini synthetici densati A pulvis 3201
Vitaminum A 3199
Vitaminum A syntheticum densatum oleosum 3200
Vitaminum A syntheticum, solubilisatum densatum in aqua dispergibile 3203

W

Warfarinum natricum 3207
Warfarinum natricum clathratum 3208

X

Xanthani gummi **6.1**-3569
Xenoni (^{133}Xe) solutio iniectabilis 1042
Xylazini hydrochloridum ad usum veterinarium 3234
Xylitolum 3235
Xylometazolini hydrochloridum 3237
Xylosum 3238

Y

Yohimbini hydrochloridum 3244

Z

Zidovudinum 3249
Zinci acetas dihydricus 3250
Zinci acexamas 3251
Zinci chloridum 3253
Zinci oxidum 3253
Zinci stearas 3254
Zinci sulfas heptahydricus 3254
Zinci sulfas hexahydricus 3255
Zinci sulfas monohydricus 3255
Zinci undecylenas 3256
Zingiberis rhizoma **6.2**-3751
Zolpidemi tartras 3256
Zopiclonum 3257
Zuclopenthixoli decanoas 3259

KEY TO MONOGRAPHS

Version date of the text — **01/2008:0884**

corrected 6.2

Text reference number

Modification to be taken into account from the publication date of Supplement 6.2

CARBIMAZOLE

Carbimazolum

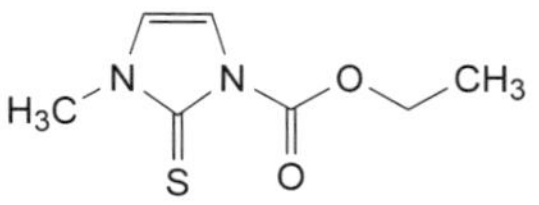

CAS number

$C_7H_{10}N_2O_2S$ M_r 186.2

[22232-54-8]

DEFINITION

Chemical name in accordance with IUPAC nomenclature rules

Ethyl 3-methyl-2-thioxo-2,3-dihydro-1*H*-imidazole-1-carboxylate.

Content: 98.0 per cent to 102.0 per cent (dried substance).

CHARACTERS

Appearance: white or yellowish-white, crystalline powder.

Solubility: slightly soluble in water, soluble in acetone and in ethanol (96 per cent).

IDENTIFICATION

Application of the first and second identification is defined in the General Notices (chapter 1)

First identification: B.

Second identification: A, C.

A. Melting point (*2.2.14*): 122 °C to 125 °C.

B. Infrared absorption spectrophotometry (*2.2.24*).

Preparation: discs.

Comparison: *carbimazole CRS.*

Reference standard available from the Secretariat (see www.edqm.eu)

C. Thin-layer chromatography (*2.2.27*).

Test solution. Dissolve 10 mg of the substance to be examined in *methylene chloride R* and dilute to 10 ml with the same solvent.

Reference solution. Dissolve 10 mg of *carbimazole CRS* in *methylene chloride R* and dilute to 10 ml with the same solvent.

Plate: *TLC silica gel GF_{254} plate R*.

Reagents described in chapter 4

Mobile phase: *acetone R*, *methylene chloride R* (20:80 *V/V*).

Application: 10 µl.

Development: over a path of 15 cm.

Drying: in air for 30 min.

Further information available on www.edqm.eu (KNOWLEDGE)

Detection: examine in ultraviolet light at 254 nm.

Results: the principal spot in the chromatogram obtained with the test solution is similar in position and size to the principal spot in the chromatogram obtained with the reference solution.

TESTS

Reference to a general chapter

Related substances. Liquid chromatography (*2.2.29*).

Line in the margin indicating where part of the text has been modified (technical modification)

Test solution. Dissolve 5.0 mg of the substance to be examined in 10.0 ml of a mixture of 20 volumes of *acetonitrile R* and 80 volumes of *water R*. Use this solution within 5 min of preparation.

Reference solution (a). Dissolve 5 mg of *thiamazole R* and 0.10 g of *carbimazole CRS* in a mixture of 20 volumes of *acetonitrile R* and 80 volumes of *water R* and dilute to 100.0 ml with the same mixture of solvents. Dilute 1.0 ml of this solution to 10.0 ml with a mixture of 20 volumes of *acetonitrile R* and 80 volumes of *water R*.

Reference solution (b). Dissolve 5.0 mg of *thiamazole R* in a mixture of 20 volumes of *acetonitrile R* and 80 volumes of *water R* and dilute to 10.0 ml with the same mixture of solvents. Dilute 1.0 ml of this solution to 100.0 ml with a mixture of 20 volumes of *acetonitrile R* and 80 volumes of *water R*.

Column:

- *size*: *l* = 0.15 m, Ø = 3.9 mm,
- *stationary phase*: *octadecylsilyl silica gel for chromatography R* (5 µm).

Mobile phase: *acetonitrile R*, *water R* (10:90 *V/V*).

Flow rate: 1 ml/min.

Detection: spectrophotometer at 254 nm.

Injection: 10 µl.

Run time: 1.5 times the retention time of carbimazole.

Retention time: carbimazole = about 6 min.

System suitability: reference solution (a):

- *resolution*: minimum 5.0 between the peaks due to impurity A and carbimazole.

Limits:

- *impurity A*: not more than 0.5 times the area of the principal peak in the chromatogram obtained with reference solution (b) (0.5 per cent),
- *unspecified impurities*: for each impurity, not more than 0.1 times the area of the principal peak in the chromatogram obtained with reference solution (b) (0.10 per cent).

Loss on drying (*2.2.32*): maximum 0.5 per cent, determined on 1.000 g by drying in a desiccator over *diphosphorus pentoxide R* at a pressure not exceeding 0.7 kPa for 24 h.

Sulphated ash (*2.4.14*): maximum 0.1 per cent, determined on 1.0 g.

ASSAY

Dissolve 50.0 mg in *water R* and dilute to 500.0 ml with the same solvent. To 10.0 ml add 10 ml of *dilute hydrochloric acid R* and dilute to 100.0 ml with *water R*. Measure the absorbance (*2.2.25*) at the absorption maximum at 291 nm.

Calculate the content of $C_7H_{10}N_2O_2S$ taking the specific absorbance to be 557.

IMPURITIES

Specified impurities: A.

Other detectable impurities (the following substances would, if present at a sufficient level, be detected by one or other of the tests in the monograph. They are limited by the general acceptance criterion for other/unspecified impurities and/or by the general monograph *Substances for pharmaceutical use (2034)*. It is therefore not necessary to identify these impurities for demonstration of compliance. See also *5.10. Control of impurities in substances for pharmaceutical use*): *B.*

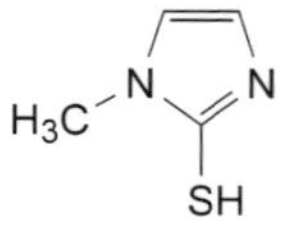

A. 1-methyl-1*H*-imidazole-2-thiol (thiamazole),